HIV/AIDS
ISSUES AND CHALLENGES

INTERNATIONAL ENCYCLOPAEDIA OF AIDS-2

HIV/AIDS
ISSUES AND CHALLENGES
Part-I

Editor
Dr. Digumarti Bhaskara Rao
M.Sc., M.A., M.A., M.Ed., Ph.D.
R. V. R. College of Education
Guntur–522 006
Andhra Pradesh. (INDIA)

2000
DISCOVERY PUBLISHING HOUSE
NEW DELHI-110 002

First Published-2000

ISBN 81-7141-524-5 (Set)

Published by:
DISCOVERY PUBLISHING HOUSE
4831/24, Ansari Road, Prahlad Street,
Darya Ganj, New Delhi-110 002 (*INDIA*)
Phone: 3279245
Fax: 91-11-3253475

Printed at:
Arora Offset Press
Laxmi Nagar, Delhi 110 092.

Preface

The HIV/AIDS is a new phenomenon in the human society. HIV destroys the immune system of human individuals, producing a defenselessness fatal state known as AIDS. The World Health Organisation has estimated that already one in every two hundred and fifty adults in the world is infected with Human Immunodeficiency Virus and according to WHO's projections a total of forty million men women and children worldwide will have been infected with HIV by the turn of this twentieth century. Visualising the devastating effects of the HIV/AIDS epidemic within our life times and beyond is difficult. Probably, no other disease in recent times has had the impact on human society generated by HIV/AIDS.

The HIV/AIDS epidemic has brought into focus many health related ethical, legal and human rights issues. This epidemic requires immediate and effective responses in new programming areas: attitudinal and behavioural changes, community-based care and support initiatives, and the maintenance of human development in the face of increasing rates of illness and deaths. At this point, education enters the scene as it can alter the HIV/AIDS situation since it brings change in the behaviour of the people.

This *International Encyclopaedia of AIDS* presents the worldwide information about HIV/AIDS, issues and challenges, reports and reviews, ethics laws and human rights, and educational activities and programmes to keep the policy makers, planners, professionals, activists, researchers, educationists, teachers and students well informed of the epidemic.

Dr. Digumarti Bhaskara Rao
26 January 1999
The Republic Day of India

Acknowledgements

I am thankful to the World Health Organisation and its associated offices for using their material namely School Health Education to prevent AIDS and STD: A Resource Package for Curriculum Planners-Handbook for Curriculum Planners. Student's Activities, Teachers' Guide, Global Programme on AIDS-HIV Prevention and Care: Teaching Modules for Nurses and Midwives, Global Programme on AIDS. Community HIV Prevention Handbook; STD care Management-workbooks 1-7, Facing the Challenge of HIV/AIDS STDs: A Gender-based Response; HIV/AIDS and STD surveillance Data Management and Use-Report, Bangkok, 1995; Carrying out HIV Sentinal Surveillance-A Guide for Programme Managers, AIDS Prevention and Care in the workplace: Enhancing the Role of Private Sector; HIV Testing Policies and Gidelines; Carrying out HIV Sentinel surveillance; AIDS Prevention; Understanding and Living with AIDS; AIDS: A Modern Epidemic; HIV/AIDS in South-East Asia: IXth meeting of the National Programme Managers, New Delhi, 1993; Information, Education and Communication: A Guide for AIDS Programme Managers, Handbook on AIDS Home Care; HIV/AIDS in South-East Asia: A Pictorial summary; etc.

I am thankful to the United Nations Development Programme, UNDP's HIV and Development Programme, and UNDP's Regional Projects on HIV and Development for using their material namely Economic Implications of AIDS in Asia; Socio Economic Implications of the Epidemic; NGOs Working with Sex workers; NGO Responses to HIV/AIDS in Asia-Case Studies; HIV in the Workplace: Dealing with the Issues-Role Plays, Development and the HIV Epidemic, Law Ethics and HIV; HIV Law and Law Reform; Issue Papers; Study Papers; Working Papers; etc.

I am thankful to the Health and Nutrition Centre, Republic of Philippines for using its material namely sourcebook on HIV/AIDS Prevention Education for Tertiary Educational Institutions.

I am thankful to the Curriculum Development Programme, Ministry of Education, Government of Thailand for using its material namely Institutional Modules for AIDS Education.

I am thankful to US Department of Health and Human Services: Whitman-Walker Clinic, Inc., USA; East-West Centre, USA; National AIDS Control Organisation, Government of India; Academy of Culture Communication Education Science and Service, Guntur, United Nations and its agencies for using their material.

I am grateful to Bhaskar Bhattacharji; V. Alexeev, Geeta Sethi, Elizabeth Reid, Mina Mauerstein-Bail, A. A. Trinidad, Palomi Cuchi, D. Pushpa Latha for their kind co-operation.

Dr. Digumarti Bhaskara Rao,
Secretary
ACCESS
D-43, S.V. N. Colony,
Guntur-522 006

Contents

1

The Global Epidemiology of HIV/AIDS

Geoff Manthey
Technical Officer WHO's
Global Programme on AIDS, Manila, Philippines.

Today, by WHO's conservative estimates, more than 12 million men, women and children are infected with HIV — the virus which causes AIDS. By the end of 1992, over 600,000 cases of AIDS had been reported to WHO; however, our estimates are that figure is closer to 2.5 million. The gap between reported and estimated cases can be explained via under reporting, misdiagnosis and reporting delays.

In the Asia/Pacific region, WHO estimates that close to 40,000 adults have developed AIDS since the start of the pandemic. But it must be remembered that AIDS takes 10 years on average to develop from the time an adult first becomes infected with the human immunodeficiency virus (HIV). So these cases reflect infections that probably occurred a decade ago.

WHO estimates that of the 12 million HIV infections, more than one and a half million people have been infected with HIV in the Asian and Pacific regions. Although 1.5 million is an enormous figure, it may not sound frighteningly large when compared with other parts of the world. After all, sub-Saharan Africa has more than 7 million cumulative infections. Unlike Africa, Asia is at the early stage of the pandemic. Here, the virus is spreading at an alarming rate. In the first six months of 1992, WHO estimates that one million new infections occurred globally. Of these infections, over 30 per cent occurred in Asia.

The problem in the Asia/Pacific region may be illustrated with some examples. HIV infection has been explosive among injecting drug users. In India's north-east states, prevalence rose from less that 1 per cent to 50 per cent in just one year. Drug injectors in China's Yunnan Province had infection rates ranging from 10 per cent to over 50 per cent in 1990, and those in Myanmar had a rate of 72 per cent in 1991.

HIV transmission due to injecting drug use has become an alarming problem in Malaysia, where prevalence in one sample of 9,000 injecting drug users in a rehabilitation centre was found to be 11 per cent in 1991 and up to 26 per cent in smaller samples. In the first 3 months of 1993, 9 per cent of injecting drug users in Ho Chi Minh City, Vietnam were found to be HIV-infected. Surveys in the Philippines, Singapore and Japan, however, have not discovered HIV infection among injecting drug users tested.

Among men attending sexually transmitted disease (STD) clinics, national rates in Thailand have grown from zero in mid-1989 to 6 per cent in mid 1992, and in Myanmar from 2 per cent to 9 per cent between 1990 and 1991. Where results are available in other countries in the Asia/Pacific region, HIV infection among STD clients remains at low levels, less than 1 per cent, except Cambodia where a recent survey found that 4.2 per cent of 72 persons were infected.

Seroprevalence rates as high as 50 per cent or 60 per cent are now being seen among female commercial sex workers (CSWs) in parts of Asia. HIV infection was first documented among female CSWs in Thailand in 1989, when the first national serosurvey detected a prevalence rate of 44 per cent among "lower class" brothel sex workers in Chiang Mai. HIV prevalence in female CSWs in India has also risen rapidly. In Bombay, prevalence has been estimated at between 30-50 per cent while in Delhi it has been found to be over 30 per cent among female CSWs.

In other parts of Asia, information suggests that spread has not yet occurred to the same degree as Thailand and India. The highest prevalence among female CSWs to date has been found in Cambodia. Some surveys have seen infection rates of 10-15 per cent. There has been a gradual increase in prevalence among female CSWs in Malaysia from zero in 1988 to 1.3 per cent in 1991.

In the mid-1980s the prevalence among female CSWs tested in the Philippines was between 1 per cent and 2.5 per cent. Surprisingly, recent surveys in parts of the country, including Cebu City, have found no infection among the 800 CSWs tested, although testing bias cannot be excluded. In Vietnam and Korea, very low levels of infection have been found. No infection has been documented recently among female CSWs in Singapore, Hong Kong, Australia and Japan.

Surveys among men who have sex with men have found relatively high levels of infection —up to 30 per cent in Sydney and 11 per cent among foreign homosexual/bisexual men in Japan.

However, studies in Singapore, Philippines and Taiwan revealed a low prevalence of HIV.

It must be remembered that by the time HIV infection is perceptible in these vulnerable groups, it has spread far and wide in the population.

Seroprevalence in the general population has reached 4 per cent in northern Thailand and 7 per cent in southern Myanmar. Cumulative infections in India totalled half a million at the end of 1991 and may have reached one million by the end of 1992—a doubling time of one year.

Statistics such as these tell us several important things. Firstly, Asia and the Pacific have the same mix of transmission routes as we have seen in other parts of the world. The same risk behaviours exist here as elsewhere in the world. In Asia and the Pacific, the number of HIV infections has tripled in the last two years. And, by the end of the century, WHO predicts that in Asia and the Pacific, over one million adults will become infected with HIV each year.

An epidemic of AIDS will follow this great epidemic of HIV infection. By the year 2000, close to 2 million adults in this region will have died of AIDS. During that year alone some half a million HIV-infected people will develop AIDS and require care.

Globally, by the end of the century, WHO projects that there will be a cumulative total of 30-40 million HIV infections in men, women and children, of which 90 per cent will be in developing countries. The projected cumulative total of adult AIDS cases will be close to 10 million, of which 90 per cent will be in developing countries. And there will be 10 million or more children less than 10 years of age orphaned as a result of AIDS, primarily in the developing countries.

But there are still facts and fiction about HIV that seem not to be fully understood by the public. Until they are, the epidemic will continue to spiral out of control. Getting these facts known and accepted, and the fiction identified and removed, are challenges facing Asian and Pacific countries.

HIV is not casually contagious. Fortunately for us, HIV is not one of the viruses that spreads through air or water, through saliva or through urine or faeces. It is spread via blood, semen, vaginal fluids and breast milk. People need to understand that they cannot catch HIV by eating food prepared by an HIV-infected person, or by sharing toilet or bathing facilities or through sneezing, shaking hands, hugging or even kissing.

Health care workers need to understand that they must carefully handle the body fluids, particularly blood, of all patients as it is always a potential source of HIV, hepatitis virus and other pathogens. And just as there is no reason to isolate HIV-infected

Cumulative AIDS cases in Men, Women and Children, Late 1992

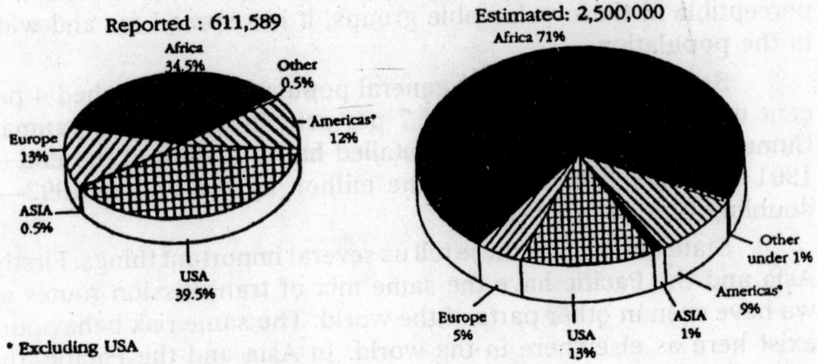

* Excluding USA

Source: Global Programme on AIDS January 1993

ESTIMATED GLOBAL NEW HIV INFECTIONS From early to mid 1992

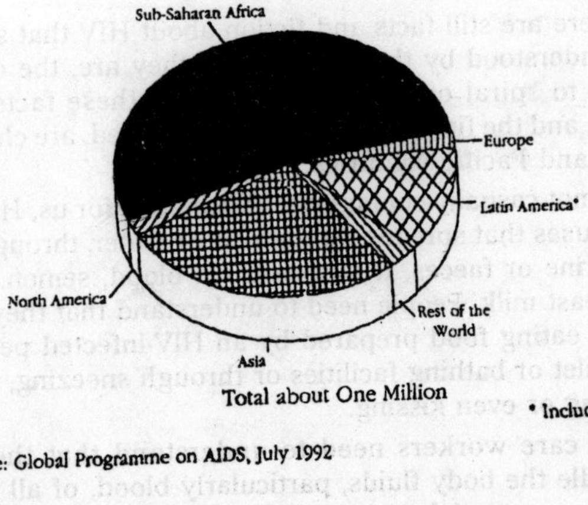

* Including the Caribbean

Source: Global Programme on AIDS, July 1992

Fig. 1.1 Estimated Distribution of Cumulative HIV Infections in Adults, by Continent or Region Late 1992

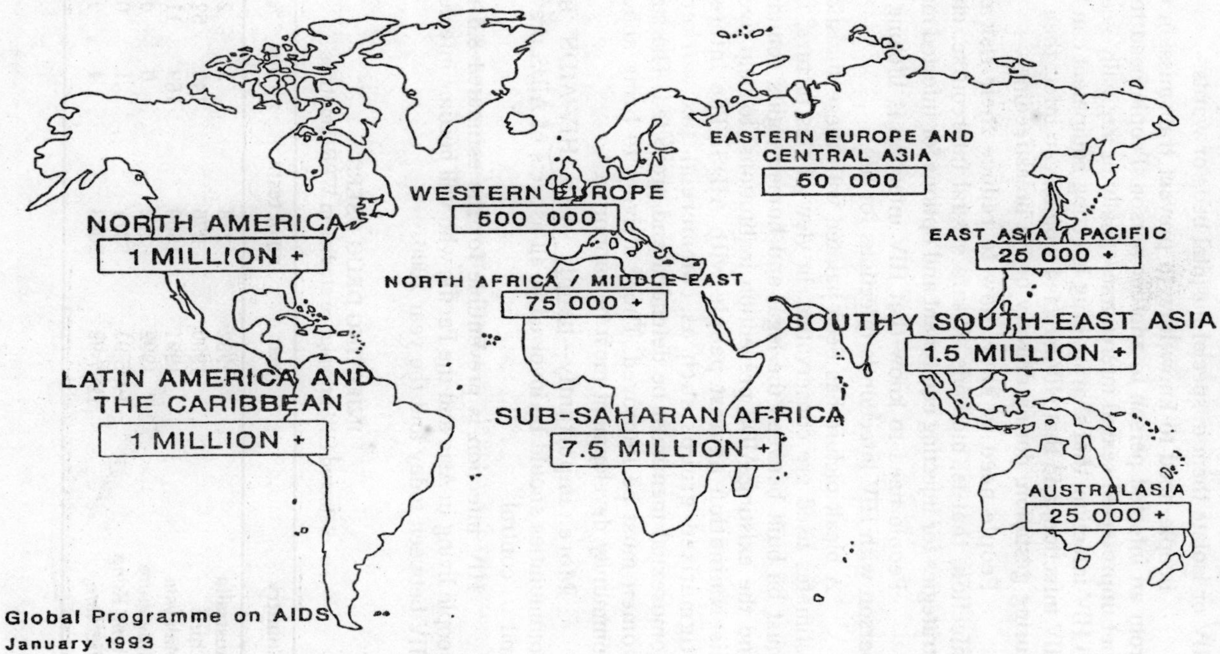

people from society, there is no reason to test hospital patients for HIV or isolate them in special hospital beds or wards.

People need to know how to prevent transmission of HIV from an infected person to another person. People need to know that unprotected sexual intercourse—anally or vaginally—can lead to HIV infection, that sharing drug injecting equipment can lead to HIV infection, and that HIV-infected women can infect their babies during gestation, during delivery or via breastfeeding.

People need to know how to reduce their risk of HIV infection, that is, methods of safe sexual intercourse, cleaning strategies for injecting equipment and options for infected mothers.

People need to know that HIV infection is lifelong and a person with HIV infection is infectious for life.

A bleak picture has been painted with these statistics. The estimates used are conservative. In view of this picture, bridges must be built between the legal and human rights communities and the existing AIDS prevention institutions, to help overcome discrimination against people with AIDS. The interests of stigmatised groups such as commercial sex workers and homosexual men must be defended and protected. The status of women must be improved. Those striving to bring about true community development must be supported.

More importantly—people with HIV/AIDS in our communities should be involved in all aspects of AIDS prevention and control.

HIV infection is preventible for the estimated 8.5 million people living in Asia and the Pacific who will become infected with HIV between today and the year 2000.

INJECTING DRUG USERS

Selected HIV prevalence studies in WPR countries

Country	year	no of tests	no pos	% pos
Australia	1992	218	5	2.30
China	1990	276	146	52.90
Malaysia	1991	1500	169	11.30
Singapore	1992	212	0	0.00
Hong Kong	1985-91	5371	1	0.02
Vietnam	1987-92	2008	4	0.20

STD CLINIC ATTENDERS

Selected HIV prevalence studies in WPR countries

Country	year	no of tests	no pos	% pos
Australia	1992	5100	17	0.33
Cambodia	1992	72	3	4.20
Hong Kong	1992	2146	2	0.09
Vietnam	1987-92	8572	5	0.06
Papua New Guinea	1992	6035	5	0.08

Source: Global Programme on AIDS, as of 6 April 1993.

FEMALE SEX-WORKERS

Selected HIV prevalence studies in WPR countries

Country	year	no of tests	no pos	%pos
Cambodia	1992	207	19	9.18
Hong Kong	1985-91	12950	0	0.00
Philippines	1992	227	0	0.00
Rep of Korea	1992	411425	11	0.003
Singapore	1992	2740	0	0.00
Vietnam	1987-92	11745	3	0.03

HOMO/BISFXUAL MEN

Selected HIV prevalence studies in WPR countries

Country	year	no of tests	nopos	% pos
Cambodia	1992	499	9	1.8
Japan	1985-89	786	24	3.1
Singapore	1992	111	4	3.6
Philippines	1992	300	0	0
FR Polynesia	1990	156	6	3.8

Source: Global Programme on AIDS, as of 6 April 1993.

2

Approaching the HIV Epidemic

Ms. Elizabeth Reid
UNDP, New York

The HIV Epidemic comes to people 's attention through the language of its texts and its spokespersons. The way it is brought to people's attention will be critical determinant of how they will respond to it. Currently, the discourse is based on metaphors of epicentres of spread identified as core transmitter groups. These are metaphors of distancing which encourage blame and denial. There are, however within affected communities, new discourses emerging of inclusion, empowerment and processes and of the complexity of the reality of the epidemic. These discourses are associated with a new way of responding to the epidemic described here as one of community mobilization.

"We are not prostitutes. It has nothing to do with us."

(Women in Latin America)

INTRODUCTION

Determining how best to approach this epidemic is neither an idle nor an academic exercise. At stake are people' s lives and well-being and the capacity of communities, businesses and economies to continue to function.

Some people are more likely to come to unsafe contact with an infected person. If they alone are targeted as transmitters or as epicentres of spread, others fail to understand that everyone must change in the face of the epidemic.

The epidemic must and can be slowed down, quickly and effectively. The first decade of the epidemic has shown us what approaches are effective and under what conditions. These lessons have been learned from the response in affected communities, be they in Sydney, Kampala or Madras. The community mobilization approach is an attempt to apply these lessons more broadly and to implement them more effectively.

For too many people, the HIV epidemic is still a distant spectre. As exemplified in the quote above, the way the epidemic is brought to people' s attention will be the critical determinant of how they will respond to it and thus whether they, personally, protect themselves from infection and whether effective and sustainable programmes are established in response to its presence in their midst.

An epidemic comes to people's attention through the language of its texts, its presentation and its programming (Watney, 1989; Patton, 1990; Siedel, 1993, for example). There are four dominant and overlapping discourses which have been constructed:

the public health discourse

the epidemiological discourse

the biomedical discourse

the educational discourse.

These discourses derive from the beliefs and assumptions about the nature and causes of the epidemic. They reflect the moral, social and institutional values of those who have constructed them and constitute the analytical framework of national responses. It is timely to cast a critical glance over the assumptions and logic of these discourses.

The Dominant Discourses: Metaphors and Misapprehensions

All four of these dominant and overlapping discourses are dominated by metaphors of small, physically locatable epicentres of spread of the HIV virus which if contained by condoms or bleach or segregation will ensure that the epidemic is held in check. Those who are assumed to fill this description are referred to as 'core transmitters'. Prostitutes, injecting drug users, STD patients and, more recently, truck drivers are the accepted target groups for intervention. In these discourses, there are no metaphors of spread which include whole populations or which include the speaker as well as the others. They are metaphors of distancing: epicentres are located elsewhere, not in groups of doctors. IEC experts or public servants. Such metaphors encourage blame and become their own justification for restrictive or punitive measures.

The metaphors of the dominant discourse have reinforced the ancient view of women as spreaders of disease, as vessels of infection for men and vectors of transmission to their infants. Women who work as prostitutes have been scapegoated by this approach and the very dangerous myth born that only such women are at risk of infection. This myth is widespread. The women whose voices began this paper are many. Patterns of HIV infection in women in general should seriously call into question the very concept of epidemic spread by a limited group of sexually active people. The HIV epidemic is propagated by accepted norms of sexual behaviour, particularly of men.

The Distortion of the Metaphors

The dominant discourse and its associated programme interventions, particularly the focus on mass education, condom distribution and STD treatment, create an illusion that nations are responding to the HIV epidemic in an effective and sustainable manner. However, there is no evidence that these approaches have been effective in slowing down the epidemic, and there is much evidence to the contrary. For example, there are studies in the US which show that HIV infection rates in female prostitutes are comparable with other women in the same geographical areas (Corea, 1992).

It is not that frequency of unprotected sexual intercourse with different partners or the existence of sexually transmitted infections are irrelevant to the analysis. Rather they have their origins in social, psychological, economic and gender relationships and it is these that determine to whom and how rapidly the virus spreads (Reid, 1992b). Furthermore, the disproportionately high infection rates in girls and young women in all populations should force us to add to this list of determining factors the biological immaturity and vulnerability of the female genital tract (Reid & Bailey, 1992).

The language of core transmitters and targeted programme approaches is drawn from STD epidemiology and control programmes. Computer models have been used to justify the claim that even a small number of highly sexually active individuals can maintain an STD epidemic in an otherwise low-risk population (May & Anderson, 1987, for example). The public health discourse has centred around the assumption that this analysis provides a basis for programme development, justifying the targeting of resources to groups assumed to be most critical for transmissions, the 'core transmitters'. It has led to the simple imperative: trace them and treat them. This orthodoxy has been transferred to HIV programming (WHO, 1992; Over & Piot, 1991, for example). This is an excellent sample of a programme fitting a model. The pressing question is whether the model fits the world.

Programming approaches targeted to 'core transmitters' are based on the following assumptions:

- # that identifiable groups of people, rather than dispersed individuals, fill this specification;
- # that all or most members of such a group are locatable and are accessible to targeted programmes;
- # that the groups of 'core transmitters' targeted in the programmes are the most active of such groups.

Core Transmitters?

It is either assumed that these models fit the world or reality is forced to fit the model like the feet of the Ugly Sisters into Cynderella's glass shoe. Thus women who work in prostitution, rather than the men who infect them, are singled out as core transmitters. Even among these women, only the more easily accessible are targeted: the bar 'girls', street workers or workers in brothels. All other women who have multiple sexual partners are unrecognized and untargeted.

Furthermore, research data have long indicated that it is not only those who have multiple sexual partners who are most prone to sexually transmitted infections (STIs) but also girls and young women. STI infection rates globally are extremely high in adolescents and young adults. Within this group, it is the young men who tend to have frequent sexual intercourse with multiple partners while the young women, who are less sexually active, are more likely to be infected with STIs (Bell & Hein, 1984), for example. These data have long been ignored (Reid 1992a). Nor is it the case that an STI programme approach targeted at core transmitters has reduced these epidemics. Indeed, the global prevalence and incidence rates of STIs are rising both among and beyond so-called core transmitters groups (Mann et al., 1992). These facts alone should cause us to pause before applying either the STD-based core-transmitter analysis or its associated programming to the HIV epidemic.

HIV programmes targeted at core groups are justified by the claim that most people are not at risk of HIV infection and that it is not possible and not cost-effective to target whole communities or populations yet the concept of being at risk relates to a person's likelihood of becoming infected. It is clear that those at risk of infection are the spouses and other sexual partners of those who are infected, when unsafe sexual intercourse takes place. Many of these people at risk are not even sexual transmitters; that is, they have no sexual partners others than those who place them at risk. They are identifiable neither as individuals nor as groups, nor are they reachable by targeted programmes.

The metaphors of core transmitters and of onwards

transmission are embedded within an over-arching metaphor of health as a battle ground and its language of surveillance, targets, control and campaigns. They distort our vision and our language. A paradigm shift is required from those who are assumed to be transmitting the virus, to those who are becoming infected and to those who are not protecting themselves from infection or who cannot do so. This shift could radically change surveillance systems, research agendas, national HIV/AIDS programme approaches and resource allocations. A simple example would be to shift to the recording of HIV infected people by age, gender and occupation as well as classification by risk situation. Such a shift would force a broadening of focus from pathogenic transmission from one individual to another, to the complex socio—economic and other conditions which lead each person to unsafe behaviour. Such a simple paradigm shift would immediately enrich the discourses and their analytical basis.

Emerging Discourses

The dominant discourses are being increasingly challenged by new discourses. A language of optimism is being developed within affected communities as they learn to live with the presence of the virus. This new discourse is about:

- # face-to-face discussion leading to changes in community norms and values relating to gender and sexuality;
- # stories of living with HIV breaking down false divisions into Us/Them and relocating the epidemic within each of us;
- # how knowing someone infected lessens fear and denial and opens up the possibility of respect for self and others;
- # ownership of knowledge, decision making and programme development leading to appropriate and sustainable responses.

This emerging discourse of optimism and empowerment is constructing a new programming discourse: a language of processes rather than interventions, of people as responsible actors rather than as manipulable objects of interventions. The approach that emerges is based on community mobilization for change. It respects and acknowledges the expertise of those directly affected, and its sources of leadership and counselling come from within the community. This new programming approach contrasts sharply with the current programming focus on impersonal technologies, condoms, STI services, blood safety kits, for example, and on directive educational interventions.

This is not to deny that the correct use of good quality condoms or the treatment of sexually transmissible infections (and other infections of the genital area) are protective against HIV infection. But these goods and services must be desired by people. People must want to protect themselves from infections, know what their protection options are and must be able to practice them. This will require radical changes in community norms and values relating to sexuality and to gender. Only when these processes are in place can the current interventions be embedded within them and only when this occurs will these interventions contribute to programme effectiveness.

The third emerging discourse links the epidemic to development (Museveni, 1991; Kaunda, 1989) and argues that the epidemic has the potential to touch every facet of human, social and economic life. It locates the reasons for the spread of the virus and the nature of its consequences in the psychological, social and economic determinants of people's daily lives. It identifies the factors which predispose individuals and populations to unsafe behaviour as including inequalities of wealth, power and autonomy, sexual norms and social values, attitudes to women, mobility patterns and the legal, ethical and human rights environment.

A country's development choices influence the speed and pattern of spread of the virus. In turn, the spread of the virus determines how the epidemic will affect national development and weaken the national capacity to respond. Those countries that are developing participative, community-based institutions, strong social cohesion and adequate redistributive policies will find the epidemic much easier to overcome.

There remain discourses yet to be articulated. HIV and AIDS evoke complex and powerful emotions and psychological states. In those as yet untouched by the epidemic, these may include hatred, anger, fear, righteousness, disgust, guilt, shame, humiliation or denial. There has been a reluctance to acknowledge the existence of this side of the epidemic and to address it. There is a deep, culturally-instilled unease which inhibits families and nations from using a language of emotions, vulnerability, sexuality and mortality.

There is silence about the dark side of the epidemic, the reality of living with the knowledge that one is infected or that someone one loves dearly is infected: the haunting presence of death, the hesitancy of desire, the longing for love, the uncertainty, the sadness. Even the emotional states, which are central to the belief that the epidemic can be overcome, are unacknowledged in its discourse. There seems to be a reluctance to use words such as 'respect', 'caring', 'compassion', 'love,', 'happiness', 'spirituality', or 'concern' in this context. These emerging and yet to be spoken discourses recognize a basic truth: to understand and respond to this epidemic, one must understand daily life and human nature in all its complexity.

Placing People and their Communities at the Centre of the Response

The language of empowerment leads to a programming approach that places people and their communities at the centre of the response to the epidemic and which builds upon the complex nature of people's daily lives. It recognizes that poverty, wealth, power, subordination and debt, to mention just a few, are essentially interlinked with the HIV epidemic.

It should be made clear what is not involved in this paradigm shift. This approach, which could be called community mobilization, is not an argument in favour of existing IEC approaches to the general population. Nor is it an argument for the geographical targeting of prevention messages or indeed any targeting. These approaches have the wrong direction of fit. The role of the outsider must be supportive, not directive. One of the starkest lessons to be learned from the first decade of the response to the epidemic is that whilst information or education may change knowledge, alone they rarely change attitudes or sexual or drug-using behaviour. It is not that information and education have no place; they must be there to be drawn upon by individuals, couples and communities. This is the correct direction of fit and is intrinsic to a community mobilization approach. Nor is this approach an argument against programmes for and within particular communities and groups, including gay men and injecting drug users. At present these programmes are amongst our richest sources of lessons relevant to a community mobilization approach. However, these group-specific programmes must be embedded in broader mobilization networks. It is not only members of particular groups who participate in unsafe behaviour but is also the case that an exclusive group-specific focus will not create conditions of sustainability. The wider community is an important source of volunteers, of workers and of financial, moral and other forms of support. However, it can also be a source of discrimination, indifference, rejection or antagonism, all of which negatively affect programmed. Hence the whole community must understand the need for and be involved in processes of attitudinal and behavioural change.

These processes are stimulated by stories of the need for support, of changing attitudes and behaviour, of concern. They consist primarily of face-to-face discussion. They require local leadership and sources of information, advice and counselling within the community. They create agents of change, people who wish to ensure that we respond effectively and compassionately.

These are the processes that are already taking place in affected communities (Carr, 1991; UNDP, 1993). However, as yet there are few such communities globally and we cannot wait for them to emerge for by then too many people will be infected. Experience in Africa and elsewhere shows that these processes can be stimulated by local organizations (Williams, 1991), by political, religious and other leaders (Hampton, 1991) and by certain research initiatives (ICRW, 1993).

A community mobilization approach will have radical implications for social research design. The research agenda must be influenced or determined by communities and reflect their needs. Social research methodologies will need to be participative and interactive and lead to a process of group and individual introspection, including reflection on socio-cultural norms and values, and on individual and collective behaviour. the process itself of carrying out HIV-related research in such cases become critical and its findings only a part of the stimulation of change.

Setting Priorities

An approach which is centred around community mobilization does not pre-empt the possibility of setting priorities. Firstly, assistance should be given to communities with higher rates of infection. More sophistication will be needed in surveillance systems in order to be able to identify such communities, occupations or locations.

Secondly, enough is now known about the physiological, social and economic causes of spread of the virus to be able to identify communities or countries where the virus is most likely to spread rapidly irrespective of present rates of infection. Their identifying characteristics include:

economically vital areas and areas with mobile populations;
communities and cultures which do not value women and which tolerate or encourage certain patterns of sexual behaviour, particularly in men;
communities which are stratified by wealth, income and/or power;
communities without strong traditions of respect and concern for others;
communities with little capacity for reflection or change.

Thirdly, assistance should be given to all groups or communities who actively seek it. These foci of assistance need to be complemented by a more general mobilization and sustained by appropriate forms of assistance, by the availability, accessibility and affordability of the required goods and services and by appropriate legal, ethical and human rights policies and practices.

The appropriate entry points for community points for community mobilization are still being explored. Approaches based on the creation of fear and revulsion have been shown to be counter-productive. We know that those who are living this epidemic in their daily lives are powerful catalysts for change. A discussion within a group about how they would react if one of their sons or husbands returned infected can initiate the concern for self and others. Mass media can also be used effectively for attitudinal change. The primary role of outside technical assistance may lie in the transfer of the concepts that are the essence of a sustainable response (Campbell, 1992):

the justifiability of faith and hope;
the interrelatedness of care and behaviour change;
the possibility of peaceful co-existence with the virus;
the language of emotions, vulnerability, sexuality and mortality;
the resources of time, compassion, labour, food and money within communities;
the reality that we are all affected.

To the transfer of these concepts will need to be added assistance in the management, monitoring and evaluation of the process and skills in drawing down the required services and technologies.

There are no methodologies yet developed for determining the cost-effectiveness of processes as distinct from discrete interventions. However, it is likely that the cost of such an approach compares reasonably with the cost of the current components of national HIV/AIDS programmes, including extended surveillance systems, KAP and similar studies, extensive mass media IEC campaigns and securing blood supplies. Furthermore this approach, based on local resources and capacities, creates the conditions for its own sustainability and for the effectiveness of other interventions.

REFERENCES

Bell, T.A. & HEIN, K. (1984). Adolescents and sexually transmitted diseases, in K. HOLMES (Ed.), *Sexually Transmitted Diseases, pp. 72-84 (New York, McGraw-Hill).*

Campbell, I. (1992), *An Integrated Response to HIV/AIDS, An Opportunity for Community Development and Change,* (London, Salvation Army).

Carr, A. (1991) *Behaviour Change in Response to HIV/AIDS. Some Analogies and Lessons from the Experience of the Gay Communities (New* York, UNDP).

Corea, G. (1992) *The Invisible Epidemic* (New York, Harper Collins).

Hampton, J. (1991) Meeting AIDS with Compassion: AIDS Care and Prevention in Agomanya, Ghana, *Strategies for Hope. No. 4* (London, Actionaid).

International Center for Research on Women, ICRW (1993) Preliminary report on the Women and AIDS Research Programme: evolving a model for AIDS prevention education among underprivileged adolescent girls in urban India (Personal communication).

Kaunda, K. (1989), Address to the 6th International AIDS Conference (Montreal).

Mann, J., Tarantola, D. & Netter, T. (Eds.), (1992), *AIDS in the World,* (Cambridge, Harvard).

May, R.M. & Anderson, R.M. (1987), Transmission dynamics of HIV infections, *Nature,* 326, p.137

Museveni, Y. (1991), New Vision, Address to the 7th International AIDS Conference, (Florence).

Over, M. & Piot, P. (1991), *HIV infection and sexually transmitted diseases* (Washington, D.C., World Bank).

Patton, C. (1990), *Inventing AIDS* (New York, Routledge).

Reid, E. (1992a), Gender, knowledge and responsibility, in J. MANN *et al* (Eds.), *AIDS in the World 1992* (Cambridge, Harvard).

Reid, E. (1992b), *The HIV Epidemic and Development. the Unfolding of the Epidemic,* (New York, UNDP).

Reid, E. & Bailey, M. (1992). *Young Women: Silence, Susceptibility and the HIV epidemic,* AIDS in Society Infold (October/November, 1992).

Seidel, G. (1993). Competing discourse of HIV/AIDS in Sub-Saharan African, *Social Science and Medicine,* 36, pp. 174-194.

United Nations Development Programme (1994). *Report on the Asian and Pacific Informal Consultation on Attitudinal and Behavioural Change,* (New York, UNDP).

Watney, S. (1989), Taking Liberties: an Introduction, in: E. Carter & S. Watney (Eds.) *Taking Liberties,* pp 11-57 (London, Serpent's Tail).

Williams, G. (1991). From Fear to Hope: AIDS Care and Prevention at Chikankata Hospital, Zambia, *Strategies for Hope. No. I (London,* Actionaid).

World Health Organization, (1992). *The Global Strategy for the Prevention and Control of AIDS,* (Geneva, WHO).

3

The HIV Epidemic as a Development Issue

Ms. Elizabeth Reid
Director
HIV and Development Programme
UNDP, New York. USA

INTRODUCTION

The immense impact of the psychological, social and economic consequences of the epidemic is already being experienced in communities throughout the world. Families have been scattered, villages abandoned, food production diminished, enterprises forced to close and public and private health care systems overwhelmed.

In sub-Saharan Africa, it is estimated that one adult in 40, men and women, are already infected with HIV and in some areas it is as many as one in four or higher. Data on communities in Asia, the Caribbean and South America show or predict similar levels of infection. Moreover, every indication is that the number of new infections will increase exponentially over the next decade. Many of these countries face the loss of whole generations of people within their communities and the decimation of their productive workforce.

Without effective responses at the community, national and international level, the efforts of the last 25 years to strengthen the human and capital resources required for national development may have been to little avail.

The Setting of the Epidemic

The impact of the HIV epidemic in developing countries must be understood in the context of the critical social and economic problems already experienced by these countries: poverty, famine and food shortage, inadequate sanitation and health care, the subordination of women and adjustment policies that allocate insufficient resources to the social sectors.

These factors create a particular vulnerability to the devastating consequences of the epidemic. Economic need and dependency lead to activities that magnify the risk of HIV transmission and mean that many people, particularly women, are powerless to protect themselves against infection. Inadequate standards of health and sanitation further exacerbate the spread of HIV and accelerate the progression from HIV infection to AIDS.

The setting of the HIV epidemic in developing countries creates a downward spiral whereby existing social and economic deprivation produces an environment in which the spread of HIV can occur and, in turn, the HIV epidemic compounds and intensifies the deprivation already experienced by those countries. Not only must the epidemic itself be directly addressed in programmes of assistance but its consequences will impact upon all existing development initiatives which themselves will need to be reformulated in order to encompass these new situations.

The Consequences of the Epidemic

The consequences of the epidemic will continue to unfold for many decades after the spread of the virus within a community. This is because those infected are productively engaged, have established households and support dependants. The cost to society, and to individuals, includes not only illness and death but also the effects of this loss on those who survive, on their communities and on nations.

Just as a stone thrown into a pond will create ripples that reach to the farthest edges of the pond, so too will the effects of HIV infection be experienced at all social, cultural and economic levels. Figure 3.1 describes the chain of consequences associated with the spread of the virus and the wide range of policy needs and concerns created by these consequences. An understanding of the full dimensions of the epidemic requires a recognition of the way in which the epidemic, while appearing first in the form of infection and illness in individuals, moves rapidly and inevitably towards a far-reaching and catastrophic impact upon communities and nations.

The invisibility of infection during its early stages and the subsequent failure to recognise its threat has allowed reluctant parliaments and bureaucracies to delay in acting to protect their populations. However, the failure to implement effective policy interventions at the earliest possible stage will result in many more serious and far-reaching consequences in the future.

Figure -3. 1 The HIV Epidemic and its Consequences

Spread of the Virus	Illness and Death	Survivors	Social and Economic Impact	Long-term Potential Impact
Description				
Initial spread hidden but increasing numbers of people becoming infected.	Spread of virus continues and infected people become increasingly ill and die.	Children, spouses, elderly and others left without support, grief and bereavement.	Depletion of the labour force, adverse impact on productive and social sectors, loss of military strength	Possibility of social and political unrest, destitution, social and economic disintegration
Policy-Context				
Behaviour change Education Prevention Legislation Other preventive measures Surveillance Human rights	Living positively Coping with fear and powerlessness Social and psychological support Employment Income maintenance Confidentiality Care and treatment Legal rights	Integration within community Emergency assistance Counselling and social support Education and health services Income generation Legal protection	Monitoring impacts Strengthening and financing health and social sectors Public sector allocations Labour market Policies Revenue generation Economic production	Minimising adverse impact on individuals, communities and nations.

Individuals and Communities

The immediate impact upon those people infected with HIV and their families is devastating. In addition to the psychological and emotional distress caused by illness and death, the HIV epidemic creates a critical need to care for those infected and to find ways of replacing their contribution to the household and the community.

Because the majority of infected people in developing countries are men and women in the age group 15 to 45 years, most will have families and dependants. There will be a decrease in family income and, at the same time, an increased need for expenditure on health care. The death or disability caused by AIDS may lead to increasing numbers of families without parents or providers, of single parent families, and of orphans, some of whom are themselves infected with HIV.

Steps will need to be taken to reorganise the division of labour within households in order to reallocate productive tasks to uninfected household members. Children may need to be withdrawn from school to assist in food production and in caring for the sick. The resulting adverse impact on children and on long-term national development may be serious.

With growing numbers of women falling ill and dying and with surviving women becoming increasingly occupied with the care of the ill, women will have less time for caring for their own children and for productive work in the fields, in self-employment, or in the paid workforce. Much of the work performed by women is not measured in cash value and therefore does not appear in economic indicators such as gross national product. Thus, it is difficult to monitor the macro-economic impact of these losses, despite their serious consequences for the survival of families and communities and the role of women within these communities.

In coping with the threat to household units, community-based programmes will be essential in order to establish support networks between households at both the emotional and economic levels. Collective action of this kind represents an indigenous, affordable response to the HIV epidemic. Community-based organizations can play multiple roles within HIV strategies, ranging from home care, counselling and emergency support for families, to training and employment programmes, income generation and co-ordination of external assistance. They permit local resources to be utilised most effectively and can assess and respond to the full spectrum of needs of their particular community.

National Level

The increasing illness and death among people formerly

productively engaged will have a serious impact upon national economies. At the national level, deaths from AIDS will lead to a loss of economic output and, hence, of national income. Many sectors of the economy may be threatened by the sudden depletion of the workforce: mining, agriculture, transport, and construction, for example. The sectors most vulnerable are those which depend on highly trained personnel or upon occupational groups which may have high rates of HIV infection, such as truck drivers, construction workers, teachers, etc.,

Because of the way that infection is clustered in families, occupations and geographical areas, the impact of multiple illness and death is much greater than the accumulated individual losses. Households and communities can quickly cease to be viable social or economic units. The trauma of grieving death after death can induce a feeling of powerlessness and an inability to act. Support systems falter with the seemingly endless demands made upon them. The lost labour becomes more and more difficult to replace and the concomitant loss of output, skills, experience and aspirations can discourage investment, force the closure of enterprises and lessen national income. Population growth rates and economic growth will be reduced.

The direct costs of the epidemic will escalate as the demands for health and social services increase creating the possibility of the withdrawal of investments in the productive sectors. At the same time, the tax base will be increasingly depleted. Foreign exchange earnings will be affected by drops in production of export commodities or crops.

In the longer term, there is the possibility of the disintegration of communities, abandoned children turning to banditry and other socially disruptive survival strategies, widespread destitution, strategic imbalances caused by the depletion of military forces, and changes in the economic bases of societies.

These long-term consequences are not inevitable. If effective steps can be taken at an early stage to minimise the spread of HIV, to provide appropriate support for the individuals and communities affected, and to implement economic and social policies that redress the harm caused by the HIV epidemic and the factors that make communities vulnerable to HIV, the potential long-term consequences may be contained. However, this requires that any denial of the magnitude of the problem cease in order to permit immediate and decisive action. The extent and seriousness of the consequences will depend directly on the timeliness and effectiveness of prevention programmes and of policies adopted to respond to the needs of the infected, the ill and the survivors.

Critical Choices

The severity of the consequences just described will depend upon how early effective policy interventions are implemented. If this is not understood, competing demands on limited national resources could mean that programmes in response to the epidemic, prevention programmes in particular, are not allocated sufficient resources.

Each different kind of consequence of the epidemic has its own set of policy and programme requirements, and these are cumulative rather than sequential. That is, as different phases of the epidemic emerge, a new set of policies and programmes will have to be developed while those already in place will need to be continued and strengthened. Further, as can be seen in Figure. 3.1, responsibility for most of these policies and programmes will lie with sectors and ministries other than health. The earlier the epidemic ceases being solely the responsibility of the Departments and Ministries of Health and begins to be a multi-sectoral concern, the greater the possibility of minimising the severity of the impact.

Along the spectrum depicted in Figure. 3.1, there are a number of critical points at which choices must be made by governments, choices which will either minimise or aggravate the subsequent impact of the epidemic. These include:

- # The type of policies and the extent of resources directed to the epidemic in its early stages. Policy decisions must be made which anticipate future needs that may not yet be visible.
- # The extent to which effective prevention programmes are implemented to minimise the adverse impact of the epidemic. These may require political courage to adopt. Programmes and information directed towards minimising sexual transmission may need to be gender specific. Different information, skills and support may be required by women and men.
- # The extent to which the community response is integrated into and complemented by the government response. The most effective national strategies will be based on the diversity of responses arising within the community.
- # The extent to which governments assist all people affected by the epidemic, that is, those infected, their families, and those that survive them, to remain an integral part of their communities.
- # At what stage communities, the government, the private sector and others begin to address the adverse social and economic impacts of the epidemic.

Human Development Challenged

This epidemic will force a rethinking of approaches to development. A focus on human development highlights the need to ensure that the benefits of growth be used to address critical needs and to improve the human condition. The modalities currently used to achieve this include credit and social investment schemes, labour market flows, employment creation and investments in education and training. These very modalities are being challenged by the epidemic.

Credit is usually seen as an instrument to achieve positive developmental objectives, for example, through public lending for low cost housing or for financing the supply of agricultural inputs. The need for low cost housing will rise as the epidemic leads to a worsening of living standards. However, the capacity to repay will be affected by illness and death and where this is widespread, the viability of such schemes will be in question. Repossession, whilst it may preserve the viability of such schemes, will worsen social stability and increase destitution. Thus, a rethinking of the use of credit for achieveing social and economic objectives will be required or a new way found of responding to these needs.

Mobility of labour too has been a positive factor in development but it is now instrumental in the spread of the virus. High rates of infection occur in most mobile or relocated populations, especially unaccompanied males. Mobility destroys both its mechanisms through the collapse of transport networks and its purpose, the redistribution of labour. Epidemiological studies have shown that truck drivers, seafarers, pilots and other transport sector personnel have relatively high rates of infection. Yet the transport sector is essential to knitting together markets, both for outputs and inputs. Lahour mobility occurs in response to labour market demands and, on a local basis, these will increase as a result of the epidemic.

Education and training play an important role throughout the spectrum of social, technical and economic development. High incidence countries will need to ensure that those infected can continue to contribute productively to the economy so that this investment is not necessarily lost.

New approaches to training may have to be devised because of increased mortality rate. one Ugandan study found an annual mortality rate of 2.5 per cent among staff of government institutions who had studied abroad between 1986 and 1988. The epidemic will also further erode the capacity to plan, manage and implement in those countries where there is little depth in trained personnel.

There will be immense costs to communities and nations. The early illness and death of the active labour force will generate a need for replacement of social investment at a time of shrinking public and national resources. The anguish of the illness and deaths of so many young adults will be difficult to bear. However, an understanding of the extent of the personal, social and economic costs will strengthen the demand for effective prevention programmes, the most effective way of minimising the adverse impact of the epidemic.

4

The HIV Epidemic and Development:

The unfolding of the Epidemic

Ms. Elizabeth Reid
Director
HIV and Development Programme,
UNDP, New York

THE DEVELOPMENT IMPLICATIONS OF THE HIV EPIDEMIC

The HIV epidemic will pose an unprecedented challenge to communities, nations and to the international community: a challenge to human survival, human rigitts and human, development. It is difficult to visualize the devastating effect of the HIV epidemic within our lifetimes and beyond.

The consequences of the spread of the virus will be inexorable and awesome. The challenge facing national and international communities is to act speedily and effectively to limit the further spread of the epidemic and to minimize its impact.

The impact of the HIV epidemic in developing countries must be understood in the context of the critical social and economic problenıs already experienced by these. countries: poverty, farnine and food shortage, inadequate sanitation and health care, the subordination of women and adjustment policies that allocate insufficient resources to the social sectors.

These factors create a particular vulnerability to the devastating consequences of the epidemic. Economic need and dependency lead to activities that magnify the risk of HIV transmission and mean that many people, particularly women, are powerless to protect themselves against infection. Inequitable power structures, a lack of legal protection and inadequate standards of health and nutrition all further exacerbate the spread of the virus, accelerate progression from HIV infection to AIDS, and aggravate the plight of those affected by the epidemic.

The setting of the HIV epidemic in developing countries creates a downward spiral whereby existing social, economic and human deprivation produces a particularly fertile environment for the spread of HIV and, in turn, the HIV epidemic compounds and intensifies the deprivation already experienced by people in those countries. Not only must the epidemic itself be directly addressed in programmes of assistance but its consequences will impact upon all existing development initiatives which themselves will need to be reformulated in order to encompass these new situations.

The important lessons learned from the first ten years of responding to the epidemic are that behaviour change to stop the transmission of HIV can and does occur but that it needs the support of community and an enabling and supportive legal environment. Behaviour change is a process which must essentially involve changes in community and sexual norms and values, the availability of voluntary and confidential counselling and testing services and the creation of an environment which creates the possibility of open and honest discussion of sexuality and dying.

We have also learned that for sustainable behaviour change to occur, there has to be a belief in the future, or at least a reason for hope. This, we have found, comes about when communities and individuals become involved in the care of those living with HIV. We know this care leads to compassion and caring, rich and valuable human attributes which are at the centre not only of the response to the epidemic but of human development itself. The coping strategies of communities must be central to national responses.

For there to be a future in the face of this terrifying epidemic, the infrastructure required by communities must continue to function. As we respond to the immediate needs of behaviour change and the care and support of those infected and affected, the need to maintain the physical, social and economic infrastructure of communities and nations must not be overlooked. The impact of the epidemic begins to affect this infrastructure when increasing numbers of people sicken and die.

The challenges posed by the epidemic to human well-being and development are so immense that collaborative and complementary action is essential for our assistance to be timely and effective. Our efforts must also be sustainable. Effective responses to the epidemic will be needed for many years to come and we must recognize this in the care with which we develop and co-ordinate our efforts.

Co-ordination occurs when there is mutual respect, a common vision, the exchange of experience and a shared sense that the policies and programmes established are effective and sustainable.

THE EPICENTRE : THE SPREAD OF THE VIRUS

The analysis presented here places people and their communities at the centre of the exploration of the repercussions of the spread of the virus. At the epicentre (Figure. 4.1) of the inexorable chain of consequences is the transmission of the virus from person to person, from adult to child. We are still struggling to understand the factors which determine to where and how fast the virus spreads and who gets infected. An improved understanding of these factors will enable us to better understand how the virus moves from place to place, person to person, day to day so that we can more effectively limit its spread and anticipate its repercussions.

Inequalities of Wealth, Power and Autonomy

The first factor is inequalities of wealth, power and autonomy. The greater the disparity, the more stratified a society, the faster and further the virus spreads. Both the rich and the poor are likely to have higher infection rates.

The rich, like the powerful, are more mobile, less constrained by community norms and can afford the lifestyles they choose, which often place them at risk of infection. The poor and the powerless alike are less able to make choices about their life circumstances, more often forced into work away from home and family, or commercial sex work. Their health and nutritional levels are low and they cannot afford to use health services.

Attitudes to Women

These inequalities and stratifications are linked to the second determining factor, namely that of attitudes towards women which are demeaning or which deny women value and. dignity. The indicators of these attitudes will include levels of domestic violence, physical and sexual abuse, abortion laws and practices, and whether women are listened to when they speak. For example, one study of couples who describe themselves as true equals shows that, whereas 97 per cent of conversations initiated by the husband succeeded, only 30 per cent of those begun by the women were continued.

Cultural prescriptions, myths and jokes all embody these attitudes to women, along with the popular and serious literature of communities and nadons. Where women are denied dignity and respect, the virus spreads.

FIGURE 4.1
The Waves of Impact of the HIV Epidemic

EPICENTRE	WAVE I	WAVE II	WAVE III	WAVE IV
Spread of the Virus	*Trauma, Illness and Death*	*Survivors*	*Social and Economic Impact*	*Long term Potential Impact*
Description Spread hidden, but Increasing numbers of people becoming infected.	Psychological trauma; HIV opportunistic diseases appear; Increasing illness and death.	Grieving and bereavement, children, elderly and others left without support.	Depletion of the labour force, adverse impact on productive and social sectors, shrinking revenues, loss of military strength.	Possibility of social and political unrest, destitution, social and economic disintegration.
Determining Factors Inequalities of #wealth #power #autonomy Sexual norms and community values Condition of genital area Attitudes to women Mobility Ethical/legal env.	Extent of spread Attitudes to affected Ethical and legal environment	Clustering of infection in households and communities Dependency ratios Attitudes to survivors Ethical and legal environment	Morbidity in productive adults Clustering in occupations and geographically Gender role differentiation Structure of labour market and economy	Effectiveness and type of earlier policies and programmes Clustering in occupations and geographically Dependency ratios

The type of attitudes that lead to the spread of the virus may co-exist with a quite high status for women in terms of access to education, training and employment.

Community Norms and Values

The third determining factor is community norms and values. Communities where the social construction of gender leads to quite different paradigms of masculinity and femininity have higher infection levels. Similarly, communities and families which tolerate or encourage male sexual behaviour patterns that separate sexual satisfaction from responsibility to others and which value passivity and self-effacement in women will be disproportionately highly infected.

Pathology and Immaturity of the Genital Area

The fourth determining factor of the speed and extent of spread is the pathology and immaturity of the genital area. When unprotected, penetrative intercourse takes place, the virus is much more likely to be transmitted if there are lesions, secretions, inflammation or scarification of the genital area. The existence of these conditions is related to hygiene practices, nutritional status, access to sensitive health services, cultural practices and reproductive practices. In women, transmission may also occur more easily at different stages in the hormonal cycle or if the genital area has not reached maturity, which does not usually occur until young women are in their twenties.

This factor is clearly implicated in the high infection rates in young women and probably in infection rates in uncircumcised men, and contributes significantly to the different rates of infections between developed and developing countries.

Mobility

The fifth determining factor is mobility. The patterns of spread of the virus follow the movement patterns of people: the criss-crossing of armies across countries, the transport routes, the commercially vigorous trading centres, job markets, seasonal flows for agriculture or for ceremony.

Mobile groups of people—senior civil servants, parliamentarians, teachers, students, migrant workers, pilots, truck drivers, the military and so on—have higher infection rates than others.

People Telling Their Stories

The final factor which determines the speed and extent of the spread of the virus and who gets infected is whether conditions exist for people to tell their stories, stories of being infected and stories of changing their behaviour to prevent themselves from becoming infected.

For this to happen, there must be a strong legal and ethical framework which will lessen the almost inevitable discrimination and stigma surrounding HIV infection. There must be community and family support systems. There must be supportive government policies relating to continuation in employment, in school, etc., Finally, there must be the courageous people to tell their stories, for the cost to the individuals and their families of speaking out is usually very high.

If we bear in mind these determining characteristics, we can now put some faces to the estimated 12 million adults already infected in the world today. We now know that soon there will be as many, or more, women infected as men. Many, perhaps most, will be couples, husbands and wives. Many, of not most, will be poor. Although there will be a not insignificant number of the infected among the rich and powerful, many will be in situations that take them away from their families and communities and most will come from communities which accept and even value the behaviour which puts men, women and their families at risk of sexual transmission. We can now begin to see our own faces amongst those 12 million.

THE WAVES OF CONSEQUENCES

The consequences of this spread radiate out over time and will continue to spread. Over time, various types of repercussions are becoming apparent. Their extent and nature are determined by many factors but there is a small number of dominant ones. The first wave of consequences follows directly from the spread of the virus: Those who are infected will, in time, start falling ill and dying.

The second wave of consequences arises from two dominant characteristics of the epidemic:

those who are infected are overwhelmingly at a stage in their lives when they have the maximum number of dependents: children, parents, others living with them, others that they are supporting; and

the virus is clustered in households and so their dependents will be left with few or no means of support.

The third wave of consequences arises from those other

dominant characteristics of the epidemic:

those who are infected are at their most economically productive and active period in their lives;

the virus is clustered occupationally and geographically; and

the rigidity of the gender division of labour, skills and responsibilities.

The extent and nature of the fourth wave of consequences is determined by two dominant characteristics:

the response of communities and nations to those infected, those caring for them and those who survive after their deaths, in particular by whether or not they remain an integral part of their communities, supported and cared for by them; and

the clustering in certain occupations and geographically.

The personal, psychological, social and economic consequences of the spread of the virus will unfold for decades after the virus has taken hold in a community and will continue to unfold for as long as the virus continues to spread.

Let us look at the overlapping waves of consequences more closely.

The first wave of impact to emerge is centered on the infected person and her or his family, partners and carers. It includes the trauma of diagnosis, community reactions (acceptance or stigma and discrimination), economic and emotional impact on their households, reaction of health care workers, illness and death. As indicated in Figure 3.2, those primarily affected are individuals and families, and the ways in which they are affected and the resources that they and others can bring to bear on their problems determine the policy and programme requirements.

In developing countries, most women and men are faced with the probability of their being infected when a baby or young child is clinically diagnosed with HIV. The lack of confidentiality, which is too frequent in these settings, often leads to the mother being singled out for blame. Fear and denial on the part of the father can lead to the woman's rejection and repudiation. The family may be torn apart and the women and her children left destitute and homeless. Strict confidentiality and the disclosure of the child's HIV status with counselling to both parents, not just the mother, can often protect the women and enable the family to continue as a basic nurturing and socializing unit for the children.

The immediate concern of infected women, and often men, is the future well-being of their children. Who will look after them after their deaths? Where the receiving family cannot be the extended family, many women would like to participate in the choice of an alternative form of care and help prepare their children for the future. Already at this stage, long before the children are left without parents, attention needs to be given to identifying or establishing forms of care for these children.

The second area of immediate concern is that the parents continue to be able to provide for and nurture their children for as long as possible. In one Kigali community, the women identified one nutritious meal a day and the treatment of any opportunistic infection, oral thrush, for example, which might impair their ability to look after their children.

As more and more children and adults fall ill, the demand for the treatment of opportunistic infection and for anti-virals will increase as will the demand on hospital beds. Whilst neglect of these demands may cause political unrest, addressing these demands may not be possible because of a lack of a basic health infrastructure and because of resource constraints. There is thus the need to achieve an informed and widespread consensus in the community, as well as in the health sector and among bureaucrats and politicians, on a treatment strategy.

The formal health care system will have to rationalise its role as it ceases to be able to provide institution-based care for all those with HIV-related illnesses. New modes of care management and collaborative and complimentary home and institutional-based care regimes will need to be designed. The increasing burden of care will be to a great extent borne by family and friends, but probably disproportionately by women and girls.

In this latter case, women's other roles and responsibilities, including child rearing and their productive roles, will be seriously affected if the burden of care is added to women's illness and death. Young girls may be withdrawn from schools to help care for the sick and for siblings and to keep the family together as long as possible.

As the burden of illness increases, household incomes and provisioning will be directly affected. Those unable to pay rent or repay mortgages may lose their homes. School fees and food requirements may become unaffordable. Furthermore, the use of household savings and assets in the futile search for a cure can seriously impoverish the family. There will need to be programmes of assistance to meet the basic needs for food, shelter, counselling and school fees in affected households.

The effectiveness of programmes for affected individuals, families and communities will ultimately depend on the legal, ethical and human rights milieu pre-existing or established to respond to the epidemic. Respect for the rights and dignity of those affected,

FIGURE 4.2
Programming the Epidemic and its Impact

EPICENTRE	WAVE I	WAVE II	WAVE III	WAVE IV
Spread of the Virus	*Trauma, Illness and Death*	*Survivors*	*Social and Economic Impact*	*Long term Potential Impact*
Level of Primary Intervention				
Individual Community	Family Community	Family Community	Workplace Nation	Nation Community
Primary Programme/Policy Focus				
Change in norms and behaviour Voluntary testing and counselling sites Legal, ethical and human rights Prevention technology Socio-economic causes	Social/sexual development Social inclusion Psychological support Legal, ethical and human rights issues Welfare maintenance Care and treatment Future planning	Legal, ethical and human rights Assistance programme social/sexual development Social inclusion Psychological support legal ethical and human rights issues	Labour market and social services planning Productivity maintenance Governance	Governance Decentralization Community survival strategies External Aid flows

guarantees of confidentiality, anti-discrimination provisions and a policy context of support and commitment that all affected people remain an integral part of their communities are sine qua non conditions for an effective response. Furthermore, without this legal framework, the affected will not speak out and tell their stories so that others may learn and change their behaviour. Such stories are amongst the most effective motivaters for behaviour change.

Often it is not until large numbers of the population are infected and many have progressed to AIDS or associated diseases such as tuberculosis that there is the possibility of a national consensus on the urgency of the matter. It is usually only at this stage that the voices of public health officials, health workers and the infected and their families finally begin to be heard.

As more adults die, the second wave of impact begins to emerge: increasing numbers of children and the elderly left without support and of single-headed households (Figure 4.1). For every adult dead, there could be on average two to three dependents. Thus the amplitude of this phase could be two to three times greater than the mortality rates in the previous phase. Poverty will also be spreading: households disintegrating; children scattered.

The most striking feature of this wave is the psychological impact on individuals and communities of so many lives lost, so many parents, siblings, friends, children, colleagues, neighbours dead. In young children this often induces an almost catatonic state, a withdrawal from the world of pain and despair. One story from the Kagera region in Tanzania is of a young girl sitting day after day at the edge of the yard, rocking on her heels and staring into space. Both her parents are dead, brothers and sisters, aunts and uncles. There is little food but she is not hungry. She rocks, grieving.

The grandmother takes time away from her overwhelming burden of care of all her other grandchildren to come and sit quietly beside the young girl. she knows she must gently draw her back into the land of the living or she will slowly die. The little girl has no will to eat, to go to school, to help out in the house. Unless programmes find a means of reaching out to such children, and similarly affected communities, other assistance programmes will be less than effective.

Grandmothers and grandfathers are bearing a crippling burden of care although, as the epidemic deepens, they too are increasingly numbered among the infected. The extent of homeless, destitute and traumatised children and elderly will be largely determined by the extent of caring environments that can be found or created for them.

Extended family and neighbourhood forms of care will soon become overwhelmed unless they, themselves, are supported. A recent study in Kigali, where the impact of the epidemic in creating dependent survivors has already become visible, shows that already one in every two households is caring for one or more children other than their own.

There are various different ways to provide assistance to the survivors and their communities (Figure 4.2): direct transfer programmes, subsidies, entitlements, credit and social services including housing, feeding and child care programmes. These must complement and support the initiatives which arise within the communities themselves. The striking feature of this epidemic is that wherever the virus spreads, individuals and communities respond. Leaders emerge, caring and coping strategies spring up and programmes are developed.

For the survivors as well as the infected, a supportive legal, ethical and human rights environment is essential if they are to be supported by their communities and if they are to be able to retain their property, inheritance and custody rights. This is particularly true for women and for orphaned children.

The third wave of impact centres around the loss of so many members of the workforce and the impact of the epidemic on household and domestic savings and on foreign exchange earnings (Figure 4.2). The epidemic will cause a reduction in the quantity and quality of labour available to produce output in both the formal and informal sectors and both measured and unmeasured activities. Women's labour, both productive and domestic, is disproportionately unmeasured. The loss of women's labour will threaten the living standards of households and communities as well as national productivity. Patterns of labour supply and demand will change, the determining factor being the clustering of the virus occupationally and geographically (Figure 4.1).

There will also be a reduction in and changing patterns of use of savings. The quantity of savings available and how this is employed influences the rate of growth of Gross National Product (GNP). Decreasing levels of savings will occur at the same time as the direct and indirect costs associated with the epidemic escalate.

Economies most vulnerable will be those that depend on a single or a limited number of sectors, agriculture alone or mining and agriculture, for example. The sectors most vulnerable will be those which require a critical number of trained personnel for whom replacements are difficult to find, pilots and mining engineers among many others, or occupations with high infection rates, transport sector workers, construction workers, senior public servants, students, for example.

The transport sector knits together producers and markets, raw materials and finished products, matches migrant labour supply to labour demand, links urban and rural economies, holds families together, enables centralised military and police control. A slow down in this sector will have extensive economic, social and political repercussions.

In the agricultural sector, farming systems which are labour intensive throughout the agricultural cycle or where labour demand peaks at certain times, as well as those with which is associated a strict gender division of labour, are most vulnerable to shortages in the labour supply. In subsistence farming systems, crop mixes are already changing, swinging away from cash crops and certain food crops to less demanding crops such as manioc. Farming systems based on the availability of wage labour, for example, plantation crops, are also vulnerable. Significant changes in patterns of production will adversely affect household nutrition and income levels as well as urban food supplies and foreign exchange earnings.

With growing numbers of women falling ill and dying, and with women being increasingly occupied with the care of the ill, women will have less time for caring for and socialising with their own children and for productive work in the fields, in self-employment or in the paid workforce.

This work is often unrecognised and undervalued. Too much of it does not appear in systems of national accounts nor is much of it included in economic measures such as GNP. It will be difficult to monitor the impact at the macro level of the loosening of these social and economic networks or parenting, providing, coping and caring. However, their absence will be widely felt. This work of women is essential for the economic and social well-being of families, communities and societies.

Increasing morbidity will eventually affect all sectors of the economy: financial institutions, education and health sectors, water and electricity supplies, industry and governance (Figure 4.2).

The fourth wave of impact is directly linked to the failure of previous interventions. If the spread of the virus is not slowed down as early as possible in the epidemic, and if those affected by it are not adequately supported, then the very survival of communities and nations will be in jeopardy. The survival tactics of the bands of destitute children could lead to the terrorization of populations. Strategic vulnerability will increase with the morbidity rates in the military. Basic services, water, electricity, road maintenance, financial services, will be impaired. Price increases and service decreases will lead to discontent and unrest. National governance could come to a halt. Households, communities and countries will disintegrate.

At this stage, even international interventions to prevent the total disintegration of the nation state may be too late. Such interventions will need to occur much earlier and in an intensive and systemative way.

These longer-term consequences are not inevitable. The extent and seriousness of the consequences will depend directly on the timeliness and effectiveness of behaviour and attitudinal change programmes and of policies adopted to respond to the needs of the infected, the ill and the survivors.

The phases identified in Figure 4.1 are not discrete; they overlap. However, there is often a time lag before the problems associated with each stage becomes visible and the phase recognised. The severity of subsequent phases will depend upon the efficiency of earlier interventions. If this is not understood, competing demands on limited national resources could mean that programmes for earlier phases, behaviour change programmes in particular, are not allocated sufficient resources. Furthermore, in each phase there are policy options which are best decided in advance, so that people can be educated to understand and accept them and planning for them commenced.

The proportional costs of delaying the start of an effective HIV programme. This displays, on the right hand side, the proportional costs at year thirty of the epidemic in a particular country. The difference in levels of cost depend on the stage that the epidemic has reached before an effective programme is implemented. The cost of starting an effective programme rises with the stage of the epidemic. This is because there will be more sectors and programme components and a greater demand for services. The different levels of cost at thirty years probably differ from each other by factors of ten or more. Thus there is a disproportionate advantage in starting effective HIV programmes early.

Each phase has its own set of policy and programme requirements and these are cumulative rather than sequential. That is, as different phases of the epidemic emerge, a new set of policies and programmes will have to be developed while those for previous phases will need to be continued. Thus the demand on human and financial resources will expand rather than change over time.

Furthermore, as can be seen from Figure 4.2, responsibility for most of these policies and programmes will lie with sectors and ministries other than health. An early understanding of this can create a broader consensus on the need for timely expenditure on effective prevention programmes. The epidemic then ceases being the responsibility solely of Departments or Ministries of Health and begins to be a multisectoral concern. The earlier this happens, the greater the possibility of minimising the severity of subsequent phases. The most powerful intervention to minimise the impact of the epidemic is an effective programme to reduce the further spread of the virus.

Thus, an effective strategic response to the epidemic would

be a phased response consisting initially in support to communities responding to the epidemic and the establishment of an appropriate ethical, legal and human rights framework. Next, the underlying socio-economic causes which determine the pattern and speed of spread need to be identified and programmes to address them established

As communities mobilize and respond, the demand for technology and services, for voluntary testing sites, condoms, health services, sterile needles, etc., will increase and, at this stage, these should be accessible and affordable. Finally, the socio-economic consequences of the spread of the virus will need to be identified, monitored and minimised.

The spread of the virus initiates an inevitable chain of consequences which will continue for decades, for generations. The nature of these repercussions is so devastating that despair and fatalism would seem to be the only rational responses. However, this bleakness is held at bay by the extraordinary response that the epidemic evokes. Wherever the virus spreads, individuals and communities respond.

THE CHALLENGES OF THE HIV EPIDEMIC

There are a number of challenges for communities and governments (Figure 4.2), choices which will either minimise or aggravate later waves of impact. The first challenge will be the type of behaviour change and prevention policies adopted and the extent of resources directed to the epidemic in its early stages.

Choices made will affect the number of people infected and hence the numbers who die and the numbers of survivors. They will determine the extent of the impact. For as long as the virus continues to spread in the community, high priority will need to be given to behaviour change and attitudinal change programmes. In the economic situation of most countries, initiating new programmes requires commitment, courage and effective arguments. Cabinet members will need to be convinced of the need for adequate financing and be active participants in policy development and planning processes.

However, even if all future cases of HIV infection could be prevented from today, every year for the next twenty years approximately five per cent of those already infected will develop AIDS and die. Thus, if in a city or country half a million people are already infected, around 25,000 people will die each year for the next two decades. In countries with an already high rate of infection, the impact would be long felt.

The second challenge will be the extent to which the

community response is integrated into and is complemented by the governmental response. Affected communities have already begun initiatives that respond to their own needs, build on their resources and use their networks and forms of social organization. They must be given the political and social space and resources to continue. Other players in the community response include community leaders, health professionals, traditional non-governmental organizations, employers, trade unions, religious and political bodies, youth groups, women's organizations and many more.

The most effective national strategies will be based on and give coherence to the diversity of responses arising within the community and will, in balancing, supporting and shaping these initiatives, command widespread support.

Another challenge will be whether and the extent to which governments assist the affected, that is, those infected, their families and carers and those that survive them, to remain an integral part of their communities. For this to occur, there need to be guarantees of confidentiality, protection against discrimination and repudiation, assistance to the infected to live positively and productively, respite and child care, access to health and education services, income and housing maintenance, assistance to families to stay together as long as a parent is still alive and programmes to keep survivors within the community.

Without such policies, increasing numbers of children and the elderly will be without the, care and support of their families or communities. The consequent lack of socialization of these children and their isolation could lead, as numbers increase, to a dissolution of social relations and the possibility of civil unrest and lawlessness. Thus the seriousness of the long-term impact is dependent upon responses to the previous challenge.

If the choice is made to assist the infected and their survivors to remain living and cared for within their communities, it will be essential for governments to create a climate of acceptance and support for this policy. People's fears and misconceptions will need to be addressed in education programmes and every means found to lessen rejection, blame and stigma and to oppose discrimination. A further challenge is whether and at what stage governments, the private sector and others should begin to plan to minimise the adverse social and economic impacts.

The epidemic has come to be in a world already shaped by a multitude of factors and these in their turn influence and determine its dimensions. Poor nations burdened with debt are unable to honour the basic rights of women and men to health care, education, shelter and employment. This has created a backlog of deprivation which both facilitates the spread of the virus and aggravates its consequences. The poverty of individuals, and of women and children in particular, has led to their increasing vulnerability to infection. Poverty caused by HIV-related illness and death deepens existing poverty, creates new poverty and increases indebtedness. This interrelatedness between the epidemic and the setting within which it is occurring will make government attempts to plan to minimise the adverse impact of the epidemic more difficult.

The challenges identified so far all occur at the level of households, communities and nations.

There is a further critical challenge which will occur at the global level: whether the world community will provide the direct foreign investment in human capital and technological development and in social safety nets to allow poor nations and nations rendered poor by this epidemic to survive.

The free working of the global market tends to increase the disparities between rich and poor nations. National governments try to offset such tendencies, nationally, by redistributing income through systems of progressive income tax. They also supplement this with social safety nets to prevent people from falling into absolute destitution.

No such systems operate at present at the global level. The closest the world comes to a global safety net is the current system of development assistance. But this system is fatally flawed, not only in the inadequacy of its extent but because its allocation at present is unrelated to the level of poverty.

Some examples. South Asia receives $5 per person while aid-receiving countries in the Middle East, with more than three times South Asia's per capita income, receive $55 per person. India has 34 per cent of the world 's absolute poor, yet receive only 3.5 per cent of total aid flows . Indeed, the 10 countries that together have more than 70 per cent of the world's poorest people receive only 25 per cent of global aid.

If overseas aid is to be able to serve as a social safety net for the world's poor, it will have to be based on principles requiring that aid should be directed to priority concerns for human development.

The final challenge rests with us. Ultimately, our hope lies in understanding the centrality of the will to live, to stay together, to cope and survive at all levels— individuals, families, communities, nations and internationally.

If we keep quiet, if we think that this is not our problem, HIV will change the world despite us. We can make a difference. We can overcome the epidemic by speaking out, by using our influence within our families and communities. By changing our lives and our behaviour, we can create a world in which we can peacefully coexist with the virus.

5

AIDS and Asia: A Development Crisis

Ever since cases of AIDS began to appear in Asia during the mid 1980s, chose involved in efforts to contain the global epidemic have warned that the spread of HIV, the virus responsible for AIDS, could inflict social devastation in the world's most populous region.

This up coming toll as yet remains in the future: there is so far no Asian city or rural area where the impact of HIV infection has reached close to that experienced in some pockets of Africa. However, AIDS is no longer a stranger in the Asian environment. Although the caseload of actual AIDS is still very low, over one million HIV infections are already thought to have occurred in Asia and the Pacific. If the rate of spread continues at its current pace, Asia can expect around one million new infections a year by the year 2000, by which time many of those now infected will have become sick with AIDS-related illnesses and died.

The relatively late arrival of HIV in Asian and Pacific countries confers on their governments an advantage not enjoyed in much of Africa, where the caseload of HIV-induced sickness and AIDS was already high by the time the presence of the virus was recognized. Governments in the region are in a position to draw from the body of knowledge and experience already accumulated about the epidemic both to prepare at the earliest opportunity to meet its many consequences, and to take urgent action to contain—so far as possible—its spread. In the absence of both a vaccine against HIV and affordable, widely applicable therapies for AIDS, at present the only means of blocking HIV transmission is to encourage people to adopt self-protective and other-protective behaviours.

Most governments have established national bodies to address issues associated with HIV and AIDS and develop strategies for prevention. Their existence can be seen as an encouraging sign that the vision of the damage HIV could wreak in the region is being taken seriously at the highest levels. However, these national AIDS bodies are not immune to the tendency which has occurred elsewhere: postponement of significant action until there is a significant AIDS caseload, by which time HIV infection levels are high and may be spiralling beyond control.

One of the key lessons from experience is that the presence of AIDS in a population has far wider implications than those exclusively concerned with health. There are a number of social and economic attributes in a given population—such as the degree of occupational mobility, the role and status of women, and taboos on the discussion of sexual behaviour and sexually-transmitted disease—which contribute to the spread of HIV. These, in turn, affect the ethical and legal environment informing responses to the HIV-affected.

Since AIDS is both incurable and fatal, the presence of the HIV virus tends to arouse fear, denial, and victimization of those infected. These emotions, operating within the family, community, and society at large, are an important characteristic of the epidemic, negatively influencing personal and official responses to it. However, there have also been positive social reactions to AIDS, within affected communities or from health or social service Non-Governmental Organizations (NGOs), which have helped prolong life and reduce social distress. There is much to be learned from these experiences.

In addition to the many social and economic factors which are part of the context of the epidemic, there are also a number of socio-economic impacts stemming from it. The most important of these is the loss to sickness, and ultimately death, of a large number of adults in the prime of their economic life: most cases of HIV infection occur in men and women between the ages of 20 and 45. This has major implications for family dependents of those with AIDS, particularly the elderly and the very young, as well as for the workforce, and ultimately for a country's productivity. The cost to social services budgets of care for AIDS patients and HIV related sickness, including paediatric cases and of the care of destitute dependents, are charges which the community and state will somehow have to bear.

In July 1991, the United Nations Development Programme (UNDP) established a Regional Project based in India to stimulate awareness of the upcoming social and economic consequences of the spread of HIV infection in Asia and the Pacifie, and to catalyze early action in response to the epidemic . The Project's authority stems from the "Alliance to Combat AIDS" entered into by WHO and UNDP in 1987, which brings to the global effort to contain HIV the strengths of both organizations, recognizing WHO's primacy in health and biomedical affairs and UNDP's international leadership in social and economic development. The Regional Project co-operates closely with UNDP's. HIV and Development

Programme, based in its New York headquarters, and with its Interregional Programme to strengthen UNDP's capacity to respond to the HIV epidemic. The Project also provides assistance to existing HIV- and AIDS-related initiatives in which UNDP is involved at country level in the region.

HIV AND AIDS

What is AIDS? Acquired Immunodeficiency Syndrome (AIDS) is caused by HIV, human immunodeficiency virus. The means of HIV transmission are few and very specific. They include the use of HIV-infected blood and blood products during transfusions; injection with HIV-contaminated hypodermic needles; and transmission from mother to child in the womb or at delivery. But by far the most important route of HIV transmission is via unprotected sexual intercourse.

HIV erodes the body's defense system, exposing the infected person over time to lung diseases, cancers, fungal infections, wasting, rashes, and sores. These eventually overpower the body's ability to fight back, causing physical—and sometimes mental—ruin and death.

There is as yet no cure for AIDS, although treatment can relieve distress from opportunistic infections. One or two new drugs slow down the rate of progress from HIV infection to serious illness, but they are very expensive and have toxic side-effects.

AIDS, a threat to humankind: AIDS is one of the most serious threats to human health and life ever faced because:

- # The major mode of HIV transmission is sexual, and the urge for physical intimacy is fundamental in all human beings.
- # An important means of transmission is from mother to unborn child, in the womb. AIDS therefore presents a major threat to bearing healthy children.
- # The period between HIV infection and onset of illness can last several years. A person with no knowledge of being infected can infect others unwittingly.
- # There is no cure. Prevention is dependent on following a self-protective behavioural code, and one which protects others.
- # Human capacity for denial is so great that the adoption of self-protective behaviour tends to become widespread only when deaths from AIDS are close to home; by which time many people have already been infected.

Responses to the HIV epidemic: The fight against HIV and AIDS at international, national, and local level requires engagement by all groups within society, not only medical scientists and health workers. These include community-based organizations and those in the business sector. Responses to the epidemic take many forms:

Research into all aspects of HIV, to understand its epidemiology and develop curative and preventive therapies against its invasion and onslaught.

Spreading information about HIV and AIDS through all possible channels to dispel stigma, ignorance, and false conceptions, and guide people to self-protective behaviour.

Providing care and counsel for those with AIDS, and for family members affected by their illness and death.

Ensuring that hospital practices, blood and blood products, and hypodermic needles are consistently HIV-free.

Challenging the immense human capacity for denial about the threat of HIV and AIDS, and lifting taboos surrounding the discussion of sexually-transmitted disease.

With the collaboration of UNDP and WHO country offices, as well as that of other local, national, and regional partners, the Project has been exceptionally active. Drawing on lessons from other parts of the world, initiatives have aimed to strengthen understanding of the full dimensions of the HIV epidemic among decision-makers in all fields, not only that of health; establish, by research and analysis, the soeial, economic, cultural, and political factors influencing the epidemic, and their implications for policy-making and the application of the law; build capacity to meet HIV infection and AIDS in a variety of sectors, within government and outside it; and harness from a number of sources the energy and creativity needed to develop preventive strategies which will work. A number of other donors have lent support, including SIDA (Sweden), USAID, ODA (UK), the UN Drug Control Programme (UNDCP), and the Ford Foundation.

All initiatives fall within UNDP's own policy framework for HIV and AIDS, articulated by the HIV and Development Programme of UNDP in New York. They are also designed to dovetail with existing country plans for the control of AIDS, developed throughout the region with assistance from WHO's Global Programme on AIDS, within which socio-economic factors are increasingly becoming a feature. The Project has also played an educational role within the international donor community, familiarizing its members with the development implications of the epidemic and embedding within tJNDP's own regional consciousness the need to review constantly efforts in other sectors in the light of HIV and AIDS.

The vely special nature of the HIV epidemic, whose life-damaging potential is almost certainly unprecedented in the history of public health, demands an unusual degree of programmatic innovation and experimentation. To help create a supportive limate towards HIV containment, the Project has enlisted many partners inside and outside governmental networks. These include NGOs, especially community-based organizations, as is consistent with UNDP's contemporary programming philosophy; and partners in the private business sector, Chambers of Commerce, and the legal and media worlds. The urgency of the HIV and AIDS situation has prompted a variety of effort. Some results may be disappointing; others may cut corners in identifying effective strategies for behavioural change—corners which must be cut if what has been described as a 'smouldering volcano' threatening Asia is to be prevented from erupting.

Already, there are signs that leading politicians, government officials, and economic analysts are taking on board the social and economic implications of HIV and AIDS. In November 1992, the 2nd International Congress on AIDS in Asia and the Pacific will be held in New Delhi. The Conference, of which UNDP WHO, the AIDS Society for Asia and the Pacific, and the Government of India are co-sponsors, indudes on its agenda a prominent concern for the economic, social, and cultural aspects of HIV, and exploration of lessons from the educational and behavioural sciences to help develop preventive strategies. This indicates a broadening of the perspective in which the epidemic and responses to it are now being addressed.

Plans are in progress for a four-year Second phase of the UNDP Regional Project. In response to the increased level of awareness in the region, a number of new project and programme initiatives are coming forward. New Strategies for communlicating the key messages about AIDS need to be thoroughly piloted and tested. New approaches for responding to the HIV-affected through community based approaches and human rights networks need support. The special challenges of protecting women from HIV need to be given extra attention.

With Project expansion in view, this publication has been prepared in the hope that the sharing of information and ideas will help to build the necessary alliances throughout the region to control the social and economic damage that HIV and AIDS will otherwise surely bring.

6

The Impact of HIV on People and Society

Up to now, the protential impact of HIV infection on people and society in Asia has largely been analyzed in terms of medical issues: the costs of testing for HIV infection, of clinical care for AIDS patients, of protecting the blood supply, of sterilization practices, and of publicizing health information about AIDS. Little attention has been given to analyzing the impact on the families of patients, or on patients' and their dependents' needs for counselling and other kinds of support.

These are elements of the much broader human and economic development perspctive conerning the HIV epidemic in Asia and the Pacific which the UNDP Regional Project is setting out to illuminate. The development of capacity to analyze upcoming impacts is pre-emptive, drawing on experience from elsewhere to identify in advance the contexts in which those impacts will occur.

AT THE PERSONAL AND FAMILY LEVEL

At presents there is little other than anecdotal evidence about the impact of HIV and AIDS at the personal level in Asia and the Pacific. However, a recent paper prepared for UNDP underlines that the dominant share of the costs of the epidemic will be borne by the affected individuals and their families; and that the onset of HIV-related illness will tend to strain the resources of those affected to a point, where they and their families become seriously disadvantaged. The costs faced at the personal and family level include the direct costs of medical are and the loss of livelihood from the death of a breadwilnner. This situation contrasts with that in most western economies where many such cost are met by state or private insurance provision and where —accordingly- there is more incentive for the institutionalized public and private sectors to invest in HIV prevention.

There is another cost, not easy it to quantify, represented by the trauma of victimization for the person with HIV. This too often follows the discovery of a person's HIV-positive status. In 1988, when a blood bank in Goa, India found HIV in the blood of a donor, he was forcibly held in isolation for 64 days under the Goa Public Health Act although he had no knowledge of his infection, was not sick, and presented no risk to society.

This case illustrates the negative impact of a legal and ethical climate which is unprepared to deal with HIV; which is governed by unjustified fear of contagion; and which inappropriately applies public health legislation designed in another era for the containment of infections with a totally different pathology, such as cholera or smallpox. In the Goa case, relatives acted on the individual behalf and the Public Health Act was eventually adjusted so that isolation for HIV-positive individuals became optional, and he was allowed home.

Another case of victimization was recently reported from a village in Kochi. A young man returned from a spell of employment in Bombay and the Gulf fell sick as an outcome of HIV infection. When the source of his illness became known, his elderly parents were made socially out cast and destitute and the young man was hounded from the village. Not only does this case illustrate the need for confidentiality in HIV diagnosis, but many other social and economic impacts and interactions: the vulnerability of migrant workers; loss of livelihood for the patient and dependents; loss of shelter and community support.

Among low-income groups, the impact of HIV related disease, or of social stigma engendered by it, is far more devastating than among those with economic reserves and social out. Poorer families have no margin to absorb the cost of health care, the loss of earnings vital to meet food bills and other basis needs. The costs of the HIV epidemic will fall most heavily on the poor in Asia, and will further entrenh their poverty thereby augmenting existing soeio-economic inequity. Thus, there is an urgent need for research into impacts at the personal and family level within all ineome groups but especially among the least well-off.

Experience from Africa, USA, and elsewhere has shown that the person with HIV needs support and confirmation of his or her intrinsic value as a human being. This is demanded not only by considerations of humanity, hut as a strategy to maximize the development of individual and family resources to offset the impact of infection. The person who is able to "live positively with HIV" can prolong his or her healthy and active life, and make provision for the future of dependents. A person reconciled to HIV infection is also motivated to protect a spouse or sexual partner from exposure, by abstinence or the use of condoms.

UNDP initiated research into the economic impacts of HIV/AIDS in Asia and the Pacific

Who is Bearing the Cost of the HIV/AIDS Epidemic in Asia? David Bloom and Sherry Glied, April 1992.

The Economic Impacts of AIDS in the Republic of Korea, Bong-minYang, July 1992.

Economic Implications of AIDS in Southeast Asia: Equity Considerations, Myo Thant, April 1992.

Economic Impact of HIV and AIDS on the Transport Sector: Developing an Assessment Methodology, Patrick Giraud, May 1992.

The implications of AIDS for the agricultural sector in Lao PDR, Anthony M. Zola, September 1992.

Overseas Contract Workers and the Economic Consequences of HIV/AIDS in the Philippines, Orville Solon and Angelica Barrozo, 1992.

The Impact of AIDS on Malaysian Industrialization, David Lim, April 1992.

The Economic Impact of AIDS, Desmond Cohen, 1992.

When family members fall sick, womenfolk provide nursing care and absorb other parts of the household maintenance burden, such as income or food provision. This is another component of the special impact of the epidemic on women, and on their daughters, some of whom may have to minister to parental sickness and death at a vely young age. When death occurs, grandparents and other relatives often have to take in bereaved offspring. Again, the additional domestic onus falls most heavily on women household members. In Africa, children in HIV-affected families are often forced to give up schooling and shoulder adult responsibilities, proscribing their life prospects one of the key impacts of HIV on atfected individuals has been the lead they have taken in providing support services. AIDS patients and their relatives have often been the courageous initiators of responses at community level which help to replace stigma with sympathy, fear and denial with correct information about HIV, despair with life-enhancement, and risky with protective behaviours. Community based action provides the best comfort for the HIV affected, and the best hope for HIV containment.

AT THE COMMUNITY LEVEL

In certain Asian communities, HIV has already made an

impact even though its full effects in telllls of sickness and socio-economic fall-out have yet to be felt. Slum communities, typified by low standards of living, significant public health hazards, a fluid populations and common resort to illegal or semilegal methods of Subsistence, are regarded by public health experts as likely 'distribution eentres' for HIV. In Northeastern India, community leaders are already aware of the need to respond to the rising level of infection among drug-users, and the UNDP Regional Project held a workshop to help them do so. This is but one example of the Project strategy to promote and assist community-based initiatives throughout the region.

Foremost among the impacts on communities of a growing toll of HIV-related sickness will be the implications of many households' inability to bear the economic loss of key productive members. Inevitably, there will be a transfer of responsibilities and e osts onto Community Coping mechanisms. In many families where men fall sick, women will not be able to manage financially on their own, or with relatives' help, and the community will be forced to provide additional child-care facilities, scholarships, and other types of support. Existing strains on available resources for community and social services, in both urban and rural areas, will deepen. Family fragmentation and the juvenile crime rate may also rise. The UNDP Consultation on the Economic Implications of HIV and AIDS in May 1992 pointed to the need for more interdisciplinary study at the community level, particularly regarding the dynamics influencing information flows and their impact on behaviour and attitudes.

At present, to place any figure on such future impacts is bound to be speculative. But certain social behavioural determinants which predispose people to HIV—such as recreational behaviours and patterns of sexual contact—are well-established, and hypothesis is practicable. The UNDP Regional Project is active in this area. Even speculative research is valuable in providing ammunition to impress upon policy-makers in all sectors the need to inject more resources into strategies for AIDS prevention. However difficult it is to promote behavioural change, there are ways to encourage it: for example, the insistence by brothel owners (with police support) on condom use by all clients, as in northern Thailand. And it is vital that, at the moment when people are prompted to change their sexual or drug-injecting behaviour, they have the means of doing so, and a clear sense of social, cultural, legal, and political endorsement.

AT THE LEVEL OF THE WIDER SOCIETY

Certain industries and sectors, notably those employing migrant, mobile or seasonal workers, have workforces particularly vulnerable to HIV infection. Industries involved in transport, tourism, entertainment, mining, fishing, and the armed forces, can anticipate economic costs as a result of HIV infection among workers. Productivity in these sectors, and in agriculture, is also likely to be affected, as has already been shown in Africa. The UNDP

UNDP support to community-based initiatives

The UNDP Regional Project places a high priority on the need to foster community-based activity for care and counselling of the HIV-affected, and containment of HIV spread. The Project acts as a facilitator, to help organizations plan, resource, implement, and monitor, their interventions; and enables them to share experiences.

Workshops

Development implications of HIV/AIDS in the NE States of India, Manipur, January 1991; a sub-regional workshop for government policy-makers and representatives of NGOs to increase awareness of strategies for limiting HIV/AIDS.

NGO writing and communications skills, Delhi, January 1992; a workshop for Indian NGO representatives, designed to help them write up their experience and "lessons learned", for use in workshops and seminars.

Promoting NGO/Business Sector Partnerships for AIDS Prevention, Thailand, June 1992; a regional consultation attended by representatives of 24 NGOs and members of the Asian business community.

Publications

NGO HIV/AIDS Project Development Manual: A manual for use by NGOs and CBOs (Community-Based Organizations) embarking on HIV/AIDS related activity; the project planning and implementation process is broken down into nine steps, from needs assessment through planning, funding and implementation, to evaluation, and is designed to help NGOs accomplish the process smoothly.

Community Responses to HIV/AIDS in Asia: Experiences from India and Thailand: Case studies of pioneering examples of community-based NGO HIV/AIDS action in

India and Thailand, for advocacy among other NGOs and CBOs.

NGO responses to HIV/AIDS in Asia: Exploring Programmatic and Organizational Issues. Six discussion cases of NGOs designed to explore the programmatic and organizational issues they face in implementing HIV/AIDS prevention and service delivery interventions. Intended for training and teaching purposes, for use in seminars, workshops or with project or programme practitioners. NGOs examined include: Southern India AIDS Action Programme, Madras; Planned Parenthood Association of Thailand; Community AIDS Service, Penang; Duang Prateep Foundation, Bangkok.

Regional Project has set out to develop a framework of research into the up coming economic impacts of HIV/ AIDS in Asia and the Pacific.

Since up to now the epidemic has mainly been seen as a health problem, its economic impact on the wider society has only been calculated— where it has been calculated at all — in terms of its burden on health care systems. Thailand is the only country in the region to estimate the up coming costs of HIV and AIDS in terms of public and private expenditures, and has found that health care costs could grow from $1.7 million in 1991 to $65 million by 2000. However, although many non-health care costs to families are noted, including the care of up to two million parentless Thai children, no attempt has yet been made to calculate the extra burden to society or the social services imposed by increased dependency ratios and the breakdown in family life.

HIV and AIDS will soon begin to have a major impact on the workplace, particularly in Thailand and India, with companies and industries experiencing losses in workdays, in trained manpower in recruitment costs, and burdens on benefits schemes UNDP-which has established its own personnel in relation to HIV - is doing its best to ensure that managers concern is directed away from responses such as exclusion or expulsion of workers whom testing reveals as HIV-positive.

Since the average period between infection and the onset of HIV-related sickness is several years, those living with the virus enjoy a long period of fitness in which they are as capable of productive work as the non-infected. Existing research indicates, moreover, that the costs of such testing, combined with the inaccuracies and short shelf-life of results obtained, disqualify workplace surveillance as an effective strategy for AIDS control. UNDP has 'begun the task of communicating this to the Asian business sector so as to avoid wastage of resources on methods of

HIV containment that not only offend human rights, but will not work.

The upcoming economic impact of HIV/AIDS in Asia and the Pacific: Towards a Framework of Research

The UNDP Regional Project hosted a Consultation on the Economic Implications of HIV/AIDS in Bangalore, India, in May 1992. A number of researchers subsequently developed proposals for action in their own environments. All focussed on HIV prevention, on expanding resources for HIV and AIDS, and on the need for epidemiological data; other priorities varied:

- The cost-effectiveness of re-orienting information campaigns towards migrants and the workplace *(Bangladesh, Malaysia, Thailand)*
- Market analysis of the commercial sex industry; socio-economic profiles of workers and clientele *(India, Nepal)*
- Vulnerability of tourists travelling overseas; promotion of AIDS-free tourism *(Korea, Thailand)*
- Cost estimates for prevention, treatment, and rehabilitation of HIV/AIDS cases *(Malaysia, Indonesia)*
- Socio-economic causes of cross-border trafficking in girls and programmes for alternative opportunities *(Nepal)*
- The need to factor into economic analyses considerations other than those purely related to cost-effectiveness; for example, the right of hospital patients to be transfused with HIV-free blood (India)
- Impact of HIV/AIDS productivity, consumption, and labour supply within the household; costs of interventions *(Philippines, Indonesia)*
- Understanding of social, economic and cultural factors to do with condom use *(Thailand)*
- Integration of existing STD programmes with HIV prevention *(Bangladesh, Vietnam)*

With the Population and Development Association of Thailand and ILO, UNDP sponsored a workshop on issues related to HIV/AIDS in the Workplace, held in Bangkok in March, 1992. Presentations focussed on familiarizing managers with the relevant personnel issues, and the creation of a supportive climate towards HIV in the workplace by personal example, by training and education of staff, by providing counselling services and at access to condoms, and by promoting open debate. The workshop

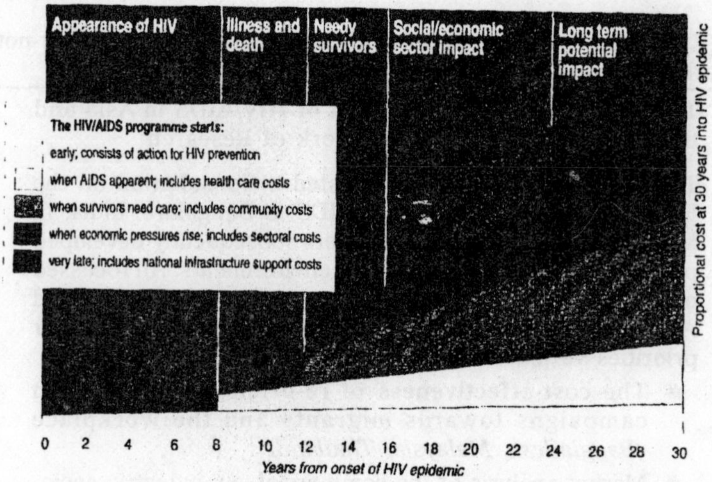

Escalating costs due to delaying the start of an effective HIV programme

conclusions placed a strong emphasis on the duty of employers to provide information services; on their obligation to desist from mandatory HIV testing of job candidates and employees; and to respect their rights to confidentiality, and to equal rights with others affected by serious illness in thus event of developing AIDS.

Certain members of the travel industry, notably hotel companies in Thailand concerned about erosion of tourist confidence, have begun to develop a workplace response. Attention is needed by other industries, such as construction companies, which similarly employ large numbers of seasonal or migrant labourers. Outflows and inflows of labour within countries and between them, are becoming a common feature of Asian economies. Between 1969-89, nearly 12 million Asians -worked as contract labour in the Middle East and in labour-short countries such as Singapore and Malaysia. In 1991, the receipts in Thailand alone from workers abroad were as high as $1 billion.

There are implications both for sending countries, and for receiving countries. Analysts in the Philippines and Thailand have already noted the possibility that their workers might be excluded from certain countries on the grounds of possible HIV infection, with implications for foreign earnings. Receiving countries will be concerned to reduce the prospect of transmission within the migrant labour community, and from it to the local population. Since migrant workers are often of low socio-economic status, their vulnerability to HIV infection is enhanced. Thus, AIDS also has the potential to reduce the labour supply, leading to higher wage levels and lowering investment from overseas.

One certain calculation about the upcoming costs of the HIV epidemic in Asia is that investment in prevention now, to reduce both the rate of HIV spread and its costs to society, is a major economy by comparison with the costs of AIDS damage control at a later stage. These costs will grow exponentially unless action is taken pre-emptively. (see chart).

Again, only Thailand has madc cost calculations based on various scenarios. If Thailand were to meet its HIV behavioural change targets (reducing sexual partners, doubling condom use, timely STD treatment) the savings by the year 2000 would amount to $5.1 billion. Even if the national AIDS control and prevention budget were to trilple in the immediate future, the cost of prevention would yield a 17 times return on investment. UNDP hopes that Thailand's example in promoting the economic advantages of HIV/AIDS prevention will have an impact throughout the region.

7

Development Practice and the HIV Epidemic

Ms. Elizabeth Reid
UNDP, New York

Development practice with respect to HIV is paradigmatically the practice of human development. This is so for two central reasons. Firstly, the focus of HIV is people's sexual, psychological and social relations and behaviour. No roads, fertilizers, procurement systems or stock exchanges are available to distract attention from or mask the fact that people are the focus of its practice. Secondly, all the classical components of development—transportation systems, labour markets, economic growth, governance, poverty and more —are within the causal framework which determines patterns and speed of spread of the virus and will also themselves be affected by the impact of its spread, its associated mortality and morbidity and the burden of dependency and social disruption it will create. No longer are failures to alleviate poverty or success in employment creation just that; they each and each of the others affect what happens with the HIV epidemic.

Thus, there is now for UNDP a double imperative: improve our development performance whilst at the same time addressing the epidemic. The tools, approaches and practices for each may well be the same. The focus must be on development practice: learning the lessons of what approaches and initiatives are most effective and of how one can catalyze and support them.

Team and Constituency Building within the Organization

Exploring new approaches to development practice involves changing accepted ways of thinking about issues and accepted procedures and practices. The inertial tendency is always towards the status quo. The HIV and Development programme has the responsibility to ensure that there is a common understanding of the epidemic and a consensus on effective ways of using development assistance to respond to it throughout the organization. As more staff are recruited to HIV specific positions, especially in the two regional projects and as HIV and Development NPOs in country offices, more resources have had to be directed to collegial team building activities amongst the HIV dedicated staff. The priorities and approaches adopted and advocated by UNDP are drawn from an ongoing exploration of and quest for effective and timely responses. It is important that all parts of the organization understand and have the human and other resources required to integrate the lessons learned about effective approaches into their work.

These team building activities have involved dialogue, guidance and skill building and the development of adequate managerial and supportive capacities in the regional bureaux. It also involves building an informal constituency throughout the organization, informed not only about HIV but also about the causal interrelationships between development and the epidemic and knowledgeable about how they take this into account in their own work: the "But what should I be doing about it?" questions. Although increased time and resources were directed to this, there was only limited success achieved and significantly more effort will need to be directed at this in 1995.

Designing Development Assistance

Many, perhaps most, country offices who have fielded HIV project design missions, whether small or large, single or multi agency, have been disappointed with the resulting proposals and documentation. As have most of their government counterparts. This should not be surprising. The issues involved are complex, and often contentious. UNAIDS and most national HIV/AIDS programmes admit that what they are doing is not having a sufficient impact on the problem.

A technological resource base has been developed—condoms, information, drugs, test kits, etc.,—but even if the problems associated with accessibility and affordability of these technologies were able to be overcome, much more is needed to protect people from HIV infection. The missing factors include areas into which development has not yet ventured: male sexuality, discourse taboos, the abuse of women, the forces of traditional patriarchy, individualism, moral corruption and others. There is no tradition to guide the development practitioner in such areas, yet this is where HIV is leading development .

However, little change will occur until those involved themselves, as individuals, as communities, as economic actors, want to change: wherever people want beer, it can be found, whatever the state of disintegration of roads or markets or the formal economy. Thus, one of the basic programming challenges is to determine how the collective will to change can be created and strengthened. Telling people to change or to behave differently or to do things differently does not work, as the history of development has taught us.

In response to the repeatedly expressed frustration of country offices, HDP has developed two alternative approaches to the traditional project design missions: the process consultancy approach developed by the MDG group in BPPS and the use of preparatory assistance to build local capacities for programme design. The former defines a different role for the outsider, the consultant who enters into a context. It is neither that of expert, source of knowledge and authority, a disempowering and ineffective role, nor one which denies to the outsider the exercise of the skills, knowledge and experience which she or he brings into the context. The process consultant is a facilitator of and contributor to processes which draw out from those involved their primary concerns and resources and strengthen their capacity to determine how themselves to achieve their self determined ends. Perhaps the most telling performance criterion for the process consultant is who writes the mission report or project document: those involved or the outsider?

In the latter approach, the whole concept of a project design mission is laid aside and ways are explored of building a national consensus on what should be done by whom with what resources. Two different approaches have been tried: a process, facilitated by external institutions or individuals, of a critical mass of key concerned nationals

- # reflecting on need and identifying areas where learning is needed,
- # learning from others and other countries (facilitated study tours),
- # applying the lessons to the particulars of the national situation,
- # programme and policy development, implementation and redesign (Djibouti)

and a process initiated by a facilitator/consultant within a country, stimulating discourse, bringing into the process all those involved and building a local consensus on what should be done (Cambodia, Bangladesh).

These approaches involve increased management and oversight responsibilities in the country office, a more profound knowledge of development practice and a capacity to work with processes rather than inputs and outcomes. Backstopping support to country offices, the role of the regional bureaux, is also more resource demanding and involves substantive as well as managerial guidance.

Identifying and Redefining the Expert

Robert Chambers, in Poverty and Livelihoods, poses the question: whose reality counts? He answers that, for an understanding of poverty, it is that of the poor and that this imperative must redefine the role of the professional. Chambers argues that the basic challenge for the professional is to learn to see things from the perspective of the poor, to allow the poor to analyze and express what they know, experience, need and want.

In the case of the HIV epidemic, this is particularly pertinent. The epidemic is new, unexperienced in the lives, personal or professional, of those normally considered as experts and development specialists. It has and will have no parallel in living or even recorded history.

Those with the subtlest and most extensive knowledge of it are those living with it as a part of their daily lives. Amongst these, those infected with the virus and those that love and care for them, there are very few leaders, public figures, elites or elders who have disclosed that they are infected. The educated, the rich and the leaders are absent by choice. Those who speak out and commit themselves to respond to the epidemic, to work for change, are mainly drawn from the ranks of the less asset or access endowed. They are the people. In donor countries, those with expertise in sexuality and HIV, in community development, are mainly, at this time in history, drawn from the ranks of the socially marginalized, from the gay men's movement and the movements of women.

These agents of change often do not have the profiles or professions that organizations like UN/OPS or UNDP are accustomed to classify, renumerate or even regard as experts. Yet experts they are because they know intimately the nature of what we are facing. And so they are becoming the trainers, consultants, speakers, partners and advocates of the response. In this way, the response becomes grounded in the reality of the epidemic. It is they who must reskill development professionals and organizations.

It has been a challenge to the programme to find ways, for example, of working with people from oral rather than written traditions, to assist those affected to develop the self-confidence and the skills necessary to use their expertise, to legitimize their presence in fora where people are unaccustomed to and uncomfortable with their being present, to work in situations of recurrent illness and dying, to deal with the loss of respected colleagues and to forge partnerships of equals within differences.

UNDP as a Development Partner

One of the emerging concepts of development practice is that of partnership. This has been formulated in reaction to felt imbalances in worth or agency between donors and recipients. This imbalance has existed in the discourse of development as well as its practices: note the acceptability of words such as "recipient".

But redressing these imbalances has not been easy. Here are the words of the Co-ordinator of the Women and AIDS Support Network in Zimbabwe:

One of the principles of partnership is equality. Can we be equal when our resources are mainly human resources and we rely on our partners for material resources? Whatever we call ourselves, partners, or donors and recipients, this inequality in money can translate into inequality in power.

... I see the dialogue that is emerging as a positive one. Increasingly, the relevance of our experience and skills is being grasped by our partners To the extent that we can exchange experiences, we build ties not only based on the flow of funds but on a recognition that we have something to offer each other.

In the response to the HIV epidemic, UNDP' s contribution has been knowledge and skill based rather than grant based. We have functioned with minimal financial resources. This has assisted the programme to develop new ways of achieving its developmental ends for, like technology, knowledge and skills cannot be transferred or shared, or even given away, unless someone wants them. Thus, we have entered into partnerships with a number of networks, consortia and institutions (LACCASO, AFRICASO, APCASO, GIPA, NAP+, GNP+, FAO, PAHO, etc.,).

The defining characteristics of these partnerships have been that the purpose of the partnership has been determined through extended discussions of each partner's priorities, capacities and ways of operating, from which a work programme was developed (or not). This has created relationships of mutual respect, based on a proper understanding of each partner's interests, roles and responsibilities, has created the possibility of partnerships of equals, equal in self esteem and self confidence, and has enabled development assistance to be an empowering rather than a disempowering set of international relations. This approach is time consuming and requires skills of dialogue and conflict resolution, but it changes the pattern of relationships from the binary and unbalanced centre-periphery or directive-receptive relations to decentralized and equitable network patterns.

Governance Capacity Building

Development practitioners have come to realize that the causes of development failure may not only reside in inadequate project design or implementation but may also exist in the actual setting of the development intervention: bureaucratic ineptitude, corruption, vested interests, lack of legal redress or safeguards, people's indifference, the suppression of dissent and such like. There is, thus, a growing awareness that development must also encompass the many elements of governance, including electoral support, strengthening of legal systems, support to legal activism, participatory politics, accountability of the armed forces, the strengthening of the institutions of civil society, decentralization and other political, legal, governmental and strategic initiatives.

There is also a growing awareness that the strengthening of the institutions of governance alone may not be sufficient to address these problems. Such institutions function best in societies where there is trust, respect and concern for others as well as self, family and kin, and where there are ways for people to come together in shared pursuits. This is referred to as the social capital of a society.

The aspects of governance critical to an effective response to the HIV epidemic include not only stable government (Rwanda, Cambodia, Zaire as illustrative) and bi-or multi-partisan support but also

- # a supportive legal, ethical and human rights framework,
- # the inclusion of those directly affected, including their non-marginalisation and non-discrimination,
- # the existence of concerned civil society organizations and groups, and
- # mechanisms and formal processes for the participation and co-ordination of all involved.

One important means of governance capacity building is the establishment and support of activist and professional networks: Ethics, law and HIV, People Living with HIV and AIDS the Global Civil-Military Alliance, AIDS support organizations and HIV researchers.

The human rights, ethics, law and HIV networks, which have been established in Africa, Asia and the Pacific, Latin America and the Caribbean, and are now beginning in Eastern Europe, draw their members from legal, governmental and academic institutions and from the organizations of civil society. They only indirectly contribute to institutional capacity building or to human resource development. Their main function is social capacity building around a common purpose, in this case,/the establishment of an agreed upon legal and ethical framework for the response to the epidemic and the provision of appropriate services to those affected.

These networks contribute to social capacity building through drawing together a diverse group of those interested or implicated to enable the addressing of issues of common interest. They broaden the base of discussion and contribute consensus building within the community sector and amongst civil society, the public and the private sectors. They contribute to governance capacity building in this way and also through advocating for law reform, changes in legal practices, the provision of appropriate services, policy and programme development and through a guardianship rule in determining the legal and ethical appropriateness of the response.

Networks of people living with HIV and AIDS are forms of social organization which assist in both building capacity for representation and participation in policy and programme development and in ensuring that their expertise and commitment contribute to the strengthening of local and national responses. Such networks are important vehicles for protecting the rights of those affected and of providing protection and sanctuary. They enable those affected to enter into partnerships collectively rather than individually and provide the possibility of a continuing organizational form and presence despite the illness and death of their founders and activists.

Social Capacity Building

Social capacity building is the facilitation of collective decision making, collective commitment to a purpose, people' s participation and the building of inclusion within communities and nations. It is a means of building the social capital identified as the neglected component of sustainable human development in the 1994 UNDP/BPPS publication *Sustainable Human Development: From Concept to Operation: A Guide for the Practitioner.*

Social capacity building provides an accountability framework for institutional capacity building and a social framework within which human resource development can contribute to the collective as well as the individual good. It provides a participatory alternative to existing sources of power within communities and nations and a more equitable mechanism for redistribution of access and benefits and for programme and policy development.

The publication *Sustainable Human Development: From Concept to operation: A Guide for the Practitioner* describes development as impossible unless people making up collectivities have a chance of engaging in activities that are meaningful to them, that build on their strength and resources and that increase their well-being, however they define that. This captures an important truth about development but leaves one grappling still with the How questions: how can a development institution like UNDP assist in bringing this about?

This question has been an important focus of HDP's work. For example, to date, virtually all HIV related socio-economic research has been "turn-key' research, the antithesis of local capacity building. HDP has been exploring ways of assisting the strengthening of national capacity to undertake socio-economic research and to use the results in programme and policy research (Senegal, Central African Republic, Kenya, Zambia, Myanmar, Nicaragua and Econet—the Asian and Pacific network of economists).

This initiative is based on the recognition that sources of learning must be local, that for ideas and programmes to take root within communities, they must spring from within, be based on the realities of the lived experiences and must be disseminated and defended from there. Participatory research initiatives support and create local processes of social learning which are an essential pre-condition for social change. These local processes of social learning must, in their turn, be complemented by strengthened national capacities for reflection and analysis so that social learning can be transformed into policy and programmes.

In addition to building local capacities for social learning, the programme aims to create new approaches to the provision of supportive technical assistance. National teams and local communities take direct responsibility for the establishment of research priorities and methodologies and the development of the ethical principles to govern the research. They set the conditions under which technical assistance is provided and determine the areas where their own research competence is in need of supplementation or strengthening. Outside expertise is fitted into local processes of social learning. The programme facilitates the drawing down of assistance from external academic and development sources, national, regional and international. The provision of technical assistance becomes more complicated but more relevant and more sustainable. The processes of learning and skills building occur within, facilitated from without.

Another challenging example of local capacity building and social learning is post-war Rwanda. HIV infection rates before the genocide were amongst the highest in the world, probably around 40 per cent or higher in the urban areas. Both the nature of the slaughter and its social and political aftermath will have significantly increased the rate of infection and spread the virus into rural populations. Now, in the post-war period, no one wants to think or talk about the epidemic. They are haunted and pre-occupied by other things. As is UNDP, in country and at headquarters. No one is listening.

How can a nation address this issue in such circumstances? The approach developed and discussed intensively with the government and civil society was based on creating mechanisms within communities to enable them to begin to talk about betrayal, pain, hatred and fear, in all their causes, supported at the national level by the development of proper governance arrangements, including the re-establishment of the legal system and the creation of national consensus on an appropriate ethical and human rights framework. It also included the provision of the required services and technology—voluntary testing and counselling services, protective technologies, etc., The government of Rwanda has presented the programme to the donors and it has generated interest. This is an important example of a development practice which creates and contributes to social capacity building: the capacity of collectivities to reflect on needs, take collective decisions, resolve conflict and plan for, indeed create the possibility of, a future.

Community and National Mobilization

The fear, the pain and the denial around HIV and AIDS are so great that they are impeding the creation of the processes of social change necessary for communities to be able to support each other and survive the epidemic.

There is a need to better understand how these processes could be stimulated. An analytical framework has been developed and broadly discussed. The right for people to be able to find out whether or not they were infected was identified as a basic but neglected right. Most Africans, and many others in the developing world, cannot find out whether or not they are infected. There are few or no voluntary testing and counselling services available. The existence of such services is essential if the silence which wraps this epidemic and its paralyzing pain and fear is to be broken and a mass movement for social change created.

The quality of people's lives is affected and often determined by how they are perceived and treated by their communities. A UNV programme in Zambia stumbled across an important way of initiating a process of community mobilization. In Livingstone, the UNV team has trained women volunteers from the compounds in basic techniques of home care. These women have few, if any, resources, often not even soap to wash bodily fluids off themselves. They are concerned about the extent of the illness and dying that is happening in their compounds. They can offer little but comfort to those they visit.

Yet the social importance of their care lies in their entering the house of someone suspected or rumoured to be dying of AIDS. Through this gesture of concern and solidarity, fear and rejection are wordlessly challenged and soon the attitudes to those infected begin changing. This gesture is an essential first step in the transition from passivity and fatalism to the mobilization of the communities own resources to care for and comfort their own. This work needs to be followed up and documented as a means whereby other communities can hear and understand the story of these courageous women. HDP has been exploring how processes of community and national mobilization can be initiated in other communities (civil-military alliance, legal and ethical networks, NGO networks, political leaders, etc.,).

Collaboration and UN System Reform

The focus on UN system reform through the establishment of the joint and cosponsored prograrnme on HIV and AIDS has created the conditions for increased collaboration between and amongst the participating agencies. Non-token collaboration presupposes an extensive knowledge of the culture, mission and modus operandi of all collaborators. It requires a great deal of staff resources, good will and mutual respect and a shared understanding of what needs to be done and how to do it. Social capital building is as essential in this collectivity of organizations as it is elsewhere.

The central elements of the HDP's contribution to the process of HIV related institutional reform have focussed on the strengthening of this social capital. It has tried to contribute to creating a common vision and understanding of the nature of the epidemic and of effective responses through discussion and analysis of the overlapping and complementary conceptual frameworks and approaches of the cosponsoring agencies. In this way, it was hoped to build trust and create the necessary preconditions for collaboration. There is a need for a similar drawing together in the wider global community.

The programme was also inward turning in its efforts to strengthen UNDP's ability to contribute to the mission of the new programme through the mainstreaming or integrating of HIV into all aspects of the work of the organization and through the mobilizing of the resident co-ordinator system. UNDP has particular responsibility within the UN system for the management of the resident co-ordinator system and for the training and capacity building of the system.

For country level activities of the new programme to be able to be effective, the UN resident co-ordinator and the country office must have the capacity to undertake those tasks critical to the operation of the country Thematic Working Groups. Strengthening UNDP's capacities in both of these areas will place new demands on HDP specifically and UNDP in general.

The issues raised by the epidemic require an understanding of the structural origins of transmission of the virus and of the epidemic's consequences for societies. As an organization whose purpose is to strengthen the operational activities of the UN system through the instilling of good development practice, UNDP's contributions will be critical to the success of the new programme.

8

Gender, Knowledge and Responsibility

Ms. Elizabeth Reid
UNDP, New York

One of the most striking features of the response to the HIV epidemic to date is how few of the policies and programmes we have developed relate to women's life situations. The daily lives of women and the complex network of relationships and structures which shape them are well known to women and well documented. Despite this, our theories, research agendas, policies and programmes have not been grounded in and informed by these experiences.

This failure to take into account existing knowledge or sources of knowledge, to seek to understand and explore relevant facts and strategies, I wish to call a failure of epistemic responsibility.

Epistemic responsibility is marked by an openness to the acquisition of knowledge and a certain kind of orientation to the world and to one's knowledge-seeking self within it.[1] Certain kinds of knowledge are contingent on experience which itself is mediated by the gender, ethnicity, class, academic discipline and geographic location of the experienced. The value of what is known is dependent upon the alternatives or perspectives considered. If assumptions have not been questioned and alternative sources of knowledge sought, then the knowledge can be faulted. Claims to knowledge can not only be verified. The claimant can be faulted for not having looked enough, for the way he or she comes to knowledge.

The concept of epistemic responsibility has already been used in the context of the HIV epidemic. It has been accepted that those in charge of blood and blood-product services in a number of countries can be held accountable for not exercising their responsibility to know, to take existing knowledge and techniques into account which could have significantly lessened the contamination of the blood supply before HIV test kits were available. Individuals, not only the systems within which they operate, can and should be held responsible for their lack of interest, commitment or sense of urgency.

Responsible knowledge of human experience in general and women's experiences in particular is essential to effective HIV-related research, policy and programme development. Since the cost of ineffectiveness in these areas is an increasing toll of human despair, destitution, illness and death, epistemic responsibility is also a moral imperative.

This article will focus on the urgent need to ensure that women's knowledge and their varying life situations are systematically taken into consideration in the formulation of responses to the epidemic. Clearly, HIV-related research, policies and programmes must be grounded in human experiences, that is, those of men and boys as well as of women and girls. However, to a great extent, the life situations of men and boys have been more accessible to those responsible for developing HIV programmes. The reason for this differential access needs exploring and provides a justification for the specific focus on women's experiences.

The strategies developed in response to this epidemic have been marked by the absence of a grounding in women' s various life situations. The cost has been high. Over 4 million women are infected, ill or dead. The majority of these women are in the age group 10 to 30, with the highest prevalence in the age group 15 to 25. In men, high prevalence occurs ten years later in the age group 25 to 35. In developing country regions, Africa, Asia, Latin America and the Caribbean, the proportion of women to men is almost equal or rapidly becoming so (China 1991). Elsewhere, the proportion is also approaching one to one, although more slowly.

Most women are at risk of infection by sexual transmission. Yet the prevention strategies advocated to prevent sexual transmission have offered women little or no protection from infection.[2] Prevention strategies in general and education (IEC) messages in particular have focused on the reduction of the numbers of sexual partners, fidelity within relationships, safer sexual practices, in particular the use of condoms, and more recently, the treatment of sexually transmitted diseases (STDs). However, these measures are grounded in men's physique, lifestyles and experiences, rather than women's, and should be directed at men. As means by which women can protect themselves from HIV infection, they are inadequate.

Advocating the reduction of sexual partners as a prevention strategy is irrelevant to the lives of the many women who have no sexual partner other than their husband or regular partner. Where women do have multiple sexual partners, this is often a choice forced on them by economic necessity. For as long as this situation and the socio-economic system that gives women few choices for economic independence remain, women will not be able to adopt this strategy.

Neither is the second strategy, faithfulness within relationships, enforceable bv women. It is estimated that between 50 and 80 per cent of all infected women in Africa have had no sexual partners other than their husbands. Having no sexual partners other than their husbands may be under women's control but their husbands' behaviour is not.

Condom usage could be an important prevention strategy for women who cannot negotiate the nature of their relationships. However, condoms are used by men not women, who can only ask for their use, and so the same structural determinant of women's lives as sketched above means that they may have no power to control the use of condoms or to negotiate abstinence.

Advocating the treatment of STDs as a prevention strategy can be faulted in a similar way: it does not adequately reflect the reality of women's lives and is, therefore, based on incomplete knowledge. Rarely are these services provided in culturally acceptable circumstances or by women. They need to be paid for by cash and are usually not easily accessible.

The probability of infection by the virus during unprotected intercourse with an infected partner may be significantly increased when there are lesions, secretions, inflammation or scarification of the genital area. In men's lives, such conditions are usually caused by the presence of sexually transmitted infections and, again, this has determined the research and intervention agendas. But even in men, it is possible that factors such as a lack of circumcision may cause conditions which increase the likelihood of infection or increase infectiousness. This needs to be better understood.

In women, the situation is more complex. Lesions, secretions, inflammations or scarifications may be caused not only by sexually transferred pathogens but as much or more by sexual practices, by cultural practices in particular female infibulation and severe forms of circumcision, by non-infectious inflammatory genital conditions or other common conditions, fistulas, for example, arising from women's reproductive role.

Few data exist indicating the incidence of these latter conditions but they are pervasive. An estimated 84 million women and girls have been infibulated or circumcised worldwide causing conditions of the genital area which could place them at high risk of infection when intercourse takes place with an infected man. More than one million women will suffer disabling illnesses and conditions from reproductive causes this year alone (Jacobsen 1991). These chronic disabilities are higher among poor women everywhere and 99 per cent occur in developing countries. The most common reproductive-related disabilities, particularly in young women, occur during illicit abortions or during childbirth and could certainly increase the efficacy of HIV transmission.

Many of these conditions, including most sexually transmitted infections in women, are treatable conditions.[3] Some will require changes in cultural practices, including child brides, pregnancies in pre-puberty girls or reproductively immature young women, assaultive sexuality, including rape and incest, and other sexual practices causing lesions or inflammation as well as in infibulation and circumcision practices.

The social, sexual and economic subordination of women places them at risk of HIV infection in different ways from men. Strategies must differ when addressed to those put at risk of infection through behaviour or circumstances over which they themselves do or could exercise control and those at risk of infection through behaviour or circumstances over which they cannot exercise control. Prevention strategies have particularly not worked for those young women who become infected immediately they commenced sexual activities. For these young women, too often the circumstances in which they became sexually active allowed them little opportunity for choice or control. The behaviours that are unsafe are determined and controlled by others.

Whilst the social construction of masculinity, reinforced by peer norms and community acceptance, may include a disdain for condoms, along with multiple sexual partners, including during marriage, these are behaviour within men's ability to change. Similarly, there may be behaviours which place women at risk of infection which are within women's ability to change.

For prevention or behaviour change strategies to be able to protect women, they must fit their lives in two directions. They must be based on the contexts in which women's sexuality is expressed and, at the level of the individual, they must be strategies that women can exercise, that are under their control.

There are few possible strategies which fulfil these conditions. The diaphragm plus spermicide may protect both women and men from HIV infection and, when necessary, can be used clandestinely by women. There is clear evidence that it protects men and women from sexually transmitted infections other than HIV (Stein 1990, Alexander 1990, Lancet 1990). However, little or no research has been done in this area. Indeed, little is known about how the virus enters women's genital tract, whether infection occurs at the level of the vagina, the cervix or the uterus or about how infected women infect men. If the virus ascends through the cervix then a diaphragm could give considerable protection but if the virus crosses the vaginal wall, it will be less effective.

The female condom effectively protects both women and men, although it cannot be used without the man's knowledge since it is visible or palpable to the man when in use. However, it has not been aggressively advocated nor means explored to make it more affordable and reusable.

All genital conditions which may facilitate HIV transmission should become a focus of attention. Those conditions which are treatable should be treated. However, the reality of women' s lives forces another question: where? Many women have genital conditions which could be treated but an insignificant number of these women attend STD services. In fact, very few women are ever internally examined throughout their life, despite repeated pregnancies (McNamara, 1990).

The protective strategy most widely adopted by women is that of talking to men and attempting to help them see the importance of protecting themselves from infection and the consequences of not so doing for their families (Mongola, 1991). This is a strategy that may best be undertaken by women collectively. Women individually may feel and be powerless but women together can both change community norms for male behaviour and change that behaviour itself (Reid, 1991).

If these strategies are not available or effective, the only other strategy that may be possible is leaving her partner. This is happening with increasing frequency in seriously affected areas. However, it is only an effective protective strategy if the woman is then able to support herself and her children, where she is able to take them with her, by means other than prostitution.

If there are no strategies which adequately fulfil the two conditions identified above, then this must be clearly acknowledged and the focus of behaviour change strategies be found elsewhere: in men's sexuality and life situations or in communities. Changing men's behaviour and changing community standards to support the required behaviour changes are the most effective way of protecting women and their children from infection.

In summary, then, we have seen that those prevention strategies advocated to date have not emerged from or responded to women's experiences; they were not even based on a responsible knowledge of human experience, of men's as well as women's. Yet all of the facts about women's and men's lives upon which this analysis is based are well documented. The failure to seek them out and use them can be measured in terms of lives lost through this irresponsibility.

Both experience and knowledge are shaped by the gender of the experienced It is, therefore, necessary to find appropriate ways of knowing women' s experiences and the structures that shape them and to develop research priorities, policies and programmes which retain contiguity with these experiences.

What men and women know differs because their experiences are different.[4] A paradigm of this would be experiences relating to biological differences between men and women. Only women can experience pregnancy, childbirth, conditions resulting from childbirth or because of her reproductive capacity. Men cannot be the knowing subject of these experiences. They can be accessible to men only through the stories women tell.

Other areas where difference in gender may preclude the possibilities of common knowledge would include sexuality, parenting, strictly gender specific tasks and, in certain circumstances, some psychological and emotional states. This is not to argue that such knowledge is necessarily or intrinsically gendered but that, where experiences are not available to one gender, the knowledge arising from these experiences is not directly available either. In many of these latter cases, the difference is a matter of cultural, social or historical contingency. Men could be knowledgeable about growing manioc, tending the sick, nurturing children, expressing grief through crying, etc., Where they are not, this can be made a matter of choice not necessity.

The need to draw upon women' s knowledge and to remain in touch with the reality of women's lives will become more critical as the epidemic deepens and increasingly people begin to fall ill and children and the elderly are left without support. As the limits of the capacity of institutionally-based services to cope become clear, community- and family-based services are being advocated (Baldwin and Twigg, 1991). The terms "community-based" or "family-based" systematically obscure the reality that these services are provided by women: caring for the sick, feeding and caring for the elderly and the young, healing the traumatised, easing grief. All the work women do in holding together families, communities and their societies. Furthermore, to the extent that caring for the sick and the dependent means women's exclusion from the labour market, this will reinforce their economic and emotional dependence on men and so their inability to protect themselves from infection.

Policies which build upon and reinforce the assumption or stereotypes of women as carers presume the availability of women to undertake these tasks, and to the extent required, as demand for the services increases with the epidemic. But at the same time that demand will increase for women's labour as nurturers, networkers, copers and carers, the economic and demographic changes induced by high adult mortality rates will increase the demand and the need for women' s participation in productive labour. The complex network of responsibilities and relationships that women exercise in families and communities may be resistant to its collapse into the single function of caring.

These considerations must be taken into account as strategies are sought to satisfy the increasing demand for care and support services and the expressed desire of the infected and the survivors to remain within their communities. We will need to recognize that care must be a collective responsibility of all involved: governments and communities, men and women, families and communities. Each has a role to play in the provision of support services to carers or in direct care provision. These strategies may vary from place to place as the details of women's lives, and men' s, vary but the responsibility for them must be collectively held and exercised for us to survive the epidemic.

It follows from this analysis that women experience and know things that men do not experience or know. The same is true for men. It also follows that it is impossible to understand the epidemic without drawing or women's knowledge and experience. We must free ourselves from the limited and limiting perspective of a particular gender, class or race.

Unfortunately, such a limited and limiting perspective has dominated the HIV research and programme agendas, irrespective of discipline: epidemiology, clinical research and trials, intervention design, biological research, behavioural research, economics and so on (WHO/GPA/91.2, Stein 1990, for example)[5]. Women have been missing from clinical trials; they have been tested without consent and denied access to the results; they have not been informed that their husbands are infected; their clinical conditions have not been included in case definitions or research priorities; stereotypes of prostitutes or wives have closed off possibilities of understanding. The primary focus of attention was elsewhere. The lack of awareness or acceptance that experience is gendered has left too many women without the possibility of knowledge of their infection status, without the capacity to plan for their children's future, with increased responsibilities and with a greatly increased chance of dying.

Because most HIV research touches experiences that are gender specific —sexuality, oppression, reproduction, labour, domestic responsibilities, etc., — it must remain continually in touch with women's lives, experiences and knowledge as well as with men's. This will require that a critical intelligence be brought to bear on it. A serious constraint to this is that women are more aware than men that experience and knowledge are gendered,[6] that social, political, moral research, policy, programme and other agendas relating to all facets of their life are drawn up on the basis of men's experiences. Daily reminders of this are rare for men, for many quite absent. As a result, the relevance of women's perspectives may not be realised by those developing responses to the epidemic and gender specificity not seen as critical to the value of the outcome. There is not a felt need to know.

This lack of a felt need to know can lead to a failure to seek further in the face of dissonant facts, to set aside stereotypes and to search to know. Let us turn to a well and long known fact, already mentioned, which should be deeply disturbing. It has been noted above that the prevalence of HIV infection is highest in young women aged 15 to 25 but peaks in men ten years later in the 25 to 35 age group. This is a consistently different pattern between women and men. It was known as early as 1986 in the earliest data sets from the epidemic, the first 500 diagnosed AIDS cases in Kinshasa. The pattern is the same in recent data sets from Uganda where the epidemic has significantly deepened and from Thailand where the epidemic is still recent.'.

However, only rarely in the literature have the possible causes of this disturbing difference been explored. Decosas and Pedneault (1991) argue that this difference is due to the fact that sexual partnerships are usually formed between older men and younger women. This is doubtlessly a contributing factor but cannot be the complete explanation, if only because it is true for women in almost all age groups and so cannot explain the striking difference in infection rates in young women compared to older pre-menopausal women.

Let us rephrase the question in order to highlight it: Why do young women (15-25) have such significantly higher rates of HIV infection than, for example, young men in the same age group? Both groups are sexually active; but young men more so than young women (United Nations, 1989). Both groups have sexually transmitted infections; but young men more than young women. Young women often have different sexually transmitted infections from young men. Both older men and young men form sexual partnerships with the women who are sexually active in this young age group. These facts are not adequate to explain why the rate of infection in young women is so steep at the onset of sexual activity and so high. The question can again be rephrased: why are more young women infected than older pre-menopausal women [8]. In one South African study, 50 per cent of all infected women were aged 15-19 years, were young women with limited sexual experience, and had significantly higher rates of infection than young men of the same age and women in all other age groups (O'Farrell and Windsor, 1991). Similar patterns are found in a study of Rakai district in rural Uganda (Wawer *et al.* 1991; Cohen, 1992).

In this case, the principle of epistemic responsibility would require urgent and high priority be given to the identification of possible determining causes of this high infection rate in young women. But this has not happened to date. Frequency of sexual intercourse with infected men is insufficient to explain the data.

Thus, it is highly probable that the condition of the genital tract in young women significantly increases the likelihood of transmission whenever unprotected sexual contact occurs. A number of possible hypotheses come to mind. The efficacy of HIV transmission to young women may be increased by.

(a) the sexually transmitted infections found in young women and/or other infections of their genital area;
(b) cervical ectopy in young sexually active women;
(c) hormonal changes at the onset of menstruation and during the menstrual cycle;
(d) the changes in the anatomy of the genital tract as young women reach puberty; and
(e) the immaturity of the genital tract in post-puberty young women.

The biology of the female genital tract remains poorly understood. We know more about the cellular structure of lungs, for example, or about the increased protection from HIV infection offered by an intact genital mucosa in monkeys (Miller and Gardner, 1991, for example). In young women, the explanation for their shocking rates of infection may be a combination of some or all of these or other factors. The research agenda is in urgent need of realignment.

Since in so many facets of the HIV epidemic experiences are gender specific, it must become part of responsible epistemic and programme practice to move on from the constraints of single gender knowledge — for both men and women — to an approach that is grounded in human experience. This is only possible if gender specific experience and knowledge can be made accessible to others and if how to let experience shape and reshape theory and practice can be learnt.

Women's gender specific experiences and knowledge can be accessible in a number of ways: by ensuring that women as well as men shape and determine the agendas, through first person narratives or through the devolution of responsibility for interventions to women and their communities.

First person narratives provide access which can be subtle and various. Some stories from the epidemic are now being told, a few by women (Rieder and Ruppelt, 1988; Willmore and Roy, 1989; Reid, 1990; UNDP, 1992). Noerine Kaleeba's moving story (1991) presents the experienced in the complex, interrelated way life usually asserts itself. First person narratives can bring to light different perspectives, different points of view and so make them accessible across gender.

Since, as discussed above, women are more aware of the dynamics of gender, the way these effect the epidemic emerge more clearly in their narratives. It is clear to them that one can understand life situations—being infected, caring for someone infected, for example—only if gender roles and relationships are taken into account. These narratives both present and interpret the relationship between the individual and society and the dynamics of power between women and men. They provide glimpses into men's lives as well as their own and relate individual agency to social and economic structures.

First person narratives increase understanding. Their truth or falsity or the justification of their knowledge claims will be determined in the same way as first person narratives in general: in their closeness of fit to reality and the extent of agreement with other stories. However, listening to and interpreting such narratives, whether as stories, on film or in consultations, is an acquired capacity. The interpreter must be sensitive to the narrator's purposes in telling her story. Interpretation demands a profound respect for the narrator, for what she says and for the lives from which the stories are drawn.

Narratives can identify new research and programme needs. A simple example: stories told by women of the discrimination and rejection that happened to them when a newborn child was diagnosed with HIV has led to the proposal that parents be counselled, informed and tested together (Willmore and Ray, 1990).

Patterns and structural factors will emerge as more women's voices are heard. The less these voices are muted or silenced, the more they will speak with authority and relevance, even when the knowledge and experiences recounted cut across the grain of received knowledge. Women know the nature and causes of their lives.

A critical strategy of this epidemic will be to ensure that women's perceptions, experiences and capacities are able to be expressed, valued, understood and acted upon. In so doing, the discontinuity between HIV—related experiences and HIV-related research and programmes will be lessened.

Narratives, however, do not capture systems of relationships which affect individuals but whose locus is beyond the individual and her realm of vision. The relationships between poverty and her infection status may form a critical part of her narrative but the relationships between structural adjustment programmes, poverty and the tragedy of being infected may not. Narratives need to be complemented by system level analyses. A full understanding of the nature and impact of the epidemic requires both kinds of analysis.

The second way in which women's gender specific knowledge can be accessible is through devolving responsibility for programme development and delivery to women. If solutions are to be found for men' s refusal to protect themselves and others, for women' s powerlessness to prevent themselves from becoming infected, bring women together to seek them (Willmore and Ray, 1990; Mongola, 1991). The strategies so decided upon may or may not integrally involve men. We may believe that this is essential but it is not ours to decide. If there is a collective responsibility for the care of people unable to survive independently, bring communities, women and men, together with governments to work out how it can be exercised. Women's knowledge and experiences are essential to the development of effective solutions.

Once it is recognised that responsible knowledge of human experiences in general and women' s experiences in particular is essential to developing effective responses to the epidemic and once people are more at ease and more skilled at acquiring or expressing that knowledge, we will be in a position to face the coming decades with some hope. We will then be able to develop programmes grounded in human experience to address the three central programming areas of the epidemic: changing attitudes and behaviour, caring for the affected and maintaining the social and economic infrastructure of seriously affected communities and countries.

NOTES

1. I am indebted to Professor Lorraine Code (1988) for an elaboration of the concept of epistemic responsibility and its relevance as a means of measuring the adequacy of theories.
2. This critique is more fully elaborated in Reid 1991 and Hamblin and Reid 1991. See also Worth 1989, Stein 1990 and Carovano 1991.
3. For many sexually transmitted infections in women, the problem is one of diagnosis rather than treatment.
4. This is not to argue that all women or all men know these aspects of their lives in the same way. It is a point about the lack of such experience and direct knowledge across gender.
5. There are three contributing factors. Firstly, that the early research populations were infected men, secondly, that male researchers have predominated in all disciplines and, thirdly, because of the severe inequalities of wealth between the developed and developing worlds, all early research populations were drawn from developed countries. It should be remembered that there were more infected women than gay men or men with haemophilia in the world at every stage of the epidemic.
6. Professor Anne Jacobson, University of Houston, Texas, drew to my attention that men may have to be reminded to worry about their daughters. It seems harder for men to believe that there is a perspective on the world different from theirs. I am indebted to Professor Jacobsen for assisting in clarifying the conceptual issues in this paper.
7. A fuller discussion of these data sets can be found in the Reading the Data module of the UNDP training material on HIV and Development.

See also, on Uganda, Cohen 1992.

8. There is some evidence that the efficacy of transmission is also high in post-menopausal women, that is, that when post-menopausal women have unprotected intercourse with infected men, the likelihood of their becoming infected is quite high.

REFERENCES

Alexander, Nancy J. "Sexual transmission of human immunodeficiency virus: virus entry into the male and female genital tract." *Fertility and Sterility*, Vol. 54, No. 1: 1-18, 1990.

Baldwin, Sally and Julia Twigg. "Women and Community Care - reflections on a debate." In Mavis Maclean and Dulie Groves (eds.) *Women's Issues in Social Policy*, Routledge, London, 1991.

Bassett, Mary and Marvellous Mhloyi. "Women and AIDS in Zimbabwe: The Making of an Epidemic." *International Journal of Health Services*, 21,1, 127-130, 1991.

Carovano, Kathryn. "More Than Mothers and Whores: Redefining the AIDS Prevention Needs of Women." *International Journal of Health Services*, 21:1, pp. 131-142, 1991.

Chin, James L. "The Increasing Impact of the HIV/AIDS Pandemic on Women and Children." Paper presented at the APHA meeting, Atlanta, November, 1991.

Code, Lorraine. "Experience, Knowledge and Responsibility." In Griffiths, Morwenna and Margaret Whitford (eds.) *Feminist Perspectives in Philosophy*. Indiana University Press, 1988.

Cohen, Desmond. "AIDS in Uganda." Report on a Programming Mission for UNDP Fifth Cycle Support to Uganda, 1992.

Decosas, Josef and Violette Pedneault. "The Demographic AIDS Trap for Women in Africa." Paper presented at the VII International Conference on AIDS, Florence, 1991.

Hamblin, Julie and Elizabeth Reid. "Women, the HIV Epidemic and Human Rights." Paper prepared for International Workshop on AIDS: A Question of Rights and Humanity, The Hague, May 1991.

Jacobson, Jodi. *Women's Reproductive Health: The Silent Emergency*. Worldwatch Paper 102, June 1991.

Kaleeba, Noerine with Sunanda Ray and Brigid Willmore. *We Miss You All*. Women and AIDS Support Network. Harare, 1991.

Lancet Editorial. "Barriers and Boundaries". Lancet 335: 1497-8, 1990.

McNamara, Regina. "Female Genital Health and the Risk of HIV Transmission." Literature review commissioned by UNDP, 1991.

Miller, Christopher and Murray Gardner. "AIDS and Mucosal Immunity: Usefulness of the SIV Macaque Model of Genital Mucosal Transmission." *Journal of Acquired Immune Deficiency Syndromes*; 4:1169-1192, 1991.

Mongola, Margaret. Interview for *Reflections on the Impact of the HIV Epidemic*, 1991. Forthcoming UNDP publication.

O'Farrell, Nigel and Isobel Windsor. "Sexual Behaviour in HIV-1 Seropositive

Zulu Men and Women in Durban, South Africa." Letter to the Editor, *Journal of Acquired Immune DeficiencY Syndromes,* 4:1258-59, 1991.

Reid, Elizabeth. "Placing Women at the Centre of the Analysis" in *Women and AIDS: Strategies for the Future.* Canadian International Development Agency, 1991.

Reid, Elizabeth. "Two Voices". *World Health,* WHO Geneva 1990.

Rieder, Ines and Patricia Ruppelt. *AIDS: The Women.* CLEIS Press. San Francisco, 1988.

Sabatier, Renee. "Women and AIDS," in *Women and AIDS: Strategies for the Future.* Canadian International Development Agency, 1991.

Stein, Zena. "HIV Prevention: The Need for Methods Women Can Use." *American Journal of Public Health;* 80:460-462, 1990.

United Nations. *Adolescent Reproductive Behaviour.* New York, 1989.

United Nations Development Programme (UNDP). Report of the Informal Consultation on Behaviour Change. Dakar, 1991. Forthcoming.

Willmore, Brigid and Sunanda Ray. *AIDS: An Issue for Every Woman.* Proceedings of the Women and AIDS Support Network Conference. Harare, 1989.

World Health Organization. Global Programme on AIDS. *Report of the Meeting on Research Priorities Relating to Women and HIV/AIDS.* GPA/DIR/ 91.2. Geneva, 1991.

Wawer, Maria J., David Serwadda, Stanley D. Musgrave et al. "Dynamics of the spread of HIV-1 infection in a rural district of Uganda." *British Medical Journal,* 303: 1303-6, 1991.

Worth, Dooley. "Sexual Decision-Making and AIDS: Why Condom Promotion Among Vulnerable Women is Likely to Fail". *Studies in Family Planning,* 20:6 November/December 1989.

9

HIV and the Challenges Facing by Men

Ms. Kathryn Carovano
The University of Michigan

INTRODUCTION

Since the beginning of the HIV epidemic, scores of men have been directly and indirectly affected by HIV. As of 1 January 1996, the Global AIDS Policy Coalition estimates that men represented 59 per cent of the projected 20.5 million HIV infected adults around the world, and their numbers continue to grow. The large majority of all people living with HIV (21.4 million; 92 per cent) are from the developing world, and men are no exception. Of the approximately 2.5 million men infected with the virus between January and December 1995, some 95 per cent were from the developing world.[1]

The Global AIDS Policy Coalition projects that by the year 2000, there will be a minimum of 38 million adults living with HIV, and possibly as many as 110 million.[2] New infections among men during 1993 were estimated at 139.73 per 100,000, compared to 99.15 new infections for every 100,000 women.[3] Sexual transmission is currently held to be responsible for 86 per cent of all HIV infections, and while men with HIV tend to be older than the women infected, they are still primarily young adults at the prime of their lives. Finally, while many men are coping with being infected with HIV, there are even more who are experiencing losses due to HIV-related illness and death among their family, friends and colleagues.

Against this backdrop, it is reasonable to wonder why, more than a decade into the epidemic, we feel it important to focus this Issues Paper on the challenges that HIV poses to men. In its simplest form, the answer is that we must examine HIV from every angle, ignoring none in order to improve our capacity to respond to the epidemic. Every day, more and more people are becoming infected with HIV, caring for family and friends who are suffering, and grieving the passing of those they have loved. While substantial efforts to respond are being made around the world, the epidemic continues to grow and to have a devastating impact on the lives of far too many of us. The need for more effective strategies to respond to HIV demands that we rethink old issues, re-examine previous assumptions, and leave no questions unasked. Michael Helquist, an expert in HIV communication based in San Francisco points out, "[h]ow we think about men—and women—affects how we try to fight AIDS."[4]

Men have always been a part of the HIV "problem", and they have played vital roles in the search for an effective response. Examples of their involvement includes speaking out as individuals livine with HIV, providing care to familv and friends, working as professional researchers, educators and care providers, and assisting in the development of local, national and global programmes and policies to respond to the growing epidemic. However, there has been no systematic examination of men's multiple roles in the epidemic, the many factors that influence them, as well as the obstacles that prevent more men from becoming involved. While many men have responded to HIV with a sense of urgency, responsibility, and compassion, they often appear to be the exceptions rather than the norm in their communities or professions.

At an individual level, there are many men who continue to engage in behaviours that place them and others at increased risk for HIV. Their actions may reflect a lack of awareness or understanding, or simply human frailty in the face of the immensely difficult task of maintaining safer sexual behaviours over time. Yet there are many others whose actions — or lack of action—can only be considered irresponsible, selfish and even cruel. These men do not heeds the warnings, do not see themselves as responsible, or seem to simply care more about their own pleasure than the risk their actions pose to themselves and others. In the extreme, they are the men who lie to their partners about their sexual history and even their HiV status, sexually exploit those with less power, and use sex as a form of violence against women, children and other men.

In many communities, the broader response to HIV has divided the infected from the uninfected, perpetuated stigmas, and aggravated the suffering of people living with the virus. Throughout the world, people have been tested for HIV against their will, dismissed from jobs, kept out of schools, incarcerated, abandoned by their families, denied medical care, beaten and killed in reaction to HIV. Because men hold most positions of power in families and communities, they must also bear the greater part of the responsibility for these misguided responses.

And finally, in nearly every region of the world, national and international governmental bodies have failed to act in a timely and effective manners. Governrnents—male dominated in nearly every country in the world—continue to bar admission to those with HIV infection, test suspect populations without consent, and simply refuse to acknowledge that those affected "matter"[5] and that something needs to be done. Many international agencies also continue to let the politics of power define their agenda and their actions, impeding the development of effective and sustainable local responses to HIV.

With this bleak scenario in mind, it is imperative to ask why this is so and what men—together with women—can do to make it different. The following discussion will focus on three primary areas of concern: HIV-related behaviour and behaviour change, illness and care, and death and its impact on survivors. The discussion in each area will attempt to illuminate ways in which men in different circumstances and different parts of the world are responding to these challenges. It will also focus on obstacles to an improved response and ways to assist men in the effort to face the challenges of HIV. The goal of the paper is to serve as a starting point for further discussion and understanding of the challenges that HIV poses to men and, hopefully, expand the capacity to respond.

HIV-Related Behaviour and Behaviour Change

We believe that individuals and whole communities have the inherent capacity to change attitudes and behaviours... We recognize that behaviour change at the individual and community level in the present HIV epidemic is a complex and on-going process.... Our experience as affected and infected individuals proves that behaviour change is possible. We believe that behaviour change is the most essential strategy in overcoming the HIV epidemic.[6]

Around the world, many men and women have made dramatic changes in their behaviour and their lives in response to the need to protect themselves and those they love from HIV, as well as to assist those infected to live full and meaningful lives. As HIV has spread across the globe, there has been a counter wave of change in attitudes and practices that has been a source of hope for all who struggle in the face of this epidemic. Yet the virus continues to spread, in large part because many people continue to hold views and engage in behaviours that facilitate its transmission. Hence, while positive changes are occurring, they are not enough.

Given that nearly 90 per cent of HIV infection is attributed to sexual transmission, conditions, norms and practices that facilitate the sexual spread of the virus must be the central focus. HIV is transmitted sexually through unprotected sexual intercourse—anal, vaginal, and oral. Because this is known, behaviours to eliminate or reduce the likelihood of acquiring HIV infection have been fairly easy to identify. People have the options of not having sex, having unprotected sex with only one other uninfected, faithful partner, or engaging in non-penetrative or protected sex (e.g., sex with a condom, dental dam, or female condom). Individuals may choose strategies involving some combination of these behaviours, either concurrently or consecutively, to meet diverse or changing needs.

Early efforts to promote behaviour change in response to HIV focused almost exclusively on identified "high-risk groups." In recent years, the focus has broadened somewhat including increased attention to understand and support change among women. While this expanded focus has been necessary and significant, it has still ignored the development of targeted efforts for most men.[7]

Because men in most cultures dominate decision-making and have greater independent control over sexual relations, it is imperative that efforts to respond to the epidemic and promote behaviour change place greater emphasis on men. As a first step, a better understanding is needed of the process of HIV-related behaviour change among men and the factors that motivate their sexual behaviour, both unsafe and safe.

There are a number of models of health behaviour that provide a foundation for understanding the process of change. All start from the premise that individuals can, and do make decisions about their behaviour and, at least potentially, have the capacity to translate those decisions into action. These decisions and subsequent behaviours are recognized as being influenced by various factors or determinants. Some are considered to be individual or internal (e.g., a person's perception of risk, their view of the costs and benefits associated with changing their behaviour, and their perception of their ability to change), while others are defined as external or societal (e.g., the quality and cost of a product or service, social norms that define expected and appropriate behaviour, laws and regulations).[8]

Behavioural theory recognizes that the determinants of safe and unsafe sexual behaviour will vary by age, culture, relationship status, sexual orientation and general life circumstances. Thc factors that motivate a young man to have safe sex with his fiancee may be quite different from those that motivate an older, married man to do so with a female sex worker, or a school-age boy to do so with a male friend. Likewise, the factors that influence a man's behaviours in a traditional African community will in some ways differ and in some ways potentially be very similar, to those that influence an urban European or Asian man. Adopting new sexual practices and sustaining them consistently over a lifetime are also understood to be distinct behaviours posing unique challenges.

While these theories provide a basis for understanding health behaviour and the process of behaviour change, they seem to fall short when attempting to explain or predict sexual attitudes and behaviours.[9] "As Damien Rwegera, a Rwandan respondent, noted, sex is "the ultimate coded and intimate exercise...."[10] Men and women engage in sexual relations for an array of reasons that range from the pursuit of pleasure, desire for intimacy, expression of love, definition of self, procreation, domination, violence, or any combination of the above, as well as others. How people relate sexually may be linked to self-esteem, self-respect, respect for others, hope, joy and pain. In different contexts, sex is viewed as a commodity, a right, or a biological imperative; it is clearly not determined fully by rational decision-making.

Health behaviour theory is limited by its focus on the individual. In fact, the factors influencing sexual decisions and behaviours involve a complex process that generally involves two people, not just one. How the threat of HIV impacts on people's behaviour is even more complex. It forces people to assess the implications of their own and their partners' past and current behaviours, as well as long-held beliefs, hopes and fears and, ultimately, it forces them to talk about these issues with their sexual partners.

Adopting new behaviours in the face of HIV is extremely difficult. To stay free of infection, individuals must adopt effective strategies and apply them consistently in some form over a lifetime: occasionally failing is only human. As Allan Berube. a historian from San Francisco, writes,

> The tragedy of AIDS. ..... is that so many people are dying random deaths for no other reason than that they took the kinds of risks we all take to lead meaningful lives.'[11]

We must keep this reality in mind as we grapple with the challenge of developing effective behaviour change strategies.

Sex and What it Means to Men

Men who responded to the UNDP request for information provided a number of insights into the meaning of sex in men's lives and the reasons why men engage in sexual relations, both safe and unsafe. There are few surprises, but their input contributes to an understanding of what motivates men to have sex, and factors that might facilitate—or obstruct—HIV-related behaviour change.

Among respondents, sex was noted as being important to men for a variety of reasons. It was mentioned in relation to the desire to love and be loved, connect with others, establish a family and perpetuate lineage, or satisfy a physical or biological need. Sexual relations were also identified as a source of pleasure, emotional bonding, and a means of expressing power, adulthood and "personhood." Respondents also noted that while sex is a commodity for some men, for those who engage in sex for pay, it is part of a strategy to survive.

As would be expected, men noted that sex and reasons for having sex change with stage of life and relationship status. Young, single men tend to have more partners and to view sex as a rite of passage, a way to establish their masculinity, a means of building self-esteem, and a process of exploration. A 24-year old respondent from the U.S. observed of himself and his peers, "We want to explore, we are energetic, and being male, we want to have sex—a lot."[12] In Zimbabwe, researchers found that "boys clearly feel that sexual experience is something of which to be proud. .... to have sex is to be a hero among one's peers."[13] A number of men from diverse cultural backgrounds commented on peer pressure among young men to "keep up" by having sex at an early age and with many partners.

Among older men and those in established relationships, sex was more often linked to the expression of love and intimacy and the desire to procreate and sustain their lineage. Damien Rwegera asserted that one of the most important things in his life is

> to participate in the perpetuation of the human species by siring and bringing up children. .... who are part of a family lineage which descends from a common ancestor and is prolonged from generation to generation. [14]

Other men also noted the continued importance of sex among older men as a means of expressing masculinity and virility. While none of the respondents mentioned it the global pattern of older men having sex with younger women, both consensually and otherwise, may also be tied to issues of prowess and control. Mohamed Osman of Somalia argued that for some older men, success in sexual relations "involves the honour and pride of men." He went on to note that "success" is defined by one's sexual performance, the ability of a man to "show his virility" and "not feel impotent."'[15]

While many respondents noted that the sexual behaviours of some men are changing in response to HIV an AIDS, nearly all felt that changes were not sufficiently widespread or rapid enough, particularly among heterosexual men. The adoption of safer sexual practices was noted by respondents to be frequently tied to the experience of knowing someone infected or affected by HIV. Concern for family members was also a significant motivating factor. Respondents gave more varied reasons for why they think more men are not adopting safer behaviours. They mentioned lack of awareness of HIV, denial of personal risk, fatalism, absence of supportive norms, perceived protection provided bit marriage or a stable relationship, the negative implications of safe sex on intimacy and trust, as well as lack of concern for the effect of one's behaviour on one's partner. Gaining a deeper understanding of why some men are changing gand why others are not is fundamental to addressing the challenge of behaviour change among men.

Implications for Behaviour Change

If uninformed, unskilled, unmotivated, unsupported or simply lacking access to "protection", men will still have sex and, more often than not, it is likely to be penetrative and unprotected. A simple truth is that it is natural to have unprotected sex. This is a fundamental barrier to the adoption of safe sexual practices, but it is important to go beyond it to understand why so many men continue to engage in unsafe sex.

A fundamental premise of most HIV prevention efforts is that understanding the risk posed by HIV and the means of protecting oneself are critical foundations for behaviour change. One respondent, sharing his personal experience, noted that;

> When I had [unprotected sex], I wasn't thinking about what sorts of infections I could get. .... I didn't even have enough information to be able to judge those things. .... it wasn't as if [protected sex] was something that I thought I should be doing and didn't.[16]

This testimony from a college educated man in the United States, reflecting on his awareness of HIV in the late 1980's, is a shocking reminder of how little even those individuals who would be expected to have access to accurate information may actually know.

Despite the efforts of HIV-related education throughout the world, numerous respondents noted that lack of accurate information continues to be a fundamental barrier to behaviour change for many men, especially in the developing world. Because men. (rather than women) generally have greater access to information about sex and assume the more assertive and directive role in sexual decision-making, targeted efforts are needed to provide diverse populations of men with information about HIV transmission and prevention.

Knowledge alone, however, is not enough to influence

behaviour. Health educators recognize that acquiring skills—or perceived skills—to correctly use condoms, say "no" to sex, or negotiate safer behaviours with a partner is also necessary for behaviour change. Studies among men in the Caribbean found that condom skills are relatively easy to teach and skill development can have a positive impact on behaviour.[17] The transfer of negotiation skills has been found to be considerably more complex.[18]

Efforts to transmit information, knowledge and skills are, in essence, designed to change the internal factors that affect behaviour, not the context in which they occur. Yet sex—and safer sex—is inextricably linked to the social and cultural context in which the behaviour takes place. Many of the reasons suggested by respondents to explain men's behaviours reflect social norms related to gender, relationships, power, and sex. Around the world, these norms have been identified as significant determinants of safe and unsafe behaviours, yet there is growing evidence that they can and do change."[19]

In many culture, norms of masculinity encourage men to deny, tear, doubts and any feelings of vulnerability. In some instances, men are urged to demonstrate their manhood by taking risks. Noting the attitudes of homeless boys living on the streets of Rio de Janeiro, Patrick Larvie writes, "the association between heterosexual masculinity and health was very clear: 'real men' do not get sick and do not need to worry about getting sexually transmitted diseases."[20] Denial of vulnerability is a powerful deterrent to implementing behaviour change; as long as men are unable or unwilling to admit that HIV could reach them, they are unlikely to have the motivation needed to change.

As noted by respondents from many cultures, norms of masculinity also encourage men to view sex as a form of conquest and expression of male prowess. According to Ernesto Guerrero of the Dominican Republic, "[i]n some regions, men have been educated under the premise that having many girlfriends (women) is the best symbol of virility and power." At its extreme, sex can become an act of violence with domination or humiliation the apparent goals. Whenever these are primary reasons for engaging in sex, respect for one's partner can be expected to be absent. Without respect, a concern for a partner's health or the health of future children, will have little impact on the behaviour of men.

In many cultures, societal norms (and human physiology) permit men to take little responsibility for the consequences of their sexual behaviour. Generally, women bear the burden of responsibility for pregnancy, often even where they are the result of rape. Because a man cannot be easily linked to his offspring — including a man with HIV — it remains possible for men to deny paternity and any responsibility. A European respondent asserted that in order for behaviour change efforts to succeed, "[w]e need to hammer in [to men] their responsibility for their dependents and themselves."[21]As it is, there are many reports of women being blamed for bringing HIV into a family (generally because their HIV status is identified first, through the illness of a child), in spite of the fact that the socially sanctioned behaviours of their male partners were more likely to have been the cause of the initial infection.

Commenting on these issues, Bob Connell notes:

> In 'Western' culture, the most honoured form of masculinity involves being authoritative. decisive, controlling other people, exerting power. This affects heterosexual relationships in damaging ways. Where sexual conquest is the main goal, a pattern of sexuality can be created where women are repeatedly at risk and have limited resources to resist this.... luntil dominant forms of masculinity are challenged and economic power shifts towards women, this isn't likely to end.[22]

This discussion offers some insights into men's sexual behaviour, and perhaps more than anything. points to its complexity and the need for a greater understanding of how men behave sexually and why.

The Impact of Development on Behaviour

While norms can have an impact on behaviour, so too can their absence. Discussing the challenges facing gay men in Poland, one respondent noted that "there is no model of how to organize their sex lives..."[23] and that this is a factor contributing to men having unsafe sex. This observation may be equally valid for men in a society undergoing a rapid transition, a situation common to many parts of the developing world. If the lifestyle of their parents and grandparent is no longer viable, men lack models of how to organize relationships and other aspects of the sexual life. Regardless of its root cause—whether rapidly changing social mores or deteriorating socio-economic conditions—the absence of viable models is likely to influence men's behaviour.

In many societies undergoing periods of transition, war or economic crisis, men are often forced to travel to other towns or countries in search of work. Male mobility and migration disrupt traditional family relations and influence male sexual behaviours in many parts of the world. One of the primary reasons given by respondents for engaging in sexual relations outside of marriage was physical separation from a spouse, and simple loneliness, both physical and emotional. Research on migrant workers who travel from Lesotho to South Africa, often for years at a time, found that "sex often becomes a source of escape and solace" from what i otherwise a lonely, harsh existence.[24] As Robert Mugemana noted, in Kenya, "[f]or men who leave their wives behind in the rural areas while they pursue employment in the cities, brothels offer an inexpensive source of sexual activity...."[25]

On the flip side of this equation are the men and boys who enter the sex industry to survive. While their numbers are small relative to the women and girls involved in commercial sex work, male sex workers enter this work for similar reasons. K.M Subhan, a Bangladesh respondent, observed that

> men and women are flocking to the cities in search of livelihood, mostly leaving their families behind...There are thousands and thousands of such homeless and jobless women and men who live on the pavements [who] take part in part-time prostitution for just a meal or so. [26]

Similar to migrant workers and men in the military, the men and boys involved in prostitution constitute a segment of the population at increased likelihood of exposing themselves to HTV as a result of their status and consequent behaviour.

Finally, another aspect of development that is likely to affect men's attitudes and behaviours is the changing status of women in many societies, and the consequent changes in relations between women and men. As more women become educated, employed and independent, men may feel that they are losing power. Research on domestic violence in Papua New Guinea revealed that many men saw the growing independence of their wives as a threat. "Men felt both excluded from development assistance efforts and resentful of their loss of dominance feelings that translated into increased domestic violence."[27] Sensitive to the potential for a similar backlash effect, Brendan Bain, a respondent from Jamaica, asserts that behaviour change efforts must be careful not to alienate men and suggests that the success of behaviour change programmes will depend partly on "the degree of care which is taken to preserve male identity and men's feelings of self-worth."[28] In a similar vein, Damien Rwegera from Rwanda asserts that,

> Behaviour change means change in culture, approach and community organization. ... Men must realize that this is a challenge to be met and managed. .... HIV infection will surely upset many commonly accepted values. ... Men must realize this and prepare themselves, not for a retreat, but for an advance into human civilization.[29]

While much of the preceding discussion focuses on why men are likely or unlikely to be motivated to adopt safer sexual behaviours, they must also have the capacity to change. Many of us working on issues related to women and HIV, have asserted that men have the power to change their sexual behaviour—something women often lack. Yet, admittedly, this argument overgeneralizes and oversimplifies the diverse experiences of men. Men—and boys—who engage in sex in exchange for money or goods often have little power in encounters with older, stronger, wealthier men. Other men may lack the power or self-esteem to reject norms and behaviours that are proscribed, in essence, by other men. For many men, the capacity to choose safer sex may be circumscribed in myriad ways depending on the socio-economic circumstances of their lives. Poverty is a recognized barrier to good health. Limited economic resources can put condoms and other services out of reach and the inability to meet basic needs may impede a focus beyond the most immediate future. Illiteracy limits access to information. Lack of intimacy, lack of security and lack of hope may all limit one's capacity to respond to the threat of HIV. The empowerment of men is seldom a topic of discussion, but needs to be considered in the effort to meet the dual challenges of HIV and development.

HIV-Related Illness and Care

The prevention of HIV and the provision of care and support for those affected are overlapping and interrelated issues. Efforts to encourage behaviour change are most effective when they incorporate people living with HIV and those directly affected by the epidemic. For men. who are traditionally less involved in the provision of care. this has significant implications.

Clearly, there are many men — and women — who have responded to those living with HIV and AIDS with compassion and concern. Among respondents who have experienced HIV related illness among their family and friends, feelings shared included deep sadness, compassion frustration, helplessness, anger, fear, and admiration for the courage and perseverance of those infected. While none of these responses are unique to men, some respondents identified factors that may affect how men in particular experience these emotions. Upon learning that his younger sister was HIV infected, Omari Kokole a Ugandan man, noted that he told her "not to worry too much and encouraged her to continue with her education. Reflecting back on that experience after he was tested for HIV, Kokole noted that "despite my external calm, I was deeply shaken.... Rather than pretend not to be worried and sad, I should have helped her to confront and deal with these very painful and unavoidable emotions."[30] While responding to news of the infection of a loved one is difficult for any person, social norms that define an "appropriate" male response may make it even harder for men to show their support and concern.

Men have been deeply affected by HIV-related illness among those they love, yet a number of respondents acknowledged that "men have a bad reputation when it comes to the topic of their support for the sick."[31] Caring for the sick is seen as women's work in most cultures, yet few things take more courage than caring for a loved one who is dying. While many men have provided care in both professional and familial roles, the burden of care for those with HIV in most societies is still being born largely by women. Robert Mugemana from Kenya has written,

> [w]hen a husband becomes ill, it is the woman who nurses him. When a child is ill, it is the woman who nurses it. But when a woman is ill, she nurses herself.[32]

The most notable exception to this pattern has been the response of gay men, initially in the U. S. and Europe, and now in numerous developing countries. As Bob Connell points out, "[h] eterosexual men have a great deal to learn from homosexual men in 'Western' countries. It is the gay communities that have made an immense effort at caring for people living with AIDS...."[33] This observation applies to many gay communities in the "non-Western" and developing world as well.

Even as some men have responded by providing care and support to people living with HIV, in much of the world, blaming and stigmatization have characterized the responses of far too many individuals, communities and governments. Respondents from every region noted the effects of this on the experiences of those living with HIV, as well as on individual and community level efforts to confront the epidemic. Mohamed Osman of Somalia noted that, "[t]he ones affected by [HIV] feel humiliated, discriminated against and abandoned, even by their closest family members, by the doctors, and by the society."[34] According to Godfrey Sealy, a Trinidadian man, "the threat of public disclosure is more frightening than the disease itself." This fear leads many men with HIV disease to deny the nature of their illness, and many friends to void visiting those hospitalized for fear of being associated with the disease.[35]

Fear of HIV-related stigmas have also reportedly had an impact on men's willingness to pursue HIV-antibody testing and counseling[36] or share their test results with others, both of which can be important in stemming the further spread of the virus. Nick Deocampo and Jomar Fleras note that, in the Philippines "[f]ew [young males] will consent to testing and fewer still will acknowledge they were infected for fear of being ostracized by their peers.[37] Describing his own HIV-antibody test experience, Omari Kokole, a Ugandan man, confessed: "I hesitated to confide in others partly because I feared I would be harshly judged and ostracized," noting a tendency in Uganda to shun those with HIV.[38] In 1989, Philly Bongoley Lutaaya, a well-known Ugandan singer was the first public figure in his country to openly acknowledge that he was living with AIDS.[39] What is shocking is she difficulty of disclosure even in one of the countries hardest hit by HIV. Even today in the Caribbean, another region with extremely high HIV infection rates, Godfrey Sealy has written: "[t]he ill and dying are faceless: we do not know who they are and society does not seem to care."[40] In addition to the painful personal burdens of secrecy and consequent isolation, the choice of those infected to remain hidden facilitates misperceptions about who is vulnerable to HIV. The unwary continue to believe that they need not concern themselves with this epidemic.

The increased involvement of men in caregiving is critical. Caring for those living with HIV is undoubtedly the best way to understand who the affected are and what the illness means. The participation of men in caregiving is also essential in allowing communities to respond adequately to the rapidly growing numbers of people living with HIV and AIDS. How people with HIV experience their illness is fundamentally determined by the support they do or do not receive from their families and communities. Martin Suarez, an Argentinean man living with HIV, links his ability to overcome the depression he experienced with his first opportunistic illness to "the affection and care of my loved ones."[41] Without question, men have the capacity to provide compassionate care to those living with HIV. Unfortunately, their involvement remains limited in many parts of the world. Why this persists appears, at least in part, to be due to gendered norms that circumscribe men's involvement in caregiving. However, these norms are being challenged and transformed by circumstances that are forcing men to assume caregiver roles. In Zambia, it has been observed that sons are often called on to care for their father after their mother has passed away. As more responsibilities shift to men and boys, they will need training and support to prepare them to take up these tasks, and enable them to gain a deeper understanding of the realities of HIV in their roles as caregivers.

Death and Loss

Around the world, men are dying from HIV-related illnesses, as well as experiencing losses among family, friends and colleagues. How men and their families and communities experience these deaths cannot be measured. The impact of any person's death will reflect the roles that individual plays in their family and community, as well as their unique experiences, talents, knowledge and skills. The experience of dying of AIDS will be defined, in some ways by both gender and the disease.

Because of the very different roles played by women and men, death is a gendered experience; the death of a man will impact families and communities in very different ways than the death of a woman. As David Nelson, an Alaskan Native man living with

HIV observed, when he dies, his family will lose "a father, a brother, a son."[42] Cheikh Niang of Senegal notes that, in many societies where men occupy the position of head of the household, a man's death "can signify the loss of economic support or a social base...."[43] In societies where women do not have access to paid work or are prohibited from inheriting or owning property, the death of a male partner and provider can have a devastating and far-reaching effect. Reflecting on the death of a fellow Kenyan, Robert Mugemana notes:

> [w]hen a forty-nine-year-old friend of mine recently died of HIV-related illnesses, he left behind two wives, one in the village with six children, and the other in Nairobi with four children. All ten children were in school. He was also responsible for his two elderly parents. ... The entire extended family was dependent on him.[44]

As men die, responsibilities such as these must be taken up by others. Tradition and norms in most cultures suggest that many will be shouldered by other men, leaving those who are healthy with increasing dependents to provide for. And while there is an understandable tendency to focus on the economic and social consequences of men's premature deaths, the loss of love and emotional support they provide will also create voids that cannot easily be filled. As the Somali respondent noted, the death of any person "leaves a great vacuum in the hearts of those who loved him or her."[45]

When AIDS is the cause of death, the impact can be even more painful and complex. In Rwanda, Damien Rwegera notes,

> [w]hen men die, their families lose their honour when the community finds out it was HIV. ... In general, they do all they can to hide the fact that it is HIV because admitting to it equals discrediting the partner and designating oneself as being HIV infected.[46]

Rwegera's comment points to two unique aspects of the epidemic:-the impact on survivors of the stigma and shame associated with HIV. and the harsh reality that. more often than not, more than one member of a couple or family is infected with the virus. Commenting on the situation in Uganda, Omari Kokole writes: "[d]ifficult as it is for a family to discover that one among them has this disease, think how much greater the tragedy when two or more of its members is stricken."[47] Under such circumstances, the impact on the family and the community is magnified, particularly for those survivors also living with HIV. As David Nelson noted,

> I have had some friends die of this illness and I feel a loss and a rip in my heart. [I feel] alone with the feelings that I guess someone who doesn't have the illness can't feel. It's different when you have AIDS and someone you know dies of it.[48]

These sentiments were echoed by Argentinean, Martin Saurez, who commented,

> [t]he experience [of having a loved one with HIV] is much harder when one is seropositive. It produces an identification with the other, which has extremely important emotional implications, since we not only see our loved one as ill, but also see our own possible evolution as sick people.[49]

Those who suffer the loss of loved ones also need to be supported in their grief and given meaningful options for the future. This will require addressing the imbalances of gendered divisions of labour and power that can make the loss of a male partner and provider a devastating tragedy for surviving women and children. Yet this response snould also include efforts to provide men with support and opportunities to acknowledge their grief and move on with hope in their lives.

Men who have lost partners, family and friends to HIV experience sadness, anger, frustration and grief. Numerous respondents argued that men experience the loss of a loved one no differently than a woman, that grief is universal, not gender specific. Others, however, noted that norms that define appropriate male behaviour may make grieving more difficult for men. Juan Jacobo Hernandez asserted that "men are supposed to be strong, stern, they're not supposed to cry or show weakness," and that, "male grieving is scarcely shown."[50] When a European man shared the experience of losing a grandparent (unrelated to HIV), he noted with regret that "...the last time I saw him,...I did not feel able to hug him and tell him I loved him, for reasons of male embarrassment or the traditions of the family and so on."[51] According to Cheikh Niang from Senegal, "[i]n general, men remarry rapidly after the death of their partners and rarely display any obvious expressions of grief."[52] This response could reflect a variety of factors, but may well be connected to social norms that proscribe how men grieve. While it may be impossible to measure. unexpressed or unresolved grief must inevitably impact the health of individuals and their communities.

Death resulting from AIDS can have a devastating impact, yet among the men who provided input for this paper, many credited HIV-related experiences of loss with mobilizing them to do something to respond to the disease. Some noted feelings of frustration and helplessness while others expressed anger at public health specialists and governments and at the "inadequate and insufficient individual and social response."[53] Perhaps most importantly, some credited their adoption of safer sexual practices and/or their decisions to become personally and professionally involved in the broader struggle against HIV to the death of someone close to them.

Allan Berube, who lost his partner to AIDS, eloquently described how the death of community members and loved ones in San Francisco mobilized that community to respond:

> many of us have decided to respond to this epidemic by making changes in our lives. We have taken responsibility for our past actions and accept the consequences without selfhate. We educate each other about safer sex and other safe practices. We ask for help and offer it. We demand the services we deserve from our governments. We learn how to live well in the present. We pay more attention to our health and explore all possible treatments. We celebrate our lives together. We face each other's deaths and our own. We remember, grieve and hope. We respond to AIDS as we would to other lifethreatening situations—by reorganizing our lives and taking care of each other.[54]

This description offers a template for others confronting the many challenges posed by HIV, a way of finding meaning in tragedy, as well as a testimony to the capacity of individuals and communities to change to meet the challenges of this disease.

CONCLUSIONS

How men respond to HIV, both as individuals and as members of communities, has and will continue to have a fundamental impact on the shape and texture of this epidemic. While men admittedly constitute a broad and diverse segment of the world's population, this paper has attempted to focus on the challenges that HIV and AIDS pose to them as a group, the ways they are responding, and barriers to a more effective response.

Profound changes are needed among men at the individual, community, national and even international level in order to respond effectively to the HIV epidemic. At the individual level, more men must adopt safer sexual practices to protect themselves and their sexual partners from infection. Prevention efforts must continue to be built on values that support communication, shared responsibility and mutual respect between women and men. These efforts will radically redefine norms that define masculinity, male sexuality, and the place of women in society.

Prevention efforts must also be built on a foundation of compassion and inclusion of those living with the virus, both because it is their right and because of the benefit it brings to those who are uninfected. Specifically this should include the increased involvement of men in the provision of care. This will help dismantle stigmas and stereotypes about those infected and affected and contribute toward a more supportive and compassionate community response. At the national and international level, policy-makers and programme planners must re-evaluate assumptions about men and the HIV epidemic. With the exception of gay and bisexual men, and some small, select target populations (e.g., truckers, incarcerated men) efforts to combat the spread of HIV have largely ignored the vast and diverse population of men. This lack of attention is intolerable at this stage in the epidemic, and men—as well as women — 2from the around the world are calling on decision-makers to reconsider and redefine their response to include men in both the definition of the problem and part of the solution to HIV.

Men must be involved, together with women, at every level and each step of this process. This Issues Paper is a first step toward soliciting and encouraging that involvement, and is written with the hope that together we can develop more effective responses to the challenges of HIV.

QUESTIONNAIRE

HIV: The Challenges Facing Men

Behaviour and Behaviour Change

1. What is most important in men's [your] lives?
2. How do men [you] experience sexuality?
3. Why do men [you] have unprotected sex?
4. Under what circumstances do men [you] have unprotected sex?
5. Are men [you] changing their [your] behaviour? If so, why? If not why not?
6. Why [or under what circumstances] do men [you] have more than one life time sexual partner?

Living with HIV Infection, Illness and Care

1. How do men [you] experience the HIV infection and illness?
2. How do men [you] experience the infection and illness of those they love [you]?
3. What care and support do men [you] provide those they [you] love who are sick or dying?

Death

1. How do men [you] experience the death of those they

[you] love? What do they [you] do when a partner died.

2. When men [you] die, what is [will be] lost to their [families] and communities?

General

1. What strategies are needed to address the challenges facing men?
2. What other issues need to be explored? What other questions need to be asked?

NOTES

1. Questionnaires were distributed to men know n to the author and staff at the UNDP/HIV and Development Programme or known to their friends. Twenty-three men from 16 countries responded mostly in writing, some via phone interviews. While the process did not involve a random or representative sample, it served to initiate dialogue on this issue.
2. European, whites married male in mid-30's. Response to UNDP request for information, March 1994.
3. 40-year old gay man from Poland. Response to UNDP request for information, March 1994
4. Connell, Robert W. Australia. Response to UNDP request for information, March 1994.
5. The Global AIDS Policy Coalition. *Status and Trends of the HIV/AIDS Pandemic*, Harvard School of Public Health. Francois-Xavier Bagnoud Center for Health and Human Rights: Cambridge, January 1996.
6. Mann, Jonathan, et al. *AIDS in the World: A Global Report*. Cambridge and London: Harvard University Press, 1992, p.29.
7. The Global AIDS Policy Coalition. *AIDS in the World: Redefining the Pandemic*. Harvard School of Public Health. Francois-Xavier Bagnoud Center for Health and Human Rights. Presented at the International AIDS Conference, Yokahama, Japan. August 5, 1994.
8. Helquist, Michael. USA. Response to UNDP request for information, March 1994.
9. The author vividly recalls a conversation with a US government official working in a Central American country who, after I had described the nature of the problem there, said in response, "But when will it hit someone who matters?"
10. Statement of Belief on Behaviour Change: A Central Issue in Responding to the HIV Epidemic. UNDP Informal Consultation on Behaviour Change, Saly Portugal, Senegal, 12-15 December, 1991.
11. The obvious exception are efforts directed toward gay and bisexual men in many developed and some developing countries.
12. See Aggleton, Peter, et al. "Risking Everything? Risk Behaviour, Behaviour Change, and AIDS." *Science*. Vol. 265. July 15, 1994, pp., 341-345; Silven, David. "Behavioural Theories and Relapse." in Focus: A Guide to AIDS Research and Counseling. Vol.8, No 2. January 1993; and Middlestadt.

Susan E. "The Challenge of Changing Sexual Behaviour." in Focus .— Guide to AIDS Research and Counseling. Vol. 7, No. 11, October 1992.

13. See Middlestadt, Susan E. "The Challenge of Changing Behaviour." in *Focus: A Guide to AIDS Research and Counseling.* Vol 7, No 11. October 1992. pp.1-4.
14. Rwegera, Damien. Response to UNDP request for information. June 1994.
15. Berube, Allan. "Caught in the Storm: AIDS and the Meaning of Natural Disaster", in *OUT/LOOK,* Fall 1998. pp.8-19.
16. 24-year old, white male, USA. Response to UNDP request for information, March 1994.
17. Bassett, Mary et al. "Adolescent Sexual Behaviour and HIV Prevention." *Report in Brief.* Washington, DC: International Center for Research on Women. September 1993.
18. Rwegera, Damien. Rwanda. Response to UNDP request for information, June 1994.
19. H.E. Ambassador Mohamed Osman Omar, Somalia. Response to UNDP request for information. March 1994.
20. 27-year old, white male, USA. Response to UNDP request for information. March 1994.
21. Smith. William and Susan E. Middlestadt. "Building Skills for Condom Use." in *A World Against AIDS: Communication for Behaviour Change.* Washington, DC: AIDSCOM/Academy for Educational Development. 1993.
22. Aggleton, Peter, et al. "Risking Everything? Risk Behaviour, Behaviour Change, and AIDS." *Science.* Vol. 265. July 15, 1994. pp.341-345.
23. Smith, William and Susan E. Middlestadt. "Building Skills for Condom Use." in *A World Against AIDS: Communication for Behaviour Change.* Washington, DC: AIDSCOM/Academ for Educational Development, 1993.
24. Larvie, Patrick. A Construcao Cultural dos '*Meninos de Rua' no Rio de Janeiro: Implicacoes para a Prevencao de HIV/AIDS.* Washington. DC: AIDSCOM/Academy for Educational Development 1999, p.40.
25. European. white, married male. mid-30s. Response to UNDP request for information March 1994.
26. Connell, Robert W. Australia. Response to UNDP request for information, March 1994. Research on these issues is summarized in Connell, R.W. *Masculinities.* Cambridge: Polity Press/Berkeley: University of California Press/Sydney: Allen & Unwin Australia, 1995.
27. 40-year old gay man from Poland, Response to UNDP request for information, April 1994.
28. Raditapole, Deborah K. "The Impact of HIV and Migration on Women in Lesotho." *HIV and AIDS: The Global Inter-Connection.* Hartford, CT: Kamarian Press/UNDP. January 1995.
29. Mugemana, Robert. "Our Future is at Stake," in *HIV and AIDS: The Global Inter-Connection,* Hartford, CT: Kamarian Press/UNDP, January 1995.
30. Subhan, K.M. Bangladesh. Response to UNDP request for information. March, 1994.
31. Bradley, Christine S. "Attitudes and Practices Relating to Marital Violence Among the Tolal of East New Britain," in *Domestic Violence in Papua*

New Guinea. Papua New Guinea Law Reform Commission, Monograph No. 3, 1985.

32. Bain, Brendan, Jamaica. Response to UNDP request for information. April 1994.
33. Rwegera, Damien. Rwanda. Response to UNDP request for information. June 1994.
34. Kokole, Omari Haruna. "We Are All Vulnerable." in *HIV and AIDS:The Global Inter Connection.* Hartford, CT: Kamarian Press/UNDP. January 1995.
35. Robert, Pierre. Canada. Response to UNDP request for information. April 1994.
36. Mugemana, Robert. "Our Future is at Stake", in *HIV and AIDS:The Global Inter-Connection.* Hartford, CT: Kamarian Press/UNDP. January 1995.
37. Connell, Robert W., Australia. Response to UNDP request for information. March 1994.
38. H.E. Ambassador Mohamed Osman Omar, Somalia. Response to UNDP request for information. March 1994.
39. Sealy. Godfrey. "We Are Our Own Worst Enemies", in *HIV and AIDS: The Global Inter-Connection.* Hartford, CT: Kamarian Press/UNDP. January 1995.
40. Undoubtedly, this can be partially attributed to lack of access to anonymous or strictly confidential testing and quality: non: judgmental counseling services.
41. Deocampo. Nick and Jomar Fleras. "To Meet the Challenge. We Must Overcome Our Fatalism." in *HIV and AIDS: The Global Inter-Connection.* Hartford, CT: Kamarian Press/UNDP. January 1995.
42. Kokole, Omari Haruna. "We Are All Vulnerable." in *HIV and AIDS: The Global Inter-Connection.* Hartford, CT: Kamarian Press/UNDP. January 1995.
43. Kokole. Omari Haruna. "We Are All Vulnerable." in *HIV and AIDS: The Global Inter-Connection.* Hartford, CT: Kamarian Press/UNDP. January 1995.
44. Sealy, Godfrey. "We Are Our Own Worst Enemies" in *HIV and AIDS: The Global Inter-Connection.* Hartford, CT: Kamafian Press/UNDP. January 1995.
45. Suarez, Martin. Argentina. Response to UNDP request for information. March 1994.
46. Nelson, David. USA. Response to UNDP request for information. March 1994.
47. Niang, Cheikh Ibrahima. Senegal. Response to UNDP request for information. March 1994.
48. Mugemana, Robert E.S. "Our Future is at Stake", in *HIV and AIDS: The Global Inter-Connection.* Hartford, CT: Kamarian Press/UNDP. January 1995.
49. H.E. Ambassador Mohamed Osman Omar, Somalia. Response to UNDP request for information. March 1994.
50. Rwegera, Damien. Rwanda. Response to UNDP request for information. June 1994.

51. Kakole, Omari Haruna. "We Are All Vulnerable" in *HIV and AIDS: The Global Inter-Connection*, Hartford CT: Kamarian Press/UNDP. January 1995.

52. Nelson, David. USA. Response to UNDP request for information. March 1994.

53. Suarez. Martin. Argentina. Response to UNDP request for information. March. 1994.

54. Hernandez, Juan lacobo. Mexico. Response to UNDP request for information. April 1994.

55. European, white, married male in mid-30' s. Response to UNDP request for information, March 1994.

56. Niang, Cheikh Ibrahima. Senegal. Response to UNDP request for information. March 1994.

57. Hernandez, Juan Jacobo. Mexico. Response to UNDP request for information. April 1994.

58. Berube. Allan. "Caught in the Storm: AIDS and the Meaning of Natural Disaster." *OUT/LOOK*, Fall 1988.

10

Young Women: Silence, Susceptibility and the HIV Epidemic

Gender as an Independent Variable for HIV Infection

There is a critical reality about the HIV epidemic which is yet to be grasped. It can be glimpsed through the following three assertions.

First, women are increasingly becoming infected with HIV. In most of the third world, there are as many, or more, infected women as there are infected men.[1] These women are wives and other partners, daughters and grandmothers, sisters, aunts and nieces.

Second, women are becoming infected at a significantly younger age than men. In areas where the epidemic is newly emerging and in areas where it is deeper, the same pattern is recorded: on average, women become infected five to ten years earlier than men.

Third, proportionally more girls and young women in their teens and early twenties are becoming infected than women in any other age group. A possible exception is post-menopausal women who also seem to be particularly susceptible to HIV infection.

The response to each of these assertions must be to ask why this is occurring.

The implications are that it is plausible that women become infected more easily than men, possibly at all ages and most definitely when they are in their teens and early twenties and after menopause. There appears to be a biological, immunological and/or virological susceptibility in women which changes with age.

Silence

The first diagnosed case of AIDS in a woman was recorded as early as 1982, in the first year of the known epidemic. In 1984, the first joint US/Belgian mission to Zaire clinically diagnosed virtually as many women with AIDS as men. Nevertheless the characterization of the epidemic by gender (male) and sexual orientation (homosexual) remained dominant.

In 1986 two critical studies, disaggregated by gender and age, became available. One from the University Teaching Hospital in Lusaka, Zambia, showed one in ten women attending the antenatal clinic infected with HIV and, amongst the hospital patients:

one in three men aged 30 to 35 were infected:
one in four women aged 20 to 25 were infected.

The other study reported the first 500 cases of AIDS diagnosed in Mama Yemo Hospital, Zaire (Figure 10.1)[2]. This data set was also remarkable in showing:

as many women as men were diagnosed with AIDS;
the diagnosed women were on average ten years younger than the men;
there was a sharp peak in AIDS cases in younger women, 20 to 29 years old.

These data were deeply disturbing yet they did not elicit a particular concern about women and HIV at the international level nor did they challenge and change the dominant discourse on the epidemic and thus the responses.[3]

Now, ten years after the first woman was diagnosed, an estimated three and a half million women are infected, the vast majority through sexual transmission. For most women, the major risk factor for HIV infection is being married.[4,5,6] Each day a further three thousand women become infected and five hundred infected women die. Most infected women are between 15 and 35 years old.

Age as an Independent Variable for HIV Infection

The profile of extremely high rates of HIV infection or AIDS in young women, first seen in the 1986 Kinshasa data set, reappears time and again in later data sets, in newly emerging epidemics, Thailand and Myanmar for example (Figures 10.2 and 10.3), in established epidemics, Uganda for example (Figure 10.4) and in industrialized countries, Europe for example (Figure 10.5)[7].

These data sets dramatically indicate that the patterns are everywhere and over time similar:

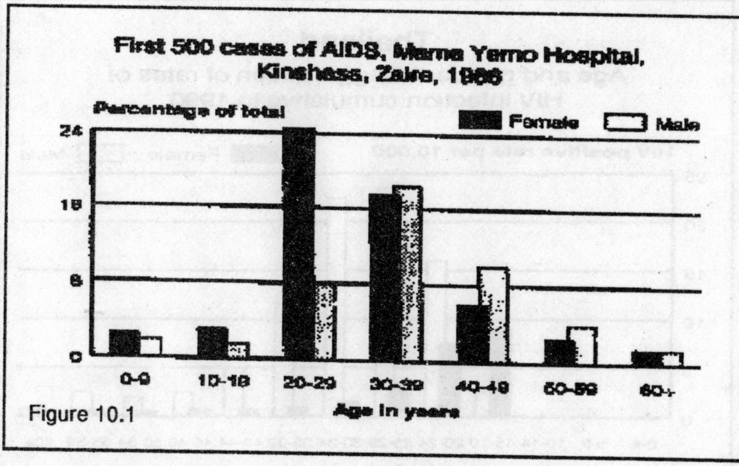

Figure 10.1

the prevalence of HIV infection is highest in young women aged 15 to 25 and peaks in men five to ten years later in the 25 to 35 age groups; and

among women, the infection profile by age has a precipitous peak in the age group 15 to 20 and declines for older pre-menopausal age groups.

Other studies[8, 9, 10] are providing dramatic illustration of the vulnerability of young women when they become sexually active early in life. Anne Chao's data from Rwanda (Figure 10.6) show that the younger the age of first pregnancy or first sexual intercourse the higher the incidence of HIV infection: over 25 per cent of young women pregnant at age 17 or younger are infected and about 17 per cent of those 17 or younger at first sexual intercourse are infected. Infection rates decrease sharply in both categories in later age groups.

It is our contention that the extent of HIV infection in young girls in their teens or early twenties shown in these data sets will be affected by all the contributory factors currently identified in the literature as increasing the rates of infection in women and men but cannot be adequately accounted. for by these factors, even in the aggregate. In the case of young women there would seem to be other influential factors. These need to be identified.

The factors identified in the literature include the incidence of sexually transmitted infections (STIs)[11,12], frequency of intercourse[13], sexual practices[14], and male/ female age differences in sexual relationships [15, 16]. To these may also be added women's nutritional status[17], and the presence of lesions, inflammation and scarification in the female genital tract from causes other than STIs[18]

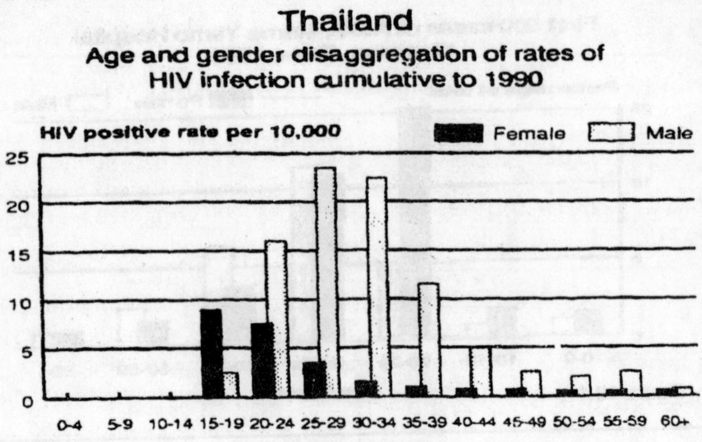

Figure 10.2

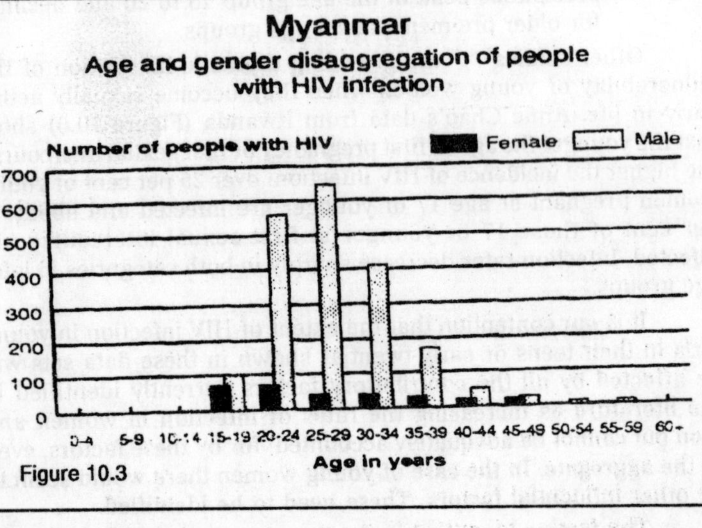

Figure 10.3

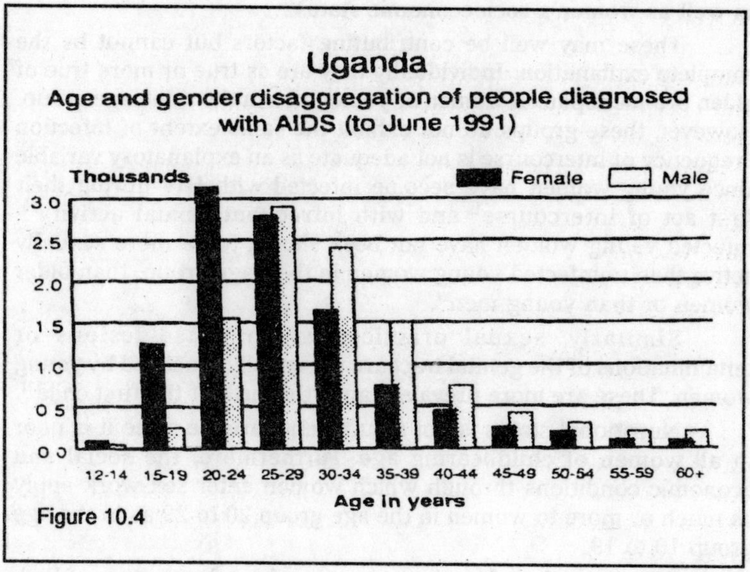

Figure 10.4

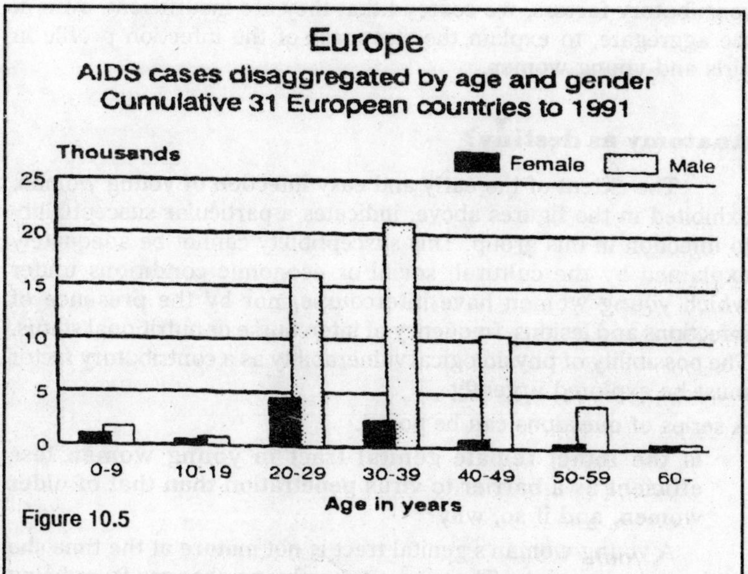

Figure 10.5

as well as women's socioeconomic status[16].

These may well be contributing factors but cannot be the complete explanation. Individually they are as true or more true of older, pre-menopausal women or young men in the same age group. However, these groups do not exhibit the same extent of infection Frequency of intercourse is not adequate as an explanatory variable since young women have become infected with HIV during their first act of intercourse[19] and with infrequent sexual activity[20]. Infected young women have not been shown to be more sexually active than uninfected young women in their age group, than older women or than young men[21].

Similarly, sexual practices which cause lesions or inflammations of the genital tract are not usually practised by young women. These are more prevalent after the birth of the first child[21].

Nutritional status is not a sufficient variable since it is poor in all women of childbearing age. Furthermore, the social and economic conditions through which women enter sex work apply as much or more to women in the age group 20 to 29 as in the age group 10 to 19.

When social explanations are offered for this pattern of high infection rates in young women, they are usually offered in terms of older men having sexual intercourse, consensually or otherwise, with younger women15 . Whilst this and all the above are clearly contributory factors, we contend that they are insufficient, even in the aggregate, to explain the steepness of the infection profile in girls and young women.

Anatomy as destiny?

The extent of the early and easy infection of young women, exhibited in the figures above, indicates a particular susceptibility to infection in this group. This susceptibility cannot be adequately explained by the cultural, social or economic conditions under which young women have intercourse, nor by the presence of infections and lesions, frequency of intercourse or nutritional status. The possibility of physiological vulnerability as a contributory factor must be explored urgently.

A series of questions can be posed.

Is the intact female genital tract in young women less efficient as a barrier to virus penetration than that of older women, and if so, why?

A young woman's genital tract is not mature at the time she begins to menstruate. The mucous membrane changes from being a thin single layer of cells to a thick multi-layer wall. This transition is often not completed until late teens or early twenties. It is

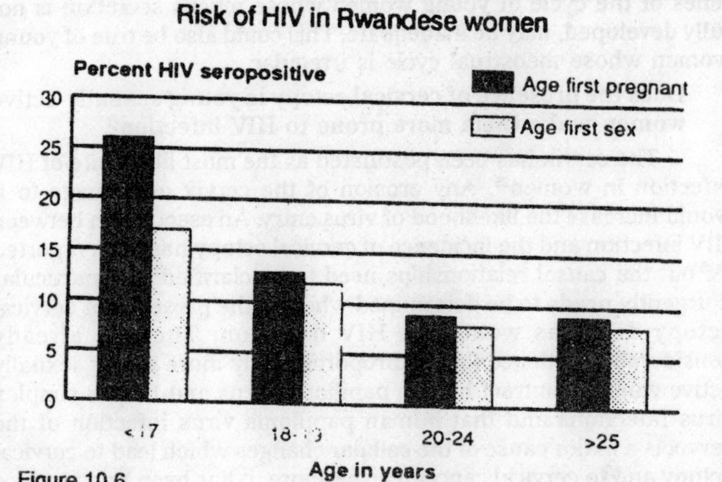

Figure 10.6

Anne Chao, 1991

conceivable there-fore that the intact but immature genital tract surface in young women is less efficient as a barrier to HIV than the mature genital tract of older women. In post-menopausal women, the mucous membrane becomes thinner and so it is also possible that the genital tract wall, even when intact, is less efficient as a barrier.

Is mucous production in young women less proficient than in older women?

Mucus in the female genital tract has four relevant roles. It acts as a physical barrier, separating semen and other material from the vaginal and cervical walls. It is a lubricant, protecting the surface of the vagina from abrasion during intercourse. It flushes the cervix and vagina in the same way that mucus flushes the respiratory tract, removing foreign material. It has an immune function[22], that is, mucus contains cells of a separate immune system whose function is to activate the immune responses of the cells in the vaginal and cervical surfaces.

If mucus production in young women, and postmenopausal women, is less proficient than in older premenopausal women, so too will these protective roles be less effective. There will be less of a barrier to viral penetration. It will provide less assistance in minimizing irritation and tearing of the genital membranes and so facilitate viral entry[23].

It is known that the hormonal fluctuations of the menstrual cycle influence the production of vaginal and cervical secretions[24]. Secretion is most prolific at midmenstrual cycle and so at other times of the cycle of young women whose mucus secretion is not fully developed, may be inadequate. This could also be true of young women whose menstrual cycle is irregular.

Does the presence of cervical,ectopy in young sexually-active women make them more prone to HIV infection?

The cervix has been postulated as the most likely site of HIV infection in women[25]. Any erosion of the cervix or damage to it would increase the likelihood of virus entry. An association between HIV infection and the incidence of cervical ectopy has been reported [20,26] but the causal relationships need to be clarified[26]. In particular it urgently needs to be determined whether the presence of cervical ectopy disposes women to HIV infection. There is already considerable evidence that disproportionately more young sexually active women contract human papilloma virus and herpes simplex virus infections and that human papilloma virus infection of the cervix is a major cause of the cellular changes which lead to cervical ectopy and to cervical cancer. Furthermore, it has been known since at least 1950 that the incidence of cervical cancer is higher in young women who began sexual activity or were married before the age of 17 [27].

Do the hormonal and physiological changes at menopause increase the vulnerability of older women to infection?

There is some case evidence that the efficacy of transmission in post-menopausal women is higher than in pre-menopausal women[28]. However, epidemiological evidence is lacking since the female population most usually tested (commercial sex workers and pregnant women) do not include them. It could be anticipated that post-menopausal infected women would usually die without diagnosis or treatment.

The biology of a woman's genital tract is poorly understood. We know more about the increased protection from HIV infection offered by intact genital mucosae in monkeys[29]. The above analysis, however, does show the urgency of developing an international commitment to providing answers to these questions.

Situational Factors

The influence on vulnerability to infection of these biologically based differences rnay be amplified by the circumstances and situations in which young women have sexual intercourse.

Non-consensual, hurried or frequent intercourse may inhibit mucus production and the relaxation of the vaginal musculature both of which would increase the likelihood of genital trauma. A lack of control over the circumstances in which intercourse occurs may increase the frequency of intercourse and lower the age at which sexual activity begins. A lack of access to acceptable health services may leave infections and lesions untreated . Malnutrition not only inhibits the production of mucus but also slows the healing process and depresses the immune system[30]. Cultural norms may favour early pregnancy, discourage the use of condoms or facilitate intercourse with older men who are more likely to be infected.

The Unheard Scream

These data show that girls and young women are excessively vulnerable to HIV infection. When will the agony of these young infected women press upon us? Anecdotal evidence from one geographic area suggests that one half of all young women there aged 15 to 19 years are infected. In other areas, the figure is one in three or one in four[8].

When will the pain and anger of these young women goad us to action? Or will we be capable of ignoring this too? There is the possibility of a disturbing parallel in the acceptance throughout the world of the loss of women's lives during pregnancy and childbirth. In Africa, as many as one woman in 21 die in the process of bearing a child. In Asia, it is one in 54; in Latin America and the Caribbean, one in 73. The tragedy and suffering of these women is too often unremarked and their deaths unmarked[31]. These deaths are needless[32].

The Prophetic Voice

The growing numbers of women infected and dying bring a deep sadness but must sound an urgent alarm. We must be aware of what the world will lose through the deaths of so many young, and older, women.

Because we live in sharply gender-divided worlds, the impact of women's deaths is different from that of men. Most, if not all, cultures raise girls differently from boys and treat women differently from men. As a result, women bring to daily life different qualities from men. Women tend to be the guardians of compassion rather than ambition, of connectedness rather than control, of healing rather than harming, of closeness rather than conquest, of mercy rather than judgment. They make possible the circle of the dance as an alternative to the ladder.

Women are the creators of new life, the caretakers of daily life and the custodians and transmitters of community norms and social values. However, in some parts of the world, one third or one half or more of all women are infected. How will the loss be borne?

Cabbage soup, writes Helene Cixous, can only warm us

passingly. To live, we need the presence of women who pay attention to life[33]. Yet even soup is usually prepared by women. It is not solely a matter of appeasing hunger of providing shelter, of resolving conflict, of raising, children, of tending fields. Women bring much more to life.

An Action Agenda

We must respond to this tragedy. There are two essential elements in the immediate strategy. First, the silence around the infection of young women must be challenged at every level: individuals, families, communities and organizations, nations and internationally. Second, a new research agenda must be established. The established hypotheses and assumptions about the nature of the epidemic, about research priorities and about gender must be set aside so that the research agenda can be reconceptualized. To do this, those responsible 'or the agenda must also change. The critically important and insightful works of Nancy Alexander[25], Bruce Forrest[22], Elizabeth Duncan[23], Zena Stein[34] and others must be acknowledged, valued and acted upon.

These two elements are necessary but not sufficient conditions for an effective strategy to protect girls and young women from being infected through their sexual and reproductive activities. An effective strategy will need to address all the factors which directly contribute to their susceptibility to infection. It must also address, in the short term wherever possible but certainly in the longer term, the indirect contributory factors[35]. There will be many elements m such an action agenda. Here we identify only a few to stimulate thought and discussion.

Neither the immediate strategy nor the broader response will be effective without political will and pressure for change. Politicians, community leaders and parents will need the courage to speak out to save these lives, to save the continuity of life. We are all responsible.

Breaking the Silence

The silence surrounding the infection of young women must be broken. Girls and young women must be able to speak out, to cease to feel silenced or powerless to change what happens to them. Others, too, must speak out.

It is critical that parents, communities and nations realize that, unless they face this issue urgently, not only will many young women be lost but so, too, will their children and their children's children. Clans and communities will cease to exist and, with them, their ancestors. Pregnancy, birth and nurturing, the continuity of life will all be placed in jeopardy.

If the silence is broken and young infected women begin to speak out and tell their stories, we must have already in place effective programmes to prevent their younger sisters from also becoming infected. If not, the breaking of the silence will add the agony of younger girls who will now know that they face a future of possible, perhaps almost certain, infection, to the agony of the young women already infected. Young girls will feel powerless to avoid the fate of their mothers and older sisters.

The psychological trauma of such a situation is virtually beyond comprehension. If we do not succeed in developing an effective, timely agenda for action, the insight and analysis which demand that the silence be broken will become a curse.

Changing the Operational Research Agenda

The mere possibility of a physiological basis to the susceptibility of infection in young women should provide the impetus for an urgent and significant research effort. Answers to questions about the female genital tract identified here, as well as others, must be found so that protective programmes can be developed.

Those who are undertaking relevant research on the female, and male, genital tracts must be supported and their findings widely and quickly disseminated. A focused effort must be made to bring together the observers of the reality and those undertaking such research and analyses together with research funders so that priorities in the bioscientific research agenda can be reset and financial support be immediately available. Doctors, nurses and social workers who are observant and understanding of the relationship between the condition of young women's genital tracts and their life situations are essential partners in the process of determining the research agenda.

Sanctuaries

Strategies must be found that lengthen the time before the onset of sexual intercourse in young women, increase the age at first pregnancy, and which increase the ability of young girls to control the situations in which they are sexually active.

Spaces must be created within which young girls can be free, and feel free, from the threat of HIV infection, within which they can pass more time before leaving to enter the world of sexual relationship and procreation and within which they can talk to one another about their coping and survival strategies, their difficulties and their successes.

Safe havens must also be found or created which would allow social and emotional interactions between girls and boys, young women and young men, and in which they can discuss and set aside the peer pressures cultural norms and gender archetypes which increase their vulnerability to infection.

The family should be the foremost of these sanctuaries. Young girls should leave their families uninfected and should be able to return to them when in fear of infection. The silence around incest must be broken, above all by mothers and those who minister to and provide service to such families. The direct price of incest is higher than ever now. The collusion of families, whether from greed or acceptance, in customs and practices which threaten the lives of their daughters must cease. Neither young women nor young men should be pressured into child or early marriages or into early pregnancies. Dowry payments or patrilocality should not prevent the possibility of a young woman returning to her family home when in fear of being infected.

Families alone cannot change cultural norms, values and practices[36]. Thus, advocating families as sanctuaries requires a complementary strategy of cultural change. Such a strategy must be led by the guardians and enforcers of culture, influential community leaders, older women, the elders, as well as by those who are now demanding such change, young men and women and their parents.

The school should also be a sanctuary from infection. However, the school is a site of non-consensual sexual activities and of HIV infection. Rape, sexual abuse and coercion by male staff and pupils combined with the exchange of sex with older men for school fees currently make the school a feared and fearful place. Community acceptance of this as normal must change. A policy of providing scholarships would obviate the need for young girls to find older men to finance their schooling. Sanctions enforced by local communities would change entrenched patterns of sexual exploitation of young girls by teachers or male students. These sanctions are now beginning to be imposed in some seriously affected areas as communities strive to keep some of their young girls uninfected.

Organizations and clubs for young women create sanctuaries where young girls can spend time without the threat of infection. They break the isolation of individual women and can lead to the creation of social support networks where young women can seek counsel and be given support to change their behaviour and to create change in their communities.

Groups working amongst street children in Brazil have opened safe houses where the girls can escape from the pressures of the street and regain a feeling of security and control over their lives. One such house is the *Casa de Passagen* (Passage house) in Recife, Brazil[37].

Such groups and organizations can also provide a refuge where infected girls and young women can come together and provide one another with support, exchange information on care and treatment and discuss issues of basic concern such as disclosure, sexuality, discrimination, pregnancy and their children's futures.

It is critical that religious organizations also create such sanctuaries for women and for men, separately and together. This would lend their moral authority to a recognition of the importance and value of young women and would help families and communities to find the courage to change and to provide sanctuary themselves.

These safe havens are critical for young girls to reach the physical maturity and the emotional and social maturity necessary to have greater control over their lives and the situations in which they have sexual intercourse.

Sanctions

The urgency of the situation may well necessitate the use of sanctions. In this respect the law can be used as an agent of social change. For example, the introduction and enforcement of laws in Southern Africa requiring men to provide financial support to all children they father, whether within marriage or outside it, have led to a significant decrease in the number of such children.

Laws against rape and incest and family law relating to the age of marriage or divorce have been less successful where there have not been concurrent changes in social and cultural values. Communities must therefore accept and decide to enforce such laws and place pressure on their members to change.

In Uganda, recent changes in governmental and community attitudes brought about by the epidemic have led to military courts trving soldiers for rape, legal services being expanded for women who have been sexually abused, vigorous reporting by the media of sexual abuse in schools and teachers being sacked for unacceptable sexual behaviour[38].

Safety

For women throughout the world, safety, that is, freedom from physical, sexual, verbal, psychological and other forms of violence, is an issue that dominates all others in their lives. The data on the extent of violence to women is quite appalling[39] but little known or acknowledged.

Abuse in the childhood or early adult lives of young women leads to low self-esteem, little ability for self-assertion and the probability of increased abuse by others, all factors which have been shown to increase the likelihood of HIV infection. In men, childhood abuse also leads to low self-esteem and to an increased likelihood of their abusing others[39].

New women's crisis initiatives exist in at least 35 developing countries[40]. All of these are dependent on external support agencies for their financing. It is vitally important to support and expand programmes to lessen violence to women and to provide refuges for abused women. This can become a significant role for external support agencies.

Restructuring Gender

The ability of young women to protect themselves from infection becomes a direct function of power relations between men and women and, in particular, of men's sexual identity. Gender is formed in families but constructed by societies[36]. Changing accepted patterns of male behaviour and expected patterns of female behaviour requires community organizing and collective action.

Individual families and societies must change how they value girls. The more women are valued, the better they will be fed and nurtured, given access to health services and education, provided with the skills required for economic autonomy and have their rights honoured, in particular to land and property, especially through inheritance.

This valuing of women will make it possible for women to value their own bodies, to improve their genital health and to have their genital infections and conditions diagnosed and treated, for cultural practices such as infibulation which increase women's likelihood of infection to be changed and for women to live through pregnancy and childbirth with minimal risk of death or lifelong disability[32].

Families must also change what they value in boys and men sc that men will be less likely to place themselves and others at risk of infection. Boys and men, not only girls and women, must become the guardians of compassion, of respect for others, of healing, connectedness and of mercy.

The Circle of the Dance

For ycung women to be able to remain uninfected, men and women, their communities and nations must want this to happen and be committed to work urgently towards it. Only then will there be hope. The priorities of the bioscientific research agenda must be changed and knowledge of all the factors which contribute to the susceptibility of young women to HIV infection deepened. Agendas for action must be drawn up locally and nationally. This will best be achieved through the creation of consultative processes which involve all those implicated in the required changes. These processes must be such that men feel able to participate, that women's insights and analyses are valued and listened to and that the external factors, the socio-economic and political climate which creates the conditions which increase women's and men's vulnerability to infection, can be addressed. Such processes are already occurring either spontaneously[41] or set in motion by concerned individuals as in the case of the Women and AIDS Support Network in Zimbabwe. They are critical if the lives of young women are to be saved . The resulting agenda for action will provide the basis for hope.

NOTES

1. Chin, James L. "The increasing impact of the HIV/AIDS Pandemic on Women and Children." Paper presented at the American Public Health Association meeting. Atlanta. November 1991.
2. Quinn, Thomas C., Jonathan M. Mann, James Curran, Peter Piot. "AIDS in Africa, an Epidemiologic Paradigm." *Science.* vol. 234, No. 957. 1986.
3. Reid, Elizabeth. "Gender Knowledge and Responsibility.," *AIDS in the World.* Harvard University Press. Forthcoming 1992.
4. Jacob, May "STDs among seropositive patients of a referral hospital in India and their role in the transmission of HIV." VIII International Conterence on AIDS/III STD World Congress. Amsterdam. July 1992. [Poster Abstract PoC 4334].
5. Hunter, D.S. Kapiga, G. L. wihula *et al.* "Risk factors for HIV-I infection among family planning clinic clients in Dar-es-Salaam, Tanzania." VIII International Conference on AIDS/III STD World Congress. Amsterdam. July 1992. [Poster Abstract PoC 4158].
6. Allen, Susan *et al.* "Human Immunodeficiency Vines Infection in Rwanda." *Journal of the American Medical Association.* Vol. 266. No. 12: 1657-1663. 1991.
7. Sources are respectively: Figure 10.2, Thailand National AIDS Control Programme.1991. Figure 10.3, Myanmar AIDS Control Programrne. 1991. Figure 10.4, Uganda National AIDS Control Programme. 1991. Figure 10.5, European AIDS surveillance. 1991.
8. Wawer, Maria J. *et al.* "Dynamics of spread of HIV-1 Infection in a Rural District of Uganda". *British Medical Journal* Vol. 303: 1303-1306. 1991.
9. Holt, Elizabeth. "HIV seroconversion in Haitian Women." Poster No. MC3010 presented at VII International Conference on AIDS. Florence. 1991.
10. Chao, Anne *et al.* "Risk factors for HIV-1 Among Pregnant Women in Rwanda." Poster No. MC3097 presented at VII International Conference on AIDS. Florence. 1991.

11. Wasserheit, J . "Epidemiological Synergy: Inter-relationships between Human Immunodeficiency Virus Infection and Other Sexually Transmitted Diseases." *Sexually Transmitted Diseases,* 19 (No. 2): 61-77. 1992.
12. Van de Perrey, Phillipe *et al.* "Risk factors for HIV seropositivity in selected urban-based Rwandese adults." *AIDS* Vol. 1:207= 211. 1987.
13. Melbye/ Mads, *et al.* "Evidence for Heterosexual transmission and Clinical Manifestations of Human Immunodeficiency Virus Infection and Related Conditions in Lusaka, Zambia." *Lancet.* :1113-1115. 15 November 1986.
14. Padian, Nancy *et al.* "Male-to-Female Transmission of Human Immunodeficiency Virus." *Journal of the American Medical Association.* Vol. 258, No. 6: 788-790. 1987.
15. Decosas, Josef and Violette Pedenault. "The Demographic AIDS Trap for Women in Africa." Paper presented at the VII International Conference on AIDS. Florence. 1991.
16. De Bruyn, Maria. "Women and AIDS in Developing Countries. *Social Science and Medicine.* Vol. 34 No. 3:249-262. 1992.
17. Bailey, Mike. Report for Save the Children Fund of V International Conference on AIDS in Africa. Kinshasa. 1990.
18. McNamara, Regina. Female genital health and the risk of HIV transmission. UNDP HIV and Development Issues Paper No. 4. Forthcoming 1992.
19. Bouvet, E. "Defloration as risk factor for heterosexual HIV transmission." *Lancet*: 615. 18 March 1992.
20. O'Farrell, Nigel and Isobel Windsor. "Sexual Behaviour in HIV-1 Seropositive Zulu Men and Women in Durban, South Africa." Letter to the Editor, *Journal of Acquired Immune Deficiency Syndromes.* 4: 1258-59. 1991.
21. Nyirenda, Meya. Oral presentation at VIII international Conference on AIDS/III STD World Congress. Amsterdam. 1992.
22. Forrest, Bruce. Women, HIV and Mucosal Immunity. *Lancet.* Vol. 337: 835-836. 1991.
23. Duncan, M. Elizabeth *et al.* First coitus before menarche and the risk of sexually transmitted disease. *Lancet.* Vol. 335: 338-340. 1990.
24. Forrest, Bruce. Personal Communication. 1991.
25. Alexander, Nancy J. "Sexual Transmission of Human Immunodeficiency Virus: Virus Entry into the Male and Female Genital Tract." *Fertility and sterility.* Vol 54, No.1:1-18.1990.
26. Mandelblatt, Jeanne S. *et al.* "Association Between HIV Infection and Cervical Neoplasia; Implications for Clinical Care of Women at Risk for Both Conditions." *AIDS.* Vol. 6: 173-178. 1992
27. Terris, Milton and Margaret C. Oalmann. "Carcinoma of the Cervix: an Epidemiologic Study." *Journal of the American Medical Association.* Vol. 174. No. 4: 1847-1851. 1960.
28. Dwyer, John. Personal Communication. 1992.
29. Miller, Christopher and Murray Gardner. "AIDS and Mucosal Immunity: Usefulness of the SIV Macaque Model of Genital Mucosal Transmission." *Journal of Acquired Immune Deficiency Syndromes.* Vol. 4: 1169-1192, 1991.

30. Chandra, R.K. Nutrition, Immunity and Infection: Present Knowledge and Future Directions. *Lancet* Vol.: 688-91. 26 March 1983.
31. Diallo, A. Boubacar. "A Tora Mousso Kele La: A call beyond duty; often omitted root causes of maternal mortality in West Africa. UNDP HIV and Development Issues Paper No. 5. Forthcoming 1992.
32. UNDP. "Safe Motherhood Priorities and Next Steps: A Forward-Looking Assessment on the Reduction of Maternal Mortality and Morbidity Within the Framework of the Safe Motherhood Initiatives (SMI). April 1991.
33. Cixous, Helene. From "Vivre l'Orange". Excerpted in *Love Poems By Women*, Wendy Mulford (ed). Fawcett Columbine. NY. 1991.
34. Stein, Zena. "HIV Prevention: The Need for Methods Women Can Use". *American Journal of Public Health*. Vol. 80: 460-462. 1990.
35. Hamblin, Julie and Elizabeth Reid. Women, the HIV Epidemic and Human Rights: A Tragic Imperative." Paper prepared for International Workshop on AIDS: A Question of Rights and Humanity. International Court of Justice. The Hague. May 1991.
36. Reid, Elizabeth. "Women and HIV." Editorial in AIDS Health Promotion Exchange. Forthcoming 1992.
37. Baker, G. Felicia Knaul and Ana Vasconcelos. "Development as Empowerment: Brazilian Project Offers Passage to a Better Life for Street Girls." *Passages*. Vol. 10. No. 4: 3-6. International Center on Adolescent Fertility. 1991.
38. Slutkin, G. "What has been Learned in HIV Prevention Programmes." Presentation made at VIII International Conference on AIDS. Amsterdam. 1992.
39. Heise, Lori. "Violence Against Women: The Missing Agenda." in *Woman's Health: a Global Perspective*. Marge Koblinsky, Judith Timyan and Jill Gay (Eds). Westview press, 1992.
40. Heise, Lori. Personal Communication. 1992.
41. Orick, George. Interview with Margaret Mwangola and Rose Mulama. Kenya. UNDP HIV and Development Programme. Reflections on the Impact of the HIV Epidemic Project. Taped 1991.

11

Young Women and the HIV Epidemic

Ms. Elizabeth Reid
UNDP, New York

The HIV epidemic is a women's epidemic: women are particularly vulnerable to infection and increasing numbers of women are becoming infected. It is estimated that one—third of all those thought to be infected—about 2 million —are women. It is also estimated that the number of infected women may overtake the number of infected men by the mid—90s. Already in sub-Saharan Africa there are more women than men infected. Studies in Central African Republic, Equatorial Guinea and Gabon show nearly three times as many women infected than men. In Honduras, Haiti, The Dominican Republic, the Bahamas and Trinidad and Tobago, the male to female ratios of reported AIDS cases, the last stage of HIV infection, have dropped rapidly in the last three years from over 6:1 to under 2.5:1.

It is also an epidemic of youth. At least half of all those infected are under the age of 25 and a large proportion of these young adults were irfected during adolescence. Recent studies indicate that the infection rates in some teenage groups is far higher than that for adults. The number of reported AIDS cases in teenagers has increased rapidly over the last two years.

Data are not available on the number of young women infected. However, women are constituting an increasing proportion of all AIDS cases and often women become infected at a younger age than men. A study from Zaire reported that among young adults aged 15 to 30 years, HIV infection was four times more common in women than in men. These are bleak and disturbing facts. Infection rates in pregnant women in high incidence countries in Central and Eastern Africa range from 10 to 25 per cent. High infection rates in women will cause a sharp increase in maternal and child morbidity and mortality rates. Maternal mortality rates in developing countries are already 12 times higher than in the developed world, the greatest gap in any human indicator.

The overwhelming majority of infected young women do not know they are infected. Most young women are diagnosed during pregnancy or at birth. To the shock of discovering their own infection status is added the fear that their baby might be infected, guilt and grief at having brought all this about and the desolation of motherhood in these circumstances.

Transmission

The HIV virus may be transmitted sexually through anal, vaginal or oral intercourse with an infected person. Sexual transmission can be prevented through the proper use of a good quality condom. Young women in most parts of the developing world are sexually active. Data on adolescent sexuality in developing countries indicate that the initial sexual contact occurs before age 17 for half of that population and by age 15 for one-third of adolescents. In Jamaica, Nigeria and Sierra Leone, more than four out of five single women aged 20 years are sexually experienced. In Mexico and Costa Rica, from about one-fifth to one-fourth of single adolescents are sexually experienced by age 20. Condom use is not common. Studies show that in four countries (Costa Rica, the Gambia, Jamaica and Zimbabwe) the condom was the most frequently used contraceptive at first intercourse. However, in general, use at first intercourse is very low. Condom usage in unmarried women aged 15 to 19 years in 15 countries studies is low but second to the pill in most African countries and in Jamaica, Peru and Thailand. Thus there are, in the developing world, many young women at risk of infection through unprotected sexual behaviour.

HIV transmission may also occur through the sharing of drug using equipment with an infected individual. Protection can be achieved through not sharing needles, through the cleaning of shared needles or through changing the mode of use away from intravenous administration. Fewer young women than young men are at risk of infection through drug injecting since in almost all drug using communities, men predominate. Young women are however at significant risk of infection through an unprotected sexual intercourse with infected current or past drug users. It is virtually impossible to know whether another person is HIV infected, certainly during the long period of infection before symptoms appear. Even HIV testing only tells the infection status of a person at an earlier period of time and not at the present. In the case of sexual behaviour and intravenous drug use, only each individual can take the necessary steps to protect themselves from infection. The responsibility of governments is to make people aware of the epidemic and the modes of transmission of the virus, to ensure that the means of preventing infection—condoms, sterile needles, bleach—are affordable and of easy access, and to minimize the possibility of iatrogenic and occupational transmission.

Young women can also become infected iatrogenically through the medical use of nonsterile needles, through the transfusion of contaminated blood or blood products and, rarely, through the use of infected human tissue or organs in surgical procedures. In many parts of the developing world, needles are commonly used in both the modern and traditional health sectors, without any or sufficient sterilization. Adolescent pregnancy can place young women at further risk of infection from blood transfusion or unsterile needles. The extent of iatrogenic transmission has not been adequately studied, but women and young children are at high risk from this form of transmission.

Vulnerability to HIV Infection

There are many factors affecting the lives of young women which make them vulnerable to HIV infection. While there are few data available to determine the extent of that vulnerability, the following discussion can serve to indicate areas for further research in this area. Prevalence patterns of HIV infection are known to be a factor of poverty, social and geographic mobility, commerce, tourism, social disruption and civil unrest.

Sexually Transmitted Diseases and Adolescent Pregnancy

The presence of sexually transmitted diseases (STDs), particularly ulcerative conditions, increases the likelihood of infection in both men and women when intercourse occurs with an infected partner. STDs are common amongst young women, particularly in Africa, the Caribbean and Latin America. They are not easy to detect in women and so most women remain unaware of their presence. Studies in Central Africa have shown that in some communities up to one-third of women in their child-bearing years are infertile, with 80 per cent of that infertility being caused by STDs. Drug use is also increasing in some parts, particularly in the Caribbean. The incidence may be much lower in sub-Saharan Africa. However, this epidemic carries within it the seeds of violence. Although rape is traditionally uncommon in sub-Saharan Africa, there are increasing reports of the rape of young women by older men in high HIV-incidence countries. This is clearly associated with the belief that the younger the woman, the more she is likely to be free from HIV infection. The raped young woman, however, is at high risk of infection, particularly since reports indicate that the attackers are usually either sexually promiscuous men who do not want to change their behaviour or, increasingly, may be men who have lost their wives, possibly to AIDS, who are fearful of taking another wife.

Sex tourism is an expression of the power of men from rich countries to purchase the sexual services of young women in developing countries. Asia is a favoured destination. The young women and their families are placed at grave risk of infection. Most data from Asia show higher levels of HIV infection in young women servicing this trade than in the general community. Similarly, studies show high rates of infection among prostitutes servicing military bases.

Geographic and Social Mobility

There is a high correlation in men between mobility and HIV infection: truck drivers, soldiers and traders in Africa have extremely high infection levels. Geographic mobility to young girls would also lead to increased risk. Again very few statistics are available but at least one study has shown that 70 per cent of rural to urban migrants are under the age of 25, and 40 per cent under the age of 16. Young girls under the age of 15 seeking schooling and employment predominate in rural to urban migration in many Latin American countries, in some African countries such as Ghana and Morocco, and in Asian countries such as Bangladesh, India, Indonesia and the Philippines. Studies of international migration show the increasing involvement of women, and of young women. A significant proportion of the young women who migrate to European countries from Asia and Africa end up in prostitution. Mail order brides are also another migratory group of young women at risk of infection.

Another particularly vulnerable group are women who live in conditions of civil unrest or war. In parts of Central and Eastern Africa, patterns of infection in women correlate with the movements over the last decade of soldiers and other military personnel.

Increased female education and increased employment opportunities for young women in developing countries have resulted in a trend towards later marriages, especially among urban, educated young women. While this may have the effect of lowering overall birth rates, it also results in an increased period of potential exposure to the risks of pregnancy and HIV infection.

Poverty and Homelessness

The group of young women most vulnerable to HIV infection are those who are homeless or living in poverty. UNICEF estimates that over 40 million young people in the world are living on the streets. Many of those have left home because of sexual abuse or poverty.

Studies from Africa, Latin America and North America show alarming rates of infection in this group. In Sao Paulo, Brazil, nearly 9 per cent of 8,000 children tested in 1988 in states institutions were HIV positive. With an estimate of 7 million homeless children living on the streets in Brazil, authorities estimate that 146,000 children may already be infected. Child prostitution is common and girls of 9 to 10 work as prostitutes, often just for comfort, food or shelter. In New York City one 1988 study of more than 1,100 young men and women aged 16 to 21 living on the street, over 7 per cent were HIV positive. Since almost none of them injected drugs, transmission would have occurred sexually. In Khartoum, a 1988 study of street boys aged 6 to 14 showed 7 per cent of them to be infected.

Increasingly poverty is becoming a female phenomenon. More women are heading households or are their main financial providers: more women and children are living in poverty. The coping options for women, young girls and children living in poverty are few and none rival prostitution as an economic survival strategy. Nowadays, however, it is in many parts of the world a virtual death sentence for the woman and the children they love and support. Levels of HIV infection among women working as prostitutes in some Central and Eastern African towns and cities are as high as 80 or 90 per cent. However there is evidence of a decrease in new infections among these women as they organize to protect themselves and to educate and protect their clients. A growing number of nongovernmental organizations, especially in Latin America, are assisting them with the education of their clients.

Even where women working as prostitutes adopt the use of condoms as a protective measure for themselves and their clients, they often fail to use them in their personal sexual relationships. This failure may arise from a belief that it is romantic love which distinguishes their commercial from personal sexual activities or from the subordinate relationship that so often exists between them and their pimps who are often their lovers.

Infected Young Women

Diagnosis of HIV infection in a young woman means not only the possibility of illness and death but also that choices about sexuality, motherhood, marriage, education and work become fraught with fear and pain. Infection too often means social isolation, loneliness and discrimination. It brings fear: the fear of losing one's job, housing, medical care a dental care; fear of losing family, friends and partner; fear for the future of one's children both infected and not infected. Disclosure of one's infection status has a high price.

For a young woman, a diagnosis of HIV infection brings with it an anguished choice to forego children or to risk giving birth to an infected baby. For young women in cultures where their social identity and acceptability is determined by their fertility, there may not even be this choice. The sexual expression of love may become difficult either for the infected woman or for her partner. Relationships become difficult to enter and to maintain.

Infected young women with an infected child will need to cope with their own fatigue and sickness as well as the child's. It is estimated that infected women in sub-Saharan, Africa have given birth to 600,000 children. Of these, about 200,000 become infected duril pregnancy: the remaining 400,000 children, as well as the others that live, will have mother that will sicken and die early in their lifetimes. One estimate is that, by the year 2000, per cent of children in 10 high incidence African countries will be without mothers as result of this epidemic. Enough is known about the impact of protracted illness and death on households to be able to glimpse the impoverishment and suffering that will ensure for these children.

This is a sad picture and reflects the reality, but not its totality. An infected young woman has years, often a decade or more, of healthy life ahead of her after infection. She and those around her, need to ensure that she can remain an integral part of the communi of social and economic use. She, and they, will have special counselling and education needs and will require supportive programmes including at a later stage child care and household services to assist them.

The Prevention of HIV Infection in Young Women

We have knowingly lived with this epidemic for a decade now. As we look back over our efforts we can identify a number of principles that have shaped our response to it.

Firstly, responsibility for prevention of infection by, or further transmission of the virus through sexual or drug-using behaviour lies ultimately with the individual. Others, family friends, governments, can only provide an environment which may assist individuals change behaviour. They cannot change it for them.

Secondly, community-based organizations, that is, organizations drawn from or based within communities most at risk of infection, have a vital role to play in responding to this epidemic by:

— drawing up education and prevention programmes appropriate and acceptable to their own members;

— providing support, counselling and care to HIV-infected people and their partners, families and friends;
— providing information, support and counselling to communities to assist them to minimize HIV transmission, and lessen discrimination and stigma.

Thirdly, prevention and care policies and programmes can only be effectively implemented where the co-operation and trust of those infected or at risk of infection are maintained.

Our challenge now is to apply this understanding to the young woman of our societies. We must acknowledge their vulnerability to infection. Not an easy task for parents, community leaders or governments. We must ensure that they themselves can acknowledge their vulnerability to infection. Maybe an even more difficult task.

Perhaps the task most difficult of all, once this awareness of vulnerability is created, will be to give young women the self confidence and skills required to change their behaviour and to choose or create relationships based on mutual concern and respect. This freedom of choice is dependent upon improving women's economic independence and upon changes occurring in the ways societies construct gender, both masculinity and femininity, and sexuality. Otherwise, for young women, HIV infection will be a direct outcome of their social, personal and economic subordination.

12

Women, HIV and Development

Ms. Elizabeth Reid,
UNDP, New York

Recognition of the need to reach women with HIV education and prevention programmes and of the need to provide care, support and treatment to infected women and children is viewed by UNDP as a particular aspect of its more general mandate, given to it by its Governing Council of member nations of the United Nations, to ensure that women are participants in, contributors to and beneficiaries from development assistance. To understand this is to understand that we, the development community, are not starting from scratch in this new endeavour within the HIV epidemic to focus attention on women and children.

We have learned many things since the governments of the world first addressed the issue of women in 1975, during International Women's Year. I wish to illustrate but a few areas of growing understanding about women relevant to our response to this epidemic.

Firstly, until data on women is collected and analyzed, women will remain unperceived, unreached and un- or undervalued. Epidemiological data on this epidemic must be desegregated by gender if we are to be able to devise and monitor programmes for women. This is not happening in all countries. WHO staff and consultants must be aware of the importance of desegregating data by gender, and the need to do so should be explicitly stated in their terms of reference.

Secondly, the impact of this epidemic on women is, and will continue to be, different from its impact on men, and different on different groups of women and children and this needs to be understood.

This meeting has been an important stimulus to understanding the emerging topography of women and children affected by this epidemic. Along with HIV-infected women and HIV-infected children, other groups are being identified as in need of understanding and support. These include the wives of infected men, Who are also women with a strong desire for children, children of an infected parent or parents who are not themselves infected, the grandmothers who care for children without parents, to which we should also add the aunts and sisters, children caring for sick parents and the widows of infected men. The differing psychological, social, sexual and economic needs of all of these groups need to be better understood if we are to be able to minimize the adverse personal and social impact of the epidemic and if prevention and care programmes are to be effective.

Understanding the impact of the epidemic on women will necessitate an extensive review of the literature on the social construction of gender and the way it influences women's access to information, services, training, knowledge, decision-making and power; of the literature on women's role in the construction and maintenance of kin and conjugal relationships and how these shape their attitudes to mothering and their economic and social, including sexual, coping strategies, particularly their strategies for caring for their children; and of the literature on women's vulnerability and powerlessness and the means of addressing and lessening these socially induced conditions.

Next, contrary to popular belief, there are fewer women than men in the world. The female to male ratio in Sub-Sahara Africa has been consistently higher than unity. In sharp contrast, in southern and Western Asia and North Africa, the number of women is substantially lower than men in the population. Amartya SEN, the Indian economist, estimates that gender differential mortality rates have created 100 million missing women in Asia. That is, if there were the same ratio of Asian women to Asian men as the African female:male ratio, there would be 100 million more women in this generation.

That the pre-HIV economic, political and cultural factors involved in such gender bias could cause so many women of our generation to be missing indicates the urgency of a better understanding of these demographic dynamics as an essential prerequisite to postepidemic demographic studies. The effect of the HIV epidemic in these cultures may well be to amplify this gender biased mortality and to lead to a disproportionate increase in mortality rates among women. This kind of finding has implications for the modelling of this epidemic since most models have not taken gender specific factors into account. This needs to be addressed.

Further, development studies have shown us just how difficult women are to reach with information, services or programmes. This is for various reasons: women are generally less literate and less educated; they spend less time in schools, work places and public institutions where information is made available; they may be less likely to read newspapers, to listen to the radio or to watch television. This does not mean that women are social isolates. They have their strong social networks but these are very often centered around other women and women's organization and institutions. Such facts must shape and determine the design of HIV education and prevention programmes for women. Furthermore, there is much evidence that many services for women are not effective unless mediated or delivered by women. Mrs. Kaleeba from TASO, Uganda, made this point strikingly yesterday.

Finally, the importance of increasing women's roles in decision-making is widely accepted but has particular implications within the context of this epidemic. Jonathan Mann made a commitment in his opening address to an equitable representation of women within the GPA at Geneva. A similar imperative holds at field level and in the recruitment of consultants. National programmes and committees will need to be reviewed and means found to ensure that women are active in decision-making throughout the programme. If women are active in decision-making throughout the programme, this will necessitate, for exarnple, the re-examination of programmes where women can only get access to condoms if they have a letter of consent from their husbands.

There are many lessons that can be drawn from the past decades of development programmes and research on women. There is an urgent need to draw these lessons together if we are to respond effectively and in a timely fashion to women and children within this epidemic.

The Governing Council of UNDP has given the Organization a strong mandate on women in development as well as a mandate to respond in a timely, effective and humane fashion to this epidemic. The UNDP was established to provide technical assistance to the developing world. It is not a loan facility or a capital development facility. Its primary focus is on human development through expert assistance. It has 113 field officers in all countries of the developing world and certain countries in Eastern Europe.

Within the United Nations system, UNDP plays a lead role at the country level regarding social and economic development. The UNDP Resident Representative in each country is, at the same time, the Resident Co-ordinator of the UN system's operational activities for development, responsible to ensure complementary, co-ordinated and harmonious action at the country level by all bodies within the system.

Because of these roles and responsibilities of UNDP in the field, WHO and UNDP, in March 1988, signed a joint WHO-UNDP Alliance to combat the HIV epidemic. This alliance combined the strength of WHO/GPA as international leader in HIV policy as well as in scientific and technical matters relating to HIV and AIDS with the role of UNDP as the lead agency within the UN system for socio-economic development. UNDP brings to this alliance four decades of accumulated experience in development assistance in all sectors.

This alliance has provided support to developing countries in developing, implementing, monitoring and evaluating co-ordinated, multisectoral national HIV/AIDS plans within the framework of the global AIDS strategy. It has also helped to ensure co-ordinated support for national plans by external agencies and to draw a broader range of expertise into national AIDS programmes.

Between ten and twelve million US dollars have been allocated by UNDP field offices to HIV prevention and control activities and to programmes of support to those infected and affected and this figure is growing. The use of national funds is a demonstration of the importance attached by developing countries to HIV and AIDS and a recognition of this relationship to their development priorities.

One focus of UNDP's assistance has been the minimization of HIV transmission through blood transfusions and through the re-use of unsterile needles in health care settings. UNDP has contributed $3.6 million to WHO/GPA to support the Global Blood Safety Initiative. Women and children have been, and remain, particularly vulnerable in developing countries to iatrogenically acquired HIV infection. Women and children are the major recipients of blood transfusions and the use of injections during pregnancy, immediately after birth and during infancy is extremely common in both the traditional and modern health systems. UNDP has also had an associated concern for the minimization of occupational transmission in health settings.

I would like to end by quoting from the statement by the administrator of UNDP, Mr. William H. Draper, drawn up for World AIDS Day tomorrow:

> *"UNDP has responded swiftly to this epidemic, but, with all that we are doing, I am concerned that much more is required of those active in development if we are to do our part to slow the spread of the virus and to lessen the associated economic and social dislocations. As UNDP approaches a new planning and funding cycle, I have asked our Resident Representatives in every country and those involved in inter-country programmes to include HIV prevention and support measures in new programmes, to measure the impact of the epidemic on their country's development and to propose ways of lessening that impact.*
>
> There can be no complacency. I pledge that UNDP will spare no effort in serving as a partner in all governments to meet this challenge with resources and resolve."

13

Why Women and HIV? It Takes Two to Tango, Safely

Ms. Elizabeth Reid
UNDP, New York

Ho hum, women again. Same words. Same images. Same stories. And, even more alarmingly, same policy and programme responses. We know that socio-economic and cultural circumstances, gender differences and biological realities all influence the length and quality of women's lives. The problem is that this knowledge has not produced the outrage and anger which would force change.

Even the starkness of the insight into women's lives that the HIV epidemic gives us has not stopped us from accepting these inequalities and injustices. We continue to take them for granted. Is the ever-increasing infection of women going to be taken for granted as well?

What is the essence of the issue? Is it a question of condoms and reducing the number of sexual partners? Is it a question of empowerment and economic independence? Or is it the more fundamental question of how we fail to value and treat one another, and women in particular, as human beings.

We should start to look for the answer by talking with women and listening to their stories. These will reveal the insights that will lead us to demand:

why we continue to rely on a strategy of information and education about HIV, AIDS and genital infections which is inappropriate for women;

why we tolerate the fact that more women than men are becoming infected with HIV (and at ages 5-10 years younger than men); and

why the burden of care generated by the epidemic is falling more and more heavily on women.

We should be ensuring that early diagnosis of HIV and genital infections is available to women and men alike and that treatment and care of women who are infected is as efficient and accessible as it is for men. We must no longer accept that women rarely seek treatment for genital infections and injuries because treatment is inaccessible due to lack of time, money and transportation, because women are often prohibited by family or cultural dictates from visiting health clinics or because the treatment available is too impersonal, immodest or threatening for them to pursue.

More than this, we must confront the way our societies and communities regard men and women, how we bring up our children, the expectations we have about the behaviour of our sons and daughters, our husbands and wives, our fathers and mothers.

It seems evident that, given the knowledge and means, men have it within their power to protect themselves from sexual and drug-use infection by HIV and that women often do not. Knowing about safer sex and safer drug use is not enough for women to avoid HIV and genital infections. It is of use only if it leads to strategies women can adopt within their particular circumstances.

Women's lack of autonomy to determine the circumstances of their lives, in particular the circumstances under which they have sexual intercourse, places them in grave danger of infection. Most infected women have become infected during sexual intercourse with their husbands or regular male partners. Men's power spreads the epidemic since it allows them to initiate sexual relationships with comparative ease. The opportunity for sexual relationships is also great for those who have mobile jobs which keep them away from home and family and which may lead to boredom and loneliness.

Women alone cannot stop this epidemic nor care for its sick and its survivors. Women alone cannot bear the burden of its psychological, social and economic impact. Nor should this be expected of them. To do so would be to build in the certainty of failure, not because of any failing in women but because the nature of HIV transmission requires a conjoint, shared response.

This then necessitates the involvement of both men and women in partnership against the further spread of the virus. This partnership can be based on men's love for their partners, children and families but it will only succeed if new patterns of communication and new patterns for the sharing of the present responsibilities and joys of women's lives emerge.

The HIV epidemic and its impact will only be overcome when men and women forge a true partnership of mutual respect and trust and of equitable sharing of the burdens of sadness, pain, care and support created by the epidemic. Men and women must seek to establish the kind of honest communication about sexuality and sexual behaviour needed to prevent the transmission of HIV and STDs in their partnerships, whether hetero- and homosexual. They must work to restructure the sexual relationships in which they take part. As individuals neither men nor women can bear the personal, emotional and socio-economic burdens of HIV alone—in partnerships, they can.

Changes in individual relationships between men and women will occur only in the context of the emergence of a new social contract, not one simply governing men's or women's behaviour but one which changes what it is to be a man or a woman. The social contract must encompass the way in which we nurture and raise our children and the way society constructs its gender archetypes. It must further allow for community explorations of the appropriateness of accepted community values and standards of behaviour. Such a social contract must be supported and reaffirmed by laws, policy, budgetary priorities and programme design and delivery.

The family in all its diverse forms thus becomes the basic nexus of change. For although individual men and women can decide on ways to protect themselves from infection, the likelihood of this happening and being sustained resides in factors which long predate adulthood and sexual activity. They have their origin in how people are brought up in family life.

It is in the family context, from birth, that personalities are formed, gender identity is created and moral values are instilled. We know that self-respect, self confidence for others and an ability to talk about personal and intimate matters are all characteristics which help people to remain uninfected. In particular, we know that it is in families that boys are brought up to be boys and girls, girls, with attendant sexual and social identities, attitudes and behaviours.

Thus it is within families that the basic prevention strategies must be but in to place. Love and nurturing must be given to both boys and girls so that they may grow into independent, confident human beings, able to form respectful and non-violent relationships, whatever their sexual orientation may be. Parental-child discourse must be developed on bodily care and sexuality and strengthened on community norms and moral values, especially with regard to respect for self and others. We must change the ways that girls and boys are raised so that as adults they will be less likely to put themselves and others at risk of infection. This will require significant changes in the social construction of masculinity and femininity.

These gender paradigms must be reconstructed in particular

ways. The new paradigms should lead to the greater valuing of compassion, concern for others and love of family in men and, for women, in a simple recognition of their value and worth. It is hard to reconcile the oft-claimed valuing of women, even as mothers, with the widespread acceptance of female infanticide or the mortality rates associated with pregnancy and childbirth (which are as high as 1 in 21 in some parts of the world: 100 million women per year).

But families individually do not determine cultural meanings, social customs or community values. They inherit, accept, respect and instill them. Thus, for families to change, communities and societies must also change. The new social contract will therefore require a radical reassessment by societies of the very way men and women see themselves and each other, of the way they relate as husband and wife, lovers, brothers and sisters, parents and children, partners, colleagues and friends.

This new social contract will also need to be embodied in law and practice if it is to exist in more than rhetoric alone. It must be reflected, for example, in the attitudes and language of judges as much as in their judgments and the prescripts of the law. Only then will it be reflected in who become the judges, lawyers, police agents and cleaners of floors. Only then will it be reflected in the wage structure, school attendance records, sporting clubs and by those who minister to our spiritual and physical needs.

Thus, changing the way people interact sexually in order to prevent further HIV infection must be a catalyst for quite radical social change. Then may be there can be a choice about who leads in the tango.

14

Women and HIV/AIDS: An Indian Scenario

Geetha Devi Ayappa
Attorney Bangalore, India

INTRODUCTION

Since the discovery of HIV/AIDS in the 1980s, which continues to spread at an alarming rate, debates and research on biomedical issues and on human rights/legal issues have gained importance. In the popular conception, medicine, and not the law, plays a leading role. But in the absence of a cure, and clear cut medical responses to HIV infection, prevention through education and behaviour modification is the only method for combating and controlling the spread of epidemic. Hence legal interventions, as a mechanism for encouraging social change, occupy the centre stage.

The legal response, which is more moralistic than rational, has paved the way for amendment of public health legislation in order to strengthen the coercive power to deal with people infected with HIV or to find scapegoats to take the blame for society's own inadequacies. However, various studies have proved the fallacy of the belief that this is the disease of 'the depraved and the deviants'. The increasing number of women being infected through heterosexual activity proves that the virus is no longer limited to the so-called 'High Risk' category of prostitutes, their clients and blood donors. There are many infected men, who due to their high-risk activity are unknowingly passing on the virus to their wives and partners.

Women and HIV Infection

Various studies in the late 1980s and early 1990s have revealed that HIV/ AIDS is increasingly affecting the poor and women, who by reasons of their socio-economic dependency are unable to take steps to protect themselves against the risk of infection. The race and gender pattern of HIV infection is confirmed in the 1991

WHO estimate that the cumulative total of people infected with HIV worldwide was in the order of 8-10 million. Of this total, more than seven million infections were estimated to have occurred in developing countries of sub-Saharan Africa, the Caribbean, and South-East Asia .

These patterns suggest that the socio-economic factor is a driving force behind HIV transmission. Poverty leads to a breakdown in rural communities and migration of labour. In addition, the lack of alternate economic opportunities often forces women into prostitution as the only available means of economic support.

HIV infection is preventable by all those who have access to information and preventive measures and the means to implement these measures. Hencc, factors such as low level of education and literacy, lack of access to adequate medical care, the low status of women and the corresponding powerlessness to control the basis upon which their sexual relationships with men take place, increase the transmission risk. Women's risk factors include poor health care (even during pregnancy), inadequate treatment of sexually transmitted diseases, lack of awareness or inaccesibility of preventive measures like condoms, lack of power to insist on the use of condoms, and other measures that are exclusively within the control of women.

In India, apart from targeting commercial sex workers, there is a total lack of focus on women in the context of HIV infection. Prostitutes are often identified as the main source for infections. Of late, there is a demand for the legalization of prostitution, not out of concern or compassion to protect such women, but out of concern for public health and as a strategy which provides compulsory health checks and screening of such women to combat the spread of HIV. Though HIV infection has entered private homes, women, due to their easy visibility, are identified as being responsible for spreading the infection.

Women are considered to be the 'reservoir' of the disease, as 'vectors' of transmission to their children and male sexual partners rather than individuals who are themselves infected or are at risk of HIV infection. They are in urgent need of information and education to protect themselves. However, mere knowledge about AIDS and knowledge of law will not ensure security and protection of oneself. Enforcing such measures is difficult in a relationship based on inequality. It is essential to recognise that the policies and strategies for combating HIV/AIDS require considering not only HIV-specific issues but also the underlying structural imbalances and the politics of physical and economic vulnerability which operate to increase women's risk to infection.

Due to the peculiarity of the transmission of the virus through sexual contact, and the moral stigma attached to "promiscuous" behaviour, many women are unwilling to be tested for the fear of being branded as 'Loose Women'. They remain unidentified, suffering silently without any care and treatment. Hence, in addition to the lack of focus on women, it is extremely difficult to ascertain the number of women already infected.

Hence, the issue of women and AIDS needs to be placed in a broader social and cultural context. Women's vulnerability to HIV is enhanced by the inequalities and discrimination they face in the society. Women are the subordinate sex, relegated to second-class status, kept uneducated, dependent, isolated and confined within the four walls of their homes. They are often denied access to education, health, independent income and property rights. All these factors combine to increase women's vulnerability and obstruct any effective prevention campaign. There is a necessity to understand the interaction between HIV infection and cultural values, the rights and needs of women and socio-economic patterns in the society which render women vulnerable to HIV infection.

The dilemma of balancing individual human rights and public rights has clearly established the importance of the legal response to HIV/AIDS. But what should the legal response be? What are the experiences of a decade of different legal response to HIV/AIDS? What are the modules by which law can be incorporated into HIV/AIDS policy? Can law, as a tool for social change, bring about the required changes in the behavioural pattern and value systems? Clear cut responses to many such questions are still evasive. A close analysis of the different roles of the law and the interaction between them is essential if law is to he used effectively to reinforce HIV/AIDS policy.

Analysing the decade's experiences of various countries one could identify three main models:

(a) Prescriptive Model

In this model the coercive laws have proved ineffective and need to be deleted.

(b) Protective Model

Here the focus is on human rights issues where one has to find a balanced approach between individualism and collectivism.

(c) Instrumental Model

Here the law focuses on combating subordination and seeks to change underlying values and patterns of social interaction. The critical point here is to determine to what extent the policies in the public spheres could enter and influence the behaviour in the private sphere of the family to bring about the desired changes.

Very often, laws are enacted in reponse to specific problems, viz. dowry, rape, prostitution, etc. But often it is found that such laws are inadequate to deal with the problem because various social structures and accompanying patriarchial values and attitudes are not tackled and mere cosmetic changes are not an answer to the problem of power structure and gender inequality. Hence it is desirable to bring about a social change in a broader social context. AIDS also presents a unique opportunity for effecting such a change, particularly for women, since it forces society to face issues that had hitherto been largely ignored, such as the relationship between poverty and prostitution etc. AIDS is also providing the impetus to examine issues of sexuality and personal relations, and thus there is potential for women to be able to take a more assertive role in personal relationships, to enable them to establish relationships based on mutual trust and respect. It highlights the need for men and women to take equal responsibilities in their sexual behaviour and concern for their children rather than placing this responsibility on women alone.

The preventive strategies offered to date provide very little protection for women from HIV infection. Enforcement of these strategies (such as monogamy and fidelity, safe sexual practice and usage of condoms) is dependent more on male behaviour. Where discussion about sex is still a taboo, it is difficult to educate women about safe sexual practices, and enforcement of such strategies is practically impossible. Law cannot necessarily resolve this dilemma. Hence, there is a need to address the broader socio-economic structure in the society and to empower women through legal intervention and policies.

Various social structures and cultural factors like religion, type of family structure and the institution of marriage ascribe secondary status to women and influence the perception about women in all other fields. A lack of priority in respect of health and education for women, lack of property rights, lack of access to finance and credit facilities, lack of supportive services in domestic chores, and the existing discrimination in all walks of life, deny women various rights which together form the greatest impediment in access to health care, education and employment opportunities. These, in turn, increase a woman's susceptibility to the risk of HIV infection.

The Indian constitution guarantees liberty, justice, and equality to all citizens of India, and prohibits discrimination on grounds of religion, race, caste and sex. It denounces practices that are derogatory to the dignity and status of women; nevertheless, sexual equality remains a far-too-distant goal. Sexual inequality and the spirit of patriarchy still pervade our personal laws which confer lower status on women.

Indian personal laws are still based on religion, but religion itself is a tool often used to victimise, separate and dehumanise women. Moreover, the diversity of personal laws for different communities is a hindrance for the democratic advancement of the country. Secularism cannot be achieved by recognising a variety of conflicting laws on the same subject. This affects the status of women because many of the reforms and policies are not implemented for fear of annoying communal sentiments.

Many of the existing laws need to be amended to ameliorate the status of women. These include laws regarding marriage and divorce, age at marriage, maintenance, matrimonial home and matrimonial property, inheritance and succession rights, sexual offences under criminal law (such as rape, adultery, prostitution, kidnapping, enticing and seducing a.married woman), employment related laws, etc.

Women perform a whole range of roles in society. They are helped or hindered in these roles according to their status and rights in society and in their family, their literacy levels and access to training, technology and professional activities, their standard of living and access to financial resources. The interaction between law and economic dependency is well established in a legal regime where women are deprived or discriminated against regarding property rights and the right to independent ownership of property. Removal of such legal barriers to economic independence through effective legislative reform can enhance the status of women within the family and in the society.

Law can be used to enhance the status of women within marriage and other sexual relationships. The double standards of sexual morality incorporated in law should be deleted. A woman's sexuality is supressed, and control over her body is denied because she is looked upon as the property of her father or her husband. In many of the Commonwealth countries, fidelity of a woman is a legal pre-requisite for claiming maintenance from her husband. The absence of any criminal sanctions for marital rape further reinforces attitudes about the sexual subordination of women. Similarly, woman do not have any freedom or right to control their reproductive functions. Hence, there is a necessity for enacting laws that ecognise the rights of women to make their own decisions about sexual relations on par with their male counterparts.

Law has a definite role to play even in broad community-based empowerment programmes, especially legal literacy. Legal literacy brings about an increased awareness amongst women and a change in their outlook which may lead to the assertion of their rights.

One effective method to ensure the improved status for women is to involve more women in the political process and in framing policies for women. Though many policies are framed for women, they are lacking in content because they have failed to incorporate women's experiences. Hence, more women should be involved in the process of policy formulation. Further, it is also imperative that more women get involved at the implementation level so as to ensure that the development benefits reach the needy.

In addition, women must form collectives to overcome their individual powerlessness and demand enforcement of their rights and changes in the existing social structures in the society.

In addition to empowering women through law, various other social structures and attitudes in the society need to be reformed, especially literacy levels and the health infrastructure. There is an urgency to ensure the equality of the sexes in the educational process and to prioritise the issue of women's health, often neglected by women themselves as well as by the society.

Women face large numbers of problems that are acute in their own way. The HIV epidemic accentuates these existing problems. Mere knowledge of what has to be done in order to protect oneself from HIV transmission is meaningless if one has no power over the circumstances that give rise to the risk.

Hence the short-term goal is that women should take greater control of their lives and make use of the existing preventive strategies that are available immediately. However, the long-term goal has to be minimising and eliminating women's subordination and to improve the status of women. For this, a fundamental change in socio-cultural values requiring reorientation of the values, beliefs, customs and the law that shape the perception and roles of women within the family and the society has to occur.

It is tme that legislation alone cannot change the values in society. However, an effective legislative policy is a necessary prerequisite for bringing about a change in socio-economic conditions. In order to overcome vulnerability to HIV, human rights considerations must look beyond the immediate concern to minimise and eliminate discrimination for the infected and address the unequal socio-economic position of women.

In this context, support can be drawn from the various international human rights instruments that offer scope to promote the human rights of women which have been neglected so far, and which are clearly highlighted by the HIV epidemic. Formal legal recognition of such international human rights instruments must be attempted by bringing about the necessary changes in domestic laws. And if such rights already exist in the domestic laws, then there is an urgency to amend them suitably so as to make them implementable.

15

Children in Families Affected by the HIV Epidemic: A Strategic Approach

Ms. Elizabeth Reid
UNDP, New York

INTRODUCTION

The concept of families is an important analytical and programming tool which is often overlooked within development theory and practice. Children do not spring untrammelled into the world. They are born with ties of blood, love and law to their families: parents, brothers and sisters, grandparents and other family members. These ties can bind generations together into a supportive and nurturing unit which provides security, care and love to its members. The ties change over time, maturing, strengthening and weakening. Such ties may be created and recreated outside of lineage groups, by street children, by adoptive families and by others.

Many of the most striking images of the HIV epidemic are of families, but of unfamiliar families: a grandparent surrounded by grandchildren, adolescent-headed families, often siblings and cousins bonded together, dying adults tended by their children and communities as families. It is timely to focus on such families rather than on children alone, or youth alone or adults. This allows for an intrafamilial and longitudinal analysis of the needs, skills and resources of families affected by HIV which provides a different basis for determining and ranking the required responses.

This analysis has already been done by a number of organizations assisting adolescents and children whose parents know they are HIV-infected, are ill or have died of AIDS. There is much to learn from them and this paper attempts to draw together some of their insights and knowledge. These programmes teach us that careful attention is needed to understand the trauma of children watching their parents sicken and slowly die and how this experience affects their long-verm development. Attention is also needed to understand how the families and communities caring for these children can be supported in sustainable ways to continue providing care to them and how the capacity for self-support of surviving families of children can be strengthened.

The forms that families take vary within and across cultures and generations. They are affected by increasing urbanization, by poverty, by political and economic migration, by changes in labour market structures, by the changing roles of women and other factors. Superimposed on all these factors now will be the impact on family life of the death of many parents and young adults.

Most of those infected are in the age group 20 to 40 years and the overwhelming majority are parents. Furthermore, the overwhelming majority of all those infected do not know they are infected. Many women are indirectly diagnosed when they are still well through the diagnosis of HIV infection in their children. Many men do not get diagnosed until they have a clinically observable HIV-related illness. In most households where there is one infected person, there will probably be three or more: both parents and one or more children.

WHO estimates that eight million adults in Africa have been infected with HIV and so possibly four million families already know that they are affected or will soon know. Many of these affected families do not cease to exist when the adults die. They live on as grandparent or adolescent-headed families, but many of them are seriously distressed, destitute or scattered. The figures for other developing regions and Eastern Europe are still much lower but in many areas are growing rapidly.

Up until now, many of the policies and programmes addressing the needs of affected children and adolescents have assumed that these needs start with the death of their mothers or parents and consist of predominantly material needs. It is important to broaden this focus. This paper argues that the needs of these young people start with the knowledge that someone in their family is infected and continue on to their social and sexual maturity. Their needs are psychological, emotional. ethical, legal and spiritual; they are for acceptance, nurturing, support, counselling and care; they include financial, material, educational, health and social development needs.

The paper also argues that the needs of these children cannot only be met by policies and programmes addressed to children and youth. There are at least three other types of interventions required: assistance to their parents, to their communities and of their governments. For the well being of their children, parents need to be able to continue working, need to be assisted in planning for their and their children's future and need access to treatment of opportunistic conditions which may lessen their ability to work and parent.

Extended family systems and communities need support in keeping these new family forms in their midst. Governments have a multifaceted role in increasing awareness, establishing an appropriate legal, ethical and human rights framework and in the provision of the required services and support.

This paper is intended to raise a number of issues which can serve as a basis for widespread discussion. It is addressed to all those interested in determining how best to respond to the epidemic. It is not a Manifesto for Children and Youth but rather another way of looking at the complex reality of this epidemic and its exigencies which may enable individuals, organizations and nations to rethink their HIV-related policies and programme priorities. It is now starkly clear in many parts of Africa that, if we do not quickly find appropriate ways of responding to this epidemic, the lives of many future generations will be bleak, anguished and often brutal.

PROGRAMME ELEMENTS

While specific programme components will vary according to the stage, the epidemic has reached and the situation, culture and resources of each country or community, five main strategic programme elements can be identified. Under each programme element, a number of programme components have been identified. These are not meant to be exhaustive nor are they operational in nature. The specific means of addressing each area may vary from one situation to another.

Certain components may already be included in a national response but may not have been seen to have linkages to the wellbeing of children in affected families. Other components may not yet have been put in place. The analysis here can provide a basis for reassessment of programme priorities, both at the national level and in community organizations.

1. Preparing Children for the Future

Most parents come to know they are HIV—infected when one of them or one of their children is clinically diagnosed with HIV related illnesses. The earlier a parent' s infection status is known, the more time he or she will have to plan for the children's future, in particular to find another family or person who can care for and shelter them. The parent will also have more time to pass on their skills and knowledge to them, to help the children be able to support themselves. Knowing their infection status when they are well will help the parents prepare their children and themselves emotionally for their deaths. The longer a parent can work and the longer he or she can be helped to stay well and nurture and raise the children, the less pain and trauma the children will experience.

Components of this programme element could include:

* **Access to voluntary, confidential and affordable counselling and testing for adults and the motivation to use it.** This would allow parents more time to plan for their own and their children' s future. Infected parents often want to seek advice on how and when to tell this to their children. Supportive services and counselling can help parents maintain a nurturing home environment for their children for as long as possible and to find future homes for them. Access to testing and counselling can also assist people in making decisions about whether they wish to have more children.
* **Disclosure with counselling of a child's infection to *both* parents.** The Women and AIDS Support Network Conference in Zimbabwe in 1989 stressed the importance of both parents being informed at the same time if that child is infected and that both receive caring counselling regarding their child's and their own HIV status[1]. In some cases where a child has been clinically diagnosed with AIDS and only the mother has been informed the father has blamed the mother and abandoned her and the sick child.
* **Continued employment.** HIV infected people who remain fit to work have the right to remain employed. If this right is denied them, their children will suffer.
* **Simple treatment of opportunistic infections.** Experience in Masaka, Uganda and Kigali, Rwanda has shown that, for many HIV-infected parents, treatment of conditions such as thrush, skin infection, diarrhoea and fever is important since it allows them to continue to work, to nurture their children and to die with dignity[2]. Providing such treatment can often help parents to remain with their children for a longer period. The parent' s suffering is eased and the children's memories of their parent's dying can be made much less traumatic. Counselling and access to appropriate low-cost or

subsidized medicines may lessen the problem ot families exhausting their resources in a futile search for a "cure".

* **Passing on to children production and income-generating skills.** The Kitovu Hospital home care team encourages parents, once they know they have been infected with HIV, to pass their production- and income earning skills on to their children[3]. In addition to helping the children to become economically independent, it can also be of emotional benefit to an infected parent who, through teaching them these skills, can do something to help their children.
* **Planning for children's future care.** The emotional stress of both parents and their children can be eased through parents planing tor the future çare and support ot their children. The importance ot this has been stressed repeatedly by infected women in all parts of the developed and developing world. Once the future guardian is identified, financial, legal and other arrangements can be made and this person or family involved in planning for the children's future.

* **Protection of children's inheritance and other legal rights.** The children's continuing access to the family house, land and goods is critical to their survival and wellbeing. Specific steps appropriate to traditional inheritance customs and/or national law may need to be taken by parents before their deaths. Discussing inheritance matters with clan elders and/or preparing and registering a will are examples. Parents need to be informed about their legal rights in relation to property ownership and how this can be passed on to the surviving spouse and children.
* **Prevention of infection while caring for the sick.** The experience of the home care and counselling teams of Chikankata Hospital in rural Zambia shows that simple techniques can minimize the likelihood of children or other family members being infected while caring for the sick and dying[4].

2. Assisting Children Whose Parents have Died

Children whose parents have died of HIV—related illnesses have often also lived through the deaths of others close to them: brothers and sisters, aunts and uncles, cousins, friends and increasingly, grandparents. Their very will to live has often been undermined. If they are to grow and develop as human beings and as members of civil society, they need love and care and the opportunity to form and maintain emotional ties with adults. Their material and psychosocial needs will have to be met; their right to remain integral members of their communities and their legal rights may be at risk and need protection. Consideration can be given to the provision of services to all children within an area heavily affected by the epidemic rather than only to those whose parents have died of AIDS. The latter approach may lead to resentment and stigmatization of children who receive targeted assistance.

Components of this programme element could include:

* **Minimizing children's psychological and emotional trauma.** The grief and loss for all living within this epidemic can be overwhelming but may be particularly so for children who watch their family members die one after another[5]. Such children not only suffer emotional pain but may also experience long-term psychosocial distress. Grief and depression may be evident or they may be expressed through behavioural problems. Children need opportunities to express and come to terms with these losses. Loving care and support can help heal the pain. Play is another important way that children do this. Experience with traumatized Mozambican refugee children. and in villages in Masaka and Rakai districts in Uganda, has shown that community-based activities such as play groups can help children recover. Normalization of daily life, like continuing to attend school. is also important. Teachers, religious leaders, nurses, healers or other adults in the community can be trained to counsel and help children recover from trauma.

Keeping survivors as integral members of their communities. This will necessitate attitudinal change where discrimination and stigma toward survivors exist. It will also require the provision of care and shelter within the children's families or communities. One significant advantage of care within the children' s own community is that relationships can be maintained which will be important as the children grow older. Children cut off from these relationships will have no one to turn to when help is needed. Where discrimination and stigma cause the isolation or rejection of children whose parents have died of AIDS. political and community mobilization for the protection of their

customary, legal, ethical and human rights will be particularly important.

Basic material needs. Direct assistance is often required by affected families. Women in Kigali asked Caritas to help them continue to be able to care for their children as long as possible by providing a nutritious meal for them and their children each day and by treating the ópportunistic infections that hindered their ability to care. TASO in Uganda[6]. WAMATA in Dar es Salaam and the Kagera[7] region' provide food and blankets and at times, financial assistance. The basic needs of affected families need to be met on an ongoing basis.

Education, training and employment creation. Formal education, vocational training, nonformal skills training and the provision of necessary tools and equipment can help children support themselves. In addition, such measures as public works programmed revolving credit schemes and other measures to create employment can benefit children directly through the families caring for them. Day care facilities, formally or informally arranged, can free time for work while ensuring that young children are cared for. Young people who have lived through the trauma of this epidemic often have knowledge skills and insights that could help other young people in similar situations. Opportunities could be created for them, for example, by apprenticing them to traditional healers or through working in outreach programmes to newly affected children.

Children's social and adolescent's development needs. To grow and develop into an adult capable of constructive social interaction, children need to be nurtured and stimulated. Younger children, for example, develop best when they have an opportunity to establish an ongoing, caring relationship with one or more adults. Such developmental needs have important implications for the type of care appropriate to provide for children and adolescents whose parents have died. Family-based care in a child's own community generally provides the best opportunities for promoting positive psychosocial development.

Children's and adolescent's sexual development needs. Sexually active adolescents generally lack

access to information services for sexually transmitted infections and to condoms, particularly sizes to fit boys. They also lack opportunities to discuss these issues with each other or others whom they respect. The Anti-AIDS clubs in Zambia or the discussion groups run by the Women and AIDS Support Network in Zimbabwe have shown that providing these opportunities can significantly change peer group sexual norms, expectations and behaviour.

Children and adolescents who have cared for and then watched the adults in their lines die one by one and who know that these deaihs are linked to the expression of sexuality may well experience problems as they move into puberty and into adulthood. There is no precedent for the extent or types of these problems. Community workers, religious leaders and others will need to be aware of these possibilities and keep communities aware of what is happening.

3. Meeting the Special Needs of HIV-infected Children

As with adults, most asymptomatic HIV—infected children do not know that they are infected. They continue to lead their daily lives. Simple infection control procedures can protect all family members or institutional workers from transmission of the virus. Testing has been advocated both mandatory and voluntary to determine the HIV status of orphans. However, there are serious ethical issues involved in testing and disclosure to children. Issues which need to be determined include: Who wants to know and why? Will it benefit the child to be tested and know?

How? Who should determine this and how? Can a child give informed consent to testing? Public policy needs to be drawn up in this area.

Infants and children with HIV-related illnesses may have special care needs. Meeting these is more difficult where one or both of the parents is also infected or has died.

Components of this programme element could include:

Support to families with a sick child. One of the most effective ways of supporting a sick child is by Providing support to the family caring for it, particularly by helping them deal with the trauma of the diagnosis. An infant with an HIV-related condition like many other sick children often suffers from chronic diarrhoea, fever and respiratory infection. As with adults, however the provision of

a healthy diet and basic medications can improve the quality of its life. A child s illness may be the first indication to its parents that they are infected with HIV .

Promotion of non-discrimination policies and programmes. Enforcement of existing laws or establishment of new ones may be necessary to ensure the rights of HIV infected children. For example, inheritance laws, both customary and modern, may have to be reviewed or enforced to ensure that infected children have access to their parents property for support, adoption laws may need to be made more flexible to facilitate care for their children and anti-discrimination laws will need to be established and/or enforced. Creating a community environment where HIV positive children can be placed with families can help reduce discrimination against these children. Families of children with an infected child should be supported if they desire to stay together.

4. Reaching Children and Adolescents who are Especially Vulnerable

Among and within families affected by the HIV epidemic, there will be some children or families of children at particular risk of destitution and of HIV infection: urban families without the support of their extended families, families who for whatever reasons lack the support of their communities, children struggling to survive on the streets, children suffering sexual abuse within families, and others. For many of these young people, survival sex, sex in exchange for money, clothing, affection, shelter, food, etc., is a basic coping strategy.

Components of this programme element could include:

Assistance to street children. Special strategies need to be developed to help children living on the street to have greater control over their lives, to have the means to avoid infection and to seek alternatives to the street. Street children and others living in marginal circumstances may not only be isolated from the wider community, they may be actively persecuted by it. Providing a broad range of measures to help increase their safety, health and well-being may help reduce their social marginalization.

Reducing the susceptibility of young women to infections.[8] Girls and young women may be particularly susceptible to HIV infection not only because they are less able to control the situations in which they have intercourse but also because their genital area provides less of a barrier to the virus and is easily irritated or torn. Communities and families need to assist young women to wait longer before becoming sexually active and to be able to ensure that all their sexual activity is safe.

5. Reducing the Number of Affected Children

This objective can be achieved by decreasing the number of adults becoming HIV-infected. Highest priority must be given to bringing about the attitudinal and behavioural change and the change in community norms and values required to bring this about. Because those with less control over their own lives are at greater risk, efforts to improve the socio-economic status of the most destitute and measures to empower women are critical to reducing the spread of the virus.

PROGRAMME STRATEGY

The breadth and diversity of the interventions required to respond adequately to the needs of children in families affected by the HIV epidemic present particular challenges to programme development and implementation. If the five programme elements just outlined are to be achieved, there must be an overarching programme strategy which is to create an environment that will encourage and support the necessary changes.

In this respect, policies to address the needs of children in affected families are no different from those directed, for example, to adults. Efforts must be made to create an environment that is sensitive to the needs and concerns of all people affected by the epidemic and which expresses care and compassion for these people rather than fear, hostility or alienation.

1. Assess Needs, Monitor the Situation and its Impact

In areas seriously affected by the epidemic, the ability of extended families and communities to provide for the basic needs of children without parents may be threatened. Those from outside the community who wish to provide support should, as an initial step, seek to understand what specific difficulties these children, families and communities are facing and how they themselves are coping with them. Cultural and socio-economic differences will result in different patterns of need as well as different survival and coping strategies both within and among communities and countries. These variations need to be taken into account in planning interventions so that the measures carried out will reinforce and not undermine constructive family and community level efforts.

An inventory and/or needs assessment can provide an initial picture of the situation of children in families affected by HIV. A system for monitoring needs and measuring the impact of interventions over time needs to be established. It can generally best be established by building upon existing systems functioning at the village level and above, such as village health or development committees or health posts. Assessment and monitoring are most effective when they are participatory processes, actively involving people from the communities most affected. Participation in assessing and monitoring needs also creates local awareness and engagement.

2. Create National Awareness and Engagement

There is a need to sensitize the public to the specific needs and problems of children in families affected by the epidemic as well as to promote a national sense of responsibility for responding to these needs. The extent and nature of the situation need to be widely understood and people committed to respond to it. The government, private organizations, nongovernmental organizations, faith communities and international organizations can all help create an environment that will facilitate appropriate responses to these children.

3. Develop a National Policy Framework

The social, legal, ethical and human rights framework of the national response as well as its administrative and co-ordination arrangements need to be in place as early as possible. The national policy framework will guide and support appropriate responses to the needs of children in affected families from the local to the national levels. Policy areas could include: measures to protect the rights and prevent discrimination against affected children and their families; the availability of affordable voluntary counselling and testing; a national drug policy that ensures the accessibility and affordability of the basic medicines needed to treat opportunistic infections; non-discriminatory personnel policies which enable infected persons to continue to work; the rights of affected families to medical benefits and insurance.

The Government of Malawi has developed a policy framework to guide responses to the needs of affected children.[9]

These establish priorities for action and define which types of services are appropriate and which are not. Existing policies and legislation should be reviewed to determine their direct or indirect impact on the well-being of affected children and on the capacities of families and communities to care for them. Some governments have waived school fees for children whose parents have died. In some cases, governments have defined clear policies regarding the kinds of services that can be provided to limit the diversion of resources into well-intended but inappropriate interventions.

4. Create Consensus on the Most Effective and Sustainable Responses

The epidemic is a new and complex phenomenon and the most effective way to respond may not be known or be widely accepted. There could be conflicting and different approaches proposed. It is important that there be widespread discussion leading to acceptance of and support for appropriate initiatives. The affected communities together with other sources of expertise should assist in the development of such a consensus. The process of consensus building will create a broader base of support if all the key actors take part and thereby develop an investment in implementing the agreed upon policies.

External support for initiatives that are not consistent with the agreed approach can be harmful. Families and communities will play critical ongoing roles in meeting the needs of affected children. Well-intentioned agencies can create problems by funding interventions that bypass or supplant these roles. It is much more difficult to try to re-establish spontaneous family and community systems of care than to support them initially.

5. Develop Mechanism to Ensure Resources are used Effectively and Equitably

Mechanisms may be needed to promote the equitable distribution of external support and to ensure that it meets local and national needs and priorities. These may be needed at both the district and national level. One example is the Uganda Community-Based Association for Child Welfare (UCOBAC), which is a consortium of local and international child focused organizations.[10] It has been instrumental in creating awareness of the problem, in facilitating the co-ordination of activities, organizing training for the staff of member groups, promoting appropriate policies and standards of care, organizing research and monitoring children's needs. UCOBAC has also established a grants bank to help ensure available donor resources are used where most needed and in appropriate ways.[11]

6. Strengthen National Capacity to Implement the Programme

Implementation requires adequate expertise, funding and clarity about roles. Governments may find, where resources are limited, that their most effective role is guiding service providers and donors regarding priorities established in the policy framework and monitoring changing needs and programme results. Bureaucratic impediments to supporting needed services should be minimized and interventions inconsistent with the national policy framework should be pre-empted. Raising public awareness and developing a consensus on needed responses can help mobilize local participation, probably the most important resource needed. Training is a crucial element in further developing capacity to respond effectively.

CONCLUSION

The ways in which HIV is transmitted ensure that, at least in the initial stages of its spread in a given country, some communities will be affected earlier and more intensely than others. It is important from the outset that the problems emerging and the services required be seen as national priorities and not just concerns of the localities and groups first affected. Equitable burden sharing is needed. Likewise, within the most affected comrnunities, the tendency is for women to be faced with a disproportionate burden for the care, nurturing and raising of affected children. Encouragement for men to share and alleviate these responsibilities should be built into programmes.

Families and communities are the first to respond to the need of children in affected families. Consequently, government and agency policies and programmes to benefit these children will need to focus primarily on how they can support families and communities to provide for their needs. The emphasis will be on supporting, and where necessary, establishing, sustainable family and community-based efforts. For this to happen an enabling environment is required in which public awareness and government policies and programmes include the full range of children's psychological, social, material, legal and spiritual needs.

NOTES

1. Willmore, Bridgit and Sunanda Ray. Report of the Women and AIDS Support Network Conference, Zimbabwe, November. 1989, Women and AIDS Support Network, Zimbabwe, 1990.
2. Sr. Ursula Sharpe of Kitovu Hospital in *The Orphan Generation.* Uganda, Small World Production, Video, 1991, and Pere Descombes, Caritas Kigali

oral report to UNIFEM on the Bill Pruitt Memorial Fund, 1990.

3. *The Orphan Generation.* op. cit.
4. Williams, Glen. From Fear to Hope, *Strategies for Hope,* No. 1, Action AID, U.K. with AMREF, Kenya, 1990.
5. Mukayogo, Christian and Glen Williams. AIDS Orphans, *Strategies for Hope,* No. 5. ActionAid, U.K. with AMREF, Kenya, AMREF, Tanzania, and World in Need, U.K.1991.
6. Hampton, Janie. Living Positively with AIDS, *Strategies for Hope,* No. 2, ActionAid. U.K. with AMREF, Kenya, and World in Need, U.K., 1990.
7. Kaijage, Theresa .J. in *Women and HIV; an International Research and Resources Book edited* by Marge Berer and Sunanda Ray, Pandora, U.K., 1993. pp. 271-274.
8. UNDP, *Young Women: Silence, Susceptibility and the HIV Epidemic,* 1992.
9. *Policy Guidelines for the Care of Orphans in Malawi and Co-ordination of Assistance for Orphans,* Task Force on Orphans, Minrstry ot' Women and Children Affairs and Community Services, Government of Malawi, July 1992.
10. Information on the Ugandan Community-Based Association for Child Welfare can be obtained by writing to UCOBAC. P.O. Box 7449, Kampala, Uganda or by fax at (256-41) 259149.
11. We wish to record our appreciation of the assistance provided to us in the preparation of this Issues Paper by John Williamson, Consultant. We would also like to thank Prof. Karen Hein, M. D., Adolescent AIDS Program. Montefiore Medical Center, New York: and Dr. Susan Hunter and Jim Sherry of UNICEF. New York for their comments.

SELECTED REFERENCES RELEVANT TO CHILDREN AFFECTED BY THE HIV EPIDEMIC

"AIDS Orphans in Africa," Sub-Working group on Exploited Children of the NGO Committee on UNICEF, meeting notes, January 14, 1992, 9 pages.

"AIDS Orphans: What Can be Done'?" *AIDS Analysis Africa,* Bank, April 1991, 58 pages.

Ainsworth, M. and Over, M., "The Economic Impact of AIDS: Shocks, Responses and Outcomes." *Africa Technical Department,* Population, Health and Nutrition Division, The World Bank, Technical Working Paper No. 1, June 1991, 41 pages.

Ainsworth, M., "Estimate of the Excess Number of Orphans in Uganda Due to AIDS and War." can attachment to a report Africa Technical Department, Population, The World Bank, July 1991, 4 pages.

Ainsworth, M. and Rwegarulia, A. A., "Coping with the AIDS Epidemic in Tanzania: Survivor Assistance," Africa Technical Department, Population, Health and Nutrition Division, The World Bank, Technical Working Paper No. 6. July 1994, 54 pages.

Alden, J.S., Salole, G. and Williamson, J., "Managing Uganda's Orphans Crisis," PRITECH, August 1991, 68 pages.

Armstrong, Jill, "Socio-economic Implications of AIDS in Developing Countries," *Finance & Development,* December 1991, pp. 14-17.

Barnett, T. and Blaikie, P., *AIDS in Africa: Its Present and Future Impact,* Belhaven Press. London. 1992, 188 pages.

Barnett, T. and Blaikie, P., "AIDS: Monitoring the Downstream Effect," *AIDS Analysis Africa.* September/October 1991, pp. 8-9.

Children and AIDS: An Impending Calamity," UNICEF, 1990. 24 pages.

Dunn, A., Hunter, S., Nabongo, C. Sekiwanuka, J., "Enumeration and Needs Assessment of Orphans in Uganda: Survey Report," The Children, U.K., April 1991. 152 pages.

Hunter. S. Bulirwa, E., and Kisseka, E., "Report of a Land Utilization Survey: Masaka and Rascal Districts," draft, October 1991, 76 pages.

Hunter. S. The Impact ot AIDS on Children in Sub-Saharan Atrican Cities. draft. 1991, 25 pages.

Hunter, S. "Orphans as a Window on the AIDS Epidemic in Sub-Saharan Africa: Initial Results and Implications of a Study in Uganda," *Soc. Sci. Med.*, Vol. 31, No. 6, 1990, pp. 681-690.

Hunter, S., "The Impact of AIDS on Children in Sub-Saharan African Cities," draft, 1992, 30 pages.

Kaduru, G., Mweige, E., and Nambi, A., "A Preliminary Report on a Needs Assessment of Rakai and Masaka Districts with Particular Reference to the Socio-economic Irnpact of the AIDS Epidemic," March 1990, 25 pages.

Lejune, A., Fogel, M-F, and Walque, E., "les Orphelins de la Ville de Kigali Rwanda." [The Orphans of Kigali, Rwanda: A Quantitative and Qualitative Study] the Red Cross of Rwanda] May 1992, original in French, English translation has been prepared, 50 pages.

Muller, O. and Abbas, N., "The Impact of AIDS Mortality on Children's Education in Kampala (Uganda)," *AIDS Care,* Vol. 2, No. 1, 1990, pp. 77-80.

Mukoyo, C. and Williams, G., *AIDS Orphans,* Strategies for Hope: No. 5, Action Aid, AMREF, and AMREF Tanzania, 1991, 35 pages.

Mulemwa, J. and Badaru, N., "A Report of the Conference on 'Managing Uganda's Orphans Crisis,' held in Kampala April 29 and 30, 1992, sponsored by the Ministry of Labour and Social Aftairs and USAID/ Kampala.

Namuli, R.M., "Programme for Orphans and Primary Health Rehabilitation Raika Birungi Byokka Project: Report of the Findings: Orphans and Foster Families Baseline Survey in Rakai District, November-December 1990".

Paloni, A. and Lamas, L., "A Duration Dependent Model of the Spread of HIV/ AIDS in Africa," Center for Demography and Ecology. University of Wisconsin-Madison, CDE Working Paper 90 -15, 1989, 31 pages.

Paloni, A., Lee. Y. J., and Lamas. L., "The Effects of HIV/AIDS on Family Organization in Africa." Center for Demography and Ecology, University of Wisconsin-Madison, CDE Working Paper 89-21, 1990, 46 pages.

Paloni, A. and Lee, Y. J., "Families and HIV/AIDS in Africa," Center for Demography and Ecology, University of Wisconsin-Madison, CDE Working Paper 90-32. 1991, 49 pages.

Poonawala, S. and Simenn off, A. Proceedings from NCIH AIDS Orphans Workshop," Nantional Council for International Health. October 17, 1990, 19 pages.

Poonawala, S. and Cantor. "Children Orphaned by : AIDS: A Call for Action for NGO's and Donors," March 31, 1991, National Council for International Health. 27 pages.

Preble, E. A., "Impact of HIV/AIDS on African Children," *Soc. Sci. Med.,* Vol. 31, No. 6, 1990, pp. 671-680

Preble, E. A., "Women, Children and AIDS in Africa: An Impending Disaster," Symposium on International and Comparative Aspects of the AIDS Crisis, *New York University Journal of International Law and Politics,* November 15, 1990, 22 pages.

Preble, E. A., "Pediatric AIDS, Child Morbidity and Child Survival Programmes in Africa: A Complex Interaction," presented at the American Anthropological Association meeting, November 28, 1990 in New Orleans, U.S.A., 18 pages.

Preble, E. A., "AIDS Orphans in Africa," Presented to the Meeting of Norwegian NGO's on AIDS, December 4, 1990, 15 pages.

Reid, E., "Young Women and the HIV Epidemic", Journal of STD, Development 1990:1. pp. 16-19.

Reid, E. and Bailey, M., Young Women: Silence, Susceptibility and the HIV Epidemic", United Nations Development Programme, 10 pages.

Reid, E., "The HIV Epidemic and Development: The Unfolding of the Epidemic," United Nations Development Programme, 16 pages.

"A Report of the Conference on 'Managing Uganda's Orphans Crisis' held at Sheraton Hotel, Kampala, 29th-30th of April 1992," Sponsored by Ministry of Labour and Social Affairs and USAID/Kampala .

"Report on a Meeting and Orphans in Africa: Florence 14/15 June 1991," UNICEF, 30 pages.

"Tanzania AIDS Assessment and Planning Study," October 1991, World Bank, 174 pages.

"The Care and Support of Children of HIV-infected Parents," World Health Organization, Global Programme on AIDS, May 1991, 38 pages.

Williamson, J., "Children Orphaned by AIDS: Unprecedented Challenges." Presented to the annual conference of the Institute on African Affairs, Washington D.C., February, 1993. 14 pages.

16

The HIV/AIDS Epidemic in Thailand

Dr. Wiput Phoolcharoen
Director, Division of AIDS,
Department of Communicable Disease Control,
Ministry of Public Health, Thailand.

EPIDEMIOLOGICAL PATTERNS

The first Thai case of AIDS was reported in 1984. The earliest recorded cases of AIDS were predominantly in homosexual men. Three years later, the importance of male to male sex as a risk factor was quickly overshadowed by the rapid increase in infection among intravenous drug users. This was immediately followed by an increase in seroprevalence among female commercial sex workers. Subsequently, the third wave of infection appeared in clients of these commercial sex workers as reflected in an upsurge of seroprevalence among men attending government sexually transmitted disease clinics. A fourth wave reflected a spread of infections among the wives and girl friends of men who visited commercial sex workers. Seropositive rates in women attending antenatal clinics continue to increase, along with an increasing incidence of reported pediatric AIDS cases. This can be observed as evidence of the fifth wave of the epidemic.

With a rather well-developed health care infrastructure, Thailand is in a position to launch and maintain an acceptable system of HIV surveillance. Information on HIV seroprevalence has been collected semi-annually in every province in Thailand since June 1990 by the Ministry of Public Health through the sentinel surveillance system.

The wide regional variations in the epidemic are particularly noteworthy. The north has the highest prevalence, while the northeast consistently has the lowest. Within the north, Chiang Mai, Chiang Rai and Phayao are the worst affected. There has been a rapid increase, for example, in Trat, Rayong and Phetchaburi. This is observed to co-relate with the number of commercial sex workers in each locality.

One of the distinguishing characteristics of the Thai epidemic is that urban and rural infection levels do not appear to be strikingly different as is the case in most African and Western settings This may be explained in part by the high mobility of the Thai population as a consequence of rapid socio-economic changes. It is also notable that the most vulnerable groups are the socio-economically backward and poorly educated labour classes in both the industrial and agricultural sectors.

Political Response

From 1984 to 1990, AIDS was perceived to be a newly-emerging public health problem. Consequently, the Ministry of Public Health was the key player in determining national policies and strategies for its prevention and control. Vigorous promotion of the use of condoms in the commercial sex settings has been an important and reasonably successful programme. Universal screening of blood and blood products was introduced all over the country in 1988. The use of universal precautions was also emphasized from the outset but has been slow in gaining widespread use.

The year 1991 can be considered a turning-point in the evolution of the Thai government's AIDS policies, strategies and programmes. The epidemic had spread to all sectors of the society and there was no sign of abatement. It became apparent that more concerted efforts and innovative strategies were essential. Hence, the National AIDS Prevention and Control Committee, under the chairmanship of the Prime Minister, was established. The Permanent Secretary of the Ministry of Public Health was assigned to act as the committee's secretariat, and the Division of AIDS, Department of Communicable Disease Control, assumed the responsibility of the office of the secretariat.

It was recognized that a multisectoral approach was highly desirable, and efforts were undertaken to involve all government agencies, non-government organizations and the business community. The National AIDS Prevention and Control Plan for 1992—96 was formulated to meet this need. The planning process entailed national level co-ordination under the leadership of the National AIDS Prevention and Control Committee. Government funding was sought to meet the initial needs of the plan. In 1993, all 14 ministries submitted funding requests in accordance with the programmes specified in the National AIDS Plan, amounting to $ 44 million. The National AIDS Programme's budget has been increasing continuously, reaching $60 million in the current fiscal year.

In 1993, the upward trend of the AIDS epidemic continued, necessitating some revisions to the National AIDS Prevention and

Control Plan for 1995-96. The increasing number of the AIDS cases and death signalled a severe erosion of the Thai social fabric. As people with HIV/AIDS began to experience stigmatization and discrimination, families, community and humanitarian aspects needed special attention. Thus, the revised plan gave priority to the following programmes:

1. Programme on Prevention for Behavioural and Social Aspects
2. Programme on Health Promotion and Medical Services
3. Programme on Provision of Counselling
4. Programme on Living with AIDS and Legal Measures
5. Programme on Research and Evaluation
6. Programme on Development of Administration, Organization and Management.

The collaboration among governmental organizations, non-governmental organizations and private sector is the key focus of the plan. There are over 200 development-oriented Thai NGOs participating in the programme against the AIDS epidemic in Thailand. The Thai NGO Coalition on AIDS, a network of 42 NGOs, was established in the late 1990s. The role of Thai NGOs in AIDS has been mainly directed towards developing models of AIDS education and social support services where government services have been relatively weak. NGOs have taken the lead in working among stigmatized social groups; developing participatory forms of AIDS education, client centered counselling and support services, campaigning on social acceptance of people living with HIV/AIDS and their rights to non-discrimination; and in training and employing people to work as AIDS educators and counsellors.

Another step has been the establishment of the Thailand Business Coalition on AIDS in 1993—a non-profit organization providing information, technical support and training programmes to Thai business in the formulation of effective and non-discriminatory measures for AIDS in the workplaces.

The Organization for the Improved Management of the AIDS Prevention and Control Programme, which was at first designed to co-ordinate the multisectoral AIDS policy, has been decentralized to ensure more efficient management. The executive board, chaired by the Minister of Public Heath, was formed in 1994. The permanent secretaries of six ministries have been appointed to lead the work of six subcommittees. These are:

1. Public Relations/ Mass Media by the Office of Prime Minister.
2. AIDS Education by the Ministry of Education.
3. AIDS Programmes for Special Target Groups by the Ministry of Interior.

These three committees will be responsible for reducing risk behaviour through changes in the social environment and community life-style, aimed at achieving both short-term and long- term objectives.

4. Medical and Counselling Services by the Ministry of Public Health
5. Social Acceptance and Human Rights by the Ministry of Labour and Social Welfare.
6. Research and Evaluation by the Ministry of University Affairs.

Achievements of the National Programme

An effective programme to prevent HIV infection must have both universal and targeted components. The universal component includes reducing HIV-related discrimination, removing social and commercial restrictions on information necessary for safer behaviour, and providing information about the risk of HIV. The targeted component involves devoting the limited resources for intensive programmes of behavioural change to situations and groups where the risk of HIV transmission is at the highest. Underprivileged communities should be specially targeted. Social action and educational measures should seek to encourage healthy lifestyles to reduce risk of infection.

Currently, there is some evidence to suggest that the National AIDS Programme has achieved significant results. A continuous decrease in sexually transmitted diseases has been seen during the last four years. Finally, the decline in the HIV seroprevalence rate among the recently recruited military conscripts, which accounts for the HIV epidemic in the majority of Thai youths, explicitly demonstrates the programme's effectiveness.

Legal and Ethical Aspects

As with other communicable diseases, the tragic epidemic of HIV/ AIDS presents the classical public health problem of a conflict between the welfare of the community and the rights of the individual, but with significant differences. Like other sexually transmitted and communicable diseases, HIV/AIDS has called for measures to prevent its spread as for the protection of the privacy and other civil rights of persons afflicted with the disease. But HIV/ AIDS poses serious and different problems because as yet there is no cure and no vaccine for prevention; and because the incidence of HIV/AIDS is concentrated in certain high-risk individuals - intravenous drug users, prostitutes and promiscuous males-who are particularly vulnerable to discrimination.

Legislation has been a significant component of the response to the HIV/AIDS epidemic. An early response to the epidemic was to prevent the influx of infected cases through migration. In 1983, under the Immigration Act, the Ministry of Interior prohibited the immigration of foreigners with HIV/AIDS. This regulation was not strictly enforced because of the lack of available tests at the time and pressure from the international community. Consequently, this was revoked in 1991.

Through a public health ministerial announcement in 1984, under the Contagious Diseases Act, AIDS was required to be reported to the health authorities. Six years later, in order to protect the confidentiality of the test results, case reporting was cancelled. Instead, AIDS was required to be notified by using a code for the purpose of epidemiological surveillance. Currently, there is no compulsory notification of those with HIV/AIDS to the authorities.

During 1990-1991, attempts were made to enact a reactionary law. An AIDS Bill which would have adopted stricter measures and punishment against those with HIV/AIDS was introduced. The purposes of this bill were to:

Establish a national committee to prevent and control AIDS.

Compel reporting of those with AIDS to the medical authorities.

Order those with AIDS to appear for a medical check-up.

Oblige those with AIDS to report their movements to the medical authorities.

Compel those with AIDS to be detained in, or to be prohibited from entering, certain areas.

Prohibit those with AIDS from spreading the disease.

Punish those who violate the law by means of imprisonment and fines.

After two years of controversial arguments, the National AIDS Prevention and Control Committee rejected this bill.

Since AIDS related legislation has been controversial and the fact that legislative aspirations may be plagued by poor law enforcement, the current approach towards those with HIV/AIDS should be informed by the National AIDS Prevention and Control Plan with its multipronged strategies. Mandatory testing without informed consent has no place in this plan because it violates the rights and dignity of individuals and is counter-productive to control of the epidemic. However, these aspirations are not reflected in the current law and practice in terms of effective redress. A key challenge will be to ensure that the AIDS Control Plan itself is able to be translated into effective remedies.

17

Are Young People in the Philippines Taking Chances with HIV/AIDS?

D. Balk, T. Brown, G. Cruz, and L. Domingo

The first AIDS case in the Philippines was diagnosed in 1984 Since then, the number of AIDS cases and detected HIV infections has climbed slowly but steadily. By the end of 1995, 234 AIDS cases and 470 HIV infections had been reported to the Department of Health Vesting has been limited, however and the number of HIV infections is undoubtedly much larger than reported.

As in most Asian countries, early infections were often associated with overseas travel or contact with foreigners. By 1990, however it was clear that the epidemic was spreading among the Filipino population.

A number of factors contribute to the potential for a serious HIV/AIDS epidemic in the Philippines. For one thing there is a substantial commercial sex industry although the National HIV Sentinel Surveillance System has detected only very low levels of HIV infection among sex workers, the system has found much higher rates of syphilis infection. This is cause for concern because syphilis and other sexually transmitted diseases not only spread through the same routes as HIV but also greatly enhance the chances of HIV transmission between sexual partners. The low level of condom use reported by commercial sex workers heightens this concern.

Secondly reports have sugested that many young men in the Philippines engage in premarital sex with girlfriends and acquaintances. Early AIDS cases were associated with men having sex with men, but more recently heterosexual transmission has increased in importance. Finally injecting drug use may provide an avenue for HIV transmission among a small number of young people.

A national Young Adult Fertility and Sexuality Study (YAFS-II), conducted in 1994, makes a substantial contribution to the information available on risk factors that could produce a serious HIV/AIDS epidemic among young people in the Philippines This issue of Asia-Pasific Population & Policy reports on key finding from the survey. More detailed information will be published in a full report.

ABOUT THE SURVEY

YAFS-II was the first nationally representative survey of youth in the Philippines that covered both men and women. An earlier Young Adult Fertility Survey (YAFS-I), conducted in 1982, included only women.

The University of the Philippines Population Institute conducted YAFS-II with a network of nine regional research centers throughout the country. The project was supported by the United Nations Population Fund (UNFPA). The East-West Center's Programme on Population collaborated in the survey with support from the United States Agency for International Development (USAID).

YAFS-II was a household survey covering men and women we 15 to 24. A total of 10,879 young people were interviewed, with separate questionnaires for men and women and for married and unmarried respondents. In addition to these questionnaires, a sealed-envelop questionnaire covering highly sensitive issues was given to a subgroup of respondents. Screening data were also collected on all households visited and on the 959 sampled communities.

The survey covered many subject areas. Several sequences of questions were designed to elicit information on sexual experience, both directly and in the context of questions about dating. Additional questions explored condom use and attitudes toward condoms, knowledge of HIV/AIDS and other sexually transmitted diseases, and levels of concern about infection.

A LITTLE KNOWLEDGE

Ninety-five per cent of all the young people covered in the survey had heard of AIDS. As would be expected, younger respondents were slightly less likely than older respondents to have heard of the disease. Still, a full 90 per cent of 15year-olds had heard of AIDS. Controlling for age, awareness of AIDS tended to be lower in rural areas, among respondents with less education, and among those with no regular exposure to the mass media. There was no gender difference in AIDS awareness.

Although awareness was nearly universal, knowledge of AIDS was more limited. When respondents who knew about AIDS were asked how it is acquired, 85 per cent correctly identified at least one sexual mode of transmission, and 25 per cent correctly identified at least one non-sexual mode. The most frequently mentioned transmission mode was commercial sex, cited by 66 per cent of these respondents. Twelve per cent could not identify a single correct mode of transmission, and 26 per cent gave at least one incorrect answer, such as having contact with the belongings of an infected person, kissing, or using public toilets.

An overall assessment of AIDS knowledge identified five characteristics associated with a good understanding of the syndrome and its transmission routes. These were age, family wealth, education, being single, and discussion networks.

Discussions about AIDS appeared to be an important factor in promoting knowledge—so important, in fact, that such discussion,s nullified the direct effect of media exposure. Young people who talked about AIDS with three or more different types of people (such as friends, partners, parents, or teachers) had a much better understanding of the disease than those who discussed it with only one type of person or did not discuss it at all. Women were more likely to have discussed AIDS with a variety of people—most young men had only discussed it with their male friends.

Most young people felt that they themselves were at little or no risk of HIV infection. Only 12 per cent thought that they were at some personal risk. Even men who had visited commercial sex workers tended to believe that they had little or no chance of contracting HIV. Among single men who had paid for sex during the 12 months before the survey and had not used a condom, only 29 per cent thought that it was likely or very likely that "someone like them" might become infected.

SOME YOUNG MEN ARE TAKING CHANCES

The risk of contracting AIDS depends largely on two factors—sexual activity and injecting drug use. In the Philippines, sexual transmission is the more serious concern. The YAFS-II survey showed that few 15- or 16-year-olds had engaged in sex, but sexual activity increased steadily with age. Among 24-year olds, 55 per cent of men and 23 per cent of women had engaged in premarital sex.

Most of the men and women who were sexually active before marriage reported that their only partner was their future spouse.

However, men were almost 20 times more likely than women to have had sex before marriage with at least one additional partner.

Reports of premarital sex tended to be higher among men who lived in urban areas and men who were Catholic. Among 23- and 24-year-olds, men with a high-school or college education were more likely to have engaged in premarital sex than were men with only an elementary education.

The survey results suggest that the longer men remain single, the greater their risk of exposure to HIV infection. By age 24, 22 per cent of single men reported having had sex with a girlfriend or acquaintance during the 12month period before the survey, and 8 per cent reported having visited a commercial sex worker. Among all single men, 13 per cent reported having had only one sexual partner, another 10 per cent reported two or more partners, and 3 per cent reported five or more partners .

Modeling studies have shown that even such small groups of sexually active individuals can greatly accelerate the spread of HIV. This is particularly true when men have sex with commercial sex workers and also with other partners. The YAFS-II survey results provide convincing evidence of such overlapping sexual networks.

Thirtynine per cent of married men reported having had at least one sexual partner before marriage other than their future wife. Seven per cent reported five or more premarital partners. As with single men, there was significant overlapping of sexual contacts. Seven per cent of married respondents reported premarital sex with their future wives, other girlfriends, and commercial sex workers Although few married men reported having visited a commercial sex worker during the 12 months before the survey 16 per cent reported having had an extramarital affair at some time during their marriage. Reported levels of extramarital sex were higher in rural areas than in urban areas.

Men who visit commercial sex workers face a particularly high risk of infection Surveys in the Philippines have sporadically detected low levels of HIV in commercial sex workers, but these levels are expected to increase over the next few years.

Eight per cent of the men interviewed during the YAFS-II survey had paid for sex at some time in their lives. The per centage that reported having ever paid for sex increased steadily with age-from 0 per cent at age 15 to 17 per cent by age 24. Men in urban areas were more likely to have paid for sex than men in rural areas, and men with a high-school or college education were more likely to have paid for sex than men with only an elementary education.

Among those who had visited a commercial sex worker during the 12 months before the survcy 26 per cent had paid for sex monthly or more frequently 22 per cent occasional and most of the remainder only once. Almost half reported changing sexual partners each time they paid for sex, while another quarter reported visiting the same partner repeatedly. The average number of paid sexual partners over 12 months was 2.5.

Male homosexual and bisexual behaviour has been strongly associated with the HIV epidemic in many countries. Among sexually experienced young men covered by the YAFS-II Survey, 7 per cent reported having had sex with other men, but only 1 per cent reported exclusively male sexual partners. An other 9 per cent gave inconsistent information or failed to answer this question. Most of those reporting some sexual experience with men had predominantly female sexual partners.

Infecting drug use has not yet made a substantial contribution to reported HIV infections and AIDS cases in the Philippines. However 2 per cent of the YAFS-II survey respondents reported that they had tried injectable drugs. This finding probably understates the true level of drug use. It suggests some limited potential for HIV transmission through needle sharing among drug users.

WHEN MEN TAKE CHANCES, THEY POLE WOMEN M RISK

YAFS-II survey results indicate much lower levels of sexual risk-taking among young women than men. Among all single women, only 2 per cent reported ever having had sex unlike their single male counteriarts, virtually all single women who reported any sexual experience had only one partner. Thirty five per cent of married women reported having had premarital sex, but nearly ad of these had only had sex with their future husbands. Only 4 per cent reported ever having had an extramarital affair.

Survey results showed no differences in levels of premarital sexual activity between rural and urban women or women with different levels of education. However, Catholic women were more likely to have experienced premarital sex than were non-Catholics

Given existing differences in social expectations, women are more likely than men to under-report their premarital and extramarital sexual experience Even taking this tendency into account, however results from the YAFS-II survey strongly suggest that single and married women are at risk of HIV infection primarily through the previous and current sexual activities of their partners.

FEW USE CONDOMS

Proper use of condoms can substantially reduce the risk of

HIV infection. YAFS-II survey results showed that knowledge of condoms was high, but actual condom use was extremely low.

When asked about their knowledge of family planning methods, 69 per cent of the men interviewed mentioned condoms without prompting, and another 18 per cent reported that they knew of condoms after being prompted. Among the women,62 per cent reported knowledge of condoms without prompting and another 25 with prompting. Among sexually active men, 98 per cent had heard of condoms, but only 58 per cent of those who knew about condoms were aware that condoms could help prevent AIDS.

Only 23 per cent of sexually active men reported that they had ever used a condom, and far fever [4 %] reported having used a condom during their most recent sexual experience Married men and sexually active single men were equally likely to have ever used a condom. Several other factors were associated with having ever used 3 condom

Residence: urban men were much more likely than rural men to have ever used condoms
Education: among 23- and 24-yearolds, men with at least a college education were three times as likely to have used condoms as men with only an elementary education
Population education in school: classes on family planning and sexually transr..ted diseases had a strong positive influence on condom use.
Regular exposure to mass media.
Knowledge of AIDS: men with the greatest knowledge of AIDS were more likely to have used condoms than men whose knowledge of AIDS was poor or moderate.

Condom use is particularly important for men who visit commercial sex workers. Men who had paid for sex were more than twice as likely as other men to have ever used condoms, but the rates of condom use for this group were still low. Only 27 per cent of those who had recently visited a commercial sex worker reported using condoms all or most of the time, 20 per cent reported using condoms some of the time, and 50 per cent said that they never used condoms at all.

In the Philippines, condoms are available in drugstores, supermarkets, and private clinics. The government family planning programme, however, has an explicit policy against supplying condoms or other contraceptives to unmarried people. When asked during the survey, nearly all sexually active men said they knew where they could obtain condoms. Most mentioned drugstores as a source, but a sizable minority—even of unmarried men—also mentioned government health centers.

Men were asked how long it took to travel from their home

to the nearest source of condoms. Not surprisingly, rural men reported more than twice the travel time (49 minutes) reported by urban men (22 minutes). In both urban and rural areas, men with only an elementary education reported more than twice the travel time (67 minutes) reported by men with a college education (33 minutes).

When asked how they felt about using condoms, 90 per cent of sexually active men expressed some negative attitudes. The most commonly expressed negative attitude (by 58 per cent) was that condoms make sex less pleasurable. Nearly half 147 per cent) said that they would be embarrassed to buy condoms at a store, and sizable minorities stated that condoms were too expensive to use regularly (34 per cent) or that condom use was against their religion (32 per cent).

SUMMARY AND POLICY RECOMMENDATIONS

YAFS-II survey results indicate that a substantial minority of young men in the Philippines are at a heightened risk of HIV infection. By the time they reach age 24, almost 40 per cent of Filipino men have had sex with at least one partner other than their wife or future wife, and 3 per cent have had five or more sexual partners. Almost 10 per cent have visited a commercial sex worker.

Young women appear to be taking fewer chances. Less than 10 per cent of single women have had sex by age 24, and most married women have only had sex with their husbands. If these results are accurate, women in the Philippines are primarily at risk through the premarital and extramarital activities of their sexual partners.

Awareness of AIDS is high, but knowledge of how the virus is spread is somewhat limited. Similarly, the perception of risk is low. There appears to be a strong perceived association of HIV with commercial sex and multiple sex partners. Young people do not seem to realize that sex with a boyfriend or girlfriend also entails a potential risk. Even among young men engaging in commercial sex without condoms, only one-third felt that "someone like them" might be likely to contract HIV.

The low level of reported condom use is of particular concern. Although most young people are familiar with condoms in the context of family planning, only a little more than half of the young men interviewed knew that the proper use of condoms could prevent HIV transmission. Only 23 per cent of sexually active young men had ever used a condom.

The policy implications of these findings are clear. Future efforts in AIDS education need to stress the possibility of risk in any sexual encounter. YAFSII survey results showed large differences in knowledge about AIDS among education groups, suggesting that AIDS information programmes need to target young people who do not have high levels of formal education. The large percentage of respondents who said that they had discussed AIDS with their friends suggests that peer education approaches may be particularly effective.

Young people are not likely to change their Behaviour if they do not consider themselves at risk. Expanded efforts are needed to inform young people of the risks of unprotected sex, perhaps through AIDS education and awareness campaigns. Among those young people who, nevertheless, engage in risky Behaviour, every effort is needed to encourage the proper and consistent use of condoms.

Although condoms are widely available through commercial outlets, the official policy limiting condom distribution at government clinics to married couples may very well be inhibiting their use. Condoms need to be made more widely available in rural areas and possibly in neighbourhoods where the less-educated tend to live. Given reported low levels of condom use among men having sex with men, any programme designed to slow the spread of HIV should also focus on condom use among male homosexuals and bisexuals.

Numerous social and religious barriers remain in the Philippines that inhibit open discussion of risk Behaviours, promotion of condom use, and training in the skills required to protect oneself from HIV. To avoid a serious epidemic, these barriers must be overcome and effective prevention programmes put into place.

18

The HIV/AIDS Epidemic in Uganda: A Programme Approach

Desmond Cohen
Former Governor
Institute of Development Studies

I. HIV AND AIDS IN UGANDA

The HIV epidemic in Uganda has its origins in the early to mid Seventies, although it was not diagnosed as such until 1984. The spread of HIV in the population has been rapid. By the end of 1991 30,190 cases of AIDS had been reported to the AIDS Control Programrne (ACP) surveillance unit, with cases from almost every District in the country. This is thought to be a significant under estimate of the true number of cases as a result of under reporting. Modelling of the epidemic suggests that the actual number of cases of AIDS is some 6 to 7 times greater than reported cases.

In 1987-88 a national serological survey was undertaken to establish the level and distribution of HIV infection in the population. In the event the survey was not fully representative, with gaps in the data for the eastern and northern regions particularly. The survey generated an estimate of an adult HIV prevalence level of 9 per cent, i.e. some 800,000 people were thought to be infected. There were wide variations between regions and between urban and rural areas. In the case of urban areas the rate was estimated to be as high as 29 per cent in some regions; much lower, but still significant, in rural areas. Because most of the population is rural [some 90 per cent] even relatively lower rural HIV rates implies high absolute numbers of people who are infected. More recent data from ante-natal clinics has yielded seroprevalence rates of 27 per cent in true urban areas like Kampala, to as low as 3 per cent in some rural areas [with the possibility that rates are even lower than this in some parts of the country]. Using the national serosurvey as the base, and applying the evidence from sentinel sites, it appears that the current numbers infected with HIV are about 1.3 million.

As noted above, the cases of AIDS which are notified to the Ministry of Health (MOH) are considered to be a massive underestimate of tne true numbers. This reflects the coverage and quality of health care in Uganda, with many persons with HIV related illnesses outside the reach of the formal health care system. Many fall back on traditional healers for assistance, and as such are never reported to the MOH. In part also, the continuing stigma associated with HIV and AIDS leads individuals and families to prefer some other diagnosis. Nevertheless, the data on AIDS as reported has some value in permitting analysis of the sex and age distribution of those identified. About a third of the reported AIDS cases are children under 5, reflecting the frequency of paediatric cases. Otherwise there is a bunching of cases in the ages 15-49, with a mean age for adults of 27 years. The elderly and young adolescents are more or less generally free of infection.

Of great importance are differences in the median ages of infection of men and women; for men this is 30 years, but for women is much younger at 25. Not only are women infected at an earlier age but there is some evidence that infection rates are higher than for men. why this is so is far from clear, and cannot simply be a reflection of males choosing more youthful sexual partners. Many other factors must also be operating, and these require analysis if there are to be effective policies for prevention, for care and for dealing with the impact of the epidemic on the social and economic system. The gender dimensions of the problem need to be constantly at the forefront of analysis and policy, and not simply, although these are important, because of the problems raised for perinatal transmission and for the general health of mothers and children.

A. TRANSMISSION OF HIV

Much is now known about HIV and AIDS and there has been immense progress made in a remarkably short time in understanding transmission of the virus. Nevertheless, there is much that is not known, and there remain major areas of uncertainty. Why women are infected at an earlier age than men is one area where research is urgently needed. It seems unlikely that a vaccine will be discovered, and be available, before the end of the decade, but even then it is improbable that in the conditions which exist in many developing countries, including Uganda, that a vaccine will be sufficient to prevent the continuing spread of HIV in the population. The potential future discovery of a vaccine thus in no way diminishes the need to put in place now effective policies for prevention and care.

Having said this the ways in which the virus are spread are now well understood. In Uganda, as in much of Africa, the major mode of transmission is sexual. Heterosexual transmission is thought to account in Uganda for about 90 per cent of cases, with the other 10 per cent of infections being from mother to child [paediatric] and from infected blood. Securing the blood supply is an important intervention, but given the relative size of the contributing factors in transmission it is of much reduced importance. Thus by far the most significant risk factor in determining the spread of HIV and the resulting size of the population which is infected, are unsafe sexual practices. This is compounded in the Ugandan case by social and cultural factors which lead many men to have multiple sexual partners, and under conditions where neither partner is protected from the virus through the use of condoms. Evidence from Uganda suggests that condoms are infrequently used; and it is reported that only about 5 per cent of women have ever used contraceptives.

There is now a well documented association between STDs and HIV infection, with the probability of infection through sexual activity being sharply increased where STDs are present. The risks of HIV infection are much higher where standard STDs are present. These risks can be substantially reduced, both of HIV and of STDs, where condoms are consistently and properly used. But this requires knowledge on the part of users, a willingness to use condoms, as well as a regular and affordable supply [conditions which are generally not met at present in Uganda]. Studies carried out in Uganda have shown that the presence of STDs in the population has been a significant factor in transmission, as well as confirming the widespread presence in both men and women of standard STDs. It is clear from these studies that STDs are a significant co-factor in the transmission of HIV, and that control of STDs needs to be an important element in any strategy for controlling HIV.

B. TRANSMISSION PROJECTIONS AND SCENARIOS

The major forms of transmission in Uganda are identified under I.A, as also are estimates of the scale and distribution of HIV infection and AIDS in the population. It is clear from these estimates, and from the discussion of the processes of transmission, that very little is known with certainty about conditions in Uganda. Nevertheless enough is known about this issue for it to be possible to model the progress of the epidemic over the next 10-15 years. Bearing in mind that such modelling is bound to be imprecise, and needs to be treated with circumspection. Any predictions have to make assumptions about future behaviour, particularly sexual behaviour, and this is inevitably fraught with difficulties. Changing assumptions does, of course, yield quite different paths of HIV infection and mortality, and quite different demographic outcomes. Of great importance for the future size of the Ugandan population is the response of fertility to rising paediatric and adult mortality, but this is an area where knowledge is very uncertain. Otherwise the most important behavioural assumptions relate to the number of sexual partners, the number of sexual acts per partner, the probability of condom use, the presence of STDs, and the extent of blood screening and blood usage.

Using the national serological survey as the benchmark it is possible to model the future course of HIV infection, and to then vary the important behavioural parameters so as to observe the relative contribution of these to the model projections. Such a set of illustrative projections has been undertaken by the World Bank (WB) [1991] [these are presently being revised to take account of the recent population census which estimated a current population that is significantly smaller than had earlier been predicted]. The worst scenario looked at by the Bank assumes a continuation of present trends, and generates a set of predictions which are highly unfavourable. In this case by the year 2010 there are 1.7 million infected adults; the proportion of adult females infected rises from 13.6 per cent in 1991 to 17 per cent; the number of HIV positive children doubles from 50,000 to 100,000; and AIDS deaths rise from an estimated 34,000 adults and 20,000 children in 1991 to 115,000 and 55,000 in 2010. Whereas in the absence of AIDS it would have been expected that death rates would have declined, in the presence of AIDS the crude death rate in 2010 is predicted as actually higher than in the late 1980s. Indeed if HIV adult infection is as high as 20 per cent then age specific mortality rates are trebled - being higher for women than for men. Similarly for life expectancy, where in the absence of AIDS this could have been expected to improve substantially over the next 20 years, under the "no change" scenario it is actually lower in 2010 than in 1985. In this model run the total population continues to rise but at a slower rate.

The World Bank explores a number of alternative projections so as to identify and quantify the effects of parameter changes. Some of these changes in parameter values reflect the impact of policies on behaviour, and thus allow some estimation of the effects both individually and in the aggregate. Thus a model run which includes changes in sexual behaviour, increased use of condoms and reduction in STDs, generates a set of outcomes for HIV prevalence, AIDS mortality, life expectancy and so on which are much more favourable. What these estimates do is to illustrate the synergistic impacts of multiple policy interventions which in the aggregate are able to substantially reduce the future levels of HIV infection and AIDS. They also illustrate the crucial role which sexual behaviour plays in transmission of HIV, and how critical for the future of Uganda is the development of effective policies in this area.

Epidemiological modelling is in its infancy, and furthermore the Ugandan data base leaves much to be desired. Much, much more research is needed into important relationships of an epidemiological and demographic nature before reaching any firm conclusions. Nevertheless, certain conclusions are more or less well-founded in the available evidence. The present level of HIV infection is high by the standards of anywhere in the world, and there are no signs of it levelling off. HIV and AIDS mortality is much higher than officially reported data would suggest. As the W B model projections suggest theta is the potential for even higher rates of HIV infection and mortality in the future. To levels which will reverse much of the improvement in social indicators, such as in infant and maternal mortality, higher life expectancy, and rising living standards.

Extremely worrying is the evidence which supports the proposition that women are more severely impacted by the epidemic than men, and that in the future this gap will widen further. This means that women will lose more healthy years of life than men; that there will be further deterioration in the rate of paediatric AIDS, and that many of the functions which women are expected to perform as both producers and carers are unlikely to be feasible. As noted above, the gender aspect of the epidemic has received little attention, both in terms of its causes, and in its implications for the development of general policies for prevention, care and socio-economic impact.

C. IMPACT PROJECTIONS

If epidemiological and demographic modelling are uncertain in their methodology and conclusions, and thus need to be treated with care, then this is even more true when attention is turned to the economic and social impacts of the epidemic. What is now generally recognised is that the effects of HIV and AIDS are certainly not confined to the health sector, but rather that the channels of effects are multiple, and the impacts extend throughout the economic and social system. This being readily accepted it follows that the policies called for by the challenges of the epidemic will be complex in formulation, necessarily be innovative both in content and implementation processes, and require a multi-sectoral approach. It is this conclusion which has guided Uganda in establishing its present AIDS strategy.

A taxonomy of the multiple ways in which HIV effects the economic system is not too difficult to construct. These can be stated in a reasonably comprehensive way, and there is widespread agreement about the channels through which HIV will effect the performance of the economy. When it comes to estimating the quantitative size of the economic effects, and the distribution of these impacts on different types of households [and within households], on different sectors of production [and within sectors], on Government as a sector of service supply and production, then there are immense complexities and difficulties. This being recognised as the position it follows that what can he stated as the probable impact both now and in the future is highly uncertain.

For Uganda at the present it is impossible to go much deeper than generalities about the likely economic and social impacts. That these are already substantial, and will become even more so in the future, is nevertheless demonstrable even given the limitations of data, analysis, and understanding. It is doubly unfortunate that these adverse impacts are being imposed on an economy whose structure has been weakened by decades of political, economic and social turmoil, and which is only now gradually restoring its productive capacities.

We have seen above that HIV primarily effects those in the age groups which are crucial in terms of their importance to society as producers, as the suppliers of social and economic support to both the young and the elderly, and as the transmitters of much of the cultural and social values which effectively defines a society. Now in trying to evaluate the economic costs of HIV it is clear that once the full contribution of individuals is recognised that standard estimates are inevitably going to be partial and far too low. It is impossible to place an economic value on the multiple and varied contributions of individuals, other than in the narrowest of terms, and attempts to estimate the economic costs of HIV suffer from major limitations. As we have seen many of the contributions of individuals to society have economic and social value but these cannot be established. Even in the narrowest of economic terms these often cannot be estimated, and many productive activities are often excluded on highly dubious grounds from calculations of national production. This is most obviously true of much of the output and many diverse contributions of women in their multiple social and economic roles.

There is a further major conceptual problem with standard attempts to measure thc economic impact of HIV, by for example trying to establish the present value of the output lost through the early death of an individual caused by HIV related illness. This approach in effect assumes that an individual's contribution to output is independent of others, which in the case of an epidemic it clearly is not. The costs, narrowly defined in terms of the measured contribution to GNP, will in the aggregate be greater than the sum of the individual contributions to the national output streams. Overall it can be readily agreed that the economic, social and psychological costs of HIV are likely to be very substantial, and much greater than those which are conventionally identified and estimated.

Persons infected with HIV will experience periods of higher morbidity which will effect their productivity. If they are in formal sector employment they may be subject to discrimination, and possibly lose their job. In any case at this stage of the illness they will have needs which are social—their relationship to their family, and their relationship to the community [defined as overlapping sets of social interactions]. Here support which is other than economic will be essential, and yet every bit as important. How to meet these needs under severe resource constraints is one of the major challenges of this epidemic. In purely economic terms, at this stage of the illness, there will be pressure on household resources, which may be diminishing, at the same time as needs will be intensifying. This stage, and the later one of AIDS, will divert resources to health and care at the expense of other less pressing wants. This increases the probability of worsening nutrition for the household, poorer housing, a reduction of schooling for children, reduced levels of health services for the rest of the family, and so on. All at a time when pressures will diminish the resources available to the household, as labour productivity is reduced, and with the certainty that women will be diverted into caring roles and away from productive activities.

These impacts are happening now in Uganda; probably on a wide scale, but in most districts largely undocumented and not measured. But the tip of the iceberg can be observed in the medical and social support activities of many NGOs, who are tackling as best they can a problem which already exceeds their capacities. Unfortunately, Uganda is only at the start of a process of rising needs, socially economic and psychological, which will inevitably intensify over the coming years as more persons already infected with HIV fall sick and die. The conditions observed in Rakai and Masaka are of massive needs relative to available resources, of intensified destitution, of increasing evidence of family dissolution. of the elderly without support. and large numbers of orphans who have multiple needs for food, housing schooling, training, care and love. Here is the future for Uganda. But the scale of these impacts can still be limited through social mobilisation and more effective policies.

The foregoing can be thought of as the impacts at the levels of the household and the community, but there will also be aggregative effects which will reduce the total output which can be produced. There are the losses due to higher and earlier mortality —the output lost to the economy through death. This will be significant, in terms of the lost contributions of men and women—particularly the loss of the latter, who have such varied roles to play in Uganda. But output will also be reduced through a diversion of savings to "unproductive" uses—particularly into health, and care for the sick. This reduction in the level, and the reallocation of savings to consumption, will take place in all sectors with Government, Business and Households all affected. National output will grow more slowly than otherwise because the savings available for capital formation will be lowered. These negative effects on national economic performance are not yet evident and will take time to come through. At this time it is difficult to predict the size of the losses of potential output, but while these are inevitable as a category, they are not inevitable in their scale. Effective policies for prevention of HIV can reduce the losses of human and non human resources, and thus minimise the adverse general impact on the economic system.

HIV is no respecter of social class, and there is some evidence that infection rises with education and income. This seems also to be the case in Uganda, where reports are now common of losses of highly trained and scarce professional human resources. True both of private and public employment, and doubly serious for Uganda given the thinness of its existing human resource base. HIV and AIDS is eroding an already depleted stock of educated and experienced labour, and as such is confounding present attempts to rebuild national capacity. These losses are not confined to urban areas. but are reported also from quite remote rural districts where HIV prevalence is generally low. The costs are, of course, not simply the losses of human capital that are entailed, but also the losses in terms of management performance as persons fall ill, and the higher health [and other social charges] which fall on employers. But the impacts are much more general than these; HIN and AIDS reduces the quality and the quantity of human resources available to the society in terms of experience, training, knowledge, aptitudes, commitment—across the board, and in all parts of the country. As HIV spreads to previously low areas of prevalence as it is presently doing in Uganda, so also do these costs become more general and pervasive.

No discussion of the impact effects of HIV would be complete without some discussion of the likely consequences for the agricultural sector and those whose livelihood is dependent on it. As noted above some 90 per cent of the Ugandan population is rural; agriculture accounts for about two-thirds of GDP, and for virtually all exports. Most output is produced on smallholdings. and women are responsible for some 80 per cent of total food supply and provide most of the labour inputs. This dependence on women's labour for both food and non-food production, under conditions where higher HIV infection rates for women are observed, is an indicator of the vulnerability of this sector. Women not only account for much of the direct inputs into production but a good deal of indirect ones as well [in marketing, processing, water supply, firewood etc.]. To these functions are added those domestic responsibilities of the household undertaken by women, which are burdensome enough, and on top of these HIV infection and AIDS impose yet further demands.

Since women are disproportionately infected with HIV, and given the dependence of the rural and household economies on their labour, there are inevitably going to be significant and serious impacts. These will not be confined to productive effects, but also extend to those functions which are integral to the survival of households. Under these conditions it is not enough to know that some farming systems are vulnerable to the losses of labour due to higher morbidity, higher mortality, and the diversion of women from productive roles to caring, but also to be able to identify those households which are most vulnerable. There is evidence that some households are already suffering extremes of destitution, e.g., in Rakai, under conditions of high seroprevalence. Other regions of the country, such as Apac and Lira Districts, where poverty is persistent and widespread, will become even more vulnerable if their HIV infection rates approach those of Rakai and Masaka. In part the policy problem is to avoid this outcome through effective programmes of HIV prevention. Whether or not HIV transmission is reduced it is crucial that vulnerable households be identified, their needs be established, and structures be created for delivering the goods and services they will require for survival. This is true both for the urban and rural populations; but in neither case will it be easy to identify the poor and most vulnerable households.

There is rather more information available about farm systems which are vulnerable to labour loss, together with data on particular crops where production is threatened. Tea, which is a minor crop, is especially vulnerable given its need for female labour inputs which are continuously applied. Coffee, which is the main export, seems also to be vulnerable to labour loss. Matooke [plantain], which is the main staple food for most of the population, seems already to be effected by falling labour supplies. Some Districts are especially vulnerable at the present, particularly those with high HIV infection rates, such as areas to the west and north of Kampala [together with Rakai and Masaka]. But all such estimates are based on fairly superficial economic data and analysis, and it would be unwise in these circumstances to base policies on these.

What is not in doubt is that HIV poses a major threat to the maintenance of food and non-food output, so as to threaten much of the rural population. These impacts will extend well beyond the rural sector, given the interactions between the rural and urban economies [in terms of labour flows, food supplies, remittances etc.,], and even into international economic relationships [given the dependence on a narrow range of export crops for the foreign exchange needs of Uganda]. This is an area of so over-riding importance as to be a priority for policy; but policies need to have a firm foundation of factual data on production conditions. It is not presently the case that such information exists; efforts need to be directed now to remedying this deficiency.

One sector is already bearing the brunt of the HIV epidemic; unfortunately for Ugandans the health care system is unable to cope with even the present level of demands. This is unsurprising given the deterioration of the system in the 1980s. Years of neglect and underfunding had by the middle of the decade turned what was once a comprehensive and effective provider of services—with integrated hospital and primary health care—into one of crumbling buildings, weak management, inadequate [if any] supplies of drugs, and a professional and technical staff which in large numbers had deserted both the system and the country. In spite of the attempts made in recent years the health system remains underfunded, understaffed and underprovided, such that rehabilitation will take many years to achieve. Not only is the health care system faced by growing demands from persons with HIV related illnesses, but it is also having to deal with a set of intensified health care needs caused by the collapse of many other programmes over recent decades [such as malarial and TB, where control programmes more or less ceased]. Many hospitals do not have enough beds, drugs and protective equipment to take care of their ever increasing numbers of patients. For example, Lira District Hospital has only 4 doctors to cater for a population of 500,000.

It is natural that HIV infected individuals and their families turn to the acute care system for help, and seek medical attention and drugs which they hope will alleviate their problems. But in doing so they add to the problems of meeting health needs generally in Uganda and in part divert resources away from treatable and curable medical conditions. This is evident from data on hospital admissions, where as much as two thirds of beds are occupied by AIDS patients and/or those admitted with illnesses such as Tuberculosis (TB) [a common opportunistic HIV infection]. This state of affairs is as much true of Government hospitals as it is of the private sector. A state exists where the care of patients with HIV related illnesses, particularly in hospitals, is crowding out other patients in ways which cannot be considered optimal from the national point of view. That this should have occurred is reflective of many factors; a health care system which at all levels already cannot cope with demands and which has been faced over a very short period of years with large scale growth in HiV and AIDS related pressures. Such processes have faced the MOH with problems it does not have the capacities to meet - neither in medical nor non-medical resources. In the event much of the burden of health care has shifted to the private sector, which is itself now overburdened, or is simply not being met at all by the modern health care sector. There is much evidence that many HIV infected persons are in receipt of little or no care from the formal system, and have turned in many cases [and in large numbers] to traditional healers. Although Uganda has been at the forefront of the national response to HIV and AIDS in Africa, it is disturbing to note that there is no STD control programme in place. This is particularly worrisome given the role of STDs as a co-factor in the spread of HIV [noted above]. What is needed is the development of a comprehensive STD programme as a matter of great urgency, but this will require putting in place a complex set of human and non-human resources to be effective.

The present position in terms of health care provision has little to commend it. The system cannot cope with present demands and is therefore double unable to deal with the projected numbers of HIV infected persons. There is no alternative to organisational reforms and the development of innovative ways of meeting the real and genuine needs of the population. To a degree these reforms have already been implemented, in some parts of the private system, where part hospital-based and part home-based systems are already operating. What is needed is an extension of what are currently small scale and pilot community based schemes to a national programme. One which is sensitive to the relative costs of alternative health provision and linking both prevention and care in the community. Here lies the challenge; but it is one which has to be faced sooner or later.

II. SETTING PRIORITIES

A. CAPACITY DEVELOPMENT: GENERAL CONSIDERATIONS

UNDP activities have as their target the building of national capacity, and at first sight this seems to be such an unambiguous concept as to need no further examination. It is as if it is self evident that this is desirable as an objective. But this presumption leaves open many important issues. At the minimum it can be assumed that donor activities aim to strengthen national capacity in ways which permit a country to achieve a preferred [better] level of development. Trying to achieve this objective seems reasonable enough as a guide to the selection of those activities which are desirable and worth supporting, and as an indicator of what ought not to be supported. But there are many problems in practice with this simplistic approach to capacity development.

1. Resources are limited so choices have to be made as to what activities are more or less important. Who defines priorities, and by what criteria are some activities given preference over others? It is unlikely that the exercise of preferences by politicians and policy makers will coincide with the selection of capacity building activities which maximise development. Indeed, and fundamental to conflict between preferences and the selection of activities, will be dispute as to the relationships between capacity building and development in general, and between particular initiatives and the achievement of selected development targets.
2. We have defined in an unambiguous way the recipient of the additional resources as "the country", and in the case of UNDP this is assumed as identical with the government of the day. UNDP deals mainly with governments, and issues of representativeness [how government came to power; does it observe civil and political rights, does it have any or much commitment to developmental objectives, and so on, may not be considered relevant]. What indeed ought to be the attitude of a development agency such as UNDP in its dealings with a government which is terrorising a segment of its population? Destroying national capacity in the process, as well as infringing basic human rights. Or to take the example of Uganda, what is the judgment to be of a government which allocates some 40 per cent of its budget to military expenditure, under conditions where real expenditures on health and education together in 1989 were only a fifth of fiscal allocations in 1970? On a per capita basis health expenditures were only 16 per cent real in 1989 compared with 1970; for education the decline was even worse to 13 per cent. Are such data to be taken as indicators of government preferences; and can it really be the case that internal and external security needs always override social and developmental priorities? Certainly such revealed allocations of budgetary resources against social sector expenditures in Uganda both contribute to the economic and social problems the country faces, and simultaneously constrain attempts through capacity building to ameliorate these.

3. What indeed is meant by "preferred level of development"? Does this mean a higher level of GNP? Is it a matter of interest how this higher level of GNP is achieved [by paying low wages to labour and banning labour organisations]? or through policies which lead to environmental degradation, both short term and long term [threatening the sustainability of the process]? Are the benefits of economic growth fairly distributed or do these accrue to an elite which abrogates the benefits of GNP growth for uses which have low social value? Or is there an acceptable set of development indicators which are the actual and real focii of government activities, with which capacity development can be aligned?
4. Is the discussion couched in terms of the short term, or is it implicit in the process of capacity building that policies are always about sustainability'? But this simply raises a further set of very complex questions. These run like this. Development is a process which takes place over time, and can be judged as beneficial where a set of social indicators can be shown to have shown improvement. There may be problems in getting agreement on what these indicators are, and there will certainly be important issues which relate to the conditions surrounding the achievement or non-achievement of the selected indicators. Also problematic is how to deal with the weighting problem. i.e., achievement of some indicators and non-achievement of others. But it could, of course, be precisely those countries [governments] who are generally non-achievers who are most in need of capacity building activities. It may be the lack of capacities, whatever this means, which prevents development as defined and measured by social indicators.
5. The object of donor technical assistance is to support and strengthen conditions in which a country can develop in a socially acceptable way, so that over time the need for transfers of resources from outside are diminished [not necessarily to zero]. in this case the meaning of sustainability, as far as capacity development goes, is as follows. Resources are made available to a country to meet those needs which are essential for development, but in a manner which over time leads to domestic changes which make the transfers no longer necessary. Transfers which are capacity building do not generate a continuing dependence on external support. This has to be one of the most important criteria to apply to TA. Only if this condition is met can capacity building unambiguously be thought of as desirable.
6. At the core of the problem is not just what is meant by

development and how it is measured, but issues of how best to bring development about. There are only too many theories, too many ideologies, too many special cases - and too many interest groups, both in developing countries, in developed countries and in international organisations [including UNDP]. At any one time there may be a dominant set of beliefs even occasionally some evidence to support these, which sets the agenda for TA and other assistance, such as those policies currently peddled by the World Bank and the IMF. These beliefs will often define what TA is actually on offer, who is delivering it and to whom, and under what conditions. Over time beliefs will be modified, relative positions of governments and organisations change, and with it the concepts and practices of capacity building [note that this is never a single valued construct but is itself one which in practice takes many forms].

B. CAPACITY DEVELOPMENT UNDER CONDITIONS OF HIGH SEROPREVALENCE

Figure 18.1 sets out in a very simplified form a structure for thinking about capacity building in Uganda — a country facing an epidemic with all its consequences [as identified in I.C above]. There are disadvantages in setting out the problem and the choices as in Figure 18.1, not least in that doing so suggests that the relationships are linear and uni-directional. They clearly are not, as will be seen later. Also implicit in this representation is the assumption that we possess sufficient understanding of what is an immensely complex set of inter-actions as to be able to delineate these into separable categories. This is acceptable, perhaps, as a device for assisting exposition of the problems and the choices, but cannot in any way be thought of as descriptive of actuality. What the Figure does is to place the policy problem within a framework which is standard for economics, but this does not prove its suitability for analysing the problem at hand. Time will tell if this way of presenting choices is useful and adds to our understanding.

The issue is that described in II.A, i.e., how to establish a set of activities that will assist Uganda in developing those capacities which will help it meet the severe socio-economic problems raised for the country by the HIV epidemic. Not in any detail, of course, but in very broad brush terms, and building on the description of the present and future position in Uganda as outlined in Section I.

Final Targets

It is perhaps easiest to start with the Final Targets, the

achievement of which is the purpose of development policy. Those which are identified in Figure 18.1 are not intended to be comprehensive, but they are the important ones. These include those targets which are most threatened by the HIV epidemic [both now and in the future]. In the ordinary course of events it would have been expected that various mortality indicators would improve, and in doing so raise life expectancy. The HIV epidemic makes it unlikely that this will occur, and that instead infant and maternal mortality, and adult mortality, will be raised, and life expectancy probably fall. Similarly with poverty, where the probability is for an increase in destitution [with accompanying worsening in other associated indicators of the standard of living, such as housing and nutrition]. The overall rate of economic growth would be lower than otherwise, with significant losses of potential output, and the external position of the economy be weaker—all because of unfavourable impacts on the level and rate of change of labour productivity, and lower rates of capital formation [both in physical capital and in human investment].

All of this was established in Section 1, and in some senses from the viewpoint of meeting the development challenge of HIV and AIDS we are not so much interested in Final Targets as such, but in the complex ways in which these are made unattainable by the epidemic. Rather the focii of policy interventions are what are called in Figure 18.1 Intermediate Targets.

Intermediate Targets

Three categories have been identified as being of over-riding proximate importance; these are the Rate of HIV Transmission, the Care of Infected Persons, and the Mitigation of Adverse Social and Economic Impacts. These are probably not all of equal social weight, and it would certainly be possible to argue that reducing the rate of HIV transmission ought to have priority in the allocation of resources [and in capacity building activities]. It would not be difficult to make this case, given the scenarios outlined in Section I.B. Far and away the greatest benefit in economic and social terms will come from those activities which reduce HIV prevalence, through the minimisation of future social and economic costs. It could also be argued that some of the effects, particularly those on macro-economic performance, will occur later and are thus perhaps less urgent. This is partly true, partly untrue, since some of the adverse economic responses are already being experienced in Uganda.

What is undoubtedly the case is that these Intermediate Targets are interconnected; thus, a mitigation of the economic losses caused by the epidemic will entail a higher level of resources for

Figure. 18.1

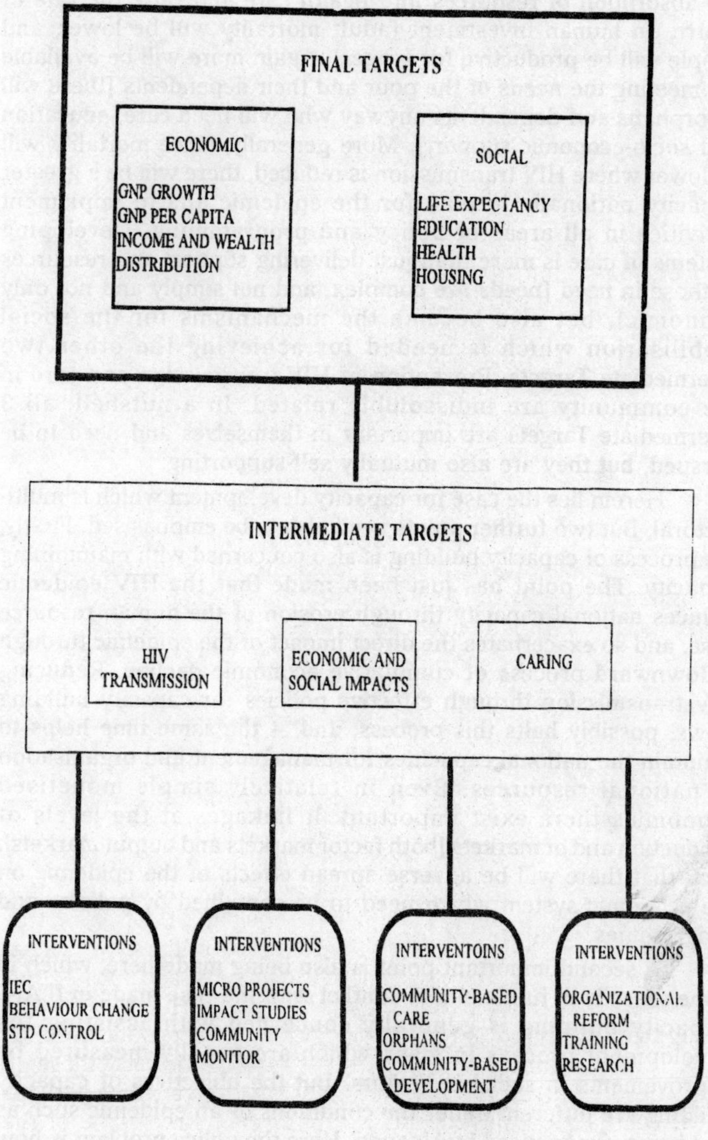
FINAL TARGETS
ECONOMIC
GNP GROWTH
GNP PER CAPITA
INCOME AND WEALTH
DISTRIBUTION
SOCIAL
LIFE EXPECTANCY
EDUCATION
HEALTH
HOUSING
INTERMEDIATE TARGETS
HIV
TRANSMISSION
ECONOMIC AND
SOCIAL IMPACTS
CARING
INTERVENTIONS
IEC
BEHAVIOUR CHANGE
STD CONTROL
INTERVENTIONS
MICRO PROJECTS
IMPACT STUDIES
COMMUNITY
MONITOR
INTERVENTOINS
COMMUNITY-BASED
CARE
ORPHANS
COMMUNITY-BASED
DEVELOPMENT
INTERVENTIONS
ORGANIZATIONAL
REFORM
TRAINING
RESEARCH

meeting the care needs of the infected and affected populations. Similarly, a reduction in the rate of transmission of HIV will reduce the absorption of resources into health care and raise the rate of return on human investment [adult mortality will be lower, and people will be productive for longer]. Again more will be available for meeting the needs of the poor and their dependents [there will be orphans and dependents anyway who will need care, education and socio-economic support]. More generally, since mortality will be lower where HIV transmission is reduced, there will be a greater capacity nationally to plan for the epidemic and to implement activities in all areas of policy and programming. Developing systems of care is more than just delivering support and resources to those in need [needs are complex, and not simply and not only economic], but also become the mechanisms for the social mobilisation which is needed for achieving the other two Intermediate Targets. Prevention of HIV transmission and care in the community are indissolubly related. In a nutshell; all 3 Intermediate Targets are important in themselves and need to be pursued, but they are also mutually self-supporting.

Herein lies the case for capacity development which is multi-sectoral. But two further points need also to be emphasised. Firstly, the process of capacity building is also concerned with maintaining capacity. The point has just been made that the HIV epidemic reduces national capacity through erosion of the human resource base, and so exacerbates the direct impact of the epidemic through a downward process of cumulative economic decline. Reducing HIV transmission through effective policies for capacity building slows, possibly halts this process, and at the same time helps to maintain the national capacities for management and organisation of national resources. Even in relatively simple monetised economies there exist important. It linkages at the levels of production and of markets [both factor markets and output markets], such that there will be adverse spread effects of the epidemic on the economic system which need to be contained by policies and programmes.

A second important point is also being made here, which in some sense is in fundamental conflict with the case made in II.A.4. Capacity building is generally concerned with assisting the development process in ways which are usually measured by improvements in social indicators. But the objectives of capacity building are different under the conditions of an epidemic such as that being experienced by Uganda. Here the policy problem is how to prevent, or limit, a deterioration in the level of development, with capacity building objectives seen in an entirely different light. Success may be gauged not by the increment of improvement in social indicators, but by the degree to which deterioration in these has been minimised. In these circumstances the whole process of project design and evaluation needs to be re-assessed. Thus, for example,to see income generation projects as a means of preventing declines in living standards under the impact of immiseration, rather than the conventional approach where projects are selected in terms of their ability to raise factor productivity and incomes.

Interventions

These are multi-dimensional activities which are capacity building. These could be about maintaining national capacity, or its enhancement. Thus a programme of workshops for different professional groups employed both by government and NGOs which aimed to improve knowledge of the HIV transmission process, and/or its social and economic impacts, would generate new insights and improve economic and social performance. These activities could be aimed at raising the efficiency of existing interventions, through for example training in management and organisation, where the aim is to improve the use of resources. Solutions in this area could themselves be innovatory, and at the same time add to domestic capacity. Thus existing NGOs, which are too small to provide internally all the skills and services they need, such as financial control and project evaluation skills, could look to other more specialised institutions. The latter might be in the public or private sectors, and the process of capacity building be about the appropriate development of service institutions where these are currently missing or ineffective. The possibilities for organisational innovation are legion; that these will be important is also self evident. Again we are back with issues of efficient resource allocation, and the need to raise factor productivity—in these cases by removing inefficiency [the failure to maximise use of resources caused by management and other internal practices which are sub-optimal] .

In evaluating national needs for capacity building, it is important not to misread signals which apparently support further allocations of resources to a particular activity. This may be best understood by looking at the example of the Kampala AIDS Information Centre. This was established to provide HIV testing and counselling services. It is about to extend its activities to other parts of the country, in response presumably lo felt needs. Most of its costs are met by USAID, and there is eftectively no cost recovery. An HIV test costs currently some $12 US, at a time when per capita health expenditures in Uganda are presently a mere $3 annually. Under what circumstances can this allocation of resources be defended? A case could perhaps be made, along the following lines. An HIV test and its associated counselling, whether the result is negative or positive, leads to such changes in behaviour as to prevent further infection [of say "n" persons]. If this is so then perhaps a case can be mafe for subsidising HIV tests at the current cost. But the case needs to be substantiated by evidence and cannot be assumed. In this example the existence of unmet demands [indeed any demand] does not prove that creating additional capacity, in the form of testing centres and in training more counsellors. is necessarily justified. Of course other arguments in favour of HIV testing centres can be made which do not depend for their validity on demonstrating any effects on sexual behaviour.

This example raises two important principles. Are resources currently being efficiently used, and does the existence of unmet demand act as an efficient signal for further resource inputs? Both of these need to be considered in decisions on future capacity building activities.

No case can be made "a priori" for or against private of public sector interventions, and in practice there are activities where in particular circumstances either or both are best able to perform. Certainly the effectiveness of certain interventions is constrained by the weakness of public provision, irrespective of whether the intervention is by an NGO or by government. A telling example of this has been the enormous decline in the quality and quantity of public educational provision in Uganda; at the present only about one-third of the relevant age group completes primary education, and very few children proceed to later stages of education. Something like one half of the total Ugandan population is functionally illiterate. This decline in educational achievement over recent decades severely constrains what can be done through policy interventions in the case of all three Intermediate Targets. Such a state of affairs not only constrains what activities can be undertaken but also requires that these factors be taken into account in their design and implementation. Thus any Micro Projects to combat AIDS have to assume as a basic fact that the target population will not be able to meet sophisticated project appraisal and evaluation requirements, and will require intensive assistance by way of training in management skills etc. Similarly with activities for reducing HIV transmission where reaching the population with relevant messages, and engaging them actively in sustained behaviour change, will entail quite different strategies [and be much more complex in design and in processes of implementation].

The final point relating to capacity building, which will repay emphasis, is that most of the population is rural, so that the balance of resource allocation in respect of all 3 Intermediate Targets needs to be focused on this group. All of the forces operating in Uganda will bias programmes against rural populations, for reasons which do not need to be explored here. The potential for disaster, both economic and social if this urban bias is not addressed, is potentially enormous. Similarly, with the gender dimensions of HIV; as we have seen in Section I.B there is an over-riding need to address all issues from a gender perspective. It is perhaps enough to reiterate that the single largest input into agriculture is women's labour, that this is the scarcest factor of production, whose availability for all uses in the society will become increasingly problematic. How to respond to the needs of women must be a major element in any choices relating to capacity building, and to resource allocation generally.

It can be concluded that the overall objectives of capacity development in Uganda, under conditions of high seroprevalence, are.

1. To improve the functioning of existing institutions through raising their efficiency in using resources.
2. To generate new insights and develop new skills in understanding and responding to the challenges posed by the epidemic.
3. To replicate those approaches and institutional structures which are successfully meeting the existing challenges to other institutions and areas of the country.
4. To support innovatory responses to HIV in all of its manifestations, and to strengthen organisational developments, in both the public and private sectors.

Knowledge Base

This is fundamental to any policies of capacity development for any purposes. All countries are resource constrained, and Uganda more so than most. Over recent decades there has been immense deterioration in the economic and social infrastructure, so that effective responses to the HIV epidemic are made doubly difficult. Even more important then in these circumstances to ensure that what is done is well done. Implicit in the approach outlined above is the assumption of known links between Interventions and Intermediate and Final Targets. In part the problem is that these linkages are only imperfectly understood. This may be because a knowledge base has yet to be established, or that where this exists it is not being effectively used.

In part, knowledge and understanding are independent of the activities being followed, and in part these are the outcome of activities. One example will suffice. The focus of much effort presently in Uganda are IEC activities to change sexual behaviour, since this is seen by Government and others as the only effective way to slow transmission of HIV. It would seem obvious in these circumstances to relate IEC programmes to what is already known about sexuality within the cultural context of Uganda. It is in fact the case that Uganda for many reasons has available a good deal of research on these matters, which ought to have informed policies for IEC. But there is little evidence that in fact these sources have been used in the formulation of policies, and in the development of interventions. Much of the IEC activity seems to have been unproductive, in the sense that sexual behaviour has not been changed in appropriate ways. There is some evidence of both poor evaluation and ineffective monitoring of IEC programmes, which has in turn led to weakness in learning the lessons of what works, and what does not.

Capacity building has to be firmly based on what is known about economic, social and cultural structures, if it is to be effective. Where this knowledge of conditions, and structural and behavioural relationships is inadequate for effective policy making then it will need to be addressed. In part capacity strengthening is about developing insights—without understanding there can be no effective policies. Such insights cannot be assumed to be present, particularly as in the case of an epidemic such as HIV, where new analytical frameworks have to be developed and tested against experience. In the case ot Uganda the early learning process is over; and now is the time to ensure the full and rapid integration of experience in policies for capacity development.

III. UNDP PROGRAMME INTERVENTIONS

OPERATIONAL PRINCIPLES

The general principles which should guide UNDP have been established in Section II on Capacity Development. These principles, in conjunction with the analysis of the HIV epidemic and its probable socio-economic impacts as detailed in Section I, set a framework for the general allocation of UNDP resources. But important as these principles are for efficient allocation of resources they are insufficient for the determination of priorities and spending decisions. The definition of operational activities requires the development of additional principles, and the application of these in taking forward a programme for UNDP assistance to Uganda.

The following are important :

* The knowledge base for interventions in many areas is imperfect and inadequate, such that a crucial initial activity will be to establish such a base. It is an important role of the Uganda AIDS Commission to define research priorities, and to direct resources into consultancies, studies, task forces etc. The output of such activities must

then inform policy formulation and the development of specific interventions.

* Policy making is a continuing process. Priorities will change because governments come and go; because the internal and external environments change; and because of learning effects, i.e., the internalisation of experience and the embodiment of this in policy.
* It follows from the foregoing that the establishment of firm allocations of UNDP resources for the period 1992-96 is neither desirable nor optimal. What are feasible objectives at this point in time are broad indications of priority areas, and identification of initial activities. In effect, what is proposed is a system of contingent allocations, where the specific activities should reflect changing needs and improved understanding [what works, what does not work]. It is important to note that a programme for UNDP requires a framework which is more or less determined; it is the activities whose relative balance should be adjusted during the life of the HIV Prograrnme, through a process of consultations, taking into account learning effects, changing needs, and so on.
* UNDP resources are limited so it is vital that these be used to maximum effect. This means, in consultation with the UAC, the identification of the points in the economic, social and political systems where activities can exert their greatest leverage; can induce changes in behaviour and attitudes; shift allocations of resources to areas of greatest need, and support appropriate institutional development. In a word, the activities of UNDP need to be catalytic. Programmes must be concentrated on the essential problems posed for Uganda by the HIV epidemic. In part, this requires a new focus—to see problems and their solutions in different ways—together with an intensification of efforts in respect of all three Intermediate Targets. Critical to achieving a new vision is a more general recognition of the developmental relationships of HIV, and the strengthening of activities for planning for, and meeting, the expected social and economic impacts.

PRIORITISATION OF PROGRAMME INTERVENTIONS

A. PREVENTION OF HIV TRANSMISSION

Certain features stand out clearly in the present efforts to reduce HIV transmission, and there are important matters here which UNDP needs to address. Much has been done to increase awareness in Uganda, and many activities are underway and planned in this area by government, NGOs, UN agencies, bilateral donors, and so on. Three observations merit separate attention.

* The presumption that awareness is generally high is almost certainly unfounded, and the admittedly partial evidence of the Mission field visit to Lira and Apac Districts suggests that there are problems in this area still to be addressed. Regions which currently have relatively low infection rates, and which for other reasons are difficult to access, are in need of communication activities to develop awareness at all levels about HIV transmission and its prevention, and to raise understanding of the deadly nature of AIDS. It is certainly appropriate for UNDP to assist others, such as UNICEF, in the identification of needs in this area, and to collaborate in the development of suitable forms of programme delivery, including strengthening institutional structures, training, etc.
* There is little evidence for Uganda that sexual behaviour has changed in the ways appropriate for a reduction in transmission of HIV. Increasing awareness has not been sufficient to induce sustained behaviour change, so how to bring this about remains the core of the problem for reducing the rate of transmission. There is work proceeding currently in this area, including a Report which is due from AIDSCOM, and there is the development of new approaches nresently underway at Kitovo Hospital. Others, such as UNICEF and DANIDA are active in this field. It is clearly appropriate for UNDP to collaborate with others in identifying why activities for behaviour change have had such little success; to support programme development, probably on a pilot scale, and to then establish joint programmes for gaining and other activities.
* Doing the foregoing would certainly be worthwhile but in crucial respects would be inadequate to meet the challenge. A point which is emphasised in Section I is the absolute need to establish a gender sensitive approach to this issue. Questions were posed above of why women are infected with HIV at a younger age than men, and why apparently there is a higher rate of female infection.

At least three directions for UNDP activities, of great importance, follow from there observations on the roles of gender in relation to the epidemic.

(a) What are the social, cultural and economic conditions which explain the gender biases in HIV prevalence? This requires detailed studies, either separately by UNDP or in conjunction with other agencies with interests in this area. It is obvious that any approach to this question would need to address not simply behaviour change but also, and crucially, the formation of behaviour.

(b) How can women protect themselves from infection? The behaviour change activities undertaken in Uganda have generally not addressed this question, but have concentrated on the ways in which men through their actions can reduce their infection rates. Thus activities have concentrated on matters such as reduction in the numbers of sexual partners, and use of condoms. Whereas most women in Africa have one and only one partner, and have little or no control over their male partner's sexual activities, and so are not able to demand changes in behaviour and insist on the use of condoms. Here there is a major role for UNDP, and one which must have high priority. The issue has received little or no attention from the programmes designed and delivered by WHO, and has been similarly neglected by the Uganda ACP. The development of understanding of the ways in which women can protect themselves from infection; the embodiment of such understanding in programmes for behaviour change, together with the establishment of service delivery activities which make it possible for women to protect themselves from infection. All are absolutely crucial for success in reducing the rate of HIV infection in Uganda.

(c) Unless (a) and (b) are successfully addressed as matters of extreme urgency, then it is difficult to see how Uganda will be able to cope with the immense problems caused by the epidemic. Women, as we have seen in Section-I, are central to almost everything—the care of the sick generally, not just those persons with HIV related illnesses; the maintenance of food and non-food production; the care and support of children and elderly dependents, and so on. It cannot be said that the crucial role of women in the economic and social life of Uganda, and the degree to which they and their contributions are threatened by HIV, have been taken on board.

UNDP has a ensure that in its programme for Uganda, through consultations with the UAC and other partners, that these failures of programme design and delivery are rectified. It follows that not only must the gender biases in transmission be addressed, through changes in analysis, policies and programmes; but that efforts be directed into the assessment of the problems of high female morbidity and mortality for the economic and social system. Both aspects of the issue are important and critical areas for UNDP programme support.

There are four other areas where UNDP could have a role in relation to transmission of HIV, possibly of secondary importance. These are:

(d) In the development of a programme for STDs which, as noted above, have been identified as a major co-factor in the transmission of HIV. Several agencies, including WHO, USAID and possibly the World Bank, are interested in establishing a programme for STDs. There is effectively no programme at present in Uganda. and given the state of general health services in the country it will be a formidable task to set up an effective system for the diagnosis and treatment of STDs. UNDP certainly has an interest in seeing such a programme established, although it would take it away from its developmental concerns, and it would seem preferable to leave the analysis of need and programme development to others. Except for a particular concern which UNDP has and which is not currently reflected in the approach of other agencies to this matter. This relates to the concerns expressed above, i.e., the high level of HIV infection amongst women and the need to reduce it. There is a good deal of evidence that STDs [together with other physiological and culturally determined factors] are important in explaining high infection rates in women. Since most women are never subjected to internal examination by medical practitioners STDs and other infections remain untreated as a consequence, and this raises the risk of transmission of HIV. It is, unfortunately, only too likely that a programme for STDs, if established in Uganda, will neglect the critical needs of women. So UNDP has an interest in being associated with the development of a programme for STDs on these grounds alone, but in order also to enable Uganda to better deal with the economic and social impacts of the epidemic.

(e) There is one important sub-group in the population who are perhaps peripheral to the main concerns of UNDP. This is the military, who may have high levels of seroprevalence and who may play a significant role in transmission. This is an area where other agencies [USAID] are active, and there may be little need for UNDP to become involved. This is, nevertheless, one area where UNDP may want to be involved in the process of training [counsellors particularly], and perhaps in the development of care. The military do have arrangements for those who are infected and who at some stage are retired from the service, but there is a need to look at how individuals and their families cope. There is a complex set of issues here; of IEC activities, STD programme development. HIV testing and ethics relating to it, condom supplies, counselling, care and medical needs. The military are important because of their relationship to the rest of the population; they are a mobile and sexually active group of young men who wield a great deal of power, and as such are in a position to do much harm to the ACP of Uganda. It needs hardly to be added that they are also deserving in their own right of a comprehensive programme for HIV prevention and care.

(f) There are some 150.000 refugees in Uganda who are the responsibility of UNHCR. Some are recent arrivals and others have been long settled in Uganda. They are a particularly vulnerable group for all sorts of reasons, and there is the real possibility that their needs in respect of HIV prevention, care and income support, will not receive the attention these deserve. Many factors are likely to combine to make refugees, and particularly women and young adults, very vulnerable to HIV infection. There seems to be little evidence that their multiple needs are being addressed by UNHCR, who do not have the capacity for dealing with these matters. This is an issue requiring inter-agency discussions and consultations with the UAC.

(g) There is a great deal of IFC activity already, and WHO has an expert in the country and is considering the secondment of another person in this field to the UAC. Others are also active in the area, and UNICEF has announced that this is a priority interest. Other UN agencies, such as UNFPA have activities in progress and planned. Also active in the area are NGOs such as The AIDS Support Organization [TASO], The Uganda Red Cross, Experiment in International Learning [EIL], and so on. There is no lack of activity, but as we have seen above there can be doubts as to its effectiveness. There are general problems here, and they are not only those which are raised above. These include constraints on the local development and production of materials for IEC purposes, and for use in training and counselling. This is raised as a matter of considerable importance at this point in the Report, rather than in the section below which deals with organisational matters. This is certainly an area where UNDP has an interest in the local development of capacity, both of technical skills in developing materials and in production, but only after a capacity needs assessment. A related matter, but one which the mission did not look at, is the role of the Media in IEC. This is certainly deserving of separate study, since capacity constraints in this area are undoubtedly important.

There remain two other areas where UNDP might have some involvement, but which are judged to be of low priority. These are:

(h) It is the case that risks of infection with HIV through contaminated blood and blood products are very high. It is also true that in Uganda only a small percentage of transmission is due to this factor and, as noted above, about 90 per cent is heterosexual in origin. At the present most blood is screened for HIV etc., and the blood supply is considered more or lass secure. Most of the costs of this programme are met by the European Community [ECI] and they are also meeting the costs incurred through the setting up of extra blood screening centres. While the EC has no firm plans for continuing support it is the case that for the moment at least the system is being financed, and is apparently working well. There is some evidence that blood is not reaching hospitals in rural districts, but this distributive problem needs to be addressed by others. The cost of a unit of blood is very high—a unit cost of 42$. This needs to be compared with per capita health costs for Uganda of about 3$, and recent estimates of the World Bank (WB) that the average cost for drugs etc., per AIDS case are approximately 14$. There would appear to be important issues here of the efficiency of resource allocation. One conclusion is that UNDP should not get involved in blood screening activities. With one caveat: the Nakasero Blood Bank hopes to establish a panel of donors [Clubs], which ought to reduce the cost per unit, and act as a vehicle for IEC. This is an interesting proposal and is one which UNDP might well assist. The start-up funding ought to be quite small, and there is the possibility of piggy-backing this activity on more general IEC and behaviour change interventions.

[i] Reference is made above to the AIDS Information Centre (AIC), and doubts were expressed about the scale of resources being absorbed into this activity. It is suggested that UNDP should not support the AIC unless it can be shown that various conditions are being met with respect to behaviour change and other benefits from testing. Carrying out such a Study would be a complex matter, but ought to be a prior requirement for any UNDP involvement. If it can be demonstrated that AIC activities do have significant and worthwhile effects on behaviour change or other important benefits then a case might exist for UNDP support. Possibly UNDP could help with limited finance for any study which is undertaken, although this could perhaps be left to USAID not AIDSCOM.

B. ECONOMIC AND SOCIAL IMPACT

The earlier Section I.C on Impact Projections more or less sets out the agenda for activities, but is no more than a brief summary of possible outcomes. It should also be noted that the WB Study [1991] has value mainly as a general statement of the issues, and does not in any way take the analysis of impacts sufficiently forward. It follows that detailed studies of the economic and social impact of the HIV epidemic are a pre-requisite for policy interventions by UNDP and others. This requirement does not preclude all activities for ameliorating the current impacts on the economic and social system, such as for example the Micro Projects Programme to Combat AIDS, but it does imply that at this stage much of UNDP activity will be preparatory rather than substantive. A constraint, which has to be removed, relates to the national capacity to develop the required insights, and to be able to undertake studies of the multiple ways in which the social and economic system is affected by HIV and AIDS. Developing these capacities and professional skills is addressed below in the Section on Strengthening Organizational Structures. Matters relating to the Health Sector are partly dealt with here but also in Section III. C. This may be confusing, but it seems, on balance, preferably to organise interventions on a functional basis.

1. Micro Projects

The Micro Projects Programme to Combat AIDS [UGAI91/005] is a pilot project which aims to reduce the adverse effects of HIV infection through the provision of financial resources and technical assistance. The target groups are those households and communities considered to be most vulnerable to the adverse impacts of HIV, and the Project involves NGOs and CBOs actively in the identification of appropriate and supportable activities, as well as in their management and evaluation. This is a project which is well deserving of support as an innovatory attempt to meet the needs of vulnerable groups through income generating and other activities. There are various ways of strengthening the Projects, including the following. Firstly it is absolutely crucial that the participation of women be a requirement for both the National Steering Committee and the District Selection Committees. This should be achieved through a minimum percentage of the membership, say not less than one-third of the total. Secondly, the performance of this Project will depend on the quality of the inputs from NGOs, CBOs etc., [the sponsoring organizations], and this is recognised through the provision for some technical assistance to these groups. This does not look as if it will be enough, and provision needs to be made for much more than is proposed. Furthermore, the planned technical assistance is too narrowly focused, and the targeted beneficiaries who are expected to identify projects, formulate and effectively manage these, are going to need much more assistance than is provided for in the Prodoc. It is well known from other income generation projects that weaknesses at the level of operation and control are a major cause of failure. Finally, there are no convincing grounds for the exclusion of Rakai and Masaka from the Project, and given that they are currently facing severe problems caused by the epidemic it is suggested that they be included.

2. Sector Studies

It is urgent that Sector Studies be commissioned on the impact effects of HIV. At present what is available are studies which largely depend on secondary information and the application of intuitive reasoning. This is no substitute for empirical research which directly addresses the important questions raised by the epidemic. There are a number of key sectors where the impact will be severe, which are critical for the performance of the economic system, and including sectors which are important for reducing HIV transmission and for providing care for those affected.

The Sectors identified are :

(a) Agriculture

This supplies most of the food and almost all the exports of Uganda; most of the population is dependent directly or indirectly on this Sector. So far the impact studies which have been done, such as Barnett and Blaikie [1990] and the World Bank [1991], provide little more than a sketch of the probable responses and distribution of effects on Agriculture. There is an immediate need for detailed analysis of the ways in which production will be affected by changing labour supply availabilities, including the effects on factor utilisation, production technologies, crop diversification, food availability, factor and output prices, and so on. In part this means collecting and analysing much new data, District by District. Plus observing the ways in which farm systems are responding already in areas with high HIV prevalence such as Rakai and Masaka. These data are crucial for the formulation of policies for meeting the needs of the agricultural sector—both in terms of production quantities; changing patterns of production [with additional needs for some inputs, such as fertilisers and pesticides]; the impacts on land use [with the possibility that land may be uncultivated and untended causing land degradation]; and the impacts on farm populations. The generation of estimates of the most vulnerable systems of production and most vulnerable households are crucial for effective policies for planning for the impact of the epidemic across a wide spectrum of concerns. The latter include issues of nutrition, food security [and food storagel, the changing pattern of labour use [and the impact of this on households dependent on rural labour markets], changing patterns of land ownership [as assets are liquidated to meet health costs in affected families, and land is redistributed at deaths. What are clearly needed are integrated studies which identify the inter-relationships, and establish the main areas where policy interventions are needed. But time is important, and it will be necessary to use Rapid Appraisal Techniques wherever possible so as to get the information and recommendations to policy makers without delay. The focii for UNDP interventions would be Ministry of Economic Planning and Development (MEPD) and Ministry of Agriculture.

(b) Health

We have seen above in Section I.C on Impact that this sector is already facing intense demands, such that many patients with HIV related illnesses are largely untreated by the formal health care sector. It seems also true that HIV-related illnesses are crowding out other categories of treatment, with results which cannot be considered optimal. This requires a Health Sector Study which looks at the strategic options, and assesses both the needs of HIV infected persons and the best ways to meet these, given the expected resource constraints facing the health sector [both governmental and private]. Inevitably the formal health care sector will be left with important responsibilities for treatment, both in terms of demands falling on different parts of the health care system [particularly on lower level facilities], on essential drug requirements, and on the training of doctors, nurses, etc. There is little point in predicting forward the present state of affairs, in that this would represent an abdication of responsibility. What is needed is a full assessment of health needs and the best ways to meet these, given both human and non-human resource constraints. To this end there will have to be a significant strengthening of the MOH in terms of its planning capacities. It goes without saying that one of the outputs of such a review would be an assessment of the impact of HIV related illnesses on the capacity of the health sector itself, given that human resources will, indeed already are, being diminished through morbidity and mortality. This is perhaps an area where WHO and the WB may be thought to have primary interests, but UNDP certainly ought to be involved both in helping Government in activities aimed at redefining strategic health care policy, and in strengthening the general planning capacity of the MOH.

(c) Education

This sector is facing huge problems and the existing challenges are already enormous. As we have seen above the performance of this sector in terms of enrollment and quality of education leaves much to be desired. Yet, like Health it is a crucial service sector with critical responsibilities for human resource development and its maintenance. As the human capital of Uganda is eroded further by HIV and AIDS the ability of this Sector to educate for replacement of lost skills will become even more important. It will, like Healths be facing the problems of AIDS mortality, so that its capacity to maintain activity will be declining. Furthermore, this Sector has to play a major role in creating awareness of HIV and in the forming of appropriate behaviours amongst a critical segment of the population—the next generation, which is as yet largely uninfected. There are multiple issues here which need attention; some are being addressed by others [such as the programmes of UNICEF], but there are important planning issues which are not. Planning for the Education Sector has to be concerned with, for example. the effects of the HIV epidemic on the school age population [the numbers to be educated], the impact of HIV related illnesses on the supply of teachers [and their training], the need at secondary and tertiary levels to plan for replacement of critical skilled and professional human resources, issues to do with the financing of the sector [under the general impact of HIV on the economy], the particular problems of groups such as children who are infected and affected by the epidemic, and increasing numbers of poor families. There is a range of important policy and programme matters where forward planning is going to be essential, and UNDP should certainly assist both the Ministry of Education and the UAC with technical and planning support.

3. Community Monitoring

Much of the foregoing reflects partial ways of measuring the impact of HIV, and while it is essential to look at effects in this way it is not sufficient to do so. What are also needed are comprehensive methods of recording impacts and social responses, i.e., some kind of cross sectional picture which integrates effects and responses within a defined space. For most households this space is going to be the community, which is itself a concept with ill-defined boundaries. In a largely rural society such as Uganda this will usually be co-terminus with the village, and what are needed are methods for observing and recording the multiple impacts at this level. Only at this level of disaggregation will it be possible to identify affected households with their specific needs, their problems as they change over time; the inter-household relationships and attitudes; the development of social caring processes, including the activities of CBOs, NGOs, churches and the like; and what is happening to rural production and the use and distribution of resources. In short to develop ways of representing and analysing communities who are facing the social and economic impacts of HIV. Since most of the adverse effects of the epidemic are going to have to be handled at the community level it follows that policy has to have detailed pictures of the problems that communities are facing, how they are coping, and what are the effective programme interventions. To achieve this objective UNDP should develop, in consultation with the UAC, a programme of Community Monitoring, with an initial set of differentiated communities as pilot studies. This will require an initial piece of research into the problems of establishing such a community monitoring programme.

C. CARING

This is in many ways the most complex issue to address, and in many ways also the most important. Many aspects of health care have been raised above, particularly those dealing with the formal health care system, both access to it and the quality of care. It is not intended in this section of the report to add further to what has already been written, for it is obvious from the foregoing that, in the case of Uganda, most of the care of the infected and the affected will have to be at the community level. Indeed one of the major challenges policy makers in Uganda have to face is how to ensure that resources do reach communities and households where they can have most impact, and where needs are greatest.

In these circumstances the activities of NGOs, CBOs, churches and other institutions have critical and vital roles to play. These institutions have already proven their value, being active in multiple directions in meeting the needs of society. The objective here is not to review their activities, and indeed much that the Report has to recommend by way of specific interventions is reserved for the following Section, where attention is directed at ways of further raising the effectiveness of the NGO sector broadly defined. But there are three very important areas where NGOs are going to be central to meeting the challenges posed by HIV, and indeed where they are already demonstrating their ability to innovate and be effective.

1. Community-Based Care

In an ideal world it would be possible to wait for the results of any Community Monitoring system such as recommended above, but the problems are too urgent for this. Actions are required now on how best to meet the medical, social and economic needs of households and communities in an integrated and sustainable way. Fortunately there are examples of how this might be done, and these cases might provide the basis for a national programme. The first step would have to be a much deeper evaluation of the two cases to be presented; to identify their strengths, and to consider the problems facing Uganda in replicating these "models" to other Districts. The initial focus of UNDP would indeed be to undertake the commissioning of such an evaluation, with the intention then of directly funding the development of those capacities which are essential for extending the programme to other Districts. This ought to be a major area for UNDP activities in meeting the challenges of HIV in Uganda.

Both of the cases are based on non-governmental hospitals. They are Kitovo Hospital in Masaka, a District of high infection and very severe social and economic problems, and Aber Hospital in Apac District where HIV infection is thought still to be low. Both hospitals have had to face the same problems: patient care needs which threatens to overwhelm the facilities, crowding out other patients; a need to find alternative ways of meeting the medical and social needs of persons with HIV-related illnesses, within the bounds posed by tight resource constraints of beds, drugs and staff; and how to integrate health care and other needs into a community framework. In part because there is no real alternative to doing this, and in part because this is actually better for the infected and affected. Integration of care, the creation of support networks, income generation schemes, IEC and behavioural change activities, support for orphans and destitute families, and mobile tearns of trained personnel [both medical and non—medical] have all formed part of their developing response. What is being achieved is remarkable, but they are of course also resource constrained in what they can achieve, and the numbers they can reach. Their capacities are clearly limited, and the constraints of space, trained counsellors, IEC materials, transport, and the like all need to be relieved. In part capacity building is about relieving these constraints, and doing so for these hospitals and others would in itself be a valuable step forward. But what is being primarily recommended is more than this: it is the evaluation of models of integrated care which have evolved over time in the face of the epidemic, and the replication of these models in their primary elements to other areas of the country, where the model can be effectively applied. This second stage will require substantive capacity building activities by UNDP and others. In a sense, it means using these cases both as models and as centres which could be given training and other responsibilities. In the latter role, they could be seen as "poles of community development", playing active roles in their own replication.

2. Orphans

This problem figures in all discussions of HIV in Uganda and as such can be briefly dealt with in this report. The number of orphans, as defined in Uganda as a child having lost one or both parents, is thought to number somewhere between 600,000 and I million. Many of these are the result of war and other factors, but this in no way changes the scale of the problem which currently exists, and which will become even larger in the coming years. There are many activities already in this area; the UAC sees it as a matter of great concern and a special committee will develop policies and interventions; and there are NGOs such as Uganda

Community-Based Association for Child Welfare (UCOBAC) and Uganda Women's Effort to Save the Orphans (UCOBAC) who have focussed their efforts in this field. The issues are highly complex and the potential solutions by no means obvious. Some of the interventions raised earlier in this Report, such as those for a Community Monitoring System and impact studies of Health Care and Education, will partially address the needs of orphans, e.g., in considering the issue of school fees. Valuable as these interventions and insights might be they are certainly not enough. This is an area where UNDP ought to be involved in capacity building, but what to do and how to do it is by no means obvious. There is a clear preference in Uganda for non-institutional solutions to the needs of orphans, although there can be no reason to suppose that this is everywhere and for all children both feasible and the best option. The national response has so far been ad hoc, and what has been done is an insufficient guide for future policy and appropriate institutional structures for the delivery of support. It is strongly recommended that before UNDP develops a programme in this area that a comprehensive study be made of the whole set of issues raised by the large and increasing number of orphans. Such a study should not focus to any degree on estimating future numbers [having some idea of numbers and their distribution is not the core of the problem], but on identifying needs and the ways in which policies and institutional structures can meet these. UNDP in consultation with the UAC should urgently commission such a study, and then develop with NGOs, government and other agencies, a programme of work.

3. Community Development

This is not a useful operational category, but it is desirable to identify it nevertheless in order to re-emphasise its importance. In practice much of the foregoing is about how to develop and strengthen community involvement in all areas, and the need to refocus the allocation of resources away from urban to rural groups, and away from formalised institutional structures to informal and localised ones. How best to do this, and the identification of priorities, will be the outcome of the recommended studies and policy related discussions in Uganda. There is much already being done at the community level, most obviously by TASO, the Uganda Red Cross and by the churches, which is extremely valuable, but highly constrained in terms of geographic and functional coverage. How to expand these activities, both spatially and in other ways, is by no means obvious. What is presently urgent is identification of needs and constraints, so as to be able, for example, to expand the numbers of trained personnel available for counselling and for behaviour change programmes. This is a matter which is also dealt with below under Organisational Restructuring.

D. STRENGTHENING ORGANISATIONAL STRUCTURES

This is potentially and actually a hugely complex problem and the following should be seen for what they are—tentative recommendations based on unscientific observations. These are thought, nevertheless, to be of value, not least in pointing in the direction of positive and productive change. For purposes of exposition only it has been necessary to identify two categories - Government and Non-Government—but obviously these are in many ways overlapping in their areas of interest, and are and should be seen as complementary. Many of the interventions above entail new functions and changing responsibilities for organisations, and the following should be seen as only a sub-set of these changes which are mainly organisational in their nature.

1. Government

The Uganda Government has recently introduced major structural changes with the establishment of the Uganda AIDS Cornrnissio n and Secretariat. This signals the commitment of the Government, and its intention that policies for the HIV epidemic be both multi-sectoral and multi-level. However, there remain unresolved issues about structure and function to which attention is turned below. The ordering of the following discussion can be considered as representative of the importance which is attached to particular levels of capacity building activities.

(a) Local Government Structures

It is a historical fact that most UNDP capacity building has been focused at the level of Central Governrnent, to the relative neglect of Local Government. In the case of the HIV epidemic all levels need to be strengthened, but the problems are much greater at the local level. This is scarcely news, and there are many existing proposals of a piecemeal nature which aim to remedy the observed deficiencies of poor policy formulation and implementation at District and County levels. There is generally too little understanding of the developmental effects of the epidemic, and too little integration across programmes—this is the familiar problem of verticality. The UAC is considering the establishment of Field Offices in a limited number of Districts; UNFPA has looked at the desirability of locating Population Officers at the same level, and there are proposals under consideration for economists from the MEPD to be located at the District. There are already many functions relating to health and development located at District level, some of these concentrating on the delivery of medical services and health education. This is also the level at which, at least in some Districts, NGOs are also operating, and need to be encouraged to operate. It is also clear that the Resistance Councils (RC) have, and are expected to have, important functions and responsibilities. but that these are not being effectively utilised. RC leaders in particular need training and especially leadership training. The importance of community action and social mobilisation is at the core of this Report, and for tnis to happen there has to be a major strengthening of LocalGovernment structures. In part this means shifting more resources, financial and human, to the local level which will require different organisational structures with new perspectives and priorities. Effective structures have to be built; in part through a comprehensive evaluation of existing and proposed systems, and support for a process of organisational reforns. UNDP has an important role to play in bringing about these very critical reforms.

(b) The Uganda Aids Commission

The Commission and the Secretariat have been in existence for such a short time that their roles functions, resource constraints needs and responsibilities, are all still evolving. The WB has been involved in needs assessment at the level of the UAC, and in respect of proposals for the setting up of AIDS Units in the various Ministries. In many senses, therefore, this is the wrong point in time for UNDP to assess what its contribution to the UAC and to individual ministries ought to be. The role of UNDP in these circumstances should be to continue with its general support for the Uganda Government's initiative, and to look positively upon requests for assistance. To a degree any response will need to be set within a framework of priorities, which is precisely the purpose of this Report. What has been argued above is that effective programmes across the spectrum of needs have to be concentrated elsewhere, particularly at the community level.

This leaves the UAC with major strategic responsibilities which are important for the development of effective policies for prevention and care, and for responding to the multiple consequences of the epidemic. To perform these functions the Secretariat has to acquire a high level of professionalism in the areas it has already identified as crucial; to utilise consultants where internal skills are unavailable, but generally to keep itself a lean and non-bureaucratic institution. UNDP should, once needs have been formulated in these terms, be willing to provide training and consultancies. For example, assisting the UAC in developing research programmes especially in the social sciences, and in helping the UAC acquire professional understanding in the areas of project development and evaluation. It being understood that these skills are needed at the level of the UAC, but not so that these activities are undertaken by the Secretariat. Thus the UAC has to be able to advise on research priorities, to be able to review research output, and to ensure that this research informs policy formulation and programme development. To become, in short, the centre in Uganda for informed discussion of HIV, and the source to whom those inside government and those outside government naturally turn for advice on policy and programme development.

(c) Ministry of Economic Planning and Development (MEPD)

This Ministry has critical responsibilities and, as such, needs to be informed and to have insights into both the causes and the effects of the HIV epidemic. As a planning ministry it has to ensure that other ministries are aware of the costs, social and economic, which Uganda is both bearing now and will inevitably also have to face in the coming years. Government needs to plan both for the erosion of its own capacities due to HIV and for the changing levels and types of services which will face Departments. As noted above the WB is considering the needs of various Ministries, including those associated with the establishment of AIDS Units. It is crucial that MEPD in particular develop a programme of training for its professionals, especially economists, so that it can modify its internai planning activities to take account of HIV, and ensure that this is also true of other Ministries in their planning roles. Since the MEPD also plays a major role in directing and co-ordinating donor assistance it is doubly important that it be aware of and understand the specific requirements for effective ACPs. To this end it is essential that senior staff and professionals be provided with the opportunity to participate m workshops, etc., dealing with HIV, and to undertake [participate in] studies of the socio-economic effects of HIV.

2. Non-Governmental Organisations

It is now readily agreed by everyone that NGOs, CBOs, churches, etc., are central to policies for prevention, for care, and for activities which aim to limit the economic and social costs of HIV. This is evident from both the analysis and the recommendations made above. Organisations such as TASO have become models for institutional developments throughout the world. An example of what can be done for the infected and affected, for prevention, for income support—across the whole spectrum of activities—by individuals of commitment and determination. Similar qualities are present in other Ugandan NGOs, with the Red Cross, the Catholic Church, UCOBAC, UWESO, and countless others, active in many directions and many areas of the country. A recent UAC inventory of NGO activities is several inches thick—a testimony to their extensive involvement at all levels.

Much has been done, which needed to be done. But the growth of NGOs has been organic, in some directions and not in others, with a regional spread which is very uneven. So also with performance, where it is evident that with growing responsibilities and programmes, in areas such as management and financial control [costing generally], and in monitoring and evaluation, there have emerged real weaknesses. This is unsurprising, and indeed some of the NGOs have already undertaken internal evaluations, restructured management, and considered strategic plans for the future.

The issue for UNDP is how can it help these organisations be more effective in meeting the challenges posed by HIV, and at the same time encourage independence and growth in response to needs. What is undoubtedly a prior requirement is an evaluation of what NGOs are presently doing; in what areas are they strong and effectivc/ineffective; what are the current constraints facing these organizations [of management, of planning, of project evaluation, of research, of cost analysis and control, etc.,] and how can these be tackled [by whom? through collaboration? through establishing specialised service agencies for management training, project evaluation, performance monitoring?]. Where is there a need for rationalisation of activity? Are there activities which are underprovided and, if so, why, and how can obstacles to provision be overcome? This is a major task to undertake such an evaluation, and to ask the questions, "What can NGOs do best?" and, "How can performance be improved?". UNDP should offer to finance such an evaluation, and then develop a programme of support for such institutions through consultative processes so as to improve their eftectiveness. These activities should have a very high priority in any ordering of UNDP activities in Uganda.

IV. OPERATIONALISING ACTIVITIES

A. PROGRAMME APPROACH

The previous Sections have dealt partly with description and analysis, and partly with principles. So far there has as yet been no explicit consideration of operational implementation of the UNDP

Programme on HIV for Uganda. The purpose of this section is to briefly rectify this omission, but to do so in a fairly schematic form. The argument for not dealing in detail with some aspects of the Programme are set out above where it was suggested that flexibility in design and in programme implementation are both desirabl. While the details of specific activities remain to be resolved and will have to be established through programme and project discussions, the overall balance of the UNDP Programme—the areas for UNDP concentration of its activities—have been strongly identified in Section III.

It is possible for there to be misinterpretation of what is being proposed by way of a UNDP Programme for Uganda, and it may be useful to state unambiguously what it is, and what it is not. The Programme is not an alternative National AIDS Control Programme (NACP); and it should not be seen as in any sense a parallel programme. Nor is it separate from the NACP, but should be viewed as integral to this, and fundamentally part of the nationally agreed Strategic Plan for responding to HIV. There is certainly no intention of supplanting, or in any way diluting, the authority and responsibilities of the UAC and the MOH [or of other actors such as WHO]. What has been attempted in this Programme is an articulated statement of UNDP's strategic assistance for Uganda which is coherent in its own terms; is founded on analysis of the changing situation in the country; and is the outcome of extensive discussions at the official and non-official levels. But the choices remain those of Government; what fits with, what does not fit with, the National Strategy for HIV and AIDS.

It is in the nature of this approach that not only has coherence been sought, as well as relevance to needs, but that other principles have been applied. These latter have included prioritisation—what are the crucial areas of actual or relative programme neglect, and how can UNDP resources be applied effectively to releasing policy and programme constraints? It is the conclusion of -this Report that UNDP' s contribution should be focused on the developmental effects of the epidemic [and especially the erosion of the human resource base of the society]. Thus activities should be identified, especially at the community level, which address these matters. But not to the exclusion of other important aspects of the national AIDS strategy, and many diverse activities which add to sustainable capacities generally are included in the UNDP Programme.

UNDP needs to see the Programme as serving a catalytic objective—to be partly about advocacy, and in part to be about social mobilisation. In the case of both of these the aims are to improve understanding and to change perception; in part to induce a larger flow of resources, and in part to induce a more effective set of policy and programme responses. To see the Programme as a means of influencing other bilateral and multi-lateral donors in their activities in Uganda. To see some UNDP interventions as "seed corn" which induce further activities by other actors; and at all times to ensure that the relative expertise of different institutions and agencies are exploited. The crucial importance of effective co-ordination of approaches and activities has been emphasised earlier, and this is rightly seen as an important function and responsibility of the UAC. The choices lie with the Ugandan Government. What has been set out in this UNDP Programme is an articulated set of activities formulated within the strategic framework established by the UAC.

Less obviously, but also important for both UNDP and Uganda, is the development of a Programme which is linked to the other priority areas of the UNDP Country Programme, particularly Poverty Alleviation and Rural Development, and Economic Policy and Management Capacity. Both in terms of the foregoing, and in what follows, coherence of the UNDP Programme for AIDS in Uganda has been an important objective; in effect to be programmatic in the many different ways which have been variously identified throughout this Report.

B. ALLOCATION OF PROGRAMME RESOURCES

Section III provides details of the main activities which are proposed, and the rationale for these. Suggested policy interventions are also made in other sections of the report, particularly in Section II. It is perhaps helpful to have more information on the proposed relative importance of different interventions within the Programme, and this is provided by the following schedule. At this stage these allocations should be seen as illustrative, and it is fully anticipated that virement will occur between both the main and sub-categories of expenditure. Nevertheless, the broad balance of expenditure between A-D should be changed only after very careful consideration and through local processes of discussion.

ALLOCATION OF IPF BY INTERVENTION AND BY ACTIVITY *(US$000)*

A. HIV TRANSMISSION

1. IEC; raising effectiveness; capacity building: training	500
2. Evaluating behaviour change; developing new models;	500
3. Low Infection areas - developing and applying interventions.	500
4. Transmission of HIV and Gender; analysis and service delivery.	500
5. STDs; programme development and gender.	200
6. HIV testing policy and behaviour change.	100
7. Refugees; evaluation of needs and HIV transmission factors.	100
8. Other activities Military; blood clubs etc.	100
Sub-Total	$2.500.000

B. ECONOMIC AND SOCIAL IMPACTS

1. Effects of female morbidity and mortality.	100
2. Social indicators; prediction and policy strategies.	50
3. Human resource balance; prediction and policy.	200
4. New approaches to modelling economic and social impact.	100
5. Micro projects.	2,000
6. Community monitoring.	750
7. Impact Studies; agriculture; health; education.	1,000
Sub-Total	$4,250,000

C. CARING

1 Community-based care; evaluation and system innovation.	2,000
2.Orphans; evaluating structures and needs; development of programmes.	500
3.Community development.	500
Sub-Total	$3,500,000

D. STRENGTHENING ORGANISATIONAL STRUCTURES

1. Local Government; evaluation and development.	500
2. UAC; professional development; consultancies; study support.	500
3. MEPD; professional development; new plarming models.	250
4. Private sector; structural evaluation and institutional innovation.	500
5. Strengthening NGO and CBO structures; training; evaluation.	1,000
6. Workshop Programme [ALL — SECTIONS A-D]	1,500
Sub-Total	$ 4,2500000

Total	$14,500,000
Management of Programme	1,000,000
Grand Total	$15,500,000

Figures 18.2—18.7 show the balance of the main programme activities in terms of interventions anal activities .

C. SEOUENCING INTERVENTIONS

It would be possible to set out a fairly precise plan for the ordering of interventions and activities, but for reasons set out above in Section III this would over-determine the content of the Programme. It was argued above that all activities should be seen as interacting and mutually supportive. Interventions, therefore, have to take place on all fronts, but not everything can be seen as of equal priority, nor in the present state of understanding capable of effective implementation. It is critically important for the success of the UNDP Programme that the knowledge base be improved in many areas, and this should be seen as a pre-requisite to policy formulation and programme design. The importance of the learning process cannot be over emphasised; this has been stressed many times in this Report and its significance for effective policy will bear repetition. Cross-learning, from experience internal to Uganda, and between Uganda and other countries, has been a target actively pursued in designing this Programme. The generalisation of the results of activities—building on experience and learning lessons—must be an essential part of the evaluation and monitoring process for all activities. This is true not merely of the Workshop Programme, where the intent will be partly to foster cross-learning, but less obviously also for all activities. It is therefore crucial that the Workshop Programme be established and be set in motion with great speed.

An important task for the managers of the UNDP Programme will be to develop a detailed plan for activities over the next five years, and to build into this plan effective monitoring and evaluation processes. Indeed, one of the activities to be pursued directly and indirectly is capacity building in these crucial respects [partly to be achieved through training, and partly through institutional development]. This has to be seen as one of the important and prior activities of the Programme. Similarly with other areas of technical assistance where it is readily agreed that the human resource base needs to be improved. Two examples of this are Micro Projects and Ministry of Economic Planning and Development (MEPD). But there are many other instances where initial activities will have to concentrate on raising understanding and on developing skills as prerequisites for policy and programme development. This does not mean that everything has to wait on the human resources being strengthened, and many activities can be started now which utilise existing skills and experience. Thus the Micro Projects can begin implementation as of now but will need to be strengthened in terms of TA; as also can some of the HIV transmission proposals, where there are existing plans and operations with which UNDP can collaborate.

As will be seen in the next part of this report there are critical issues of management of the Programme and of its implementation which need to be resolved. In many senses getting these things right will determine how successful the Programme is in meeting the problems facing Uganda. It is worth devoting both time and other resources to resolving these aspects of the problem as an initial activity, and only then to develop the detail of the UNDP Programme. This is an important and cnucial element of the Programme, and one where the UAC, the MEPD and UNDP all have valuable contributions to make in defining effective structures.

D. PROGRAMME IMPLEMENTATION

Section IV.B summarised a complex programme of activities for the period 1992-1996. It is proposed that 19.5 per cent of the Country Programme IPF be allocated to AIDS, i.e., some 15.5 million US. This is a large and very significant proportion of the Country Programme (CP), and it is absolutely essential that in the conditions facing Uganda that these resources be effectively managed. Government has, in agreement with UNDP, an important role in the determination of the implementation process for the Programme. It is an objective of UNDP policy to strengthen Ugandan expertise and increase the use of goods and services supplied by or through national governmental, non-governmental and private institutions in programme development, implementation and management. It is fully recognised that the capacity for government execution has been raised by the establishment of the Government Execution Unit [GEX] in the MEPD.

However, while it is the ultimate objective that national institutions implement both programmes and projects, and the establishment of GEX is an appropriate step in this direction, it is certainly not presently the case that this is feasible. Uganda will continue to need expertise, services and other inputs from external sources during the Fourth CP, including UN system sources. In this respect the Specialised Agencies of the UN system will continue to have a critical supporting role, but with the proviso that over time their contribution will increasingly be in the form of external specialists to complement local expertise. In terms of the UNDP Programme for AIDS it would readily be accepted that ILO, for example, should have an important role to play in the measurement of the erosion of the human resource base caused by HIV, and in the development of policy and programme responses. In a similar way FAO has or ought to have the relevant expertise for assessing the impact of changing labour supplies on agriculture, and in establishing the effects on the level and mix of farm output. It is appropriate that WHO have a continuing and central role in the setting of health policy, and in particular in the development of a multi-sectoral framework for HIV policy. Thus WHO remains the most important technical resource in many areas, most obviously in health.

The experience of the UNV Programme will also be invaluable in the implementation of UNDP's activities. At the national level UNV support can be provided to the UAC, the MEPD, and sectoral ministries, in the fields of monitoring and evaluation, and in research and training. At the District level UNV could assist in training and in planning, monitoring and evaluation and much else. They have particular expertise, technical and administrative, which could be valuable to NGOs and CBOs, particularly in roles

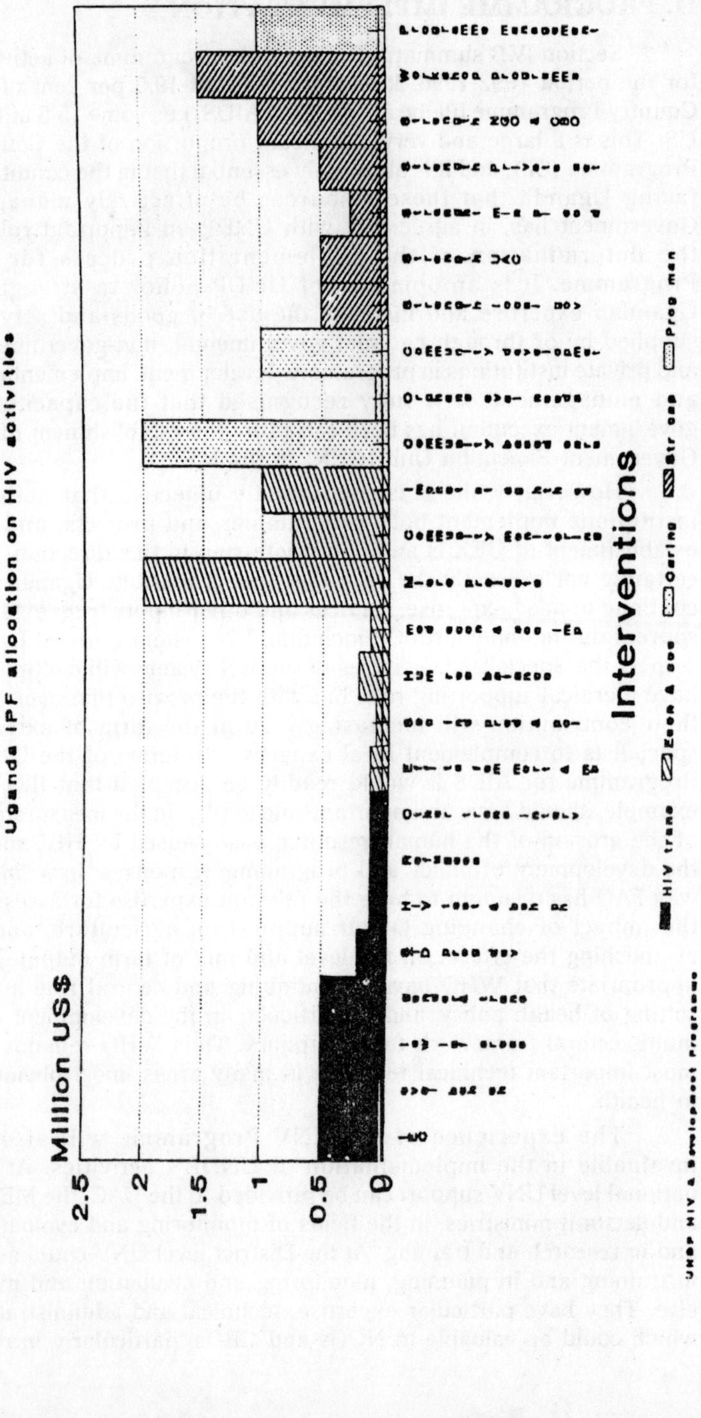
Uganda IPF allocation on HIV activities
Million US$
2.5
2
1.5
1
0.5
0
Interventions
HIV trans
Caring
Prog man

Fig. 18.2

Fig. 18.3

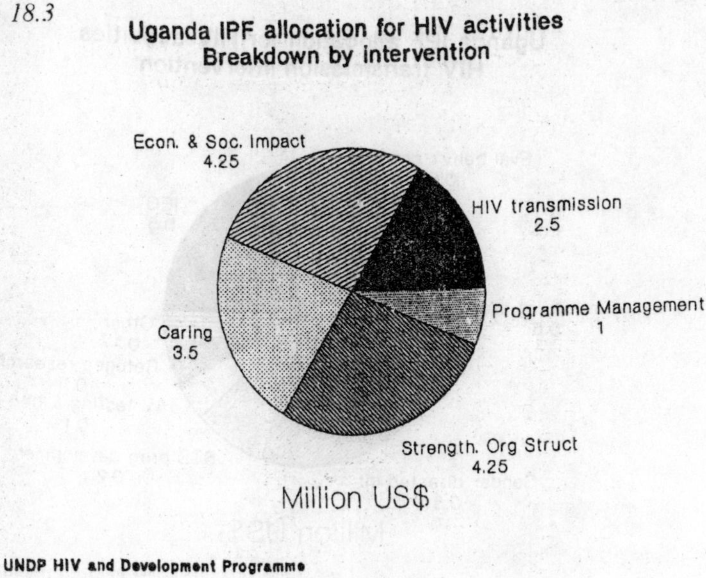

Fig. 18.4

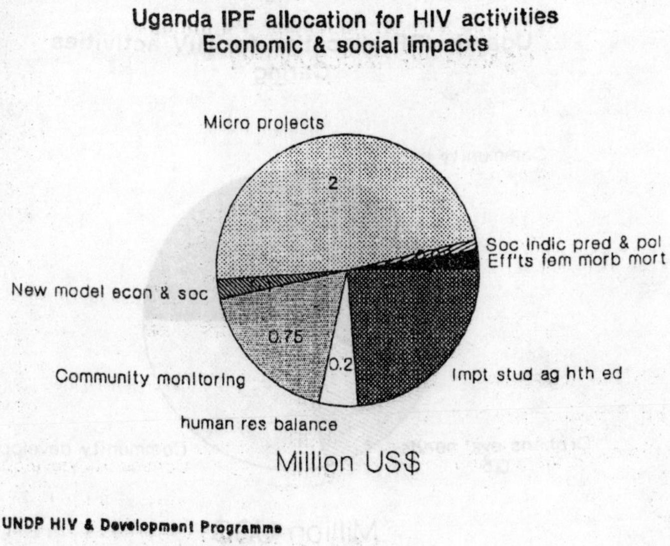

Fig. 18.5

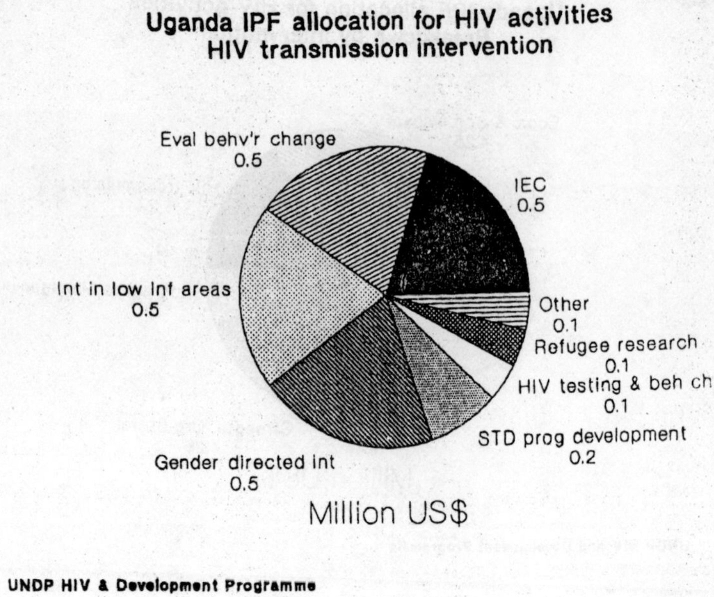

Fig. 18.6

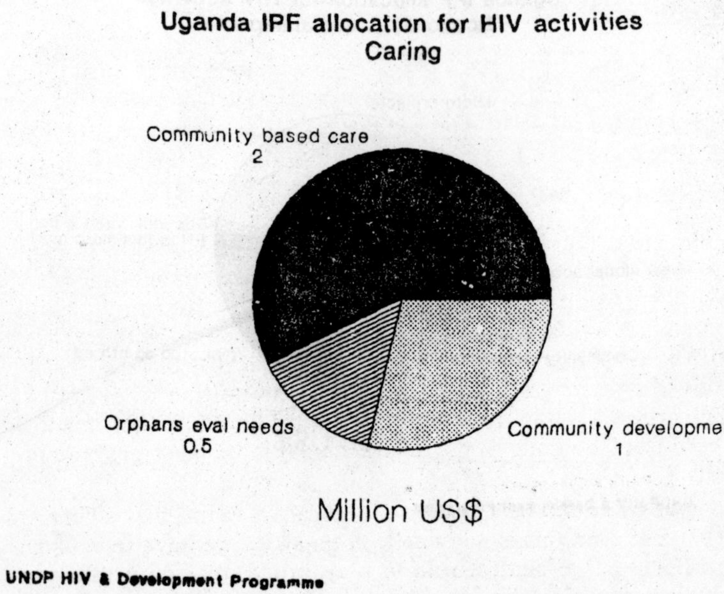

Fig. 18.7

Uganda IPF allocation for HIV activities Strengthening organisational structures

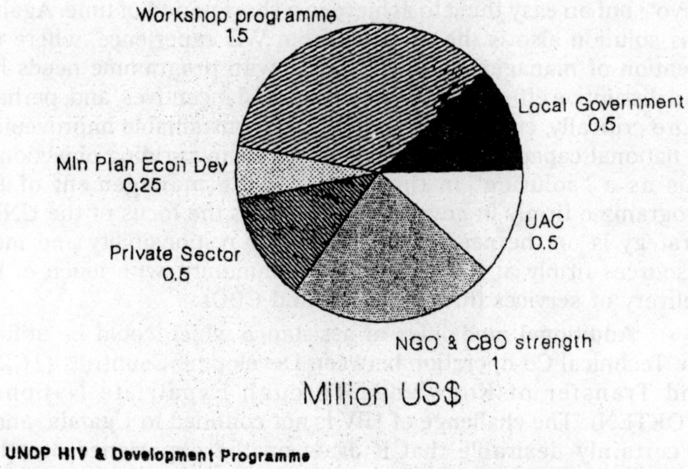

relating to the mobilisation of effective activities at the local level, where technical expertise and experience are major constraints.

The options in respect of implementation are fairly straightforward and in some senses this is not the core of the problem. Some institutions, such as the UAC, are ruled-out by the fact that they are not an implementing agency. For other fundamental reasons to do with the nature of the multi-sectoral approach it would be inappropriate for the MOH to be responsible for overall implementation of the UNDP Programme. One possibility is to lodge management of the Programme with an NGO, which is essentially the option chosen by USAID. But this has its disadvantages too, not least in the high proportion of overheads which are charged by EIL, which substantially reduces the quantity of resources actually applied and available to meet programme needs.

Possibly the best option is to locate a Manager, or Unit, in MEPD, but even this is not wholly optimal. As we have seen above the MEPD has a central role to play in external co-ordination, including planning the use of external resources which directly and indirectly are related to the national AIDS strategy. Its position at the core of Government has been increased by its amalgamation with Finance, so that Planning and Finance functions can now be fully integrated. On the other hand the MEPD has no expertise in the area of HIV and AIDS, and this would have to be created "de novo": not an easy thing to achieve in a short period of time. Against this solution also is the evidence from WB experience, where the creation of management units to deal with programme needs has had disruptive effects on pay structures and incentives, and, perhaps more critically, created no long term and sustainable improvement in national capacities. There is perhaps an over-riding objection to this as a "solution" in that it places the management of the programme firmly in government, whereas the focus of the UNDP strategy is on the need to locate greater responsibility and more resources firmly at the level of the community, with much of the delivery of services through NGOs and CBOs.

Additional modalities of assistance which could be utilised are Technical Co-operation between Developing Countries (TCDC) and Transfer of Knowledge Through Expatriate Nationals (TOKTEN). The challenge of HIV is not confined to Uganda, and it is certainly desirable that it draw on the experience of other countries and institutions through TCDC. There are also additional resources of experience, knowledge and commitment to be drawn on through the TOKTEN programme. This permits Uganda to add to its resources through the repatriation of trained nationals who left the country in the 1970s and 1980s. Their contribution, under conditions of a worsening human resource endowment, has become even more critical in meeting the challenges of the present and following decades.

REFERENCES

Barnett T. and Blaikie P. M. [July 1990]. Community Coping Mechanisms in the Face of Exceptional Demographic Change. Report to the Overseas Development Administration (UK).

World Bank. Uganda: The Economic Impact of AIDS [June 1991].

19

Placing Women at the Centre of the Analysis

Ms. Elizabeth Reid
UNDP, New York

There is a growing consensus in the development assistance world that human development should provide the framework for development assistance in the 1990s. Yet, while this is widely welcomed by women, there are few, if any, grounds for assuming that this ideology will benefit women any more than any of the previous development assistance ideologies, be they economic growth, growth with equity, basic needs or whatsoever.

The literature on women and development extends back almost as far as the literature on development itself. The mandates and directives have long been in place. Yet, the success stories are anecdotal rather than systemic and this is causing a growing questioning of past approaches.

There are those amongst us, serious but with a sense of humour, who, in response to this chronic failure, are now proposing two new but linked approaches: the radical procedural approach and the radical analytical approach. The first approach consists in developing a set of procedures that might better bring about the achievement of our women in development objectives. For example, all missions that are responsible for programme or project formulation, implementation teams and evaluation missions must be predominantly or exclusively composed of women. All hose consulted during such missions must be predominantly or exclusively women, and so on. Such procedural directives, if issued by UNDP or CIDA, for example, would undoubtedly be greeted by great discomfiture if not outrage. But it is interesting to note that the obverse, which is the present situation, is not.

The radical analytical approach places women at the centre of the analysis; that is, in any development-related activity whatsoever, the analysis should begin at where women are, whatever they are doing, and should aim to get them (women) where they want to be and bring about the changes they want the rest of the world (men, children, social institutions, financial institutions, economies, etc.), are to be drawn into the analysis primarily on the basis of how they relate to women or how they can contribute to achieving women's goals. Again, radical only in that the obverse is the accepted modus operandi.

Today is not the occasion to elaborate on these approaches, but it is the occasion to understand the cost if we do not place women at the centre of the HIV analysis. The failure to do so has already brought an immense cost in women's lives, a cost which is forcing an understanding that, for the 1990s and beyond, human development will be conditional upon human survival; that is, human survival, not human development, may well become the primary focus of our development assistance.

Let me elaborate on this, taking the example of HIV/AIDS. The main focus of HIV/AIDS programmes to date has been the prevention of the further transmission of the virus. I will focus on sexual transmission since, for women, this is the overwhelming way in which women become infected.

The three main prevention strategies for sexual transmission that are being advocated, particularly in developing countries, are: one, the reduction of the number of sexual partners; two, condom usage; and three, faithfulness in relationships and celibacy and abstinence outside of them. To these, a fourth has recently been added, namely, the treatment of STDs.

I do not wish to discuss, today, the merits of these strategies, per se, bur rather to look at their adequacy as prevention strategies for women and those who people women's world.

Let's take the first, reduction of sexual partners. Preliminary data from African studies indicate that 60 per cent to 80 per cent of all infected women have one and only one sexual partner. Therefore, this strategy has no relevance to their lives. Nor is it relevant to the lives of those women who, because of economic circumstances, are forced to sell or exchange sexual intercourse. Thus, for the majority of women this strategy is inapplicable, irrelevant strategy.

Secondly, condom usage. Men use condoms. Results from programmes with sex workers have clearly shown that some women can successfully negotiate condom use. However, this remains a rare skill among women. Most men do not use condoms, and most women do not have the ability or the leverage to protect themselves in this way. This is a strategy for men.

Thirdly, faithfulness, abstinence and celibacy. At the current stage of the epidemic, it can be estimated that every day, each day now, 1,500 faithful women are infected. That is, every day, just now, there are 1,6500 women who have no sexual partners other than their husbands who are becoming infected. This number will increase as the number of infected men increases. There are some indications that the incidence of rape, particularly of young girls, has increased and there is no reason to believe, in fact, on the contrary, that this is not also true of incest. For most women, abstinence and the faithfulness of both partners in a relationship is not within their power to bring about. For a growing number of girls and women, sexual assault is a reality. So this strategy is inapplicable.

These are grim facts. But they are the realities that lie hidden behind the epidemiological data. The strategies that are being advocated are strategies that men, now women, have under their control. This is the area why one in every 40 adult women in Africa is infected. It is the reason why there are as many or more women in Africa that men as infected. It is also the reason why, in the Latin American and Caribbean regions, the male/female infection ratio has dropped so precipitously over the last couple of years.

Is there no hope for women? In the longer term, the power imbalances in relationships and society which create women's subordination must be changed. But what, in the short term, can women to do save their lives and those of their children?

If one lays aside for the moment the current strategies and begins the analysis with the reality of women's lives, then the first question is: Is there any protective measure that a woman has under her own control which will offer her protection from infection?

Protective measures can be divided into two types: those which prevent contact with an infected person and transmission of the virus and those that decrease the efficacy of transmission when unprotected sexual contact occurs. The first, for example, includes condom usage, faithfulness and abstinence. Then measures are much more efficacious than the second type. However, the second type may overall be just as effective, or more effective, if more people can act upon them.

There are, in fact, in each of these two categories, some measures that an individual woman can use. It is important that we start naming them.

One of the most efficient know means of reducing the efficacy of transmission of the virus, that is, when you have unprotected sexual intercourse with an infected person, is unbroken genital skin. This is the advice we give to health workers: The most effective barrier is unbroken skin. If you are covered in blood, wash it off. In the genital area, unbroken skin is also protective.

Transmission of the virus can be facilitate by the presence of genital lesions, inflammation, secretions and scarification. The causes of these conditions in women include genital urinary tract infections, STDs, sexual practices and traditional infibulation practices. All genital conditions which may facilitate transmission should now become a focus of attention. Not all of them do women have the power to change. A number are treatable. Others, in particular, sexual and infibulation practices, will require longer term solutions. However, there are many conditions that can be improved, through improved hygiene or through treatment.

Women may be culturally or socially constrained from using STD-dedicated services, or even from seeking treatment for a genital condition. This is often not culturally or socially sanctioned. If we want to enable women to avail themselves of this means of protection, it becomes important to know whether the diagnosis and treatment of these conditions can be combined, for example, with other consultations requiring an internal examination. That is, if women cannot go to be treated for these conditions, can we locate services where they are already being externally examined.

This analysis will lead to a broader emphasis on, then an exclusive focus on improving STD services. STD services are mainly used by people, men and women, with multiple sexual partners. Most women do not use these services and most women suffer from genital conditions other than, but also including, STDs. Thus, a woman-centred analysis in this area would focus on the diagnosis and treatment of those genital conditions in both men and women which place them at increased risk of infection and would focus on the delivery of services at points where these people go.

Another strategy for reducing the efficacy of transmission may be to ensure that the change sin a person's infectivity over the course of infection are widely known. A person's infectiousness, the ability to infect someone else, increases as he or she progresses from asymptomatic infection to symptomatic infection. Whereas an individual woman may not be able to refuse sexual intercourse in general, she may be able to find a way if her partner were ill. In other words, she may be able to do this in a short period of time although not over a long period of time. This knowledge about infectivity is an important element in the counselling of discordant couples in our societies. In societies where the virus is diffused throughout the population, this information should be widely known so that those who can, can use it as a protective measure.

Apart from the above, there are at least two strategies for preventing contact with an infected person, the first type of measure, which are under a woman's control.

Little attention has been given to barrier methods which, unlike the condom, are under a woman's control. The literature on the sexual transmission of diseases other than HIV to women indicate that diaphragms protect women from, for example, gonorrhoea, to the same extent that condom usage does. There is no reason to assume that condoms protect women more than diaphragms do, with or without a spermicide, in the case of HIV. Yet, no attention has been given to determining the adequacy of diaphragms as a protective measure.

The second strategy under women's control for preventing contact with an infected man is, in the absence of any known alternatives, becoming more widespread in high incidence areas. This is desertion, that is, just moving away, walking away from home and relationship. It is an option often with tragic consequences for the woman who may well find herself unable too support herself and, when she is able to take them, her children. In such cases, prostitution, and so infection, may be her only coping strategy.

There is a pressing need to further explore and identify the strategies which a woman may have under her control. However, at the same time it must be understood that the most efficient and effective prevention strategies are those that men have under their control. Thus, every effort must continue to be made to change men's behaviour.

In this area, also, there has been a great neglect of a woman-centred analysis. There are at least two very powerful instruments that have not yet been fully identified in the efforts to change men's behaviour the first is women's collective action. The second is the law.

While women individually may feel and be powerless to change men's behaviour, women collectively can effect extraordinary changes. The literature on the global movement of women over the last couple of decades abounds with examples. The women of Maharastra who decided to no longer tolerate drunkenness in men, in their husbands, formed themselves into vigilante groups. As a group, not individually, the went out looking for the stills and for drunken men. They changed drinking men's drinking patterns. The Chipko women tied themselves to trees to prevent environmental degradation in Nepal. Mexican women in the mid- to late seventies formed an alliance across all types of women and women's groups to bring down the incidence of rape and sexual assault of women. Kenyan women, also tired of drunkenness in their husbands, came together to devise strategies for stopping that behaviour. And the models go on and on.

There is a need to look for models of women' s collective action which have changed men's HIV-related behaviour. The collective voices and actions of women to be called upon can range from the national machineries for women and national women's organizations, all the way to groupings of women at the village level. We learnt in Kenya that if you wish to increase women's income, you cannot give a goat to an individual woman.

Traditionally, goats are owned by men. If you give a goat to a woman, the man will slaughter it when he chooses and take the money. What the women did, then, was to come collectively together. If women collectively owned a goat, no individual husband could make such a decision. We need analogues to face this epidemic.

The second instrument is the law. There is now an extremely effective and very active Women and Law in southern Africa project. At the initiation of this project and for quite different reasons, it was decided that one important area of study would be the newly introduced laws relating to child support. These laws required men to pay for the upkeep of any children that they fathered. What the women and law project has found is that there have been striking changes in male sexual behaviour. Men are now fathering fewer children. Now that they are required to provide for and support those that they father, they father fewer.

This provides an important model. We have tried for a long time through direct legal intervention in the area of rape and incest to change men's behaviour but with varied success. Here is an example of the use of the law to bring about behaviour change which has been extremely effective.

While the primary analysis so far has focused on prevention, a similar analysis is needed to determine the potential impact of this epidemic on individual families, communities and economies and, hence, to plan effective and timely responses. Even in, so to speak, the malecentred analysis, we are not very far along the road to understanding, describing and finding effective strategies. But the point I am making is that what we need to do is to start elsewhere, in this area too, to start in women' s spaces.

Let me give you some glimpses of what a woman-centred analysis would reveal.

Firstly, most women do not know that they are infected. Most women do not want to know. Infected or otherwise, they must still continue with their daily lives. There is no one to take their place.

For many women who know that they are infected, there is no privacy, no confidentiality. Disclosure is not in their hands. Most women find out that they are infected during pregnancy or when a young child falls ill and is diagnosed. The diagnosis of the child makes public the women's infection status.

For women who know that they are infected, what dominates virtually every minute of the day are two primary emotions: anger and guilt. Anger towards the person, usually their husband and the person with whom they have so often infected one or more of their children.

The reality of the lives of these women is that, although, as stated above, probably up to 60 or 80 per cent of infected women were not infected though their own behaviour, they are blamed as the source of the transmission. The stigma and the discrimination associated with this disease rests too often with women.

Next, the supportive services required by seropositive women will be more than drugs and medical care. They will range from household care for ill women, child care for their children, emotional support to lessen discrimination, and financial support, as so often they will not have an income coming into the house. The dominant concern for many infected women is the present and future support for and care of their children, particularly since the fathers of those children will often be sick or dead.

The displacement of women's work from patenting, from productive activities and from community work to care for the sick will have immense consequences within those families and communities. This deplacement, coupled with the high mortality rates in women, could well lead to the disintegration of family structures. This can be seen already in parts of Africa. It will lead to changing patterns of agricultural production and the possibility of decreased food production, and to a decrease in informal sector trading where women trade mainly food. It will lead to shortage of personnel in those formal sectors where women predominate, which still include health and education.

If one includes in one's analysis of the HIV epidemic an analysis centred on women, whether it be with respect to prevention or with respect to developing strategies for minimizing the impact of this epidemic. It is my contention that different strategies and priorities will be identified which may end up being more effective than the present strategies. This is not an academic or a feminist exercise. For women it is a matter of life and death.

Putting women at the centre of the analysis leads to quite different approaches and strategies. For women today, the lack of this analysis for the HIV epidemic has already cost perhaps millions of lives, their children. The price is too high to continue with the blindness of the past. We must change.

20

Creating the Possibility: A Movement for Social Change

Ms. Elizabeth Reid
UNDP, New York

For a movement for social change to come about, there has to be a shared cause or vision, a collective will to change and a sufficiently large group of people as its base. In Africa today, one of the most important challenges is to bring about a will to live, a will to live as an infected person, the will to remain uninfected and the will to live with and despite this virus which is silently and invisibly invading its communities.

This first meeting of the network for African people with HIV and AIDS is the kernel of this social movement, embodying individually and collectively this will to live, a will to live the life that one has richly and fully, the collective will to bring an end to the stigma, rejection, discrimination, neglect, isolation, pain and fear that each of us has had to bear.

The question I would like to pose is: how can we turn this gathering here today from a meeting into a movement, a movement for the changes that we talk and dream about, a movement of activism, of solidarity, of empowerment, a movement sweeping Africa, changing the fatalism and indifference to passion and concern?

There are, perhaps, 220 million adolescents and adults in Africa today living in fear, the fear that they may be or soon will be infected. This is an awful lot of fear, a fear that need not be there. Among the 220 million, there are only, perhaps, at a guess, a quarter of a million who know their infection status, perhaps, only one-tenth of a million. Yet there are at least 8 million people in sub-Saharan Africa who are infected. Among those who know that they are infected, there are even fewer who have come to live with that knowledge.

Most people in Africa die without knowing whether or not they are infected, even if they silently fear so. Reflect upon how you yourself came to know that you are infected. Few men get diagnosed as being infected. Some young men and women get diagnosed, still too often without their consent, when they are granted scholarships for overseas study, when they enter certain professions or vocations or donate blood. A number of women get diagnosed indirectly through a diagnosis of AIDS in one of their children. Most of the few men and women who know that they have AIDS are diagnosed clinically when they are quite close to death.

Very few people in Africa have access to voluntary testing and counselling services. Very few people who know that they are infected have access to counselling, peer groups and other support services to help them learn to live with this knowledge. Very few countries have created the supportive ethical, legal and human rights environment required in order to be able to provide such services.

Programmes of care and support are, for the most part in Africa, programmes for the terminally ill. They are to assist with the dying with HIV, not with dle living with HIV. They are emotionally draining for the counsellors and carers since they work almost exclusively with the dying and those close to them, people often rendered destitute by illness and with few or no coping strategies. The kind of care and support that they can be given is limited. Most people are too sick to take care of themselves or their families. to provide for them or to feed them. They are too ill to be able to do anything to prepare their children for the future, to set their affairs in order, to pass on their knowledge to their families or colleagues or to be activists for change.

Assistance to the dying is not widely balanced by assistance to those living and well with HIV, by programmes to assist people to live with the knowledge that they or someone they love are infected, yet well. There are so few people who have access to voluntary counselling and testing services or who wish to find out. Thus few National HIV/AIDS Programmes achieve the synergy and the energy which can arise when the infected well are included. Furthermore, those that are struggling to learn to live with this knowledge, to become the activists, are too rarely the politicians, the church leaders, the educated or the articulate. This epidemic requires a seemingly rare form of courage, a form of courage which each of you has. But there are too few people yet to create the base of a movement for social change.

How can we change this, break through the stifling silence that has wrapped itself around Africa? Is this silence and paralysis inevitable where people cannot find out their infection status and do not even want to? Does it increase the fear, the anguish and the apathy? Do others feel like the women farmer in Uganda who described herself as "crippled" by not knowing? Does not being able to find out increase an individual and collective sense of powerlessness?

Why might a person want to know their infection status? Statements glibly made that people in Africa do not want to know their infection status have made me think back over my own experience. My husband, Bill, and I were living in Kinshasa, Zaire, when we began to suspect that he might be infected. He had grown up in rural Zaire and had spent much of his life in Zaire or elsewhere in Africa. We had been married less than two years and we had a baby son, John-William. Bill was a fine and much loved person. He was my companion, colleague, lover and husband. We had a very close and loving relationship. It was 1983 and there was no test and, in Kinshasa, virtually no access to information about progression, symptoms or treatment and little, mostly wrong, about life span.

We lived with fear as a constant companion. Which means to say that we lived as if it were not true that he might be infected. We went about out daily lives as before the fear. Except in our lovemaking where the fear that he might be infected haunted us. Except in our love for each other where this fear kept confronting us with the possibility of the loss of this deep and satisfying love. Except that we would look at our little son and wonder how, if true, this might affect him. Except that we had planned to have more children.

To others it was as if nothing had changed. They could not see the fear and we certainly could not have shown it or spoken about it without losing everything we valued outside of ourselves: our work, our friendships, our dignity. And anyway we lived in the hope that it might not be, that the fear was ungrounded. Fear and hope were tangled up inside us. It was a terrible time, living as if he were infected and as if he were not, unable to speak about these fears, dreading and hoping. We were in the same position as about 220 million Africans are today. It was cruel.

As soon as he had begun to fear that he might be infected, Bill went out and bought condoms. I did not have to suggest, beg or negotiate and I may not have been able to if it had been left up to me. I have not been brought up to do such things easily. But, fortunately, I did not have to struggle with the fear of death in the act of love. Neither the knowledge that he might be infected nor the possibility of condom breakage had any place in our lovemaking. I was not making love to a virus, or to an infected person. I was making love to Bill.

Yet sometimes the fear of pain and loss was unbearable and

it was I that drew back his hand as he reached for the condom.

I can understand those who have said to me that the condom becomes a symbol and a reminder of the death to come. I can understand those who have said: "I love him. What does it matter if I become infected too?" Or those for whom the edges blur, who sometimes, living so much within the epidemic, feel that they are already infected.

Finally, a test became available and we decided to challenge the fear, to allow for the possibility that the hope might be justified. We wanted to know.

In those parts of the world where testing and counselling is widely available, many people will choose not to know. Their right to this knowledge is respected, they could know if they wanted to, but they choose to live protectively of themselves and others, without this knowledge. This is a different psychological setting from a world where few, if any, can gain access to this knowledge. For many years after Bill's death, I choose not to know. I knew that I could not live with the knowledge that I was infected and facing the same future. I feared that I would give up, even take my life. But I had a son to raise who had already lost his father. I chose not to know.

What happened when we found out that Bill was infected? The finding out was brutal. No counselling. No support. Just the result. There was no more hope.

The feeling of hopelessness was overpowering. Bill was infected and there was nothing we could do about it. We were left with a sense of deep bewilderment, of absolute powerlessness.

We struggled, mainly separately and alone, the only time in our life together that we were so far apart, to learn to live with this knowledge.

Eventually it became clear to us that the only way to live with this knowledge was to go on living. We had stumbled through helplessness, distress, turmoil, impotence. We stumbled into living.

How did we make that transition from the trauma of the diagnosis to living? Much of it had to do with the sort of person Bill was. He believed that life was worth living, that we together had much more happiness to find and that we had worthwhile work to do. He realized that not taking his life into his own hands was leading to a death wish, a sense of helplessness and hopelessness. It also had to do with my family and our friends. They too had to learn how to live with this knowledge and so they understood what we were facing. We helped each other.

The living we found was simple enough: we did those things that we would have been doing anyway. We led full and happy lives. The reality of his infection had been acknowledged but placed in its proper perspective. And life continued.

We had come back to living but our lives had essentially changed.

I was never again to be without the knowledge that Bill was infected. It was not incapacitating, just constant; not a fear of death, not an anticipation of death, not any state of mind with respect to death. Just something intractable inside me as I went about living my daily life, a constant call to courage.

We had made the journey to living within the epidemic. Pity had no place there. It is an emotion from outside looking in. We were involved, absorbed, challenged, laughing, learning, bickering together.

Bill is dead and has joined the ancestors. His son and I keep him living with us, in our memories, in our hearts and in our lives.

This is just one story of moving from the cruelty of fear to knowing that someone one loves dearly is infected, to learning how to live with that knowledge. It is a story of the will to live, of the ability to influence the quality and, perhaps, the length of one's life, of activism, of solidarity and of sexuality.

The more stories we have the more we will know about the critical questions facing us: why would a person want to know their infection status? What happens when they find out they are infected? How can they be supported in making the transition to living with that knowledge? How can the group of people who are infected, active and well be expanded? And how can it be formed into a movement for social change so that we can all, the infected, the uninfected and the affected, live peacefully with this virus and with each other?

These stories must be told but will not be if the story tellers or their children or families are rejected or in any way harmed by their telling.

These questions are a part of what you are here to talk about: the processes of empowerment and change through solidarity, activism and self-organization.

Thank you for the honour you have given to me in inviting me to be with you on this momentous occasion, the birth of this Africa-wide movement for social change, a movement towards living with HIV and AIDS.

21

Breaking the Silences

Ms. Elizabeth Reid
UNDP, New York

A blanket of silence has wrapped itself around Africa, smothering the voices, the fear, the pain, the cries for help. There are some brave voices, including those of a number of courageous women who are with us today. But, still, few couples are talking to one another about staying uninfected, few parents are talking to their children, few colleagues are talking about the future management of their work places, few leaders about the future of their countries.

Why this blanket of silence? Is it because there seems to be a difficulty in living in a present where people do not themselves know whether or not they are infected, where they can only watch to see if those they love - spouses, daughters, parents, siblings—start growing thinner, where each day there are more funerals?

There is even more silence surrounding the future. Few seem to be willing to address the question of how they will live in a future, perhaps only five to ten years away in some countries, when they will be surrounded by people dying, where the normal expectations of daily life will be more and more disrupted, where the devastating impact of this epidemic will be more visible in the faces of children on the streets, in the empty seats in offices, in the scarcity of public services.

Yet if people do not begin thinking about and planning for the future now, the impact of this epidemic could cause civil and economic disintegration as people flee or turn against their leaders or turn against each other. Just because the pain and the silences are no longer bearable.

To prepare people for a less bleak future, a future which could mix pain with hope, grief with love, today's silences must be broken and people start talking about HIV in the way they talk about the effects of devaluation on their lives, or who will win the soccer or when the rainy season will come.

Breaking the silence is critical for keeping families together. Without couples and families talking, there could be a breakdown in trust between men and women, a reluctance, particularly on the part of women, to marry, to have sexual intercourse or to have children. Many women and men may decide not to marry, not to establish families.

Breaking the silence is critical for preventing more people from becoming infected. Experience in responding to this epidemic has taught us the profound importance of dialogue, of discussion between sexually interacting people.

Such a dialogue presupposes a desire to remain uninfected and not to infect others. Thus it presupposes not only awareness but also self esteem and mutual respect. But it requires something more. It requires a capacity to talk intimately about sexuality, desire and protection from infection. Seemingly, and for different reasons, talking things over, breaking the silence, is not easy either for women or for men.

There is also a need for greater insight into, and discussion about, why and how men and women enter into sexual relations.

For women, this may have to do with cultural imperatives which place high value on motherhood and on the continuation of the lineage. Or the reason may have to do with economic imperatives, an inability to survive economically without the support of a man or except by commercial sex work. Or with a need for protection, a critical social role that men play.

For both women and men, factors which are causative or contributory include:

— the impact of poverty, particularly as women seek to care for husbands and children;
— the impact of the structures of the labour market on family structures through, for example, mobility and migration;
— the impact of a lack of employment opportunities, including for the young and for women;
— the incidence of war, civil conflict and violence;
— cultural practices such as child-brides and female infibulation;
— the impact of an upbringing centered around relations of authority, control and coercion on male sexual practices;
— the cultural role of sexual relations, particularly as a cleansing of the past, or a freeing of a person's spirit or as a safeguard against bad luck; and
— the influence of alcohol or drugs on sexuality.

All of these factors have to be discussed in the context of national HIV/AIDS programmes if the spread of the virus is to be slowed.

The second programme focus of most national HIV/AIDS programmes is the care and support of those infected and those who care for them.

Most people in Africa die without knowing that they are infected, even if they fear so. Those who do know, particularly if they are men, know because they are diagnosed with AIDS when they are quite close to death. Some women get diagnosed indirectly through the diagnosis of a child with AIDS. Few blood donors choose to know their results. Few people in Africa have access to affordable voluntary testing and counselling sites.

Thus programmes of care and support are, for the most part, programmes for the terminally ill. They are to assist in the dying with HIV, not in the living with HIV. They are not programmes to assist people to live with the knowledge that they or those they love are infected.

Many counselling, care and concern programmes are volunteer based. They are built on the widespread concern and commitment that exists in African communities towards those who are experiencing misfortune. Most but not all those who volunteer are women who are already burdened by their other roles and responsibilities. Many of the men who volunteer know themselves to be infected with the virus.

Home-based care programmed in particular, play an important role in breaking the silence around this epidemic. They lessen fear and stigma in communities. They help men and boys learn how to care for the sick and the dying. They help protect those for whom they are caring from abuse and neglect. They help in making AIDS a part of everyone's daily life. However, their effectiveness and sustainability is often limited by a lack of integrated planning. There are often no associated systems that guarantee the timely provision of basic necessities such as soap, food for starving households, protein supplements for the sick, simple medicines, especially for the treatment of opportunistic conditions, transport to and from the hospital or health centre or services for children.

They are also emotionally wearing for the counsellors and carers since they are working almost exclusively with the dying and their families, often rendered destitute by the illness and often with few or no coping strategies. Assistance to the dying is not counter balanced by assistance to those living and well with HIV.

Further, because on the whole these programmes are for the terminally ill, the range of support and counselling that can be given is narrow. Most people are too ill to take care of themselves or their families, to provide for them or to feed them. They are too sick to be able to do anything to prepare their children for their future, to set their affairs in order or to pass on their knowledge to their families or their colleagues.

Thus most national HIV programmes are stretched between prevention and the care of the terminally ill and few achieve the synergy which can arise when the infected well are included. Most programmes do not reach the majority of those affected by this epidemic—the infected well and those who love them. These people remain untouched, unacknowledged and without help. In some countries they constitute 20 or 30 per cent of the adult population, in some communities 40 or 50 per cent.

In Africa today there are possibly seven or eight million or more HIV-infected and well men and women who do not know their infection status. The majority of them are married and supporting families. Most are productively active. Most do not want to know their infection status. However, a number of studies are now showing that a significant exception to the latter statement are widows and many youth.

The questions I want to pose today are: Is it in the national interest to motivate people to know their infection status? Could it be in people's own interest to know? If these questions are answered in the affirmative, then there will be a need to radically revise national priorities and donor policies.

What happens when people do not know their infection status and do not want to know? Is this a significant contributory factor to the blanket of silences? Does it increase fear, anguish and apathy? Do others feel like one rural woman in Uganda who described herself as "crippled" by not knowing? Does it increase an individual and a collective sense of powerlessness? Do all these essentially psychological conditions prove a serious constraint to behavioural and attitudinal change? As of yet there are only partial answers to these questions since few studies have raised them. But those that have would seem to indicate that they may be answered in the affirmative by many people.

However, a number of studies have shown that not knowing and so not talking has meant that children are unprepared for the loss of their parents and that parents have not planned for their future. Studies recently carried out by FAO in Eastern and Southern Africa have shown that where people do not have access to this information, where they feel unable to talk about the eventuality of their deaths, whole bodies of knowledge relating to agricultural practices and agricultural processes can be lost. Anecdotal evidence from a number of countries have shown that fear of their status coupled by a reluctance to speak has meant that skills and experience relevant to industrial and financial management of firms and government departments have been completely lost and the opportunity for training of replacements missed.

Thus, particularly in more seriously affected countries, it could be in the national interest to create a milieu in which people Would be able to find out their infection status and feel able to discuss this with their colleagues. This would make it possible to train replacements for those infected, to create opportunities for them to pass on their knowledge and experience, to restructure workplaces to make them less dependent on the skills of particular individuals. Furthermore, if there were evidence that knowing one's infection status could make it possible to live longer as a well infected person, this would assist in increasing their productive lives, increasing the return of the investment of their parents and the State in their education and training and, equally importantly, decrease the likelihood of future civil unrest, since these people could remain caring and providing for their families longer.

Should the State decide that it wishes to motivate people to know their infection status, it would have to ensure that those who knew and were prepared to disclose this information were protected from stigma and discrimination before ensuring widespread access to voluntary testing and counselling sites.

Why might a person want to know? For many women and men the overwhelming reason is a desire to stay alive and well as long as possible to care for, raise and support their children, to plan for their children's future and to provide for their spouses. In Uganda, men and women have used the time while they are well to pass on to their children their own income generating skills: subsistence or cash crop farming, beer brewing, weaving and cloth making, carpentry, and so on. Parents, particularly in urban areas, have opened bank accounts for their children and both men and women have made wills, often discussing their wishes with village or political leaders or with their family elders. They have taken the time to put their affairs in order before God and men. They have also used the knowledge of their infection status in sexual and fertility decision making.

Often knowing one's infection status creates a will to live as long and as well as possible, particularly when one knows others who are living well and happily and as these long-term survivors of HIV infection become more known and studied. The creation of this will to live well and long is, perhaps, one of the greatest challenges that this epidemic offers to Africa.

The length of time a person will live after infection is also influenced by whether or not they prevent themselves from being reinfected and by nutrition, exercise and lifestyle, including alcohol and drug use. It is directly influenced by the support and care they receive after being tested from their families, their carers, their friends and from other infected people and by whether they are in productive employment. Often HIV-infected people become HIV educators and counsellors.

The length and quality of their lives will also be dependant on whether they have access to the treatment of common infections such as pneumococcal pneumonia, salmonella and TB. Hence their ability to live long and well as HIV infected, to continue in productive employment and to care for their families is directly dependent on the health care sector and its priorities.

There are very few African studies on the impact that being tested for HIV has on people's lives. But a small recent study in Zimbabwe showed a gender difference in the impact, in particular in communication with one's partner after getting a positive HIV result. All the men who were married and living with their wives informed their wives of their results. All of their wives accepted their diagnosis, that is, accepted that their husbands were infected. All of the wives then went, themselves, to be tested. Both the husbands and the wives reported consistent condom use after diagnosis. Only those marriages with a previous history of marital discord broke up.

All except one of the married women in the study informed their husbands of their diagnosis but only half of their husbands accepted the diagnosis and only half of the husbands went to be tested. Less than half of the husbands consistently used condoms after the diagnosis. As with the men, almost a quarter of the marriages broke up. Almost none of the single women tested told their partners since they were afraid of being stigmatised and of having their infection status known all around town.

Less than five per cent of the women in the study earned enough money to support themselves.

Tnis small study would seem to show the importance of motivating men to be tested and counselled. Their wives are more accepting of the diagnosis and there is more consistent condom use after diagnosis.

Thus, creating a desire among people, and perhaps especially men, to know their infection status could help break through the barriers of fear and denial, could decrease the powerlessness of women to prevent themselves from becoming infected, could make people more active participants in national HIV/AIDS programmes and could lead to their greater empowerment, whether their results were negative or positive.

In breaking the silences that surround this epidemic, families may better survive and cope and nations better control their destiny.

22

A Call Beyond Duty

Mr. Alpha Boubacar Diallo
Co-ordinator, UNDP's Regional
Project in Sub-Saharan Africa

It is one of the merits of the Nairobi (1987) and Niamey (1989) conferences on Safe Motherhood to have brought to the attention of the international community the true dimension and nature of the long neglected and tragic problem of maternal mortality. Their call for action has produced an encouraging mobilization of international and national institutions and organization, with new studies of the problem being undertaken and new national programmes being developed.

While there is a consensus that the most appropriate approach to solving the problem of maternal mortality has to be multisectoral and multidisciplinary, most of the strategies developed so far have put the major emphasis on a medical solution, with sometimes limited socio-economic supporting interventions. By contrast, the socio-cultural dimension has so far received very little attention in both referenced studies and in the development of national programmes. In most cases, socio-cultural conditions have been lumped in with the socio-economic factors.

One of the reasons for this situation could be the bias of research towards quantitative methodologies. Another reason is the understandable caution required in handling cultural values, together with a judgment that these are difficult to change.

Is the omission of the socio-cultural dimension justified for any understanding of such a sensitive, intimate, complex but also important phenomenon as is human reproduction? In doing so, are we running the risk of overlooking some key primary causes in the pursuit of symptoms and secondary causes? This has serious implications for the effectiveness of strategies designed to bring about the conditions essential and necessary for assuring safer motherhood for millions of women, particularly in the developing world.

It was during a 6000 km journey through rural Senegal in 1989 to collect data for a study[1] on maternal mortality that the importance of the socio-cultural dimension was clearly illustrated. We were privileged to a wide spectrum of rich experiences. Some were unusual, many were dramatic and most were deeply moving. From this mass of data, impressions and feelings, two critical impressions stand out.

First, a strong connection was established with the women we met. The success of our approach was thus predicated on an ability to explain the purpose of the study, and consequently to gain the active support of the host community through an equal partnership. One outcome was our strong sense of moral obligation to improve the fate of these women, and to help them avoid the tragedy of maternal mortality, a risk they face during each and every pregnancy.

The second observation is that, while the team felt that the findings of the study had made some significant contribution to the understanding of factors affecting maternal mortality through a systematic investigation of factors contributing to maternal death in both the health system and the community; including the modelling of demand and supply for obstetric services; the development of an index of obstetric risks; the correlation between risk and knowledge; the distance from a health centre, etc., our Report could only capture a small fraction of the reality that we had experienced.

Beneath the reality open to study with the tools and methodologies generally used to analyze the phenomenon of maternal mortality lie other crucial determinants. Understanding these could be essential if one is ever to develop effective strategies which reduce rates of maternal mortality in West Africa.

Let us explore the nature and consequences of these determinants and their implications for the development of effective strategies for substantially reducing maternal mortality.

These determinants are best summarized by the expression: *"a tora mousso kele la"*, which in Bambara is an expression used for the loss of life of a woman in childbirth. The equivalent is: *"she fell on the battlefield in the line of duty"*.

The internal logic and corresponding concepts embodied in this expression are an integral part of a larger reality, namely a system of societal beliefs developed through the ages to manage a major event: the procreation process. As with any such system, society also develops a related set of practices, customs, and normatively sanctioned behaviours within its accepted values which become elements of its culture.

From the onset and throughout the field trip we were to discover the importance of the socio-cultural dimension.

The initial indication came from our first community

interview. To compensate for the small size of our sample and improve the reliability of our results, we chose to collect the data from three independent sources. For data on maternal deaths we used the local government official census documents, the health services statistics, and the community official records, and then carried out our indepth interview of community leaders. We then checked for inconsistencies and discrepancies.

We soon discovered that for the collective memory of the community[2] that maternal death was a "non event". We could not get data from a direct question such as, How many maternal deaths occurred during a given time period? We had to devise a four-step approach. We started with the total number of deaths for the period. From this total we got the number of deaths to women. Then from the latter the number of deaths within the age bracket 15 to 45. Finally we correlated this number to known pregnancies and births.

Many significant determinants of maternal mortality can be attributed to a large extent to the "logical" implications of the Bambara expression.

Let us examine some of these implications and their consequences for maternal mortality. Finally we can see how these elements will affect the choices for an effective set of strategies for the development of programmes for safer motherhood.

The implicit assumptions underlying the Session are:

(1) Childbirth is assimilated to a battle.

(2) Any battle, in essence, has inherent and unavoidable associated risks. Among the risks are casualties and deaths.

(3) It is the duty, not to say destiny, of women to have to go through this battle in order to achieve the ideal family size required by the norms of society.

(4) As a "warrior", the pregnant woman is valued for her bravery, expressed in terms of stoicism.

(5) In preparation for the battle, the major emphasis is centered around psychological coping strategies for achieving the stoic stance.

(6) Society, for its part, develops strategies to transcend the adversity of an eventual casualty; in this instance, maternal death.

(7) The phenomena of both is beyond our power to understand: being supernatural.

(8) It is also beyond our abilities to defend ourselves against this phenomenon through ordinary measures.

(9) Thus traditional interventions will be on the plane of metaphysics.

In most of West Africa many key issues related to the ways devised by society to manage the phenomenon of reproduction have serious impact on a number of determinants of maternal mortality. A fuller understanding of the problem would thus require consideration of the socio-cultural context. From this perspective, a key cultural parameter is the importance given to the continuation of lineage. It is deeply rooted in the world view of the society and shapes its value system.

> **Using a battle as a metaphor for childbirth emphasizes the recognition by society of the high level of risk associated with giving birth. The women are called upon to fight this risky battle as a matter of DUTY. The fate of women is thus subordinated to the realization of the requirements for the continuation of the lineage.**

The first requirement for the continuation of the lineage is the value placed on childbearing. In the scale of social values childbearing is elevated to a virtue which confers high social status. On the other hand, a stigma is attached to a childless woman who is often regarded as tainted with sin and, at worst, with evil. In parts of West Africa, where funeral rites play an important function in social relations, the ultimate punishment is reserved for barren women and for those losing their life in childbirth They are denied normal funeral rites and are buried secretly at night outside the village. It is a case of the society reserving it harshest punishment for its innocent victim.

By focussing on fertility to satisfy the continuity of the lineage, women are under strong pressures to bear children. Most studies have shown that it is only after 6 to 8 surviving offspring that a substantial majority of African women wish to stop childbearing. But under prevailing conditions of high infant mortality, to insure the probability of survival of the desired optimum family size condemns women to repeated and frequent pregnancies. In part, this may explain the high fertility rates still observed in most of Africa and the associated high maternal mortality.

I was recently alerted to the strength of the value attached to childbearing even in a non-traditional urban environment. A well traveled and western educated professor of social sciences at an institution of higher learning, out of sympathy for the "desperate" situation of her sister who has been unable to bear children, decided to get pregnant for her sister. This is viewed as a proof of deep love. Her sister will raise the child as her own.

The consequences of numerous and frequent pregnancies in order to attain a socially determined ideal family size expose African women to a higher lifetime risk of maternal death (1 in 21) compared with women in northern Europe (1 in 9.850).

The responsibility for the fulfillment of the requirements for the continuation of the lineage is vested in the clan. This exclusive social organization is characterized by a strong interrelationship of mutual support and obligations binding the members together. It is governed by the principle of subordination of individual interests to those of the group. The notion of duty is toward the group: the extended family. The role of women in the reproduction process is subordinated to the requirement of maintaining the "viability" of the extended family. She is a passive actor called upon to fulfill with "dignity" and "modesty" her ascribed duties.

I have often been baffled by the extravagance of naming ceremonies in West Africa. Even in periods of deep economic crisis, these are grandiose festive events requiring lavish expenditure way beyond what the majority of the population could afford. In this always well-attended event, the mother of the newborn is conspicuously anonymous in the group of women. What is being celebrated is not even the newborn but first and foremost the lineage and, secondly, its strengthening through the name given. This is amplified by the *"griot"*[*] in his litany on the pedigree of the extended family. This glorification calls for lavish rewards to the benefit of the griots.

While preparing this paper, I had a discussion with a medical doctor friend. She related a recent incident and how hurt and angry it made her. While recuperating from a cesarian section in a private clinic, the aunts of her new-born burst into her room. She was barely greeted and all the attention was focussed on the baby. They had come to take the baby for the naming ceremony. She was left by herself to endure both physical and emotional pain. *"She was only doing her duty"!*

One consequence of this subordination of the individual to the "greater good" of the group, the extended family, is that the major decisions during the reproduction process which affect the whole life of women are outside their control. Society is depriving them of the authority for autonomous decision making in this vital event in their lives. They are *powerless* in making the decisions that shape their fate. During our field trip we came across over and over again cases requiring an urgent medical evacuation to a nearby health center being unduly delayed or not acted upon because the husband, whose consent for such a decision was required, was either working in the field or absent.

While this could be expected in a traditional social setting, women do not fare better in the modern health delivery system. Here they are subjected to mutually reinforcing sets of unfavour able circumstances. While the health providers have acquired the medical skills based on scientific knowledge, their behaviour is shaped by the prevailing traditional social values that they have retained. They operate in a health structure model inherited from the former colonial power in which the decision making process is the exclusive, unchallenged privilege and prerogative of health providers. It should be remembered that the bulk of expatriate medical personnel was then made up of military health providers. Finally the maze of bureaucratic hurdles with unpredictable rules changing according to the mood, personality or personal interest of each agent can severely limit the access of health services in emergencies for those without connections or wealth.

It has been estimated in a major urban center that in the great majority of the SMI (MCH centers) it took only six minutes for most of the midwives to conduct a normal prenatal consultation with a predominance of one-way communication[1]. It is also not uncommon to see visiting teams being taken through the delivery room while a woman is in labour without ever seeking her prior permission or consent.

The study project offices were located in a major urban SMI. I once witnessed the heroic efforts of a caring resident doctor to secure admission for an emergency case patient into the hospital. The patient had been shuttling back and forth between health facilities. Finally, as a last resort, the supervisor advised the doctor to deposit the patient at the entrance of the hospital and hope for a miracle, so that she could at least attend to her heavy case load at the SMI.

In order to fulfill their ascribed "duty" to the extended family, the whole life cycle of women is affected. From childhood she will be prepared to play her roles of wife and mother. At a very tender age she will be initiated to demanding domestic work while her brothers are spending most of their time playing children's games. In any compound it is common to see little girls helping their mothers while the little boys are roaming free of responsibilities. In most cases she will be eating with the women. A well-bred wife is expected to reserve the best portions for her husband. The little girl will share the meals with the women and most probably receive less in terms of nutrition than her brothers. Because her destiny is first and foremost to be a good wife and mother, she will have less chance for formal education or training than boys. In our study, only 7 per cent of the women could read. Because of the very strong social stigma attached to the status of unmarried women, the family is under strong pressure to marry her to the first convenient party. In most cases, this will be at an age when her body is not yet ready for childbearing. In our study, 7 women out of 10 had their first birth before they reached 17 year . Because of the dishonour on the family name attached to pregnancies outside marriage, unwanted pregnancies are kept secret and preferably terminated through clandestine abortion under less than optimal sanitary conditions — a major cause of maternal deaths.

The preparation of young women for safe motherhood is totally inadequate. In terms of acquisition of a useful knowledge base, this is most often limited to reassurances about the menstrual process along with advice on personal hygiene. Pregnancy, delivery and care of the newborn is seldom explored in detail. If it is, it will be in the form of metaphors requiring guesses at the true meaning. Further, the code of behaviour set up by society does not allow for frank discussion between a mother and daughter on reproductive matters. Even if this was possible, its usefulness would be limited because the society does not seem to have accumulated a practical knowledge base to systematically pass on from one generation to the next. The information transmitted takes the form of "stories" among peers or parables from the older generation which are very difficult to decipher for a young woman with little life experience.

In our study we attempted to determine the knowledge base of our target population on indications of a normal pregnancy, complications during pregnancy and delivery. On the scale of the knowledge index we developed, 58 per cent scored low, 36 per cent average and only 7 per cent high. We did find a correlation between a higher score and having experienced the event themselves and also being at a greater distance from a health center. When presented with facts indicating a probability of a severe hemorrhage some of the women we interviewed indicated that they believed this to be a good sign because the body was eliminating the bad blood to be replaced by new blood.

Contrary to the inadequacy of preparing young women for safer motherhood in terms of useful factual information, the psychological preparation receives a major emphasis. The desired outcome is to increase the threshold of tolerance to physical pain. This is to be demonstrated through stoic behaviour. A common example is the advice given to young women to be prepared to endure a level of effort equal to that which would be required to produce water by pressing hard enough on a stone. The pains of delivery are endured in expectation of harder moments to come. One is surprised and relieved after delivery not to have gone through the dreaded anticipated level of pain. The desirable heroic stance is usually rewarded by lavish praise for the demonstrated courage and admiring compliments from the women attending the new mother and also from the family members and the community. A less than "heroic" behaviour is the subject of verbal abuse and scorn. At this point a paradox is worth exploring. The midwives in maternity wards are notorious for their ill treatment of their patients. One would have expected a more supportive behaviour because of their training, the ethics of the medical profession and the fact that they also are mothers. On close examination one can see that their behaviour is quite similar to that of the traditional birth attendants when confronted with similar situations. Their behaviour is culturally determined and is guided by the norms requiring the mother to maintain a stoic stance. Because of this stoicism, vital life threatening signals that require urgent and immediate action are suppressed and not communicated until too late, leading to tragic loss of life.

In place of a body of practical knowledge capable of insuring safer motherhood, traditional society has developed a supernatural set of explanations for the phenomenon of reproduction. This has led to the attitude that the phenomenon is beyond the power of rational understanding. This being so, there are no concrete steps that can be taken to modify a predetermined outcome. The interventions to secure a favourable outcome will be in the realm of metaphysics and call for traditional para-psychological therapy.

The consequence of these attitudes is a large number of non-assisted births. Our findings indicate that only 2 out of 5 women received assistance from a qualified birth attendant during delivery. It is worth noting that traditional birth attendants usually intervene only during the last phase of delivery — the expulsion. Further if they intervene in case of complications, they are more likely to increase the risk to the life of the mother and baby by ill-timed, unsafe and intrusive interventions to speed up the process.

Society has developed coping strategies of *"denial"* for dealing with maternal mortality which is treated as a "non-event" in the collective memory of the community. This attitude of *"denial"* is also found among health providers at all levels of the health services. As pointed out by Pr Fadel Diadhiou of the Dantec Teaching Hospital, maternal death is too often viewed as "daily occurrence dramatically common".[5] He has been working with great dedication to bring about a change in this prevailing attitude. He keeps emphasizing to his students and staff that each maternal death should be regarded as a dramatic event which should mobilize the conscience of each health provider so as to make it an event as rare as possible.

Those who are advocating caution on the ground of sensitivity or respect for the integrity of the host culture have to weigh this against the fact that any delay in ACTING NOW is to condone the avoidable cruel and unjust death of millions of innocent women (one death every minute).

A closer examination will show that methodological considerations are not a real obstacle to the inclusion of socio-cultural variable in our study of maternal mortality.

These quantitative methodologies do not necessarily always lead to effective policies and programmes and qualitative methods can yield valuable results in terms of effective strategies. While quantitative methods demonstrate possible relationships between dependent and independent variables, as well as the strength or significance of the relationship, qualitative methods allow a more general understanding of the phenomena under investigation by analyzing it within the sub-system of which it constitutes an element. This requires first an understanding of the internal logic of the sub-system along with its relation to the larger system. Only then can the logical sequencing of the chain of causality be established. From this chain the key variables can be identified along with their relative significance in explaining phenomena. In our case study, we focussed on the dominance of the centrality of the continuity of the lineage in the socio-cultural value system as a key element in understanding maternal mortality.

The results of our analysis of the system can be used for programme development. Identification of key parameters permits the design of effective strategies so as to affect events along the chain of causality in order to achieve desired outcomes. Programme effectiveness will be enhanced by testing the consistency of a selected strategy with the internal logic of the system.

For example, in the case of socio-cultural values affecting some important determinants of maternal mortality in West Africa, we can for the purpose of programme design consider two enabling factors. These are the moral duties of children toward their mother, and the web of mutual obligations required from the members of the extended family.

While society in West Africa confers status to women bearing children, this translates into worship of mothers by their children. As a rule of thumb, insulting a peer could lead to a quarrel; if it is someone's father, this could escalate to a serious conflict. Insulting someone' s mother, he will have to fight if he is a man of honour, even if he is sure of loosing the battle. The implied moral foundation of mother worship is the debt of gratitude owed to the one who has given us the gift of life. Mother worship is an important element of the values system. Since society requires a fight to preserve the honour of one' s mother, to be consistent it cannot require less to preserve her life particularly when she is giving the gift of life. Therefore, society will have to promote safer motherhood. This, in turn, implies the need to remove the *"denial"* surrounding the tragedy of maternal mortality. This will necessitate that society finally come to terms with this tragedy and give it the too long overdue priority it deserves. Only then can we have genuine community mobilization of conscience, will and resources to address the problem.

This would be a major area of strategy design for programme development. Some immediate outcomes of this social mobilisation would be a substantial reduction in the workload presently required from pregnant women, the removal of food taboos for better nutrition and reallocation of financial resources from name giving ceremonies to pre-natal and natal care. An example is the practice on the island of Goree for friends and family to contribute for every pregnant woman toward acquiring a layette. The island is linked with the mainland by a ferry boat only during the day. The maternity is lacking the bare essentials, as is often the case. The layette is meant to solve these problems; it will usually have the minimum required supplies for safe delivery and post natal care for the newborn. As far as accessibility is concerned, the great majority of the rural population in West Africa lives on "islands".

The web of mutual obligations characteristic of extended family translates in the area of health into a system of continuous support through physical presence of relatives and friends. In sharp contrast to the western need for privacy in such circumstances, in West Africa this would be perceived as a form of punishment through isolation and exclusion from the group. With some exceptions, the layout of health services has not yet come to terms with the reality that the family will move in with the patient.

Curiously, a notable exception to providing this network of support through physical presence is with birthing. Tragically it is when the woman is most in need of physical, material and emotional support that she is left by herself to cope with the challenges of childbearing. This is even more tragic with the case of a large number of inexperienced young women with their first child.

A second major area of strategy design for prograrnme development could be the extension of this support system to childbearing. Again, society, to be consistent with the value accorded to childbearing cannot deny the necessary support required to achieve the desired outcome. To this end, two basic premises in the belief system which hold that—the phenomenon of childbearing is beyond our understanding and, secondly, that it is beyond our power to modify the course of events, have to be shown to be no longer valid. The realization by society of the possibilities for ACTION which would enhance favourable outcomes will give the necessary purpose to extending the support system to childbearing and safer motherhood.

This new knowledge and understanding of the attitudes of the community could impact now on several determinants of maternal mortality. Thus, identifying the web of the family support system could promote a more systematic follow-up of each pregnancy and an earlier identification of problems. It provides a mechanism for more rapid decision making in case of emergencies, even in the absence of the husband. Most importantly, it could drastically reduce the number of unattended deliveries. Finally, the positive psychological impact on pregnant women cannot be underestimated.

A major element for the success of the extended support system would be the role to be played by traditional birth attendants since they are already an integral part of the community. The experience of Professor Fall in Khombole, Senegal has shown that trained and supervised birth attendants over a period of years have achieved significantly better results in reducing maternal mortality than midwives in the formal health service. This opens up the possibility of solving the problems resulting from unattended deliveries in a very short time period. The role of traditional birth attendants in this strategy should not be one of an inexpensive substitute for para-medical personnel but should be that of an active agent of social change within their community.

One important result of the Nairobi and Niamey conferences is the Safe Motherhood Initiative. Since then, there has been an increase in interest for the problem of maternal mortality. More research has been undertaken. Some countries have initiated programme development activities. A broad approach was recommended in recognition of the fact that a combination of factors: medical, socio-economic and cultural, affect maternal mortality.

So far, most of the studies and corresponding programmes have put most of the emphasis on strategies based on medical solutions. This bias can partly be explained by the choice of variables. These studies are centered around intermediate and proximate factors affecting maternal mortality but underlying factors such as socio-cultural parameters have been notably neglected. This approach has serious shortcomings and inevitably limits the effectiveness of the corresponding public policy strategies. Analyzing only some elements of a phenomenon in isolation can lead to erroneous conclusions when used as a basis for decisions affecting the whole system.

An illustration is the study by Harrison in Northern Nigeria[6] on the effect of the health care and intensive nutrition programme for pregnant women in relation to operative delivery due to fetopelvic disproportion. He concluded that, for a generation or more, for small women (150cm or less) there will be a rise of the-operative delivery rate for fetopelvic-disproportion due to gain in weight of the foetus. The absence of a programme to treat the increase in obstetric complications could lead to an increase in maternal mortality.

For programme development does this mean that health care and intensive nutrition only benefit the foetus? Unless there are adequate health services capable of treating the obstetric complications, should the nutrition programme be abandoned for small women?

Another shortcoming of an exclusively medical solution is

an implicit assumption that an effective demand exists and that the problem is primarily from the supply side. This is often not verified by the field realities. In our study, the analysis of demand and supply for obstetric services gave the following results: 83 per cent felt the need for the services, 79 per cent wanted them but only 39 per cent actually sought the services.

We visited 43 health facilities, including a newly built regional hospital. None could compare in cleanliness and comfort for the patient to a community built health post run by a dynamic group of women' s organizations but we were surprised to find out that it was seldom used. The reason was that the door was in full view of a regular meeting place for men. This lack of privacy discouraged many women from using the facility. After a meeting of community leaders, it was decided to move the meeting place.

This is not to imply that the medical solution is not essential to the solution of the problem of maternal mortality. It is a necessary but not sufficient condition. Medical and non-medical solutions are not mutually exclusive; in fact, they are complementary and allow synergy among activities. Without strategies dealing with the socio-cultural constraints and involving the active partnership of the community, health services even if they are appropriate and adequate, which is often not the case, will continue to be overwhelmed by the scope and complexities of the problem. For any programme to be effective, there is need for an optimum mix of strategies taking into consideration all the major factors in the chain of causal events that affect maternal mortality.

In the West African context, the problem of maternal mortality is deeply rooted in the socio-cultural value system of society. Since along the path all the factors that contribute to maternal health are interrelated, a viable programme has to take these into consideration for strategies to be effective. It is therefore essential not to omit the root causes. As one moves down the path, opportunities for effective interventions are missed while the probabilities of unfavourable outcomes increase. Unfortunately, this is too often the case with a great number of women reaching the health facilities too late to be saved, as is shown by higher maternal mortality ratios from most hospital service statistics.

"A tora mousso kele la"! If society is going to send the women to battle, then it must remove the mines from the battlefield. The necessary knowledge about the nature of the mines, their location and how to remove them is now available. It must also provide full support: material, physical and emotional. Finally, it should honour those who have been willing to give the precious gift of life sometimes at the risk of their own. It is a moral obligation for society to minimize casualties on the 'battlefield' of motherhood. One fundamental human right is the right to life. Safe motherhood is a

fundamental human right. There is no democracy without fundamental human rights being respected. The new hope for democratization in Africa will never be fulfilled as long as half of the population is denied a fundamental right: *safe motherhood.*

AND THE TIME FOR ACTION IS NOW!

NOTES

1. DIA, A., et a.l., "Rapport de la Deuxieme Mission D'Identification Pour la Reduction de la Mortalite Maternelle au Senegal".
2. The collective memory of the community is significant, particularly in societies with oral traditions. It constitutes a driving force of most social events.
3. Griot: Caste of traditional musician-entertainers of West Africa. They have an uncommon mastery of the spoken word. They are the depository of the history and traditions of the clan as well as the genealogies of important extended families.
4. Aissatou Lo, "Impact of Surveillance of High Risk Pregnant Women in Urban Areas".
5. Dia. A. et al. op. cit.
6. Harrison, K.A. "Predicting Trends in Operative Delivery for Cephalopelvic Disproportion in Africa". Lancet, April 7, 1990.

23

Behaviour Change: Some Analogies and Lessons from the Experience of Gay Communities

Adam Carr
Journalist and
HIV Consultant, Australia

1. The Gay Community and Behaviour Change

The HIV epidemic first made itself known to the world when it appeared among gay men* in the United States in 1979 and 1980: the first published account of the disease, in July 1981, described cases seen among gay men in Los Angeles, over the following three years AIDS appeared in the gay communities of all the developed countries. Although as early as 1982 cases of AIDS were seen in people other than gay men (male and female injecting drug users, recipients of HIV-contaminated blood products, heterosexual men and women including female sex workers and infants born to HIV-infected women), the great majority of diagnosed AIDS cases in most of the developed countries during the 1980s were seen in gay men.

The appearance of the HIV epidemic had an enormous impact on the gay communities** of the developed countries, and

* *The term "gay men" is used here to mean all men who have sex with other men, regardless of whether they identify as homosexual, bisexual or heterosexual.*

** *The term "gay community" referred originally to the community of gay men and lesbians. Lesbians increasingly do not accept that they share a community with gay men, and the term "gay and lesbian communities" has been adopted. Accordingly, I use the term "gay community" here to refer to the community of gay men.*

organisations to respond to the epidemic were formed in most countries by 1985. One of their most urgent tasks was to advise gay men how they could avoid contracting the disease. Before the discovery of HIV as the cause of the disease in 1983/84, the reason gay men were developing AIDS was unclear. It was therefore very difficult for gay men to protect themselves from it. Since, however, it was evident that HIV was sexually transmitted, gay community organisations (and government health authorities) recommended to gay men that they reduce the number of sexual partners they had. Many gay men followed this advice, some to the extent of ceasing to have sex at all.

In retrospect, though, it is evident that this advice was ineffective. Reducing the number of sexual partners does not significantly reduce the risk of contracting HIV infection in a population where infection is already widespread. It just slows the process down somewhat. In any case, men are extremely reluctant to accept advice even at the risk of their own lives. In this respect, at least, gay men are no different from man in general.

The discovery of HIV and the subsequent determination of the exact mechanisms of HIV transmission during sex between men enabled gay community organisations to make more specific recommendations to gay men. It became clear that unprotected anal intercourse was responsible for virtually all HIV transmission among gay men, and the correct and consistent use of condoms and water-based lubricant during anal sex would reduce the risk of HIV infection for gay men to close to zero.

These discoveries made it possible for gay community organisations to make recommendations to gay men which were both effective in preventing HIV infection and capable of being adopted in a sustained way by the majority of gay men. Few men enjoy using condoms, but the use of condoms for anal intercourse was a compromise between fear of HIV infection and fear of giving up sexual gratification which most gay men were prepared to accept and able to implement. While compliance with even this fairly minimal modification of sexual behaviour has been far from universal, it has been sufficiently widespread to reduce greatly the incidence of HIV infection among gay men in most developed countries.

I have referred to gay community organizations making "recommendations" to gay men about changes in sexual behaviour. In fact, of course, the process of bringing about behaviour change among most gay men was vastly more complicated than simply issuing recommendations. The populations of gay men in the developed countries are very diverse, and include a significant group of "submerged gay men (few of whom actually identify as gay) who are not in contact with the organised gay community. The gay communities are divided along lines of race, ethnicity, age, place of residence, educational level and social/economic status. Patterns of sexual behaviour among gay men differ considerably along these lines, and are further complicated by issues such as injecting drug use, use of alcohol and other recreational drugs, the sale of sex for money, trans-sexualism and other behavioural influences.

These considerations made the task of bringing about sustained and appropriate behaviour change among gay men an extremely complex one, and a task made more difficult three further factors: the great urgency imposed by the rapidly expanding number of gay men acquiring HIV infection, the lack of previous research into the sexual behaviour patterns of gay men, and the lack of models of successful campaigns to bring about rapid and widespread changes in personal behaviours. When gay community organizations undertook in the early 1980s the task of bringing about rapid, radical and sustained changes in the sexual behaviours of a large and diverse population of sexually-active men, they undertook to do something which had never been done before, in a very short period of time, and bereft of the usual resources, research data and analytical tools which usually accompany such major campaigns of social engineering.

2. Factors Influencing Behaviour Change Among Gay Men

By the late 1980s, however, these deficiencies had to some extent been addressed. A number ot major research projects had been carried out among gay men to find out more about their patterns of sexual behaviour, to monitor the speed and extent of behaviour change, and to determine the social and cultural factors which facilitated or impeded the process of behaviour change. One of the most far-reaching of these projects has been carried out in Australia. This is the Social Aspects of Prevention of AIDS (SAPA) project, a joint undertaking of the AIDS Council of NSW (a gay community non-government organization) and the School of Behavioural Sciences of Macquarie University, Sydney.

In 1986 and 1987, SAPA researchers conducted extensive interviews with 535 Australian gay men, and have been analyzing the results since, issuing their findings in regular instalments since 1988. Report No. 7, The Importance of Gay Community in the Prevention of HIV Transmission, appeared in April 1990. The report consists mainly of a statistical analysis of the relationship between the interviewees' attachment to the gay community (measured by several criteria) and the degree, appropriateness and speed of the changes in their sexual practices in response to the HIV epidemic.

The report's conclusion is worth quoting at length.

"In general, gay community attachment and locale are important predictors of change. These data speak to the importance of informed social support. It appears that educators who stress the need to address communities from the point of view of the communities themselves are correct. Gay community and locale are also implicated in the relationship between knowledge and change. Knowledge of "safe sex", something that to some extent only the gay communities dealt with in their media and educational campaigns, is also implicated in change.

This study does point to the importance of gay community attachment to sexual behaviour change ... sexually-confident, well-educated (about safe sex) gay men ... who are sexually and socially engaged with gay community ... are more likely to have changed their sexual behaviour than gay men who are not attached to gay community.

It is evident that education campaigns should continue to be informed by gay communities and that the men who perhaps are most at risk are those who are not reached by gay community campaigns. Men who for whatever reason are separate from any form of attachment to gay community need special attention.

In general, men who have contact with others, via attachment to gay community, sexual, social or cultural/political, are most likely to have changed their sexual practice. They have the informed social support necessary to modify their behaviour. Men who are isolated from others like themselves and (who) are unattached to gay community in any form are those least likely to change."

The SAPA research demonstrates that the most important component of preventing HIV infection among gay men is their willingness to identify themselves as gay, and to become "sexually-confident, well-educated gay men, who are sexually and socially engaged with community". Other Australian research has supported this view. Sinnott and Todd (1988) found that the most important source of accurate information about HIV transmission and prevention available to men who have sex with men is the material produced by gay community organizations and distributed within the gay community. Bennett et al. (1989) found that men who find male sexual partners in public places such as parks ("beats"), and who have a low rate of self-identification as gay and a low level of contact with the gay community, also have a much higher rate of unsafe sexual practice and therefore a higher risk of HIV infection.

The conclusion of this research seems clear. Men who identify as gay, who are confident in that identification, who are socially, culturally or politically active in the gay community and who find their sexual partners in the gay community, are much more likely to have accurate knowledge about HIV infection, than are men who have sex with men who are not attached to the gay community. They are also much more likely to act on that knowledge by making appropriate and sustained changes to their sexual practice.

It is therefore clear that bringing about appropriate and sustained behaviour change among gay men has not just been a matter of producing information about HIV and safe sex and distributing it to individuals. Behaviour change among gay men has resulted from a community wide response to the epidemic, which has sought to use the existing communication networks and value systems of the gay community to influence the collective behaviour of that community. New community values about acceptable and unacceptable sexual behaviours have been established, and have been enforced by community opinion, a far more effective way of enforcing standards of behaviour than coercion by the state.

The experience of the gay communities in the developed countries is not uniform. The Australian gay community, on which the SAPA research is based, has had certain advantages not enjoyed by some other communities: a high degree of racial and linguistic uniformity, concentration in a small number of cities, government funding, a supportive social and political environment to carry out prevention work, and access to a cadre of skilled community activists to design and carry out both the programmes and the research which has guided them. But in broad terms the experience of the Australian gay community has echoed those of the other developed countries. Rapid and massive behaviour change can be brought about through community-based programmes.

Since 1985 or so a number of studies have been undertaken, in the United States, Australia and other developed countries, to determine the reasons why some gay men have adapted to the demands of behaviour change in response to HIV and AIDS more readily than others.

The SAPA studies have cast some light on this subject, as have American studies such as the Multi-Centre AIDS Cohort Study (MACS), which has followed thousands of gay men over several years to monitor their behaviour and the factors influencing it.

The findings of these studies and others like them, taken together, show that a number of identifiable groups of men are at continuing risk of HIV infection. These are:

men under 25

men with low educational and literacy levels

men from non-English-speaking backgrounds

men who use alcohol and recreational drugs while having sex
men who do not identify as gay or as part of the gay community (this factor has already been discussed above.

An additional, perhaps more surprising, finding was that gay men in relationships were more likely to be at risk of infection than were men who were not in relationships.

These groupings reveal distinct social co-factors for HIV infection among gay men.

Age is clearly one of the most important of these factors, because it relates to several of the others. Many younger people are likely to use alcohol and "soft" drugs while having sex. Many young gay men have low incomes. Young people of all sexual orientations are prone to the opinion that nothing bad can happen to them, and this is aggravated in the case of HIV risk by the fact that, because of the eight to ten year incubation period of HIV, few gay men under 25 have many friends with diagnosed AIDS. Young men are also less likely to have formed firm sexual self-identifications or to have developed strong gay community links, which are important in building a sense of the immediacy of the HIV threat and of responsibility for one's own and one's partner's health.

The issue of the relationship between social and economic status, of which educational levels and literacy skills are generally assumed to be indicators, and sexual behaviour among gay men is a complex and controversial one, and has been bedeviled by a politically-motivated preoccupation with identifying (or creating) a category of "working-class gay men". Gay men have a peculiar occupational structure, heavily weighted to white collar and service occupations, with many transient, part-time and shift workers. This blurs traditional distinctions of class. In addition, many young gay men from working-class backgrounds find that the gay community offers contacts and opportunities, and a ladder to higher-status occupations and incomes.

Nevertheless, many gay men still have limited educational levels and poor literacy skills, partly because of the alienation that many gay men feel from their peers during the period of accepting a gay identity, which coincides for many with the years of higher secondary education. Low literacy cuts many gay men off from the gay print media and print-based HIV educational campaigns waged by gay community organisations, which, as Sinnott and Todd showed, have been the most important sources of information about HIV and AIDS and about sate sex. and are also an important source of positive reinforcement for gay identity and community involvement.

In Australia, which does not have the deep racial divide which characterises the United States, issues of ethnicity and linguistic background are still important factors influencing the ability of gay men to adopt and sustain behaviour change. Most developed countries now have large populations of first or second-generation immigrants, many of them from developing countries, and many of them maintaining cultural and religious traditions which mark them off from the culture of the host country.

Gay men in these ethnic communities, who often do not identify as gay, suffer a double crisis of identity, in that they are violating their communities' accepted standards of behaviour by being gay, while being isolated from the host countries' gay community by cultural or linguistic barriers. This cuts many men off from the behaviour change messages which the gay community organisations are producing, usually in English and usually using an imagery and a vocabulary derived from the majority culture.

Alcohol and other recreational drugs have been identified as among the major villains of the HIV epidemic in the gay communities. Alcohol, it is said, lowers self-control, heightens self-delusion and makes previous decisions about safe sex harder to stick to. The fact that so many gay men find their sexual partners in places where alcohol is served make this a chronic problem. Many health educators, however, argue that the belief that alcohol makes men incapable of controlling their sexual behaviour is a myth, and a myth which serves the interests of men in many contexts. They argue that men use alcohol as an excuse to engage in sexual (and other) behaviours which they know to be socially unacceptable.

It may seem contradictory to say that gay men in relationships are at higher risk than gay men who have multiple sexual partners. There are two factors operating here. The first is that most highly sexually-active gay men have been acutely aware that they at high risk for a long time. They were the first to be targeted, and many long ago adapted to the discipline of safe sex. The sex-centered, antiromantic "culture of promiscuity" that exists around the saunas and sex clubs has served as an effective agent of behaviour change for many of these men. On the other hand, many gay men who think of themselves as relationship-centered and "not promiscuous" have been slow to perceive their own risk.

3. Lessons of the Gay Communities' Experience with Behaviour Change

It may seem a heroic leap to try to use the experiences of gay men in affluent societies to find lessons for reducing the impact of the HIV epidemic among the majority of people at risk of HIV infection in the world: men, women and children in the developing countries. But it is not an impossible task. Despite the enormous differences in circumstances and contexts, there are some underlying similarities in the experiences of the two populations which can be usefully studied.

This is particularly so when we remember that it is the sexual behaviour of men which is the fundamental behavioural problem in preventing the further spread of HIV infection in most parts of the world. The HIV epidemic in the developing countries is increasingly being understood to be a consequence of the sexual and social subordination of women in those countries. This is evidenced by a pattern of infection in which men are the vectors of infection and women the principal subjects of infection: married men who have multiple sexual partners are infecting their wives, who are prevented by economic and social restraints from protecting themselves from infection.

There are those who may feel that it is impossible to induce men to forgo sexual gratification and adopt socially responsible behaviours. The experience of behaviour change in the gay communities suggests that this is not so. The gay communities are, after all, communities of men. The gay communities offer a unique opportunity to study the sexual behaviour of men.

That the behaviour change campaigns mounted by gay community organisations have succeeded to the extent that they have in bringing about rapid and sustained change in the sexual behaviours of gay men, without resort to any kind of coercive mechanism, offers hope that changing the sexual behaviours of heterosexual men is not beyond the scope of human ingenuity.

It is difficult to judge how far the social and behavioural risk factors which have been identified as making some gay men more likely than others to engage in behaviours likely to expose them to HIV infection are applicable to other risk populations, and particularly to people in developing countries. Clearly HIV infection in heterosexual populations raises issues around gender and power imbalances between men and women which do not arise in the gay communities. It seems clear, too, that the sale of sex plays a greater role in the proliferation of HIV infection in these countries than it does in the gay communities. Nevertheless, it may be possible to draw some analogies from the research about the risk factors which have been identified among gay men.

Among the more likely candidates for social risk factors among heterosexual populations in developing countries are drug and alcohol use and relationship status. Men in all cultures use alcohol and recreational drugs of various kinds as social disinhibitors, and drinking or drug use frequently accompanies sexual activity. The extent to which alcohol abuse by heterosexual men contributes to the subsequent HIV infection of women, both sex workers and wives, is something which can be determined only by research on the spot, but it seems a fair bet, on the analogy of the experience of the gay communities, that a link will be found. If it is, it is important to remember research in the gay communities: that the link between alcohol use and unsafe sexual behaviour is not that alcohol deprives men of the ability to control their sexual behaviour, but that it gives them an excuse to behave in ways which they know would be otherwise unacceptable. The exposure of that excuse goes a long way to ending the ability of men to use alcohol in this way. Gay community HIV organisations have run campaigns stating this explicitly, such as the "Drugs and Alcohol: No Excuse" campaign of the Victorian AIDS Council.

The analogies between the transmission of HIV within gay male relationships and its transmission within marriage in developing countries is harder to develop, because of the obvious fact that a gay relationship is a voluntary and informal (in a legal sense) relationship between two men, and any power dimensions that exist within it have been largely invented by the participants, whereas a marriage is a relationship between a man and woman, contracted in law and carrying with it the legacy of centuries of accumulated tradition and assumption about gender power distribution. A marriage is usually an economic relationship as well, involving the economic dependence of the woman. Nevertheless, it may be pointed out that the belief among many gay men that participation in a monogamous relationship somehow confers immunity from HIV infection may have some parallels in heterosexual relationships. It has been pointed out that, biologically, HIV in women is a disease of fidelity, not of promiscuity, since most women who contract HIV infection sexually do so from repeated exposure to a single infected man, usually their husband, rather than from single exposures to many infected men. Behaviour change campaigns which seek to promote monogamous relationships and marital fidelity will therefore be singularly inappropriate in places where a high proportion of married men are already infected.

There are a number of lessons which may be drawn from the experiences of the gay communities in designing HIV behaviour change and prevention programmes in societies which may appear to have very little in common with those of the developed countries where most gay men live.

Information and Motivation

The first point is that the provision of information is not enough. In the early 1980s both governments and community-based organisations in the developed countries engaged in large-scale mass media and community campaigns to disseminate basic facts about HIV and AIDS and to stimulate community awareness of the disease. Some of these campaigns were restrained and confined to giving information. Others were frankly alarmist, such as the British "tombstones" campaign and the Australian "Grim Reapers" campaign. What they all had in common was their failure to bring about any significant changes in behaviour in their target populations.

Research shows that people do not change deeply-entrenched behaviour, such as sexual practices, simply on the basis of unintellectual awareness that the behaviour may be dangerous to them. A study of gay men in Los Angeles showed that those who were continuing to engage in unsafe sexual practices had exactly the same level of knowledge about HIV and safe sex as those who had adopted and maintained safe practices. The differences between the two groups were those of identity with the gay community, as discussed above. This reinforces the point that behaviour change among gay men in the developed countries has been brought about by community-based campaigns which promoted safe sex practices as a community standard of behaviour.

By contrast, populations at risk of HIV infection which have been subjected only to information-based mass media campaigns have failed to show any significant change in behaviour. An obvious example is sexually-active young heterosexuals, whose risk of HIV infection is substantial but who have failed to respond to media campaigns aimed at influencing their behaviour. There is an obvious and positive lesson here for developing countries: expensive and high profile media campaigns are ineffective in bringing about behaviour change. This is an important point for countries with limited resources and poorly developed mass media structures, and particularly those which do not have linguistic or cultural unity (such as Papua New Guinea, for example) which would find national media campaigns even more difficult.

Individuals and Communities

The second lesson is that behaviour change is not so much a process of individuals absorbing information and making rational decisions about their behaviour. It is much more a process of individuals changing their behaviour as a result of their membership of a community which is changing the standards of behaviour it expects from its members, because they identify with that community and wish to remain members of it.

The best example of this is condom use. Most gay men dislike using condoms, but have accepted that they should do so, not so much from a rational decision to use condoms because this is the best way to avoid HIV infection (although this is probably how the decision would be articulated), but because they are aware that the community of gay men to which they belong, from which they derive a sense of identity and of personal worth, and to which they wish to continue to belong, has now adopted condom use as its standard of behaviour, and condemns those who do not use them. The sanction for failure to use condoms is not so much HIV infection, a long-term and somewhat nebulous threat, especially for younger gay men who do not have personal experience of HIV, but disapproval and possible ostracism by their peers.

It follows from this that campaigns based on mobilising loyalty to and identification with specific communities offers the best hope for influencing the sexual behaviours of heterosexual men. While the gay community is a community of men who share a sexual orientation, and thus has certain unique advantages as a vehicle for influencing the sexual behaviours of its members, there is no reason why any pattern of community identification could not be adapted to the same purpose.

This is in fact precisely what has been attempted with other risk populations in the developed countries, such as female sex workers and injecting drug users. Some rudiments of community organisation and identification already existed among these populations before the advent of the epidemic. HIV organizations have sought to build on these foundations, creating a community infrastructure, and communications network to build a sense of community commitment to safe behaviours and a sense of solidarity in achieving and enforcing behaviour change in the emerging community. While the results of this strategy have been mixed, they have been at least partly successful in some places; notably in Australia, where the incidence of HIV infection among injecting drug users and female sex workers is extremely low by world standards.

Once again, of course, this is a strategy of building or, if necessary, creating communities based on an identity that relates directly to the risk behaviour involved; a community of female sex workers all share the risk behaviour of exchanging sex with men for money, and a community of injecting drug users all share the risk of behaviour of injecting drugs.

Whether it is possible to mobilise the identity of heterosexual men with other kinds of community, for example a religious community, a sporting community or a neighborhood community, to reinforce the need for changes to sexual behaviours is difficult to determine. But it is certainly possible to suggest that the mechanism of community identification and loyalty, and thus the need and desire to retain membership of the community by conforming to the expected pattern of behaviour of that community, still operates regardless of the nature of that community, and this mechanism is the mainspring of bringing about behaviour change through community-based programmes.

Greater and Lesser Evils

The third point is that behaviour change messages must give people realistic and sustainable choices. Few people welcome large-scale changes in their lives, particularly when these changes involve sacrificing behaviours which people find gratifying and which play a large role in forming their identities and sense of worth. When gay men were advised that they should abstain from sexual activity or radically reduce their number of sexual partners, most failed to respond, because these changes were too great to absorb into their lives. When the message was refined, and concentrated on the adoption of condoms for anal sex, there was a high level of acceptance, since this was a change which most gay men could accommodate without radical disruption to their lives.

The debate within gay community HIV organisations about oral sex is an instructive example of this. There have been a small number of documented cases of HIV transmission between gay men following the intake of semen during oral sex. Some gay community organisations feel that oral sex should therefore be included on the list of unsafe sexual practices which gay men should be advised to abstain from. Others have argued, however, that the risk of HIV infection through oral sex is so low, certainly many times lower than the risk of infection through unprotected anal sex, that making a recommendation against it would be counter-productive. Many men, it is argued, would look at a list of "prohibited" practices and conclude that they could not make such radical changes, and would therefore make no changes at all. It is better, in this view, to accept a continuing small risk of infection through oral sex in order to persuade the majority to abandon the really high risk activity, unprotected anal sex.

The analogy for developing countries may be that, since the really radical changes in behaviour needed to completely eliminate HIV infection cannot be achieved in the necessary time, because the intensity of community-based education needed to bring them about is too resource intensive, prevention efforts must focus on changes may be less effective in preventing HIV infection but which have a relatively low level of impact on people's lives and which thus have a greater chance of being adopted quickly.

Thus, in countries in which condoms are neither readily available, cheap nor culturally acceptable, that is, where men will not use them and women cannot compel them to do so, the best option may be to enable women, and particularly sex workers, to improve their level of genital health so that their risk of infection through unprotected vaginal intercourse is reduced to a level comparable to that of women in developed countries, where HIV infection among heterosexual women is spreading much more slowly than it is in developing countries. This strategy will buy time for a more comprehensive strategy, based perhaps on large-scale voluntary testing and partner notification, to be developed and implemented.

Horizontal and Vertical Education

The fourth point is that the source of information and education must always be as close as possible to the people who are the targets of the education campaign. Ideally, the source of the information and education should in fact belong to the population at risk of infection. This was a lesson which the gay communities in the developed countries learned only after some costly errors in the early years of the HIV epidemic. The initial educational campaigns mounted by gay community organisations were heavily media-based: they consisted of print materials such as posters and leaflets, and display advertisements in the gay print media.

As noted earlier, these campaigns were deficient in that they failed to communicate effectively with gay men who did not speak or, more commonly, read the language in which the campaign was being conducted or who lacked the literacy skills to take in the messages being put forward. But they were deficient in a more fundamental sense as well. Even though the source of these materials were gay community organisations, set up by gay activists who lived and worked in the gay community, they were still a form of vertical education: self-appointed experts were addressing messages to their communities through the impersonal medium of print. While these campaigns achieved considerable success, they failed to influence the behaviour of a large number of gay men in a sustained way.

By 1986 gay communities in some countries were evolving a more sophisticated form of HIV educations based on peer education models. While the gay activists and health professionals who worked for gay community organisations were in a sense the peers of the gay men they were seeking to educate, the techniques they were using were the same as those traditionally used by governments and other sources of authority to influence behaviour and guide opinion. Gay men, as a marginalised and in some senses oppressed group, tended to be sceptical of messages seen as deriving from sources of authority: This was particularly true of men who shared the social and behavioural characteristics discussed above which made them less likely to readily adopt appropriate behaviour changes.

The peer education strategies adopted by some gay community organizations were based on a philosophy of empowerment of individuals within the context of developing a stronger gay community. "Ordinary" gay men, that is, gay men who were not already HIV activists and were not professionally qualified were recruited to organise meetings of their friends, at which HIV and safe sex were discussed in the context of their own lives and relationships. In these small group discussions, gay men could discuss freely the difficulties and challenges of adapting to safe sex, could freely admit failures and lapses, and could offer each other support in sustaining behaviour change.

Men who "graduated" from these meetings were in turn recruited to organise more meetings, thus penetrating wider and wider strata of the gay community, and of the population of men who have sex with men but who do not identify as gay. Particular attention was paid to young men, to older men, to men from non-English-speaking backgrounds, to bisexual men, to men who injected drugs, to trans-sexuals and to male sex workers: all groups which had been identified as having particular difficulties in adapting to safe sex. More ambitious programmes were developed in some places: The "Gay Now" programme of the Victorian AIDS Council in Melbourne, Australia, organised large-scale meetings involving hundreds of gay men at which facilitators led discussions and activities both in small groups and for the whole meeting. Several thousand gay men participated in these meetings during this campaign.

While these peer education programmes were naturally uneven in their degree of sophistication and in their organisation, there is no doubt that they carried behaviour change messages to a much wider network of gay men than were being reached by more traditional behaviour change campaigns, or that these messages were being communicated more effectively in the highly personalised context of smallf group meetings than they could ever be through even the most sophisticated print campaigns.

The key to the success of gay community peer education campaigns was that behaviour change messages carry more impact when conveyed horizontally, by peers, than when they are conveyed vertically, by sources of authority to "the masses", and that individuals who are given the power to make decisions about their own lives in the context of a supportive community are far more likely to adopt and maintain appropriate behaviours than those who are spoon-fed behaviour change messages as passive and socially-isolated consumers. In this, of course, the gay communities simply rediscovered the techniques by which all knowledge was conveyed in periods before the evolution of mass communication systems.

There are models even more directly analogous, since HIV peer education campaigns have been mounted among female sex workers in some developed countries, including Australia. Their success has been less marked than that of the gay community campaigns, mainly because it is more difficult to empower female sex workers, who are usually young and economically marginalised, than it is to empower gay men, many of whom enjoy a degree of class and gender privilege. It is also much more difficult to construct a genuine community of female sex workers than it has been to construct a community of gay men. Few women positively want to be sex workers: it is harder to engender a sense of pride in being a sex worker than it is to spread a sense of pride in being a gay man. Nevertheless, HIV peer education campaigns among female sex workers have achieved some successes, and could serve as a model for campaigns among sex workers elsewhere.

4. Conclusion

In summary, there are a number of important lessons that can be drawn from the response of gay communities to the HIV epidemic. The first is that people do not change their behaviour on the basis of an intellectual awareness that the behaviour may be dangerous to them. Rather, one of the most important determinants of sustained change is membership of a community organization which actively promotes and supports such changes.

Secondly, behaviour change is less a process of individuals deciding to change than one of communities changing their standards of behaviour and values. Thirdly, behaviour change messages must give people realistic and sustainable choices from amongst which individuals and couples can choose according to their preferred sexual practices and the circumstances of their lives.

Finally, the source of information, advice and counselling should be as close as possible to the community, preferably within the community. Behaviour change messages carry more impact when delivered by friends and colleagues than by authorities. Further, having and being encouraged to exercise the power to make decisions about their own life within a supportive community is critical.

The relevance of these experiences to people at risk of HIV infection in developing countries should be obvious. The application of these lessons is independent of access to modern communication technology. Further, in countries where governments and other authority structures are either weak and ineffectual, or authoritarian and mistrusted, it is most unlikely that government directed behaviour change campaigns will have a great impact. A strategy which has at its centre the empowerment of oppressed and marginalised individuals and the development of strong and autonomous communities will enable women and men to protect themselves against HIV infection.

24

Carrying Out HIV Sentinel Surveillance

WHO-Regional Office for South East Asia, New Delhi

1. INTRODUCTION

During the past decade, the world has seen what appeared at first to be an illness largely confined to homosexual men and drug injectors in developed countries, become a pandemic affecting millions of men, women and children on all continents. The problem predominates in sub-Saharan Africa, Asia and much of Latin America and, by the year 2000, the infection rate among women will be equal to that of men. AIDS came later to the South-East Asia Region. The first reported AIDS case was in 1984 and HIV infections in most countries were reported in 1986 or later.

In order to better characterize the nature and the magnitude of the epidemic, HIV surveillance can play a very important role. HIV surveillance studies in India, Myanmar and Thailand documented an exceptional increase in HIV infections among female commercial sex workers, injecting drug users (IDU) and other population groups. Such data are essential for advocacy as well as planning purposes. Good surveillance data can be used not only to estimate the current magnitude of the problem and make future projections of HIV/AIDS, but also to assist decision-makers in instituting appropriate and rational intervention programmes. This paper describes the steps in establishing an HIV sentinel surveillance system and the use of data so obtained for programme purposes.

2. AIDS SURVEILLANCE: PROS AND CONS

AIDS surveillance refers to the collection of data on AIDS cases. However, because of the very long latent period (average 10 years) of the disease, the incidence of AIDS provides an indirect description of the underlying and preceding HIV epidemic.

Moreover, many AIDS patients may not be correctly diagnosed or some of them may not have contact with health services/facilities. Thus, the completeness of AIDS case reporting varies widely under different settings. The data generated by this "case reporting" system may therefore not be able to help recognize the current magnitude of the problem in the country or fully understand the dynamics of HIV transmission.

Nevertheless, AIDS is a notifiable disease in most countries and the surveillance of AIDS cases and deaths at national level can give information relevant to and necessary for organizing clinical management of patients with AIDS. Notwithstanding some of the constraints mentioned above, every attempt should be made to report AIDS cases. The diagnosis of AIDS is based on clinical and laboratory evidence. WHO case definition should be used according to the available diagnostic facilities.

Voluntary HIV testing should be offered to patients with symptoms compatible with AIDS. After having provided appropriate counselling, the serum from the patient would be first tested vith one ELISA or rapid/simple assay with higher sensitivity, and reactive samples retested with a test having higher specificity and using a different assay technique (based on different antigen preparations and/or different test principles). Serum reactive in both the tests is considered HIV antibody positive. Serum that is non-reactive in the first test is considered HIV antibody negative and that which is reactive in the first test and non-reactive in the second test is also considered HIV negative.

All health institutions at primary health care level should know how to diagnose a case, and those meeting the WHO case definition should be reported to the appropriate health authority. The national AIDS progxammes in turn should report summary data to WHO using the quarterly surveillance form (Annex 1).

3. HIV SURVEILLANCE

HIV surveillance can be defined as a collection of epidemiological information of sufficient accuracy and completeness regarding the distribution and spread of HIV infection to be relevant to the planning and implementation of HIV/AIDS prevention and control programme activities. Its objectives are to:

(1) determine the geographical spread of HIV infection;

(2) monitor the trends of HIV epidemic;

(3) provide information for estimates and future projections of HIV/AIDS in a country;

(4) use such data to mobilize the national political and social

leaders as well as to generate external support for the programme; and

(5) more importantly, provide useful data for appropriate planning of health and medical care services.

Since the primary objective of surveillance is to monitor trends in HIV infection over time and place, sen-surveys need to be conducted at repeated intervals using a consistent methodology in the same population group so as to demonstrate true change, if any, in HIV prevalence. The following epidemiological aspects should be considered while designing the surveillance procedure:

(1) HIV infections are not uniformly distributed in any population. The distribution of HIV infection in the population depends on the prevalence of certain behaviours or practices associated with an increased risk of HIV infection;

(2) There are limited major modes of HIV transmission, and not everyone in the population runs the same risk of HIV infection; and

(3) HIV infections were introduced into different geographical areas and populations at different times.

Sentinel surveillance is the method of choice for obtaining data on HIV infection rates in various population groups and thereafter for monitoring trends. It is therefore recommended that all national AIDS programmes establish HIV sentinel surveillance as soon as possible.

3.1 HIV Sentinel Surveillance

Sentinel surveillance means canying out cross-sectional studies (also known as prevalence surveys) of HIV prevalence rates at regular intervals among selected groups in the population known as "sentinel groups". In other words, with sentinel surveillance trends in HIV infection are monitored over time, by group and by place. Sentinel HIV surveillance can theoretically be community-based or clinic/health facility-based; the latter is much more convenient and hence should always be preferred.

The following procedures can be used for the plaming and implementation of HIV sentinel surveillance and for analysis of the data so obtained:

Planning

(a) Selection of the Sentinel Population and Sites

The first step towards the development of a sentinel

surveillance is the selection of the sentinel population. The population can be divided by transmission pattern into higher and lower risk groups.

Some examples of groups with higher risk behaviour include:

- # those having sexual intercourse with multiple partners; for example, patients with sexually transmitted diseases,
- # those sharing inadequately sterilized needles, syringes and other skin-piercing instruments, for example, injecting drug users, where this is a problem.

An example of population groups with lower risk include pregnant women. However, it should be kept in mind that initiating surveillance in lower-risk groups may be relatively unproductive unless a critical level of HIV prevalence among those with higher-risk behaviour has been reached. Hence testing of pregnant women may not be very useful in low-prevalence countries and should, as a general rule, not be carried out if HIV prevalence in higher risk groups is below 2 per cent.

It is important to emphasize also that data from donated blood screening should also be analysed to get an indication of HIV prevalence in the lower risk population. Although not a sentinel population *per se*, such data provide valuable information to monitor blood transfusion safety. The results should however, be disaggregated, where possible, by voluntary and remunerative donations.

As far as possible, easily defined and consistently accessible groups should be selected as sentinel population. For this reason, the sites should be chosen where blood is already being drawn for some other purpose and a part of it could conveniently be separated and tested for HIV in an unlinked anonymous manner. From the programme point of view, it is preferable to select sites in such a manner that all important transmission categories in the country are covered e.g., sexual transmission, injecting drug use and blood transfusion in Thailand, India, Nepal and Myanmar, and sexual transmission and blood transfusion in all other countries. Furthermore, sites should be accessible, convenient, have sufficient numbers of patients, and have staff willing to participate in the surveillance activity. Therefore, the sites which meet these criteria include STD clinics, drug treatment centres, and antenatal clinics.

(b) Sampling

The next step during planning is to decide about the sampling methodology. For convenience, it is advisable to collect consecutive blood samples till the predetermined sample size is reached (consult (c) below for sample sizes) or, from the operational viewpoint, take all samples consecutively over the eight-week period provided the minimum sample size has been obtained.

Often patients attending a site are referred to the laboratory for blood testing and some of them opt to drop out. This leads to participation bias and therefore the drawing of blood should be arranged at the clinic site, if possible. Double counting, viz., a patient considered twice or more in the same blood collection series should be avoided. If the period of data collection is short, the possibility of double counting becomes minimum. The other method to eliminate double counting would be to include only "new" patients.

(c) Sample Sizes

The fact that HIV occurs in an epidemic form means that large differences in HIV prevalence can exist between geographical areas. As a result, the minimum sample size required for surveillance purposes should be determined for each sentinel site. The following sample sizes are considered to be appropriate for sentinel surveillance:

Patients attending STD Clinics:
250 or more over an eight-week period

Injecting drug users attending treatment clinics:
250 or more over an eight-week period.

Antenatal clinic attenders:
As the prevalence of HIV among clinic attenders is likely to be lower and change more slowly than in STD clinic attenders, a large sample size is required, e.g., 400 or more over an eight-week period. This sample size gives a greater precision, and thereby small changes in the prevalence rates can be detected.

Tuberculosis (TB) patients:
HIV surveillance in patients attending TB clinics does not give pure trend data *per se*. It does, however, give important information on HIV related disease morbidity (e.g., TB). Increased HIV prevalence in patients with tuberculosis is the effect of both increase in HIV as well as increase in TB because of HIV.

As the prevalence of HIV among tuberculosis patients is increasing in many South-East-Asian countries, a sample size of 250-300 is suggested at the initial stage. This sample size may be covered within an eightweek period. In a high priority area, surveillance should be done even if no one site can provide a sample size of >250.

(d) Frequency of Survey

As described above, sentinel surveillance should be carried out using the sample sizes given above and repeated once a year to look at HIV infection trends. Experience suggests that it is better from the programmatic viewpoint to carry out surveillance in more sites and repeat them once a year instead of fewer sites every six months. However, every possible attempt should be made to obtain good quality data. On consecutive surveys, the methodology and laboratory procedures must be similar to those used previously so that data from the various surveys could be compared to each other. If possible, in each laboratory the same technician should be made specifically responsible for running tests in order to avoid human error.

(e) Testing Methodology

The unlinked anonymous testing method must be used, where possible, as it minimizes participation bias. In this type of testing, a part of the blood sample originally collected for other purposes is used for testing for HIV. For example, at an STD clinic, when blood sample is collected for VDRL or hepatitis B virus, a part of it can be separated out and sent to the laboratory after removing all personal identifiers, namely, name, address, etc., so that the HIV test results cannot be linked with the individual. The sentinel sites should, however, be encouraged to refer the clinic attenders, when necessary, to the centres where voluntary HIV testing and counselling could be provided.

(f) HIV Testing Strategy

For HIV surveillance, WHO recommends the following testing strategy depending on the expected HIV seroprevalence in that population group:

Areas with HIV seroprevalence >10 per cent:

The serum is tested with one ELISA or rapid/simple assay. Serum that is reactive is considered HIV positive.

Areas with HIV seroprevalence <10 per cent:

The serum is first tested with one ELISA or rapid/simple assay with higher sensitivity. Any serum found reactive on the first assay is retested with a second ELISA or rapid/simple assay with higher specificity based on a different antigen preparation and/or different test principles (e.g., indirect versus competitive). Serum that is non-reactive on the first test is considered HIV antibody negative. Serum that is reactive on the first test but non-reactive on second test is also considered antibody negative.

Implementation

It may often not be possible to initiate an HIV sentinel surveillance programme simultaneously in many regions/areas of a country. The surveillance programme should initially be introduced in one or two sites, preferably in a priority area, and extended later to other areas or sites once adequate experience is gained.

After having decided on the type of population groups to test, and the sites (summary given in Annex 2), the next step is to initiate collection of blood samples, retaining minimal epidemiological data and conducting laboratory tests. In order to do so the responsible individuals at each site should be trained to carry out the following activities:

(a) Data Collecnon

While every effort should be made to unlink the HIV test result with the individual concerned, the data collection form for each serum sample should include the following information:

- # general location of the sentinel site (not the name of the clinic)
- # population group,
- # month and year of serum collection,
- # age group,
- # HIV laboratory test result.

Collection of any additional information should be carefully weighed against the fact that too much information may allow individuals to be identified. The data collection form and the laboratory result should be linked only by a unique code number.

(b) Storage and Transport of Blood Samples

At the sentinel sites, the specimen tube for HIV testing must contain a minimum of 0.5 ml of serum. These should be properly labelled and stored in the freezer compartment of the refrigerator and sent to the HIV testing laboratory in batches of not less than 50 samples. When a few samples are sent and tested, there may be a danger that a positive laboratory result could still be linked to the individual.

(c) HIV Testing

All sera collected at any one sentinel site in any one sampling period should be tested in the same laboratory at the same time, using testing strategy outlined under *HIV testing strategy.*

As described earlier, care should be taken not to test a "few" samples at a time because this may lead to potentially identifying individual(s) who might have tested positive. The intention is to make the tracing of the HIV testing results to the individual virtually impossible.

Analysis

Data collected at each HIV sentinel site and for each senitinel group at that site should be analysed and compared separately to make meaningful interpretation Primary data will be the number of sera examined for a particular group at a particular site and the proportion positive for HIV. It is advisable not to aggregate the data but try to monitor trends separately for each population group at each site. Differences in prevalence over time can be tested for significance by a chi square test, if required.

Interpretation and Use of Data

The HIV surveillance data should be interpreted to assess how rapidly HIV prevalence is increasing in different groups and areas. This helps in determining which population groups need priority attention with respect to interventions and what differences exist between sentinel sites. Also, surveillance data can be used to estimate how many people may be currently infected and how many are expected to develop AIDS in the future. The results of sentinel surveillance should be disseminated not only to those responsible for fomulating policy but also to health care providers at sentinel sites. The data should also be reported to WHO using the quarterly surveillance form (Annex 1).

3.2 Use of Other Sources of Data

Sentinel surveillance is the method of choice for assessing HIV prevalence and for monitoring trends. However, if any *ad hoc* surveys have been carried out by other researchers, these sholild be taken into account in assessing the overall picture of the HIV situation. When the data on donated blood screening are available, these should also be analysed periodically to monitor the blood transfusion safety in an area or the country.

Annex 1

WHO HIV/AIDS SURVEILLANCE REPORT

WHO AIDS Surveillance Report
(Quarterly)

I.

Country:

Report Date	____ / ____ / ____ Day Month Year

II.

Responsible Officer	
Unit/Department	

III.

Reporting Period Ending	____ / ____ / ____ Day Month Year
Total cumulative AIDS cases	

IV. Indicate Period of Diagnosis

	Number of Cases
Cases diagnosed prior to 1987	
1987 Jan-Jun	
Jul-Dec	
1988 Jan-Jun	
Jul-Dec	
1989 Jan-Jun	
Jul-Dec	
1990 Jan-Jun	
Jul-Dec	

	Number of Cases
1991 Jan-Jun	
Jul-Dec	
1992 Jan-Jun	
Jul-Dec	
1993 Jan-Jun	
Jul-Dec	
1994 Jan-Jun	
Jul-Dec	
1995 Jan-Jun	
Jul-Dec	

V. National Definition of AIDS (check all that apply)

- ☐ CDC/WHO (1987)
- ☐ WHO Definition
- ☐ WHO Definition with HIV anitbody positiv results
- ☐ Other (Specify ____________________

Current Reporting Period:

From: / /	To: / /

VI. Age/Sex Distribution of AIDS Cases Reported during the Reporting Period

Age	Male	Female	Not Specified	Total
0 – 4				
5 – 14				
15 – 19				
20 – 29				
30 – 39				
40 – 49				
50 – 59				
60 +				
Note Specified				
Total				

VII. Risk/Transmissioin Categories

	Male	Female	Total
Adult			
Heterosexual			
Homosexual		N.A.	
Bi-sexual		N.A.	
Injecting Drug User			
Blood Transfusion/Blood Products			
Other			
Not Specified			
Children			
Perinatal			
Blood Transfusion/Blood Products			
Other			
Not Specified			

WHO HIV Surveillance Report
(Quarterly)

Country

Report Date	/ /
Reporting Period Ending	/ /

1. HIV Sentinel Surveillance

Sentinel Site/Region	Population Group	Number HIV Tested	Number Positive	Percent Positive	Study Methods*

Please choose one i.e. unlinked anonymous, voluntary, mandatory, compulsory

2. HIV *Ad-hoc* Survey Results

From: ____/ ______ Month Year	To: ____/ ______ Month Year

Survey Site	Population Group	Number Tested	Number HIV Positive	% Positive	Study Methods

3. Screening of Donated Blood for HIV

From: ____/ ______ Month Year	To: ____/ ______ Month Year

Region	Number Tested	Number HIV Positive*	% Positive

*On ELISA or any rapid test used.

Annex 2

SUMMARY PROCEDURES FOR HIV SENTINEL SURVEILLANCE

Procedures	Higher risk population		Lower risk population	
	Injecting drug users	Patients with STD	Pregnant women	Patients with tuberculosis
Sentinal site	Drug treatment centres	STD clinics or general clinics	Antenatal clinic	Hospital/Chest clinic or TB clinic
Sample size	250 or more	250 or more	400	250 - 400
Period of completion	8 weeks	8 weeks	8 weeks	8 weeks
Frequency of survey	Once a year	Once a year	Once a year	Once a year
Sampling	Consecutive	Consecutive	Consecutive	Consecutive
Selection criteria	New patients	New patients	Primi, 17-30 years	New patients, 15-45 years
Testing methodology	Unlinked anonymous (UA)*	UA*	UA*	UA*

*Where possible, i.e., blood is aleady collected for other purposes.

25

Women and AIDS : Agenda for Action

The Fourth World Conference on Women is talking place at a time when women are increasingly becoming infected with HIV, the virus that causes AIDS. From being almost absent from the AIDS epidemic in the 1980s, women infected with HIV now number more than seven million—with another one million women becoming infected this year. By the year 2000 over 14 million women will have been infected and four million of them will have died. Women worldwide are asking why a virus that infecs both men and women is increasingly affecting women in a disproportionate manner.

The bleak reality is that the sexual and economic subordination of women fuels the HIV/AIDS pandemic. In order to break the cycle of neglect which affects women across their life span and across generations, it is essential to undertake actions which will allow women to make informed choices and enable them to improve the quality of their lives. Women must empower themselves by networking forming alliances, and advocating for change. Top-level political commitment is needed to reduce the social vulnerability of women to HIV infection by improving their health, education, legal and economic prospetcs. Effective HIV/AIDS prevention and care efforts along with sound policies and programmes targeting women affected by HIV/AIDS need to be developed and integrated into existing national structures, particularly at the community and family level. Because such social vulnerability cannot be effectively challenged by women as individuals alone, or even as groups, building effective alliances between women and men based on mutual respect, remain the greatest challenge, but also the best hope, for the lives of tomorrow.

I. INTRODUCTION

In the space of just one decade, AIDS has turned into a pandemic affecting millions of men, women and children on all continents. WHO estimates that 4.5 million AIDS cases had occurred by late 1994 and foresees that this cumulative total will triple by the year 2000. The number of people infected with HIV—the virus that can lead to AIDS-is much greater. According to WHO's conservative estimates, as of late 1994 more than 18 million adults and over 1.5 million, infants have been infected with HIV since the start of the pandemic (Figure 25.1). By the year 2000, there will be an estimated 30-40 million infections.

To what extent has the epidemic affected women? Enormously. A decade ago women seemed to be on the periphery of the epidemic. Today they are at the centre of concern. WHO estimates that almost half of all newly infected adults are women. This means that the number of women acquiring HIV each year cannot be counted in the thousands, or even in the hundreds of thousands. In 1994, more than one million women were newly infected. Already, 7-8 million women have been infected with HIV worldwide (Figure 25.2) and this figure is rapidly growing. Estimates are that over 14 million women will have become infected with HIV by the year 2000, and about four million of them will have died.

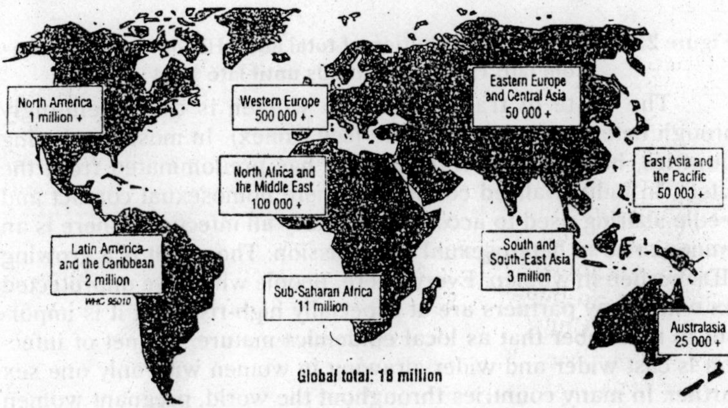
North America
1 million +
Western Europe
500 000 +
Eastern Europe
and Central Asia
50 000 +
East Asia and
the Pacific
50 000 +
North Africa and
the Middle East
100 000 +
Latin America-
and the Caribbean
2 million
WHO 95010
South and
South-East Asia
3 million
Sub-Saharan Africa
11 million
Australasia
25 000 +
Global total: 18 million

Figure 25.1. Estimated distribution of total adult HIV-infections from late 1970s/early 1980s until late 1994.

Among both men and women, the hardest-hit group is youth. WHO estimates that half of all infections to date have been in 15-24 year-olds. However, in nearly all parts of the world, the peak age of infection is lower in girls than boys. In many countries, 60 per cent of all new HIV infections are among 15-24 year-olds, with a female to male ratio of two to one. An analysis of reported AIDS data from several African and Asian countries suggests that young women under 25 account for nearly 30 per cent of female AIDS cases and young men for approximately 15 per cent of male cases.

As infections in women rise, so do infections in the infants born to them. To date, these total about 1.5 million, of whom more than half a million have already developed AIDs. Overall, about one-third of babies born to HIV-infected mothers become infected themselves.

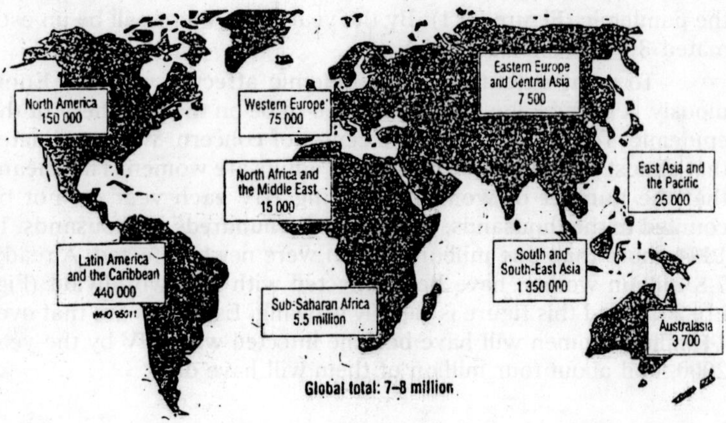

Figure 25.2. Estimated distribution of total adult HIV-infected women from late 1970s/early 1980s until late 1994

The route of transmission to women is overwhelmingly through heterosexual intercourse (see Annex). In most developing countries, heterosexual transmission has predominated from the outset. In industrialized countries, where homosexual contact and needle-sharing used to account for nearly all infections, there is an ominous rise in heterosexual transmission. The result is a growing AIDs burden in women. Everywhere, people who have unprotected sex with many partners are at especially high-risk. But it is important to remember that as local epidemics mature, the net of infection is cast wider and wider, drawing in women with only one sex partner. In many countries throughout the world, pregnant women attending antenatal clinics are showing a high prevalence of infection. Studies of women attending antenatal clinics find that many are monogamous and have been infected by their one partner—their husband.

The sexual and economic subordination of women fuels the HIV/AIDS pandemic. In order break the cycle of neglect which affects women across their life span and across generations, it is essential to undertake actions which will allow women to make informed choices and enable them to improve the quality of their lives. Given the growing dimensions of the HIV/AIDS pandemic, the need for change is literally a matter of life of death.

II. HOW HIV/AIDS IS SPREADING AMONG WOMEN?

Sexual Subordination Leads to HIV Vulnerability

In many societies, there is a significant power differential between men and women, supported by social and cultural systems that posit the control by males. Males are expected to initiate relationships, and sexual assertiveness in women is often stigmatized or punished. The gender power differential is compounded by age differences. Women typically marry or have sex with older men, who have been sexually active longer and hence are more likely to have become infected themselves. In countries with high HIV infection rates, men justify the selection of young adolescent girls, even female children, on the grounds that they are less likely to be infected with HIV/AIDS.

> **"For example, a situation like this develops. If your man comes home at 3 a.m. smelling of a perfume you don't recognize, that's the time he's going to ask for sex because he's trying to clear his conscience by making you think he hasn't alreay had it. But if he goes out drinking with the boys, he comes home and goes straight to sleep peacefully. You have to go along with what ever he asks, even if you're smelling this strange perfume, because you can't say 'no'."**

Many countries which promote monogamy and mutual fidelity, and discourage multiple casual partners as a societal norm, have also encouraged these values as a primary AIDS prevention strategy. Some societies, however, expect women to adhere strictly to this norm while tacitly condoning male deviation from it. Women are expected to have one lifetime sex partner while men are expected, or even encouraged, to have more than one partner. As a result, women are more likely to be monogamous than men and to have fewer lifetime partners. Reliance on "monogamy" or "mutual fidelity" as a principal solution can be misleading for women, as fidelity protects against HIV/AIDS only if it is completely mutual and life-long. It creates an illusion of safety for individuals who are monogamous but who cannot be certain about their partners.

In some cultures, women don't have the "permission" to talk about sex with men, or to negotiate safer sex practices. To do so many have serious repercussions, ranging from stigma to fear of violence or abandonment. Despite this, many HIV/AIDS prevention and family planning programmes have expected women to assume responsibility for the prevention of both pregnancy and sexually transmitted diseases (STDs), including HIV infection, in a context in which they have limited control over when, with whom, and how they engage in sexual activity.

Male resistance to condom use and women's inability to negotiate safer sex puts women (as well as men) at greater risk of

HIV infection. For men, the rationale for resisting the use of condoms includes concern about reduced sensitivity, ignorance about how to use the condom properly, and fear that using it will permanently interfere with fertility. In addition, within marriage or other long-term relationships, the very suggestion of condom use carries with it an indication of "infidelity" or other behaviour that could threaten the security of the relationship, making it difficult for both men and women to introduce condoms into an existing relationship.

Some countries have statutory or *de facto* restrictions based on age or gender regarding access to information about sexuality, contraception, disease prevention, condoms and lubricants, and health care. In many communities, schools and other institutions that work with adolescents are wary of providing sex education or otherwise discussing issues related to sexuality, due to social and cultural concerns about "protecting" young women from sexual experience. As a result, young women and men lack adequate information and skills to protect themselves if they are sexually active. In addition, children and adolescents, in some countries, must have a parent's permission to obtain health care services. This is a particular problem for young people who have left home or are homeless.

Women are also vulnerable to coerced sex, including rape and other sexual abuse, in and outside of the family, and forced sex work. Any non-consensual penetrative sex can carry an increased risk of transmission of HIV and other STDs, particularly as men who rape are not likely to use condoms. Moreover, even when sex is non-consensual, women are often stigmatized and blamed, causing them to be ostracized from family and support networks. The problems associated with rape and other forms of violence against women are often intensified in war situations, in which occupying or invading armies, systematically rape women as part of a strategy to intimidate the local population.

In all countries there are customs related to women's sexual activity. Some have become deadly.

Economic Subordination Leads to HIV Vulnerability

In virtually every society, women face discrimination in education, employment, and social status, resulting in economic vulnerability to HIV/AIDS. This includes, for example:

discrimination that girls face in both educational institutions and the family; for example, girls who are encouraged to take different subjects from those taken by boys have less access to financial and other family resources,

and are often withdrawn from school to assume domestic responsibilities;

- # occupational segregation of women into low-paying clerical and service jobs, unequal pay and fewer promotions (vis-a-vis men), fewer workplace benefits and concentration of women in the informal sector;
- # lack of access to technical assistance, training and credit; for example, in agricultural sector development, policies have traditionally provided funds and technical training to men involved in cash crop farming and not to women, who have been more likely to be engaged in subsistence farming.

Households headed by women are much more likely to be financially poor than those in which there is a working resident male. Women's economic dependence on male partners in order to avoid poverty for themselves and their children makes it difficult for women to negotiate safer sex practices to protect themselves from infection.

Some national laws reinforce women's economic dependence on men. Laws that restrict property ownership and inheritance to men, and in some cases limit women's ability to enter into independent contracts or obtain credit under their own names, impede women's ability to control income and property, and reinforce their economic dependence on male relatives. This dependence makes it difficult for them to refuse sexual practices that put them at risk of STDs and HIV infection. Laws regarding marriage, divorce, and child custody can impede women's ability to leave relationships in which they or their children are physically or sexually abused, or exposed to the risk of HIV infection.

Worldwide, many women rely on prostitution, or sex work, for economic survival. The proportion and the number of women who do so, in both developed and developing countries, is often directly related to the economy and the level of unemployment. In many parts of the world, prostitution is illegal and underground, which means that prostitutes my have to work without adequate control over the conditins of the sex work transaction.

"A woman in Asia put in a nutshell the dilemma faced by so many women like herself across the world: "AIDS might make me sick one day," she said. "But if I don't work my family would not eat and we would all be sick anyway".

Migration as a result of war, famine, political oppressin or poverty, can increase a women's vulnerability to HIV infection if she is isolated from community structures, and does not speak or read the local language. Furthermore, women who are migrant workers, refugees or returnees are often more vulnerable than other women to some kind of sexual barter, (e.g., to obtain entry or residence permits, in exchange for transport, or to obtain or hold onto jobs), receiving financial support from men with whom they have sex, or engaging in formal prostitution. Similarly, when men migrate to urban centres, leaving wives and girlfriends at home, they may have other partners in cities.

There is often a lack of social and financial support to help women with HIV infection plan for the care of their surviving, and often healthy, children. This lack of support increases the emotional and psychological stress among women who understand that they are going to die while their children are still young. In some countries, as the number of children orphaned as a result of the epidemic has increased, some women have assumed responsibility for these children, taking them into their homes, often without any financial or other support, and often with inadequate space, food, or other supplies.

Female Biological Vulnerability to HIV

AIDS is essentially a sexually transmitted disease (STD), which like some other such diseases can also be spread through blood and blood products, and from an infected women to her unborn or newborn child. Women are biologically more vulnerable then men to HIV infection and other STDs. Studies in many countries have found that male-to-female transmission of HIV appears to be 2-4 times as efficient as female-to-male transmission. Postulated as the major factors responsible for differential transmission are the larger mucosal surface areas exposed to virus in women and the greater viral inoculum present in semen compared with vaginal secretions. Male-to-female transmission of some STDs is at least 15 per cent more efficient than female-to-male transmission. Young girls are particularly vulnerable. Their immature cervix and relatively low vaginal mucus production presents less of a barrier to HIV, making them biologically more vulnerable to infection than older premenopausal women.

Other data suggest that STDs— especially those, such as chancroid and syphilis, which cause ulcerative lesions—greatly facilitate both the acquisition and transmission of HIV. However, women with STDs are often asymptomatic and fail to recognize any infections. As a result, women are more vulnerable to HIV infection because they are more likely to have untreated STDs. Often their vulnerability to STDs is the result of their partners' behaviour rather than their own. This increases the likelihood that they will not recognize lowgrade infections. At the same time, women tend to avoid STD clinics for fear of being recognized and stigmatized. Women who do seek medical services often choose to go to primary health, family planning, and material and child health clinics for their care. Unfortunately, such facilities are often less well equipped to diagnose and treat STDs or may be unsympathetic or judgmental towards women with STDs.

Finally, women are disproportionately the receipients of blood transfusions and other blood products (e.g., for anaemia or childbirnt complications). In the absence of adequate blood screening, women's vulnerability to blood-borne HIV transmission increases.

Impact of HIV/AIDS on Women

Because women are sexually, economically and biologically vulnerable to HIV/AIDS, they are often stigmatized and blamed for "causing" HIV/AIDS and other STDs. Women are frequently identified as "reservoirs of infection" or as "vectors for transmission" to their male partners and their offspring. This inaccurate view is iactually harmful in a number of ways: it fails to focus on men's equal responsibility to prevent HIV/AIDs; it prevents programmes from developing services which meet the needs of women; and it underlies some research and intervention strategies which have been designed more to protect men from women than to enable women to protect themselves.

> *"All the gender issues we had never tackled came up at once", says Theresa Kaijage, a founding member of the Tanzanian AIDS Service Organization called WAMATA. "Initially we ignored them or thought they were irrelevant. We thought it was Eurocentric to tackle them in Africa. We thought our African culture was different and dealt with things in a different way. All the agendas that we had ignored- legal, educational and health problems, inequitable gender relations—suddenly we are dealing with these multiple issues, which people have not learned to analyze in a way that promotes equal sharing of both resources and power at all levels. In order to deal with AIDS, we have had to confront these."*

Many people assume that if a woman has HIV infection, she has had multiple partners or engaged in prostitution and that such behaviour marks her as a "bad woman". As a result of this social stigma associated with HIV infection, women known or thought to be infected have been dismissed from their jobs or not hired, evicted from their homes, abandoned by their husbands or other long-term partners, and denied the custody of their children. In addition, women perceived to be at risk of HIV infection have been denied health insurance, and health care personnel have refused to treat women they thought were or might be infected.

Some countries have implemented mandatory testing schemes targeting women. Women who test positive or who are suspected of being infected suffer from increased discrimination, random and institutional violence, arrest, incarceration, and deportation. Most often such testing is without the women's informed consent, and without appropriate pretest and post-test counselling.

Most societies rely on women to be voluntary caregivers for their families, as well as occupational caregivers for the community. Older women may be expected to assume a major caregiving responsibility at the same time that adolescent daughters may be kept out of school to care for younger children or other family members who are ill. The expectation that women will provide most of the care for people with HIV infection and AIDS results in high stress, especially if such care must be provided in addition to other work, including paid work outside of the home and family-centred work, such as subsistence farming. Such stress is compounded when the women become ill themselves, often with no one to care for them.

If the vulnerability of women to HIV infection is to be reduced, both men and women must work to counter gender discrimination and the subordination of women. Policy makers, community leaders and other people in positions of power must recognize the connection between women's economic and social status and their vulnerability to HIV infection. Men and women need to reassess the way they see themselves and each other, the way they relate as husband and wife, partners, lovers, brothers and sisters, parent and child, coleagues and friends.

The inequality between men and women fuels the spread of HIV/AIDS. Unless the interaction between HIV infection, cultural values and the rights and needs of women is reconized, the fundamental change required to stem this pandemic is unattainable. While women require urgent consideration in the response to the epidemic, interventions must mobilize all sectors of society, including, and in particular, men.

It is important therefore, to develop complementary and interlined strategies for action, incorporating a gender analysis of the socio-economic and cultural causes and effects of the pandemic. Specific activities are listed below.

> *"To enable women to protect themselves there are three issues at stake : improving the social and economic status of women: providing a method over which they have sufficient control: or getting more men to adopt safer sex. This is not an academic exercise in setting priorities, but a question of-life. and death for many women".*
>
> *Dr. Eka Esu Williams, Nigeria*

Reducing the Vulnerability of Women to HIV/AIDS

Preventing HIV Infection Among Women

Support the development of HIV/AIDS prevention interventions that provide the necessary messages, skills, and support services to men and women, including marginalized or hard-to-reach groups, such as migrants, the wives and non-marital partners of migrat.ing men, women and men in prison, and adolescent girls and boys both in and out of school:

- # increase girls' access to education including access to scholarships and other financial assistance;
- # support programmes that target both men and women with informed messages about the importance of using condoms to protect both partners from HIV and other STD, and about their mutual responsibility to engage in safer sex practices;
- # support sex and HIV/AIDS education for young people (male and female) in school and out of school to iricrease their understanding and skills in human sexuality;
- # support the development of sound HIV/AIDS work-place polices and effective workplace educations programmes;
- # remove obstacles to women's ability to earn money and engage in productive labour'by supporting' child care services, equal pay for equal work,employment training programmes, as well as small business and agricultural-development programmes;
- # ensure a safe blood supply through blood donations from low risk,' voluntary, non-renumerated blood donors'and test all blood for HIV.
- # reduce unecessary blood transfusions by improving women's nutrition, preventing anaemia, treating infections, preventing the loss of blood due to complications in pregnancy, and using blood substitutes wherever possible;

Reduce the incidence and prevalence of STDs among women by increasing their access to and utilization of appropriate STD services:

- # develop appropriate educaticnal programmes that target both men and women concerning the increased risk of acquiring HIV infection in the presence of an STD;
- # fund activities that educate women how to prevent and recognize signs and symptoms of STDs and to seek appropriate health care services;
- # provide high quality condoms through effective social

marketing programmes and promote the use and distribution of lubricants and other agents that reduce the likelihood of microscopic vaginal lesions associated with sexual intercourse;

improve the provision of STD diagnostic and treatment services for women, regardless of age or marital status;
Support research to better understand women's biological vulnerability to HIV, and the impact of contraceptives and other means of fertility regulation, and of pregnancy, on HIV infection and disease progression;
advocate that biomedical scientists and. private industry give top priority to developing a vaginalvirucide or microbicide active against—HIV and other STDs.

Reducing tbe Impact of HIV/AIDS on Women

Reduce the stigmatization and discrimination of women regarding HIV infection:

encourage countries where mandatory testing or routine HIV screening programmes exist to replace them with voluntary, confidential testing supported 'by counselling services;
support programmes that work with families and communities of women with HIV/AIDS in order to reduce the likelihood that women will be ostracized due to their HIV status;
plan and implement HIV/AIDS prevention interven-tions with sex workers, and support self-help and advocacy organizations for sex workers;
review the impact of laws and regulations relating to prostitution on working conditions as well as on the ability of HIV/AIDS and STD prevention activities to operate effectively.

Caring for Women with HIV/AIDS

Increase the availability of support services for HIV positive women who want help with reproductive decision-making and for women with children who need help with planning for their care:

ensure that women have access to voluntary, safe and affordable contraceptive measures;
support programmes—to assist women with HiV/AIDS . in family planning decisions and planning for their surviving families;

ensure that HIV-positive women are not pressured or forced to be sterilized, and that pregnant women with HIV infection are not pressured or forced to terminate pregnancies.

Ensure that women do not carry the entire burden of care for people with HIV/AIDS:

encourage men and women to share in the caregiving role, and support interventions that provide training for women and men in basic health care procedures;
support community-based institutions that can provide professional alternatives to home care and respite care for primary caregivers;
encourage families to keep their daughters in school, and discourage them from relying on adolescent girls for caregiving responsibilities,
support programmes and interventions to assist women and men who provide foster care to children orphaned as a result of HIV/AIDS and other diseases.

IV. CONCLUSION

The sexual and economic subordination of women continues to fuel the HIV/AIDs pandemic. Women are increasingly becoming infected with HIV and at a significantly younger age than men. At the same time, proportionately more girls and young women are becoming infected in their teens and early twenties than women in any other age group. Today, the stakes are higher than ever. The ways in which we respond to the pandemic now will influence the ways in which women participate and contribute in the twenty-first century.

26

Female Genitile Health and Risk of HIV Transmission

Dr. Regina Mc Namara
Assistant Professor of Clinical Public Health Centre for Population and Family Health, Columbia University, New York City.

INTRODUCTION

This paper is concerned with preservation of the intact surface of the female genital tract as a defense against heterosexual transmission of HIV. If the vaginal epithelial mucosa, the female's normal barrier against infection, is not intact when the male deposits infectious semen, susceptibility to HIV transmission may be significantly increased. STIs are one source of damage to that barrier and their association with HIV transmission is well-documented. (See e.g. Wasserheit, 1990; WHO, 1990.) Other causes of genital trauma and infection in both women and men that may open a pathway to HIV infection have been given little attention. For women, cultural conditions and inadequate health services compound the disadvantages of sexual and social inequality, increase their vulnerability to infection and limit their resources for treatment.

This discussion of genital infection and trauma is intended to convey the widespread nature of the problem and its roots in the social and economic context of the lives of women in developing countries. Barriers to diagnosis and treatment of genital conditions are often specific to women varying in different cultures but with common themes: lack of information; differential access to health care; violation of norms of personal modesty; and ignorance or denigration of women's needs. These barriers can be lowered with education, economic opportunities, better and more available health services and preventive methods that women can control themselves. To accomplish this, the health and well-being of women must be prominent on national and international research and aid agendas.

GENITAL INFECTION AND TRAUMA

In—the following discussion it is understood that: intact vaginal epithelial mucosa alone may not be sufficient protection against HIV transmission during intercourse; the use of condoms is important even in the absence of a sexually transmitted infection or other genital condition; and the study of HIV continues and current knowledge indicates that genital health can decrease, but not eliminate, susceptibility to infection.

Sexually Transmitted Infection

Genital ulcers caused by syphilis, chancroid and herpes are believed to facilitate penetration of HIV through disruption of epithelial mucosa or through the increased local concentration of lymphocytes which are target cells for HIV. A World Health Organization (WHO) expert committee meeting in 1989 concurred that it is biologically plausible for all STD pathogens that cause genital ulcers or inflammation to be a factor in increased infectiousness or susceptibility to HIV (WHO, 1989). Other sexually transmitted infections, such as gonorrheal, chlamydial and trichomonal infections, may also enhance susceptibility (Oxtoby and Gayle, 1990). Trichomoniasis may be a far greater risk than genital ulcer disease because of its extensive prevalence in many parts of the developing world (Wasserheit, 1990).

The term sexually transmitted infection extends the list of traditional venereal diseases (gonorrhea, syphilis, chancroid, lymphogranuloma venereum and granuloma inguinale) to cover more than 20 organisms and syndromes, including chlamydia, genital herpes, and human papillomovirus infections. The major primary manifestations of sexually transmitted infections throughout the world include urethritis in men, cervicitis and vaginitis in women and genital ulcers, genital warts and enteric infections in both men and women. With infections of the lower reproductive tract, women can experience abnormal vaginal discharge, a burning feeling with urination, abnormal vaginal bleeding and genital pain or itching.

The prevalence of sexually transmitted infections, and thus the patterns of disease, vary greatly among and within world regions and within countries. In western countries, at present, the Herpes Simplex Virus (HSV) is the most common cause of Genital Ulcer Disease (GUD); in many developing countries, syphilis and chancroid appear to be the most common causes (Hatcher *et al.*, 1989). Infection rates are approximate since facilities for testing and treatment are scarce in developing countries, private physicians in developed countries frequently do not report their patients' sexually transmitted infections, population-based studies are rare and much of the research is subject to biases inherent in studies of selected groups (e.g., commercial sex workers, STD clinic patients, prenatal and family planning clients).

Although a female is more likely than a male to be infected from a single act of intercourse with a partner who has a sexually transmitted infection (Hatcher et al., 1989), women are seriously undercounted in sexually transmitted infection data in all countries, in part because their conditions are often asymptomatic, but also because services they can or will use are not available. Clinical diagnosis or screening for infection is rarely incorporated into services offered at family planning antenatal or maternal and child health (MCH) clinics. Sexually transmitted infection clinics, when they are available, are usually not acceptable to women. Consequently, estimates of the gender distribution of the incidence of sexually transmitted infections cannot be made with any confidence.

Wasserheit (1989), in an international review of female reproductive tract infections, found greater prevalence reported in African-studies than those conducted among Asian or Latin American populations. The median of the rates of gonorrhea was 10 per cent in the studies in African countries; 1 per cent in Asian countries and 6 per cent in Latin America. Median rates of trichomoniasis were 19 per cent, 11 per cent and 12 per cent for African, Asian and Latin American studies, respectively (Dixon-Mueller and Wasserheit,-1991).

Although a female is more likely than a male to be infected from a single act of intercourse with a partner who has a sexually transmitted infection, women are seriously undercounted in sexually transmitted infection data in all countries, in part because their conditions are often asymptomatic, but also because services they can or will use are not available.

Since the major immediate causes of infertility in women are probably gonorrhea, chlamydia and other reproductive tract infections, infertility serves as an indirect measure of sexually transmitted infection prevalence. Untreated, these infections lead to pelvic inflammatory disease, which leads to tubal inflammation, damage or distortion, which leads in turn to inability to conceive or to spontaneous abortion (Sherris and Fox, 1985). The measure of female infertility used in most population studies is childlessness at the end of the reproductive years. However, this incorrectly assigns all childlessness to female rather than male infertility, and misses infertility that follows first or later births. The indices vary widely, from as low as 1.0 to 1.5 per cent in Korea and Thailand to as high as 13 per cent in urban areas of Colombia and 23 per cent in one rural area of New Guinea (Belsey, 1980).

In sub-Saharan Africa, the highest levels of childlessness have been found for the most part in three zones: southwestern Sudan and northwestern Zaire; Cameroon and Gabon; and south-eastern Angola and northeastern Zambia. These areas, and regions in Burkina Faso and Uganda, have reported infertility levels of over 21 to 40 per cent. In adjacent areas, levels of childlessness are still well above 3 per cent which is considered a normal fertility bench-mark. (Frank, 1983). A large multicenter study conducted by the WHO found tubal occlusion, often resulting from sexually transmitted infection, as a cause of infertility in 11 per cent of infertile women from developed countries, 16 per cent from non-African developing countries, and 49 per cent from African countries (cited in Hatcher et al., 1989). Differences in the prevalence of sexually transmitted infections, or in access to treatment, may well explain differences in infertility rates.

Genital Trauma

Sexually transmitted infections are a major but not the sole source of damage to the female genital tract. Additional sources of infection or trauma that could damage the epithelial barrier include female genital mutilation, childbearing, insertion of objects into the vagina and trauma during sexual intercourse. Maintaining cleanliness of the genital area under the harsh conditions of nomadic life, drought or life-long water scarcity requires heroic measures. Infections probably caused by inadequate cleansing—of cloths used to absorb menstrual blood are also reported (Wasserheit et al., 1989).

Female genital mutilation is a plausible cofactor for HIV transmission which has not been adequately studied. Of the three types of operations performed on young girls, the gravest is infibulation, also called pharaonic circumcision. The clitoris, labia minor and parts of the labia major are removed and the two sides of the vulva are fastened together, leaving a small opening for urination and menstruation. Consequences of infibulation, such as inflammation of the genital area, partial closure of the vaginal orifice, abnormal anatomy or friable scar tissue are conditions that, according to the WHO, may increase susceptibility to HIV (WHO/GPA, 1990). Long-term consequences of infibulation are chronic urinary retention, urinary tract infections, incomplete healing and excessive scar tissue (or keloids) which can cause vaginal obstruction. Childbirth (when the infibulated section is cut open for passage of the infant) can be severely traumatic with consequences as grave as rupture of the vagina. Complications caused by these female genital operations are not reported with any regularity, in part because of the reluctance of the women to expose their genitals for medical examination (Gordon, 1991).

In northern Sudan, according to preliminary reports from the demographic and health survey, 82 per cent of married women had undergone pharaonic circumcision. A additional 15 per cent of the married women underwent Sunna circumcision, the "mildest form in which the tip of the clitoris is removed or an intermediate type of excision when the whole clitoris and often adjacent parts including the labia minor are removed (Ahmed and Kheir, 1990). The intermediate and Sunna forms are practiced more widely in subSaharan Africa and the Middle East than is the pharaonic (which is reported mainly in southern Egypt, Ethiopia, Somalia, Djibouti and in other Red Sea coastal areas). Current estimates of the total number of African women who have undergone some form of circumcision or infibulation approach 100 million (Women's International Network, n.d.).

The Safe Motherhood Initiative launched in Nairobi in 1987 brought to the fore of international discussion the problems of maternal mortality in developing countries. Research and interventions have focused on the risk of death yet, during each delivery, women confront the risk of damage to the genital tract. Tears or incisions during childbirth, with potential for infection, are common traumas of childbirth and massive infections can result from induced or spontaneous abortions. Very young women are especially vulnerable to risks associated with delivery (especially when childhood nutrition has been poor, infections are frequent and growth is stunted). Childbirth at very young ages is not a rare event. In Mauritania, for example, 15 per cent of girls have given birth by age 15; in Bangladesh, 21 per cent have had at least one child by age 15 (United Nations, 1991:59).

When the pelvis is immature or underdeveloped, cephalopelvic distortion and prolonged obstructed labour can cause damage as severe as vesico-vaginal fistula (VVF). With VVF, there is an opening between the urinary bladder and the vagina and the afflicted women continuously leak urine, wetting their clothes and excoriating their mutilated vulvae and vaginas. Reports on VVF from Egypt, Ghana, India, Kenya, Nigeria, Pakistan, South Africa, Sudan, and Turkey indicate obstetric causes for 80 to 100 per cent of the cases identified (Tahzib, 1989). In one Nigerian hospital, 30 per cent of those suffering from VYF were under age 15; 59 per cent were under age 18 (Ampofo, et al., 1990). The number of women with VVF is not known; many are believed to be suffering quietly out of sight, shunned as pariahs by family and community and without protection.

Other causes of genital trauma abound and include such traditional practices as the 'gishiri' or 'salt cut' in Nigeria which involves incision of part of the interior vaginal wall by a traditional birth attendant, traditional healer or occasionally by the woman herself. The purpose is to cure a variety of vaginal conditions and infertility (Adebajo, 1989).

Herbs, traditional preparations and foreign objects inserted into the vagina can cause inflammation, abrasions and infections, and so increase risk of HIV transmission. Practices may be intended to increase the male partner's pleasure during intercourse. Among pregnant women studied at a hospital clinic in Malawi, 12 per cent reported using one or more of the following to tighten the vagina: herbs, aluminum hydroxide, cloth or stones (silica gel, potassium permanganate or pumicelike stone). Not surprisingly, stones were found to have an irritating and erosive effect on vaginal mucosa and the data reported suggest that they may facilitate entry of HIV (Dallabetta et al., 1990).

Globally, women are known to insert objects into the vagina as medication, for contraception or to induce abortion. The array of items used for these purposes in Mexico for example, includes herbs, pills, soap and lime (Shedlin and Hollerback, 1981). A more complex process is described in Nigeria:

> To prepare [the abortifacient], leaves and seeds from certain local trees (ejirin seeds and itu leaves) are ground and the juice from another tree (epin) added to form a paste. The paste is then made into small balls and dried. As they become dry, more juice is added two or three times. The balls are inserted into the vagina and, according to our informants. they have the effect of destroying the foetus (Adebajo, 1989:14).

A cross-cultural study of indigenous fertility regulation conducted in seven countries illustrates the diversity of potentially damaging objects (Newman, 1985). In Afghanistan, women reported intravaginal insertion of wooden spoons or sticks treated with copper sulphate to cause heavy bleeding and abortion (Hunte, 1985). Egyptian women use aspirin, lemon juice, black pepper and plant stems (Sukkary Stolba, 1985). In other countries, bamboo leaves. grass. the midrib of the coconut palm, water pumped under hiah pressure, hangers, knitting needles and umbrellas are used as abortifacients (Ngin. 1985; Low and Newman, 1985).

Genital conditions conducive to H1V transmission may also result from sexual intercourse especially in the absence of foreplay when the unlubricated surface is irritated by penile penetration. Among older women, atrophic vaginitis may cause mucosal tears during sexual intercourse (Peterman. 1990). The contraceptive sponge may absorb vaginal secretions excessively and cause dryness (Hatcher *et al.,* 1989), and drying out the vagina before intercourse to increase penile friction has been reported in Zambia (S.K. Hira, cited in Feldman, 1990).

Damage to the female genitalia and increased susceptibility to HIV infection can result from rape or other modes of violent assertion of sexual supremacy by men. This is a risk factor, especially for sex workers who have repeated encounters with drunk and violent clients. In a Harare, Zimbabwe study, half the sex workers interviewed said that their most recent client was drunk (Wilson et al., 1989). An additional genital hazard comes with the use of condoms for frequent acts of intercourse in a short time period. According to recent reports from focus groups with sex workers in Thailand, the customer with a condom takes a longer time to ejaculate, the lubricant wears off, and friction and irritation follow (Sittitrai et al., 1989).

DIAGNOSIS AND TREATMENT: THE OBSTACLES

Recognizing the major role played by the integrity of the female and male genitalia in reducing heterosexual transmission of HIV can be an important contribution to global prevention efforts, but diagnosis and treatment are possible only when women and men can present themselves to someone with the skills and means to identify correctly th(conditions and supply appropriate medications .

Utilization of Health Services

Little is known about what use women in developing countries make--of health services for themselves. They are usually questioned only about their use of services that are related to reproduction or to their children's health. The most recent, comprehensive source of information on use of services related to pregnancy is the demographic and health surveys conducted in the 1980s in 29 developing countries. They indicate that many of the women interviewed had at least one visit to a trained midwife or physician at some time during pregnancy, but far fewer delivered with trained assistance. Table 26.1 shows socio-economic and geographic differentials within countries, as well as between countries, in prenatal visits and delivery assistance in Egypt, Ghana, Guatemala, Mali and Thailand.

The obstacles many women face in access to health care are caused by poverty, lack of education, inferior position in society, and inadequate health systems, among others. The result is that, if a woman does not have prenatal care, or if her one or two visits do not include an internal examination, she may pass through her entire life and bear her children, yet never have an internal examination.

TABLE 26.1: PERCENTAGE OF WOMEN WITH PRENATAL VISITS AND TRAINED ASSISTANCE AT DELIVERY, IN SELECTED COUNTRIES, BY RESIDENCE AND EDUCATION

	EGYPT %	GHANA %	GUATEMALA %	MALI %	THAILAND %
Residence					
Urban					
Prenatal	69	94	58	70	95
Delivery	57	70	60	77	96
Rural					
Prenatal	42	78	26	19	73
Delivery	70	26	13	26	46
Education					
None					
Prenatal	42	72	18	27	49
Delivery	20	26	13	26	46
Primary					
Prenatal	55	—	40	—	79
Delivery	34	—	34	—	59
Complete primary					
Middle					
Prenatal	65	92	64	—	79
Delivery	49	55	64	—	59
Secondary					
Prenatal	81	97	86	95	97
Delivery	78	79	87	98	95

* Educational levels for Thailand: 0-3, 4-7. 8+

Sources: Demographic and Health Surveyes: Egypt. Ghana, Guatemala. Mali and Thailand.

In Egypt, 42 per cent of rural women receive some prenatal care from a physician or trained nurse or midwife; yet only 19 per cent deliver with trained assistance. Seventy-eight per cent of rural women in Ghana have at least one prenatal visit; only 29 per cent have trained assistance at childbirth. In rural Guatemala and Mali, fewer than 20 per cent have trained help at delivery and percentages with prenatal care are scarcely greater. In all countries, urban women are more likely than rural women to use these services.

Strong upward trends in utilization of trained assistance are seen as women ' s educational levels rise from no education to secondary school education. In Guatemala, for example, prenatal care increased from 18 to 86 per cent, in Mali from 27 per cent to

95 per cent in Mali (Chayovan, 1988; Sayed, 1989; Ghana, 1989; Guatemala, 1989; Traore, 1989).

Distance from home to the health facility, lack of transportation and lack of funds undoubtedly explain some of the births not attended by trained personnel, yet the differential between source of care for prenatal visits and deliveries also suggests that deliberate choices are being made. The value given to a natural and familiar setting and the spiritual and material support for the cosmological conceptions of the patient offered by traditional birth attendants strongly influence a decision to give birth in the home community (Twumasi, 1987). These factors weigh heavily against the lack of privacy in a health facility, the use of unfamiliar positions during childbirth, shame at crying out before others and the indignity of exposure (Auerbach, 1982; Rehan, 1984; Schuler et al., 1985; Beeson et al., 1987; Kerns, 1989).

The statistics on utilization do not take into account the quality of care (training and skills of the provider or shortages such as supplies or equipment, including specula and gloves for internal examinations). In a typical prenatal examination, the woman is weighed, blood pressure is taken, the abdomen may be palpated, urine may be tested and sometimes blood may be drawn for testing. The woman may be asked about vaginal discharge, itchiness or other symptoms, but a pelvic examination is not always performed if it is not indicated by her history or condition. Even a woman using a modern family planning method, unless it is an intrauterine device (IUD) or tubectomy, might not be examined internally.

Women often are not aware they have vaginitis and cervicitis, which are the most common syndromes in lower tract infections (Hatcher et al., 1989; Wasserheit, 1989). It is estimated that 10 to 50 per cent of women with trichomoniasis, 25 to 30 per cent with gonococcal cervicitis and probably over 50 per cent of women with chlamydial cervicitis or bacterial vaginosis experience no symptoms (Wasserheit et al., 1989 citing Holmes et al., 1984). Such symptoms as vaginal discharge may be taken to be a fairly normal condition, not requiring medical attention (Orubuloye et al., 1990). The discharge and even a substantial degree of discomfort are often ignored (McFalls and McFalls, 1984).

Access to Health Services

Differences in access to health care between men and women, as widely reported, are acute with regard to conditions affecting sexual organs. A man with symptoms might go for STI treatment, at least at an advanced stage; his wife is more likely to remain untreated. This is not always because women are unaware of what is happening-to their bodies but because their bodies are devalued and are not seen as requiring care. Preferential health care for male children —is documented— in Asia, principally in Bangladesh and India, and in the Middle East (Cook, 1987). This apparently leaves its cultural mark on the adult female.

In the rural areas throughout developing countries, women doctors are rare; in the Moslem culture especially, women are not allowed to be examined by a male doctor. Distances to health facilities can be very great, and women lack autonomy and money. They are often not released from household and child-care duties to go to a clinic during office hours or to wait at hospitals or dispensaries. Travel outside their immediate community may be forbidden (Kloos, 1987) or inhibited by lack of education and the confidence needed to deal with the official systems. More efficient means of transportation — such as bicycles, motorbikes, horses and donkeys — may be for use only by males (Stock. 1983).

Where they are confined to purdah, as in Hausa society, a woman must obtain the permission of her husband before leaving the home compound. Many men are reluctant to allow their wives to make long, unescorted journeys for health care, particularly if the husband perceives the wife's illness to be non-threatening and amenable to traditional treatment (Stock, 1983).

Men are often the intermediaries between women and health services and assessment of the severity of a condition and the choice of an appropriate source of treatment, if any, may be made by the husband or by senior male members of the family. In Zaire, sufferers retain decisionmaking rights only if they are adult, capable of walking and travelling, financially able to pay for care and, usually, male (Janzen, 1978).

The obstacles many women face in access to health care are caused by poverty, lack of education, inferior position in society, and inadequate health systems, among others. The result is that, if a woman does not have prenatal care, or if her one or two visits do not include an internal examination, she may pass through her entire life and bear her children, yet never have an internal examination.

Personal Modesty

Even if symptoms are recognized, and even if services are available, obstacles remain. For women, a strong deterrent is reluctance to undergo a pelvic examination. This was emphatically demonstrated by a survey on female genital operations in the Sudan. Ninety-five per cent of the sample population, 3,210 women, were interviewed, but only 12 of the women were willing to be examined (Gordon, 1991). Some of the women may have wished to conceal the evidence that they had undergone mutilation; the majority were more likely to be expressing a strong sense of personal modesty.

Reluctance to expose the genitals is not unique to women in developing countries. In the United States, for instance, fear of a pelvic examination was cited by 25 per cent of adolescents queried as to their reason for— not coming sooner to a family planning clinic (Zabin and Clark, 1981). As Scrimshaw states emphatically: "Any woman from just about any culture who has ever had a pelvic examination knows how undignified and embarrassing it feels" (1973: 10).

Embarrassment or shame has particular force in some cultures, as is evidenced by the unpopularity of contraceptive methods that require genital exposure and contact. Injection, for example, has been recommended for women in India so that they might avoid both the mortifying experience of exposure to medical scrutiny and the need to handle their genitals when using a method (Marshall, 1973). Embarrassment with genital exposure associated with IUD insertion is reported from Indonesia where the Islamic religion plays a major role in choice of contraceptive method. Many Moslems object to the intimate physical contact between IUD providers and their clients, despite recent rulings from high Moslem councils conditionally endorsing IUD use (Molyneux et al., 1990).

Modesty as a value central to the image of womanhood is notable in the care taken to cover the genitals of females even in infancy, as in Latin America, while male children are free to expose their genitals until they approach puberty. Douches and coitusdependent contraceptive methods which violate standards of modesty are rarely used by women in Colombia (Browner, 1985) and never among the Aguarunas in Peru, who interpret any viewing or manipulation of female sexual organs as erotic (Berlin, 1985). Some Mayan women in Guatemala do not remove their skirts even for childbirth (Beck, 1991). Mexican women asked to name the parts of their bodies could find no word for the vagina except "la parte" (the part), and that was uttered with manifest embarrassment (Shedlin, 1982).

The depth and force of modesty is exemplified by the pregnancy and childbirth practices of rural Hausa/Fulani women in the northern region of Nigeria. Muslim women in purdah do not openly admit to their pregnancies. They often labour alone in their compound (with other women keeping within hearing distance in case assistance is required). The traditional birth attendant (TBA) is called in after the child is born to cut the cord and look after the mother and baby (Sokoto Maternal Health Project, 1990).

Fear and stigma surround problems relating to the sexual organs and women suffer in silence. In India, inhibitions about drawing attention to the body can be so great that even female health workers must rely upon verbal accounts of the symptoms of women who will not subject themselves to a physical examination (Ramasubbam, 1990).

Feelings of "verguenza", or shame, and their influence on attendance at family planning clinics, were examined by Scrimshaw in detail (1973). Many of the women interviewed in Guayaquil, Ecuador, who never undressed completely before their husbands, were forced to expose themselves to male doctors at the clinic without even a drape over their legs during the pelvic exam. With a drape, at least, the woman cannot see the doctor and has some illusion of privacy.

Moroccan women report feeling inhuman when they are ordered to take off their pants and sit in a drafty hall where people walk by while they are waiting to see the service provider for family planning (Mernissi, 1975). This study, the Scrimshaw work also from the 1970s and a much earlier study by Stycos in Puerto Rico (1955) gave serious scientific attention to a subject that is still acutely and universally felt by women, still a grave problem and still for the most part ignored.

> *. . . when men are infected, their wives are suspected of infidelity; when women are infected, they are assumed to have strayed...*

Sexual Inequality and Stigma

Restrictions on travel, fear of pelvic examination and violation of the sense of personal privacy are formidable barriers in themselves, without the added stigma of a sexually-related infection. An association of STIs and promiscuity, references to sexually transmitted infections as the woman's disease in popular parlance in some languages and common use of the term reservoirs of infection to describe prostitutes place the onus solely on the female, regardless of the male's multiple relationships. Research in Zaire found that when men are infected, their wives are suspected of infidelity; when women are infected, they are assumed to have strayed (Schoepf, cited in Bledsoe, 1989:11). The image of women as the source of disease is reinforced by the media and public health announcements, as in the Zambian advertisement: —Avoid AIDS. Take Time to Know Her (Bledsoe, 1989:11).

Counseling women about prevention and the need for treatment of their partners may presume incorrectly that they are free to discuss sex and condom use without jeopardy. Discussion of this emotionally charged topic is rare in many cultures. A survey of spousal communication in Asian countries, for example, found that close to one third of the women interviewed in the Philippines never talked to their husbands about sexual matters, nor did 47 per cent in Singapore or 53 per cent in Iran (UNESCAP, 1974). In sub-Saharan Africa, sexual activities are rarely discussed either between spouses or between the generations (Caldwell et al., 1989). In Latin American culture, communication between men and women (or parents and children) regarding sex is not the norm (Worth and Rodriguez, 1987; Santos Ortiz, 1990). In a study of decision-making on the use of family planning in Mexico, 35 per cent of the survey sample had never discussed the subject of birth control with their spouse (Folch-Lyon, 1981). In focus groups, women expressed the difficulties they experienced in any discussion of sexual relations with their husbands. Castro de Alvarez (1990) observed that cultural norms in their patriarchal society dictate that Latin American women appear naive about sexual matters and that a woman knowledgeable about and prepared for a sexual encounter is considered loose. It is thus very difficult to realize the necessary conditions for promoting condom use and persuading a partner to be treated for a sexually transmitted infection. They are: relative sexual equality between men and women; the possibility that other sex partners can be acknowledged; and options other than motherhood to define self-identity or self esteem (Worth, 1989).

When there is no communication about sex, and when women fear that their relationships will be jeopardized by asking for safe sex practices, promotion of condom use among women is likely to fail.

When there is no communication about sex, and when women fear that their relanonships will be jeopardized by asking for safe sex practices, promotion of condom use among women is likely tofail. The anger at being made to feel responsible for men's sexual behaviour expressed by women in a New York City study probably has near universal application. Women claimed men decide what is going to happen sexually and that if the staff wanted men to wear condoms, they would have to talk to them, not to women (Worth, 1989). Prevention strategies that place the onus on women ignore the subordinate position of the many who are economically and emotionally dependent on their male sexual partners. For these women, negotiation, even perhaps discussion, is not an option (Maldonado, 1991).

Among the socio-cultural and psychological constraints to overcome in promoting condom use in Zaire are strong beliefs and feelings about the contribution of semen to women' s health and the importance of reproduction (Schoepf et. al, 1988). The decision to use a condom is a decision not to reproduce as well as not become infected. The general use of condoms may. therefore, be in direct conflict with the desire of women to fulfill their reproductive roles and with the expectations of their partners and families that they do so. It is also a decision that must be made for each act of intercourse. Women must repeatedly address the issue of sexual decision-making and sexual control, and each time this is done they are emotionally, sexually, physically and economically vulnerable (Worth, 1989).

SUMMARY AND RECOMMENDATIONS

The causes of damage to the epithelial barrier that allows vaginal transmission of HIV are numerous: sexually transmitted infections insertion of objects into the vagina, trauma during sexual intercourse and genital mutilation practices, among others. Obstacles to prevention. diagnosis and treatment are also numerous. Most are embedded in the cultural and economic context of women's lives and can be overcome only with concerted effort at the level of both local communities and the national health systems. These issues must be given priority in national and international research and aid agendas.

Recommendations in this section are given with the caution that a change in women' s knowledge. and behaviour is necessary but women alone do not carry the responsibility for prevention of HIV transmission. Men, in their political and economic positions of power as well as in their sexual partnerships, are responsible for change, as it is women's subordination -lack of control over their bodies and their lives — that is the primary HIV risk factor (Hamblin and Reid, 1991; Carovano, 1990).

Community Level

On the level of the local community, the starting point for education of women and men is the message that women's health is important for reasons other than childbearing. Knowledge about their bodies ability to speak of sexual organs and processes without shame, hygienic practices (especially as regards menstruation) and signs and symptoms of genital-urinary problems must be communicated through social networks in the community. By whatever means, women must be helped to talk of these things together in their own-idiom, without embarrassment, and to help each other devise strategies for raising these issues with men. Men must be helped to be at ease speaking of their own and women's sexuality, with each other and with women, candidly and not crudely. Role models must come forth who in their knowledge of and attitudes toward women can redefine the masculine image.

> *Women's groups are a near universal resource and women can use them to learn to speak of their bodies, sexuality and genital health in their own way, according to their own customs.*

Knowledge about sexuality and reproductive biology is transmitted by older experienced women, in many societies, especially where social separation of sexes emphasizes communication between women rather than between partners (Newman, 1985). The local setting may suggest other rules for discussion of sexually-related matters, as in Tunisia where women never speak of family planning with their daughters or with anyone of a different age group (Huston, 1978). Women's groups are a near universal resource and women can use them to learn to speak of their bodies, sexuality and genital health in their own way, according to their own customs.

Preferences for local, familiar and predictable midwifery services for childbirth suggest that traditional midwives can play an important role in developing awareness of threats to genital health and the ability to recognize symptoms of STIs and in providing advice on resources for treatment. Training TBAs for safe delivery and health education is a fairly widespread practice. Although the trainers usually discourage midwives from performing internal examinations, in order to avoid infections, and their curricula do not usually cover sexually transmitted infections and other genital conditions, midwives can be trained to ask about symptoms, to advise and, when linked to a health service system, to refer women for diagnosis and treatment.

Research on traditional medicine rarely examines conditions other than pregnancy that motivate women to seek care. However, evidence generally supports the view that traditional practice is popular and addresses a broad range of women' s conditions. Traditional medicine co-exists with modern medical practice, and it is not uncommon for consultations with both systems to occur serially or concurrently (Janzen, 1978; Cosminsky and Scrimshaw, 1980; Heggenhougen, 1980; Green and Makhubu, 1984; Cleland and van Ginneken, 1988; Good, 1988; Ingstad, 1990).

In Malaysia for example two traditional systems (Ayurvedic and Chinese) and the local Malay folk medical system, accepted as parts of general Malaysian culture and society, are linked to the official health system and used widely as additions or alternatives to modern medical practices (Heggenhougen, 1980). A Guatemalan plantation population can have simultaneous access to folk curers (curanderos), herbalists, midwives, spiritists, shamans, injectionists, pharmacists, private physicians, public and private clinics and hospitals and home remedies (Cosminsky and Scrimshaw, 1980). Good (1988) estimates that most African rural areas have at least one part-time traditional healer for every 200 to 300 persons; in the towns, there is one healer for every 400 to 800 persons. In Swaziland. at least 85 per cent of the population is believed to make use of the services of traditional healers (Green and

Makhubu, 1984). Many of these opinion leaders and therapists are female. While the role of traditional healers in communicating information on genital health and its protection is not universal, they are an ubiquitous and influential resource.

Health Systems

Strengthening health service systems for prevention and treatment of genital infections and other conditions must be a major national and international priority that should go beyond traditional categories of service. The narrow focus of public health programmes concerned with women is apparent in their labeling as maternal and child health services. The rationale for this lies in the belief that improving women's health is an important precondition to child health. A recent variation on this reasoning focuses on the woman as a potential transmitter of HIV to her infant and as a caregiver to people with HIV infection and related illness and orphaned children.

Health systems reflect this limited view of women's lives and potential and the pervasive gender inequalities which deny women control over their own bodies. Expansion of the concept of women's health to encompass the breadth of their activities and concerns is an immediate public health responsibility. Grants for study and research, support for networks of organizations, forums, training, policy analysis, advocacy and new and improved programmes are all required to bring attention to the restrictions on the health services women are now offered. These health services are restrictive both because they are difficult of access in many areas and because they respond only to a narrow range of women's health needs.

Prenatal services provide a good opportunity for health care workers to counsel women on protection of the genital tract and to diagnose and treat genital-urinary tract infections. Training of clinical personnel to be alert to adverse genital conditions is necessary; equally necessary are respect for the patients' sense of inappropriate or shameful exposure and care to ensure privacy to the maximum degree possible. Screens constructed from local materials, drapes made from local cloths—to shield exposed areas, minimum time without full clothing—these are in themselves indications of concern for feelings as well as relatively simple measures to make services more acceptable to women. Increasing the supply of female medical personnel on all levels is essential. In the prevailing absence of educational opportunities for women from the earliest grades through university degrees, more women must be given scholarships.

Much of the work needed does not require advanced training and extensive employment. In-service training of local women in health centres and in the community can reduce barriers while extending the availability of services. Primary health care and family planning services have amply demonstrated the value of recruiting and training paramedical personnel from the local population. If there is genuine community participation, especially of women's organizations, in facility and service planning, then needs, perceptions, problems and expectations can be freely expressed, respected and addressed.

Family planning providers can lead the formal sector in exploring how health services can reduce the institutional obstacles women encounter. Their programmes could provide services for diagnosis and treatment of genital lesions, inflammations and infections, and could be the only available source of health care for sexually active women, especially poor women. Functions that would be relatively easy to integrate into family planning services, given appropriate training and supplies and a commitment to genital as well as reproductive health are as follows: substituting modern contraceptives for objects damaging to the vagina (which will also diminish their use as abortifacients); educating women and men about risks; and diagnosing, treating and counseling sex partners.

The scarcity of resources for health care in developing countries is glaringly evident. There is a shortage of laboratories and supplies for diagnosis, as well as medication for treatment of STIs. In the shorter term, rapid expansion of laboratory testing is not feasible. However, it is possible to develop and subsidize distribution of supplies for inexpensive, relatively simple diagnostic techniques using cervical swabs, vaginal KOH odor and dipstick assessment of vaginal pH, as demonstrated in a study of reproductive tract infections in Bangladesh (Wasserheit, et al., 1989). As appropriate tests are developed, the health systems must undergo the changes necessary to put them to use.

Research and Aid Agendas

Priorities for research and development assistance are not easily set for a topic so seldom examined in its personal and social complexity. It is urgent that technological advances be made to develop and provide inexpensive diagnostic tests for women in developing countries. Female providers in traditional and modern sectors must be trained to educate, diagnose and treat. Their work should be evaluated through operations research.

The dilemma, or paradox, of condom use as the main strategy to prevent women from contracting HIV stems, of course, from the fact that it is a strategy for men. Since it can not be used when the male is dominant and resistant, alternative means of mechanical or chemical barrier protection must be found quickly, they must be distributed widely at little or no cost and they must have appeal to women.

> *A vaginal virucide which would offer protection against transmission without preventing conception is vital for women who desire children and who need to have them in societies where their status and economic security depend upon procreation.*

Spermicides and diaphragms shift the focus of control over prevention to the woman, a preference demonstrated by women who were given the choice in studies in Cameroon and Ghana (Spieler, 1990) and Rwanda (Allen et.al., 1988). Barriers that depend on the woman alone may be less effective than condoms, yet more effective in the long run if they are consistently and widely used and the condom is not (Stein, 1990). Laboratory and clinical studies indicate that vaginal spermicidal contraceptives which place a chemical barrier between infected fluids and vulnerable mucous membranes offer women considerable protection against STIs (see North, 1990, for a literature review), although use with a condom is more certain. Nonoxynol-9 (N-9), the most widely used spermicide, has been tested as an HIV virucide and laboratory findings suggest that it offers some protection. However, it has not been determined whether spermicides alone, without any mechanical barriers, protect against HIV infection (Cates and Stone, in press). Problems encountered in interpreting results of clinical studies have stemmed from a research focus on special populations (e.g. prostitutes with rates of sexual activity far exceeding the general population) and confounding factors such as use of N-9 with a vaginal sponge, which could itself cause microlesions or irritation from high concentrations of N-9 (Gollub. 1991). Female condoms (e.g., pouches made of polyurethane or latex) are being tested although they are not now in a form that is likely to have wide acceptability.

A vaginal virucide which Would offer protection against transmission without preventing conception is vital for women who desire children and who need to have them in societies where their status and economic security depend upon procreation (Stein, 1990). A promising avenue for the research is the possibility that concentrations of N-9 lower than recommended as a spermicide may be effective as a virucide (Stein and Gollub, 1991). The urgency of the need to investigate this and other virucides and the necessity for rapid development of a method women can use to protect themselves cannot be overstated.

The literature on the possible association of female mutilation with HIV transmission is sparse and speculative. Infections of the mutilated area, trauma caused by sexual intercourse, and blood transfusions necessitated by excessive bleeding at childbirth are plausible reasons. The universality of the practice in some African regions suggests that there may be a group of women at risk of infection of appalling dimensions as the epidemic expands geographically. A vigorous investigation of the relationship between female mutilation and HIV transmission must be undertaken.

Societal Transformations

> *Collectively, women are developing strategies to stand up to the official systems, to change men 's behaviour and to realize the strength of unity for survival. They must be assisted with information, with legal aid, with health services and with opportunities for education and economic independence. A woman 's lack of control over the resources for her own physical and mentul health and well-being is a violation of human rights that constitutes a direct threat to her life.*

The place of women in society is a primary cause of exposure to risk of HIV infection and a primary barrier to use of health services. Some of the consequences of this role of women are: little or no information; restrictions on movement outside the local community; fear of strange environments that are often with justification perceived as hostile; and the role of the men as mediators between women and the health system. The changes that must be made in the legal, economic and cultural spheres over the long term are immense and must be made largely by those who are favoured by the present inequities.

Yet over the short term there are collective actions women can take in their local communities. Women working together are learning to develop strategies for communication with their sexual partners about HIV, sexually transmitted infections, use of condoms and other sexual behaviours, finding as well the courage and determination to face opposition. Collectively, women are developing strategies to stand up to the official systems, to change men's behaviour and to realize the strength of unity for survival. They must be assisted with information, with legal aid, with health services and with opportunities for education and economic independence. A woman's lack of control over the resources for her own physical and mental health and wellbeing is a violation of human rights that constitutes a direct threat to her life.

REFERENCES

Adebajo, Christine Olufunke (1989). "Traditional practices that are harmful to health." Paper presented at a meeting of the Inter African Consultative Expert Group on the Possible Link between Traditional Practices and the Transmission of HIV. Addis Ababa, Ethiopia. 911 May.

Ahmed, Samira Amin and E. Haj Hamad M. Kheir (1990). "Sudanese sexual behaviour in the context of socio-cultural norms and the transmission of HIV." Paper presented at the IUSSP Seminar on Anthropological Studies Relevant to the Sexual Transmission of HIV. Sonderborg, Denmark, 19-22 November.

Allan, Susan et al., (1988). "Acceptability of condoms and spermicides in a population based sample of urban Rwandan women." IV International Conference on AIDS. Stockholm, Sweden, 12-16 June. Book 1, 1989:349, Abstract 5137.

Ampofo, E. Kofi et. al., (1990). "Risk factors of vesico-vaginal fistula in Maiduguri, Nigeria: a case control study." *Tropical Doctor*, July. pp. 138-139.

Auerbach, Liesa S. (1982). "Childbirth in Tunisia: implications of a decision-making model.' *Social Science and Medicine* 16. pp .1499- 1506.

Beck, Diane et al ., (1991) . American College of Nurse-Midwives. Personal Communication. May .

Beeson, Diane et al., (1987). "Client-provider transactions in family planning clinics." In *Organizing for Effective Family Planning Programmes,* edited by Robert J. Lapham and George B. Simmons. Washington, D.C. National Academy Press, pp.435-456.

Belsey, Mark A. (1980). "Infertility: etiology and natural history." *In Workshop on the diagnosis and treatment of infertility*, Nairobi, Kenya, 21-22 February 1979, edited by P.J. Rowe and S.R. Raharinosy-Ramarozaka. Bath, England. Pitman Press, pp.11-42.

Berlin, Elois Ann (1985). "Aspects of fertility regulation among the Aguaruna Jivaro of Peru. In *Women's medicine: a cross-cultural study of indigenous fertility regulation,* edited by Lucile F . Newman . New Brunswick, N .J . Rutgers University Press, pp .125- 146.

Bledsoe, Caroline (1989). "The cultural meaning of AIDS and condoms for stable heterosexual relations in Africa recent evidence from the local print media." Paper presented at the IUSSP Seminar on Population Policy in Sub-saharan Africa: Drawing on International Experience, Kinshasa. 27 February - March 2.

Browner, C.H. (1985). "Traditional techniques for diagnosis, treatment and control of pregnancy in Cali, Colombia." In *Women's medicine: A cross-Cultural study of indigenous fertility regulation,* edited by Lucile F. Newman. New Brunswick, N.J. Rutgers University Press, pp. 99-123.

Caldwell, John C., Pat Caldwell, and Pat Quiggin (1989). "The social context of AIDS in sub-Saharan Africa." *Population and Development Review* 15(2) pp.185-234.

Carovano, Kathryn (1990). "More than mothers and whores: redefining the AIDS prevention needs of women." *International Journal of Health Services* 21(1)pp.131-142.

Castro de alvarez, Virginia (1990). "AIDS prevention programme for Puerto Rican women." *Puerto Rican Health Science Journal 9*(1)pp.37-41.

Cates, Jr., Willard and Katherine M. Stone (1992). "Reproductive Tract Infections and Contraceptive Use. Safely." In *Reproductive Tract Infections in the Third World: National and International Policy Implications,* edited by A. Germaine, K. Holmes, P. Piot, J. Wasserheit. New York. Plenum Press, in press.

Chayovan, Napaporn, Peerasit Kamnuansilpa, and John Knodel (1988). Thailand Demographic and Health Survey 1987. Bangkok. Institute of Population Studies, Chulalongkorn University and Demographic and Health Surveys, Institute for Resource Development/Westinghouse. May

Cleland, John G. and Jerome K. Van Ginneken (1988). "Maternal education and child survival in developing countries: the search for pathways of influence." *Social Science and Medicine* 27(12)pp.1357-1368.

Cook, Robert (1987) . " Current knowledge and future trends in maternal and child health in the Middle East." *Journal of Tropical Pediatrics,* 3 (Suppl. 4) pp. 3-10.

Cosminsky, Sheila and Mary Scrimshaw (1980). "Medical pluralism on a Guatemalan plantation." *Social Science and Medicine,* 14B, November, pp. 267-278.

Dallabetta, Gina et al.. (1990). "Vaginal tightening agents as risk factors for acquisition of HIV." VI International Conference on AIDS, San Francisco California, 20-24 June 1990. Vol .1, p. 268, Abstract No. TH .C. 574.

Dixon-Mueller, Ruth and Judith Wasserheit (1991). *The Culture of Silence: Reproductive Tract Infections Among Women in the Third World.* New York. International Women' s Health Coalition.

Feldman, Douglas A. (1990). "Sexual practices in traditional Africa: planning for culturally appropriate HIV-related interventions." Unpublished. p.19 pages.

Folch-Lyon, Evelyn, Luis de la Macorra, and S. Bruce Schearer (1981). "Focus group and survey research on family planning in Mexico." *Studies in Family Planning* 12(12) pp. 409-432.

Frank, Odile (1983). *Infertility in sub-Saharan Africa.* Center for Policy Studies Working Papers, No. 97, June. New York, The Population Council.

Ghana Statistical Service and Institute for Resource Developmenti Macro Systerns, Inc., (1989). *Ghana Demographic and Health Survey 1988.* Columbia, Maryland. Ghana Statistical Service and Institute for Resource Development/Macro Systems, Inc., September.

Gollub, Erica (1991) . School of Public Health. Columbia University and HIV Center for Clinical and Behavioural Studies, New York State Psychiatric Institute. Personal communication, June.

Good, Charles (1988). "Traditional healers and AIDS management." In *AIDS in Africa: the social and policy impact,* edited by Norman Miller and Richard C. Rockwell. Lewiston, NY, Edwin Mellen (published in association with the African-Caribbean Institute and the National Council for International Health), pp.87-95.

Gordon, Daniel (1991). "Female circumcision and genital operations in Egypt and the Sudan: a dilemma for medical anthropology." *Medical Anthropology Quarterly* 5(1) pp. 3-23.

Green, Edward C. and Lydia Makhubu (1984). "Traditional healers in Swaziland: toward improved co-operation between the traditional and modern health sectors." Social Science and Medicine 18(12)pp.1071-1079.

Guatemala Ministerio de Salud Publica y Asistencia Social (1989). *Encuesta nacional de salud materno infantil 1987.* Columbia. Maryland. Instituto de Nutricion de Centro America y Panama and Institute for Resource Development/Westinghouse, May.

Hamblin, Julie and Elizabeth Reid (1991). "Women, the HIV epidemic and human rights: a tragic imperative." Paper prepared for the International Workshop on "AIDS: A Question of Rights and Humanity, International Court of Justice, The Hague, May.

Hatcher, Robert A. et al., (1989). *Contraceptive Technology: International Edition.* Atlanta. GA., Printed Matter, Inc.

Heggenhougen, H K. (1980). "Bomohs. doctors and sinsehs—medical pluralism in Malaysia." *Social Science and Medicine* 14B, pp. 235-244.

Holmes, Kino K. et al. (eds), (1984). *Sexually transmitted diseases.* New York. McGraw Hill.

Hunte, Pamela A. (1985). " Indigenous methods of fertility regulation in Afghanistan." In *Women's Medicine: a Cross-Cultural Study of Indigenous Fertility Regulation,* edited by Lucile F. Newman, New Brunswick. N.J., Rutgers University Press, pp.43-75.

Huston, Perdita (1978). *Message from the village.* New York, The Epoch B. Foundation.

Ingstad, Benedicte (1990). " The cultural construction of AIDS and its consequences for prevention in Botswana." *Medical Anthropology Quarterly* 4(1) pp. 28-40.

Janzen, John M. (1978). *The Quest for Therapy: Medical Pluralism in Lower Zaire.* Berkeley, University of California Press.

Kerns, Virginia (1989). *Women and the Ancestors: Black Carib Kinship and Ritual.* Urbana and Chicago, University of Illinois Press.

Kloos, Helmut et al., (1987). "Illness and health behavior in Addis Ababa and rural central Ethiopia. " *Social Science and Medicine* 25(9) pp.1003-1019.

Low, Setha M. and Bruce C. Newman (1985). "Indigenous fertility regulating methods in Costa Rica." In *Women's Medicine: A Cross-Cultural Stud} of Indigenous Fertility Regulation,* edited by Lucile F. Newman. New Brunswic};, N.J., Rutgers University Press, pp.147-160.

Maldonado—Nugyekuba (1991). "Latinas and HIV/AIDS." *SIECUS Report* December 1990/January 1991. pp .11-15.

Marshall, John (1973). "Fertility regulating methods: cultural acceptability for potential adopters." In *Fertility control methods: strategies for introduction,* edited by G.W. Duncan et al. New York, Academic Press, pp. 125-132.

Mcfalls, Joseph A. and Marguerite Harvey McFalls (1984). *Disease and Fertility* New York, Academic Press.

Mernissi, Fatima (1975). "Obstacles to family planning practice in urban Morocco." *Studies in Family Planning* 6(12) . pp .418-425.

Molyneaux, John W. et al., (1990). "Correlates of contraceptive method choice in Indonesia. Population studies in Sri Lanka and Indonesia based on the 1987 Sri Lankan Demographic and Health Survey and the 1987 National Indonesian Contraceptive Prevalence Survey. The Population Council and Demographic and Health Surveys, Institute for Resource Development, Demographic and Health Surveys Further Analysis Series, No. 2, March.

Newman, Lucille F. (1985). "Context variables in fertility regulation." *In Women's Medicine. a Cross-Cultural Study of Indigenous Fertility Regulation,* edited by Lucile F. Newman. New Brunswick, N. J., Rutgers University Press, pp.179-191.

Ngin, Chor-Swang (1985). "Indigenous fertility regulating methods among two Chinese communities in Malaysia." In *Women's medicine: a cross-cultural study of indigenous fertility regulation,* edited by Lucile F. Newman. New Brunswick, N.J., Rutgers University Press. pp. 25-41.

North, Barbara B. (1990). "Effectiveness of vaginal contraceptives in prevention of sexually transmitted diseases." In *Heterosexual transmission of AIDS,* edited by Nancy J. Alexander et al. New York, Wiley-Liss, pp.273-290.

Orubuloye, I.O., John C. Caldwell and Pat Caldwell (1990). "Sexual networking and the risk of AIDS in southwest Nigeria." Paper delivered at the IUSSP Seminar on Anthropological Studies Relevant to the Sexual Transmission of HIV. Sonderborg, Demnar;. 19-22 November.

Oxtoby, Margaret J. and Helene D. Gayle (1990). "AIDS in women and children." *Outlook* 8(4)pp .2-6.

Peterman, Thomas A. (1990). "Facilitators of HIV transmission during sexual contact." In *Heterosexual transmission of AIDS,* edited by Nancy J. Alexander et al. New York, Wiley-Liss, pp. 55-68.

Ramasubban, Radhika (1990). "Sexual behaviour and conditions of health care: potential risks for HIV transmission in India." Paper prepared for the IUSSP Seminar on Anthropological Studies Relevant to HIV Transmission, Sonderborg, 19-22 November.

Rehan. Nagma (1984). "Knowledge, attitude and practice of family planning in Hausa women *Social Science and Medicine* 18 (10) pp. 839-844.

Reid, Elizabeth. Women, HIV and Development. Paper presented to the Conference on the implications of AIDS for Mothers and Children, Paris, 27-30 November 1989.

Reid, Elizabeth. "Young Women and the HIV Epidemic". *Development,* (Journal of the Society of International Development), No. 1, 1990, p. 16.

Santos-Ortiz, Maria del Carmen (1990). "Sexualidad femenina antes y despues del SIDA." *Puerto Rican Health Science Journal* 9(1)pp.33-35.

Sayed, Hussein A. et al., (1989). *Egypt Demographic and Health Survey 1988.* Cairo, Egypt, National Population Council and Institute for Resource Development/Macro Systems Inc., October.

Schoepe, Brooke Grundfest (1988) . ' AIDS and society in Central Africa: a view from Zaire. " in *AIDS in Africa: The Social and Policy* Impact, edited by Norman Miller and Richard C. Rockwell. Lewiston, NY, Edwin Mellen (published in association with the African-Caribbean Institute and the National Council for International Health), pp. 211-235.

Scheler, S. et al., (1985). "Barriers to Effective Family Planning in Nepal." Studies in Family Planning, 6(5) pp.) 260-270.

Scrims Law, Susan, C. (1973). *Lo de Nosotras: Pudor and Family Planning Clinics in a Latin American City.* New York. International Institute for the Study of Human Reproduction. January.

Shedlin. Michele G. (1982). *Anthropolog and Family Planning: Culturally Appropriate Interventions in a Maxican Community.* Ph.D. Dissertation, Columbia University.

Shedlin Michele, G. and Paula Hollerbach (1981). "Modern and traditional fertility regulation in a Mexican community: the process of decision making." *Studies in Family Planning* 12(6/7) June. July, pp. 278-296.

SHERRIS. Jacqueline D. and Gordon Fox (1983). "Infertility and sexually transmited disease: a public health challenge." *Population Reports.* Series L, No. 4, July (reprinted July 1985).

Sittitrai, Weerasit, Rapeepan Sujaritraksa, and Anchalee Wisuttimak (1989). "AIDS education materials for Thai commercial sex workers; preliminary report." Center for AIDS Research and Education. Science Division, Thai Red Cross Society, January.

Soko to Meternal Health Project (1990). "Report of planning activities." Usmanu Danfodiyo University Sokoto. and Ministry of Health Sokoto, Report of maternal health project for prevention of maternal mortality June.

Spieler. Jeffrey M. (1990). "Summary discussion" (remarks of Dr. Lamptey). In *Heterosexual transmission of AIDS* edited by Nancy J. Alexander et al. New York, Wiley-Liss. pp.419-426.

Stein, Zena A. (1990). "HIN prevention: the need for methods women can use." *American Journal of Public Health* 80. pp.460-462.

———and Erica Gollub (1991). Testimony submitted to the National Commission on AIDS. Denver. Colorade. 5 June.

Stock. Robert (1983) Distance and utilization of health facilities in rural Niveria." *Social Science and Medicine* 1 7(9) pp.563-570.

Stycos, J.M. (1955). "Birth control clinics in crowded Puerto Rico." In *Health, Culture and Community*. edited by Benjamin D. Paul. New York, Russell Sage Foundation, pp.189, 210.

Sukkary-Stolba, Soheir (1985). "Indigenous fertility regulating methods in two Egyptian villages." In *Women's Medicine: a Cross-Cultural Study of Indigenous Fertility Regulation,* edited by Lucile F. Newman. New Brunswick, N.J., Rutgers University Press, pp.78-97.

Tahzib, Farhanq (1989). "An initiative on vesicovaginal fistula." *Lancet* June 10, pp. I316, 1317.

Traore, Baba, Mamadou Donate, and Cynthia Stanton (1989). *Enquete demographique et de sante au Mali 1987.* Columbia, Maryland: Centre d'Etudes et de Recherches sur la Population pour le Developement, Institut du Sahel and Institute for Resource Development/Westinghouse, January.

Twumasi, P.A. (1987). "Traditional Birth Attendant Review Programme in Ghana." Commissioned by Ghana Ministry of Health. October.

United Nations (1991). *The World's Women 1970-1990: Trends and Statistics.* New York United Nations Publications, Sales No. E.90.XV11.3.

United Nations Economic and Social Comission for Asia and the Pacific (UNESCAP) (1974). "Husband-wife communication and practice of family planning." *Asia Population Studies Series. Bangkok.* 16, pp .26-27.

Wasserheit, Judith N. (1989). "The significance and scope of reproductive tract infections among third world women." *International Journal of Gynecology and Obstetrics* Suppl. 3 pp.145-168.

———(1990) . " Reproductive Tract Infections . "In *Special Challenges in Third World Women's Health.* Presentations at the 117th Annual Meeting of the American Public Health Association, Chicago, October 1989. New York, International Women's Health Coalition, March, pp. l-15.

———et al., (1989). "Reproductive tract infections in a family planning population in rural Bangladesh." *Studies in Family Planning* 20(2)pp.69-80.

Wilson, D.P., C.S. Lavelle, and C. Mutero (1989). "Sex workers, client sex behaviour and condom use in Harare, Zimbabwe." *AIDS Care* 1(3) pp. 269-280.

Women's International Network (n.d.). "Women and health summary facts: genital and sexual mutilation of females (1)." *News.* Lexington, Maine.

World Health Organization (WHO) (1989). "WHO consensus statement: sexually transmitted diseases as a risk factor for HIV transmission." *Journal of Sex Research* 26(2) pp. 272-275.

————(1990). Consensus statement from the consultation on global strategies for co-ordination of AIDS and STD control programmes, Geneva, World Health Organization, WHO/INF/90.2.

World Health Organization/Global Programme on AIDS (WHO/GPA) (1990). *AIDS Prevention: Guidelines for MCH/FP Programme Managers. II. AIDS and Maternal and Child Health.* Geneva, World Health Organization, May, WHO/MCH/GPA/90.2.

Worth, Dooley (1989). "Sexual decision-making and AIDS: why condom promotion among vulnerable women is likely to fail." *Studies in Family Planning* 20(6)pp.297-307.

————and Ruth Rodriguez (1987). "Latina Women and AIDS." *SIECUS Report* January-February. pp.5-7.

Zabin, Laurie Schwab and Samuel D. Clark Jr. (1981). "Why the delay: a study of teenage family planning clinic patients." *Family Planning Perspectives* 13(5) September/October, pp.205-217.

27

Sharing the Challenge of the HIV Epidemic

Ms. Elizabeth Reid
UNDP, New York

Conceptual Complexity

There are two important characteristics of the HIV epidemic which need to be acknowledged and understood, by national leaders in particular, for they will affect and determine the nature of the response to the epidemic in the Asian and Pacific region.

Firstly, the epidemic is at one and the same time both a crisis and an endemic condition. It is a crisis because the speed of spread of this virus can be so awesome. Infection rates can, and have even in this region, increased from two per cent to 25 per cent in adult populations in less than four years. There is no reason to assume that this is not happening in this region. Before people are even aware that they are surrounded by infected family and friends, their communities have been deeply penetrated. This fact alone should be sufficient for the epidemic to be viewed as a calamity, albeit too often invisible in its early stages, as much in need of an immediate response as the invasion of one country by another. For war nowadays rarely has the toll in human lives that this virus is causing and will cause.

That it is an endemic condition may best be simply illustrated by the fact that even if in an affected country there were to be no further cases of infection as from today, the pain and trauma of the deaths of those already infected will continue for the next twenty years and the social and economic repercussions of their deaths will continue on for decades and generations after that. We know that nowhere in the world is the spread abating or even slowing down. Each day of continuing spread adds to the ramifications and duration of its devastating impact.

Both dimensions, the epidemic as crisis and the epidemic as

endemic, need to be recognized. leach has its own appropriate responses.

Secondly, the epidemic manifests itself both as a specific problem but also as a pervasive one. Its specificity is revealed in its associated morbidity and mortality, in increasing numbers of people, mostly healthy, productive young women and men, getting sick and dying. The response of the first decade of the epidemic addressed this quality of the epidemic. It focused on the epidemic as a health crisis and on its ramifications for health service delivery.

However, the repercussions of these deaths will permeate and affect every facet of human life and national development, more so in countries where men and women are infected in more or less the same numbers. The causes and the consequences of the spread of the virus embrace poverty and wealth, disempowerment and influence, wellbeing and disease, deprivation and development, trust and bad faith; the very way we are as human beings.

Both of these dimensions of the epidemic, its particularity and its ubiquity, must also be recognized. Each of these too has its own appropriate responses.

Thus this epidemic is conceptually complex: at once a crisis and an endemic condition; at once a specific issue and a permeating one.

Programme Imperatives

These two characteristics of the HIV epidemic impose a set of imperatives upon us:

the imperative of an effective response;
the imperative of a sustainable response; and
the imperative of a co-ordinated response.

The prerequisite of an effective response is a common understanding of the nature of the epidemic, which takes into account the above two characteristics, and a shared vision of the way forward. This we do not yet have. This should not surprise us for the epidemic is a new and complex phenomenon for which there is no likeness in living memory, not one drawn from war, not from disease, not from natural disasters nor from man-made ones.

This is not to say that we are blindly groping. We are doing what we know needs to be done while we search for new and more effective ways to respond. The more we share a vision of an effective way forward, the more co-ordination and the building of partnerships will naturally follow.

The second imperative is that of a sustainable response. The commitment and contributions of affected individuals and communities have yet to be recognized or valued but they are extensive.

They lie at the heart of a sustainable response to this epidemic but in most cases they need to be supplemented by further human and financial resources. The closeness of these individuals and communities to the problems and needs created by the epidemic generally ensures that their responses are appropriate. Similarly, governments are increasingly beginning to allocate national resources to the epidemic although in most cases they still have to be persuaded that it affects all aspects of societal development both now and in the future.

The required human and financial resources must be available for effective responses. However, these responses must also be ranked in order of effectiveness since resources, whether of individuals, communities, nations or of external support agencies, will continue to be limited and will themselves be reduced by the epidemic.

Thus priority must be given to strengthening national capacity to ensure that these resources, and that of the external support agencies, are used in the most effective manner. There is not time and there are not sufficient resources for illconceived, inappropriate or ineffective responses. The selection must be ruthless for the demand on resources, both human and financial, will continue and increase inexorably for decades. Communities and governments must have the ability to monitor, assess and evaluate their interventions and to modify, redesign and expand them.

Where the response to the epidemic is effective and sustainable, hope is brought into being that the desolation and distress of this epidemic can be eased, a hope that can turn back the tides of fatalism and despair

The third imperative. that ot a co-ordinated response, means that we must build the partnerships required to ensure that the search for effective and sustainable policies and interventions is an ongoing process and that duplication is minimized. Such partnerships are needed among the community groups responding to the epidemic, between such groups and government, among government ministries, between the public and the private sectors, among external support agencies, especially within the UN system, and between donors and countries.

The Challenges to be Shared

Before we elaborate further on the partnerships required by this epidemic, we need to identify the challenges facing the Asian and Pacific region that we are being called upon to share.

I want to identify just three such challenges;

the challenge of making the invisible visible;

the challenge of creating an ethic of compassion; and
the challenge of placing people and their communities at the centre of the response to the epidemic.

The first challenge to make the invisible visible, is a clear imperative in this region. We must find the means to belter understand and make known the speed and the surreptitious patterns of spread of the virus. Surveillance systems tell us where the virus has been but we need predictive systems that map out for us where it is likely to go. Understanding the factors which determine this will enable us to put faces to the figures, to see ourselves in its path or in its wake.

But more than just numbers and silhouettes of those affected need to be made visible. Those living within the epidemic, those at the forefront of change, must create a new language that makes more visible the new realities of life in the post-HIV era.

This is already happening in two important aspects of the epidemic. Firstly, we are beginning to develop a language of optimism: affirmations of the possibility of behaviour change, of the centrality of compassion and concern, of care and commitment. Secondly, we are developing a language of process rather than of interventions, of people as responsible actors rather than manipulable objects. It is a language of empowerment, of participation, of listening and talking, of counselling of deciding together.

However, there is still a silence, an inarticulateness, about the dark side of the epidemic: the doubt, the trembling, the uncertainty, the distancing, the denial, the fear. We do not yet have a language that reflects the reality of living with the knowledge that one is infected or that someone one loves dearly is infected: the constant companion of mortality, the sadness, the tentativeness of desire, the longing for love, the stripping raw of self by death after death after death of partners, of children, of childhood friends, of companions.

There is another silence around a central reality of this epidemic: that it evokes a wilderness of emotional and psychological states with whose very existence we are uncomfortable, for which our vocabulary is too limited and which we are reluctant to acknowledge and express. These include hatred, anger, shame, guilt, humiliation, grief, indignity. There is a deep unease which permeates families and societies about using a language of sexuality, of mortality and of vulnerability.

Even those emotional states we value and which are central to our belief that the epidemic can be overcome, we hesitate to publicly acknowledge and express. We lack a familiarity of usage of words such as care, compassion, happiness, humility and wonder.

For that which is invisible about this epidemic to be made

visible we must spin this language, weave it into our lives and grow strong in the courage to use it.

The second challenge we face is to create an ethic of compassion. Let me begin by delineating what this is not. Compassion is not pity, which strips one of dignity and individuality. Compassion cannot be expressed in authoritarian relationships structurally based on inequalities of power: doctor and patient, men and women, parent and child, caste and class. For this reason an ethics of compassion will threaten conventions of distancing and objectivity, norms of control and domination, prerogatives of position and wealth.

An ethic of compassion will value concern over ambition, connectedness over individualism closeness over control mercy over judgment. An ethic of compassion will require the presence of men who pay attention to daily life.

An ethic of compassion is not a matter of appeasing hunger, of providing shelter, of resolving conflict. These are as compatible with charity or pragmatism as with compassion. Rather it involves seeing ourselves as one with others, our lives essentially intertwined with their lives.

An ethic of compassion will bring a particular focus to our work. It will add a sense of urgency to keeping people uninfected. It will place high importance on keeping those affected by the epidemic, the infected, those who love and care for them and those who survive them, within our families, workplace and communities.

Keeping those infected alive for as long as possible will be not only an economic imperative but also a human imperative for even when sick and dying, those infected can nurture their children, touching them smiling, talking, keeping them company and can pass on to them their own skills for economic survival, be they farming, brewing, fishing, street selling, cobbling weaving, repairing or whatever.

Helping those infected to die with dignity through, for example, the treatment of opportunistic infections or the provision of shelter and assistance, will reduce the psychological trauma of the children left behind. Their memories will be of the person they loved not of their unseemly condition.

The third challenge is that of placing people and their communities at the centre of the response to the epidemic.

Again this can be defined by contrast. It means that primary focus will not be placed on technologies (condoms, test kits, etc.) or on interventions (education campaigns, STD services, for example) but on the initiation of processes whereby both individuals and communities can change and through which agents of change are created. The technologies and interventions will become the handmaidens of, not the masters of, change, there to be called upon as required.

Placing people at the centre of the response to the epidemic will enable that response to reflect and build upon the complex nature of people's daily lives and to address their needs in a cohesive manner. It will begin the process of breaking down a compartmentalized development approach to essentially interlinked conditions: poverty, disempowerment, disease, subordination, illiteracy, land ownership, to mention a few, and HIV infection. It recognizes and accepts that little is simple in the face of this epidemic

An approach that values and builds on the vagaries of human life and human nature will lead to realistic and therefore sustainable responses. It will provide the basis for the hope. the belief, that we are not powerless in the face of this pathogen and that we will indeed overcome the epidemic and its consequences.

The most striking feature about this epidemic is that individuals and communities have been mobilized and empowered by it. People are speaking out; community groups are coming into existence. We see this already in this region. This conference has honoured Dominic de Souza. There are many other courageous men and women like him in our communities, speaking out, working with others. However, in a non-supportive environment, too often the impact of such individual initiatives wanes over time as people move on or die or groups lose their initial momentum.

The Partnerships to be Built

The energy, vision and commitment of these agents of change needs to be transformed into an active force for change, a force which can transcend the particular and permeate communities and nations. For this to happen, four social contracts or partnerships must be built.

The first partnership must be a new social contract between men and women.

The HIV epidemic and its impact will only be overcome if men and women begin to forge true partnerships of mutual respect and trust and of equitable sharing of the burdens of sadness, pain, care and support created by the epidemic. Men and women must seek to establish the kind of honest communication about sexuality and sexual behaviour needed to prevent the transmission of HIV in their partnerships. They must work to restructure the sexual relationships in which they take part.

Women alone cannot stop this epidemic nor care for its sick and its survivors. Women alone cannot bear the burden of its psychological, social and economic impact. Nor should this be expected of them. To do so would be to build in the certainty of failure. Not because of any failing in women, but because sexuality, love and coping are essentially shared experiences.

Changes in individual relationships between men and women will occur only in the context of the emergence of a new social contract, not one simply governing men's or women's behaviour, but one which changes what it is to be a man or a women. The social contract must encompass the way we nurture and raise our children. the way society constructs its gender archetypes. It must further allow for community explorations of the appropriateness of accepted community values and standards of behaviour. Such a social contract must be supported and reaffirmed by laws, policy budgetary priorities and programme design and delivery.

The family in all its diverse forms thus becomes the basic nexus of change. For although individual men and women can decide on ways to protect themselves from infection, the likelihood of this happening and being sustained resides in factors which long precede adulthood and sexual activity. They have their origin in how people are brought up in family life, whether that be an extended or nuclear family or another environment.

It is in the family context, from birth, that personalities are formed gender identity is created. moral values are instilled. In particular it is in families that boys are brought up to be boys and girls, girls, with their attendant sexual and social identities, attitudes and behaviours. We know that self respect, self confidence, respect for others and an ability to talk about personal and intimate matters are all characteristics which help people to remain uninfected.

Thus it is within family contexts that the basic prevention strategies must be put into place. Love and nurturing must be given to both boys and girls so that they may grow into independent, confident human beings, able to form respectful and non-violent relationships, whatever their sexual orientation may be. Parental-child discourse must be developed on bodily care and sexuality and strengthened on community norms and moral values, especially with regard to respect for self and others. We must change the ways that girls and boys are raised so that as adults they will be less likely to put themselves and others at risk of infection. This will require significant changes in the social construction of masculinity and femininity.

These gender paradigms must be reconstructed in particular ways. The new paradigms should lead to the greater valuing of compassion, concern for others and love of family in men and, for women, in a simple recognition of their value and worth. It is hard to reconcile the oft claimed valuing of women, even as mothers, with the widespread acceptance of female infanticide or the mortality rates associated with pregnancy and childbirth, as high as one woman in 21 in some parts of the world: 1 million women per year. New patterns for the sharing of the responsibilities and joys of women's lives must emerge.

But families individually do not determine cultural meanings, social customs or community values. They inherit, accept, respect and instil them. Thus, for families to change, communities and societies must also change. The new social contract will therefore require a radical reassessment by societies of the very way men and women see themselves and each other, of the way they relate as husband and wife, lovers, brothers and sisters, parent and child, as partners, colleagues and friends.

The second partnership must be a social contract between the affected and the not yet directly affected.

The infected and those close to them are amongst the most powerful agents of change in the world today. They can give us glimpses of how we can peacefully co-exist with the virus, of how we can become empowered through the trauma and the tragedy of the epidemic. Within the desolation of this epidemic, they give us snatches of laughter and happiness. They can help us explore and better understand the nature of intimacy, desire and sexuality in the age of the virus.

But these insights of the affected will not be shared, this gift will remain ungiven, if, in the sharing, the affected are stripped of their self esteem and dignity, subjected to humiliation and discrimination, left alone in a hostile limelight without support and companionship.

These insights, these glimpses of the world within the epidemic. must be shared if our response is to be grounded in human experience, if this experience and knowledge is to shape and reshape theory and practice.

The stories of the affected provide access to lives which are subtle and various, which present the experience of living within the epidemic in the complex, interrelated way life usually asserts itself. The stories bring to light different perspectives, different points of view and so make the understanding of how to live with the epidemic accessible across class, gender, educational and lifestyle barriers.

Women are more aware of the dynamics of gender in their daily lives. Thus how gender affects the epidemic emerges more clearly in their stories. Life situations such as being infected or caring for someone infected can be understood only if gender roles and interrelationships are taken into account. Women' s stories both present and interpret the dynamics of power between women and men and the relationship between the individual and society. They provide glimpses into men's lives as well as into women's lives and relate individual agency to social and economic structures.

Stories, however, do not capture systems of relationships which affect individuals but whose locus is beyond the individual and her or his realm of vision. The relationships between poverty and infection status may form a critical part of the story but the relationships between structural adjustment programmes, for example, poverty and the tragedy of being infected may not. Hence, stories need to be complemented by system level analyses. A full understanding of the nature and impact of the epidemic requires both kinds of analysis .

This partnership between the affected and their communities is critical. It is an acknowledgement within the community that the epidemic concerns the community as a whole and not just certain individuals perceived or assumed to be at risk. The absence of this social contact favours discrimination, marginalization, denial and infection. The Them/Us mentality which dominates in the absence of this partnership has, sadly, too often characterized perceptions of and responses to the epidemic. There is no other in the shadow of the epidemic. We are all there.

This second partnership or social contract, once in place, will enable the creation of a supportive milieu that encourages the affected to speak out. tell their stories, reflect on their lives and hopes and help us all to live peacefully with this epidemic.

The third social contract must be between communities and government.

The responses we have seen occurring within affected communities provide us with the hope that the epidemic can be overcome, and the insights into how this can come about. These responses are universal. Wherever the virus has spread, communities have responded, to provide care and support, to stop further infection, to assure the rights of the affected to minister to spiritual, emotional and physical needs.

But individuals, families and communities cannot carry this epidemic alone. There must be a social contract, a partnership, between governments and affected communities. Governments must provide an enabling environment that will evoke, nourish and sustain these responses. This enabling environment must include national policies that acknowledge the centrality of community responses, a body of legal and human rights laws that respect the principles of non-discrimination and respect for the rights and dignity of affected individuals, mechanisms for interaction between government and communities, and assistance, as required, for programme design, delivery and financing by communities.

The need for additional resources for this epidemic is frequently mentioned. Whilst it is clear that external resources are needed, it is important to stress that the initial financial resources mobilized to respond to this epidemic are invariably those of individuals, families and communities. As yet, these remain unrecognized and unquantified. We must name these contributions and quantify them for, sadly. this is the way that most people recognize and establish the value of such actions.

These resources—peoples' volunteered time, the food, means and insights they share, the transport provided, the labour contributed, the funds raised—lie at the heart of a sustainable response.

Yes, the resources must be supplemented. They are not without end. They themselves are depleted by the epidemic. They are not, always or usually. sufficient. Communities know what additional resources, human or financial, they need for sustenance and growth. They need to be empowered to be able to define their external support requirements, select them, manage them and account for them in appropriate ways whether these resources come from national or international sources.

Mutual trust and respect is a sine qua non for a social contract between communities and their government. This may not be easy for either but it must come about.

The fourth partnership must be a global contract.

As the epidemic deepens, its devastating potential impact on all aspects of human life and national development is becoming better understood. Certain nations may be brought towards the threshold of destitution. Will the world wait until this stage is reached in some countries? When will there be a global response? Will the world community provide the resources for investment in the education, health and social welfare of people and in the technological development required to enable these nations to continue to function? Will there be global social safety nets to allow nations rendered poor by this epidemic. and the poor within nations, to survive?

The working of global trade agreements and markets have increased the disparities between rich and poor nations and rich and poor individuals. At the national level, many governments try to offset such tendencies by redistributing income through systems of progressive income tax and by supplementing this with social safety nets to prevent people from falling into poverty and absolute destitution. No such systems exist at present at the global level.

The closest the world comes to a global safety net is the current system of development assistance. However, this system is fatally flawed, not only in the way it is programmed, but in the inadequacy of its extent, and because its allocation is unrelated to levels of poverty. Less than 7 per cent of global aid is spent on human priority concerns of basic education, primary health care, family planning, safe drinking water and nutritional programmes. Only a quarter of overseas aid flow is earmarked for the ten countries containing three-fourths of the world's absolute poor. In fact, India, Pakistan and Bangladesh contain nearly one-half of the world's poor but get only one-tenth of total aid.

Twice as much development assistance per capita is given to high military spenders among the developing world as to more moderate military spenders. The international financial institutions, like the World Bank and the IMF, are now taking more money out of the developing world than they are putting in, adding to the reverse transfer of around $50 billion per year to the commercial banks.

If overseas aid is to be able to serve as a social safety net for the world's poor, it will have to be based on principles requiring that aid should be directed to priority concerns for human survival and human development.

These four social contracts or partnerships are essential to an effective sustainable response to this epidemic. They will be difficult to forge and will not come about without the commitment and courage of our leaders and friends. There is an ever increasing urgency to embark upon the endeavour to build them.

The Way

At the heart of this epidemic, either there can be violence and fragmentation or there can be stillness. In the hearts of those yet personally untouched by it, it is the same. It is the same in the hearts of those affected.

For all of us, knowing how to live with HIV can bring a certain stillness to the centre of our lives. It can still the violence and the fragmentation the fear and the denial. It is this stillness which creates the possibility of living.

We need to reach out to each other, as one human being to another. There can be no Them and Us if this epidemic is to be overcome. We are all seeking to pass from untruth to truth, from darkness to light, from vulnerability to ease.

There is a special truth and light, a special love and laughter, which can be given to us by those who are courageous enough to tell their stories. We must learn to share in their sadness and hope, their tears and laughter. We must partake of their dignity and courage.

That we have gathered here at this Congress bears witness to the tact that we are pilgrims, engaged upon a voyage of understanding.

This voyage will require from each of us truth, compassion, faith wisdom, respect for others and courage.

It will be a voyage of understanding what is, of understanding reality, not of asserting what we would like to be the case, what we would prefer to believe.

It will be a voyage of sharing, the sharing of a sense of mystery, of a burden of sadness, of the pain of care, of the laughter of life.

It will be a voyage to change for each of us, for none of us are untouched by this epidemic.

It will be a voyage of the heart and the mind to communities of concern and commitment.

It will be a voyage through pain, through the dark side of the epidemic, with hope.

28

Responding to the Challenge of HIV and AIDS

The UNDP Regional Projeet for Asia and the Pacifie Region will have completed its initial phase by the end of December 1992, leading to a new four-year Project in 1993. The response to the Project, initially enthusiastic but guarded, indicates that the socio-economic implications of the HIV epidemic have already moved closer to the centre of policy-making concern. Organizational and bureaucratic barriers have begun to crumble, leading to dynamic partnerships across operational sectors.

The challenge now is to build on the increased level of awareness. New initiatives are coming forward from NGOs and business sector allies; government departments and policy institutes. New strategies are emerging for improving HIV awareness, communicating information and advice, counselling those affected, combating prejudice, and promoting behavioural change. New service delivery approaches, such as some just starting in the hotel and transport sectors, need to be monitored for application elsewhere. The human rights lobby is starting to defend people with HIV from discrimination and privacy invasion. This mushrooming volume of activity needs encouragement and concrete support.

Consciousness-Raising Among Decision-Makers

There is still much to be done in changing the policy climate towards HIV. AIDS as a subject exerts a powerful fascination. Unfortunately, even hightly educated and relatively well-informed people tend to believe that AIDS is confined to special groups and that HIV must—and can—be kept at bay by isolation of people known to be infected. Familiarization with a less alarmist, more positive approach so that it becomes embedded in policy-making attitudes cannot be achieved overnight. Many politicians, government officials, academics, NGO leaders, and captains of industry and commerce, still need to be introduced to HIV as a social and economic phenomenon. The existing concern of others needs reinforcement if it is to be translated into action.

The UNDP country and regional workshops have provided all opportunity to identify researchers keen to make a contribution to the analysis of the epidemic participants from a variety of disciplines have become resource persons for further workshops, or for the preparation of new components in AIDS country plans. A regional network is developing or socio-economic expertise in the field of HIV and AIDS related studies. Data and authoritative analysis is not only vital *perse*, but of great importance in providing the evidence needed to persuade the sceptical that HIV and AIDS are, indeed, a threat in their own country and will reach their own social milieu; and that something can be done to reduce this threat both by health professionals and others.

Country workshops and regional consultations are primarily aimed at consiousness and knowledge building, they also have an advocacy function. When individuals participate, for example, in discussions on education about HIV in the workplace, they are also confronting—often for the first time in their professional capacity - the need to take the personal, social and economic consequences of the epidemic seriously. The intent is to create a snowball effect of HIV concern, which will be taken forward during the new project phase.

Support to Community-Based Initiatives

UNDP's guiding principles for policy development in the field of HIV and AIDS emphasize the importance of enhancing the capacity of community-based organizations (CBOs). As a result of the presence of AIDS in Asia, new CBOs have emerged spontaneously to address various aspects of the epidemic. Other NGOs, mostly those concerned with health, but also some concerned with urban community development, or with human rights, have added concerned about HIV to their existing agendas.

The role of the NGO sector vis a vis the HIV epidemic is very special. Whether interest.-, creed-, or profession-based, NGOs exist to address preoccupations shared by a specific group of human beings. They are driven therefore, by human motivation and experience; not by the constructs familiar to professional planners and policy-makers.

Those that are community-based are, by definition, close to their constituencies. The connection between HIV infection and intimate behaviour make this a difficult subject to address at a personal level—where all behavioural change takes place. To bring about such change requires eliciting people's confidence and empathy, which is especially difficult among those engaging in behaviour which is 'not respectable' or illegal. Helping people to avoid H1V infection will require a process of building alliances with organizations and authority figures people trust. These are most likely to be found in the NGO and CBO community.

The UNDP Regional Project therefore playes a strong emphasis on these groups. It. keeps abreast of new developments, initiates contacts, and networks between organizations enabling them to learn from each other's experiences. Organizations that have sprung up in response to HIV and AIDS have high motivation but little experience, and need organizational and management skills. In the ease of existing NGOs, the challenge is to find common ground with their own agendas so that they can be persuaded to undertake HIV-related initiatives among their own membership or clients. UNDP has already held a number of formal and informal consultations for NGOs.

The inspirational role of NGOs is also an important tool for HIV prevention. Case histories, both of HIV-related human predicament, and of effective nurturing or preventive strategies, can have a profound effect on the caring human conscience and are important in dispelling prejudice and rallying resources. The impact not only on the public at large, but on decision-makers, of people's courage in the face of AIDS has had a major effect on the overall campaign, world-wide and in their own societies. During the next four years, the Regional Project will offer support to up to six innovative community-based pilot projects. These will be fully documented with a view to cross-fertilization of information and the stimulation of similar approaches, where suitable, in other environments.

A promising area of partnership for NGOs is with the business sector. A recent regional consultation organized by UNDP brought together NGOs and CBOs with representatives of the hotel, advertising, retail, and pharmaceutical industries and Chambers of Cormmerce of India and Thailand. This was the first ever occasion on which the business and NGO communities have met together in a structured context to discuss how they can work together on AIDS related projects.

The need to shed preconceptions and find common ground between corporate and NGO agendas as a pre-requisite of joint action was the theme underlying the consultation proceedings. The business perspective is that NGOs are unprofessional and have little to offer; the NGO perspective, that companies' objectives are barely cormpatible with social concern and they can best be seen as an occasional source of funds. NGOs need to learn how to target their approaches by analyzing the corporate culture, offering services appropriate to the employer and employee setting, and building up personal contacts.

Hua Hin Consultation to promote NGO/business sector partnerships for AIDS prevention, June 1992

The objectives of the Consultation were to increase awareness of successful NGO/business partnerships in programmes relating to HIV and AIDS; to share guidelines for establishing such partnerships; and to identify and develop the skills required to make such partnerships work. Among the topics addressed at the meeting were the following:

Characteristics of Partnerships: the Business Perspective (Bill Timmerman, Saatchi & Saatchi, Singapore)

Characteristics of Partnerships: the NGO Perspective (Teresita Bagasao, Kabalikat, Philippines)

Partnerships: Lessons Learned (Royal Garden Resorts/ Population Development Association, Thailand)

HIV: Social Security and Insurance Schemes (Nikom Chandravithun, Thamasart University, Thailand)

HIV and Workplace Personnel Policies (Lee Dilokvidhyavat, Chulalongkorn University, Thailand)

Seeking Business Sector Support: Presentation Techniques (Margie Maciolek, Northwest Airlines, Thailand)

HIV: Labour Law and Other Legal Issues (Vitit Muntarbhorn, Chulalongkorn University, Thailand)

Marketing NGO Services to Business (James Reinnoldt, Northwest Airlines, Thailand).

Among the outcomes of the consultation was a new sense among the representatives of the commercial world that NGOs can provide a useful technical resource for workplace initiatives; and that there is a need to develop policies and prepare management for coping with HIV, as well as to educate staff concerning all aspects of HIV infection. Progress was also made towards developing strategies across the NGO-business divide. Although there is no quick-fix method of partnership development fruitful relationships are practicable if NGOs develop the skills and confidence to form them.

Action for AIDS Prevention

'The UNDP Regional Project will maintain as a primary focus the need to prevent further HIV transmission. At present, the only sure guard against the spread of HIV is the observation, throughout society, of a strict personal sexual code. (Drug users will also need to use sterile needles for drug-injection.) For people to adopt such behaviours, they have to be both properly informed and motivated. This requires an open discussion on sexual mores.

In most, societies of the region the topic of sexuality is not openly discussed, even between husbands and wives, parents and children. However, the challenge of AIDS has brought a realization that as long as sexual behaviour remains a taboo subject, correct information about how to avoid HIV will remain locked away. In this context, the work of many NGOs in breaking down communications barriers needs to be encouraged and emulated.

Compounding the dangers inherent in the silence surrounding sexual affairs are certain cultural practices which increase the vulnerability of the entire population. These include the assignment to sex workers of the task of initiating male children into sexual activity; and the dedication of certain women to a state of sexual servitude, often under the guise of traditional marriage, and their subsequent sale or abandonment. to the commercial sex market.. Both the silence surrounding sex, and the practices in question, have to be sensitively addressed. In this context, further research is required, and the work of NGOs concerned with women's and children's rights needs to be supported.

Particular audiences - the young, workers in occupations which take them far from home, those in the entertainment industry have to be targeted and reached persuasively. All media need to be used in advertising; television; group and individual counseling through NGO's, religious congregations, and personnel net departments. More attention will in future be paid by UNDP to the role of the communications media in reporting HIV and AIDS. Most people derive their notions about AIDS and HIV from newspapers and television. Ghoulish and sensational reports, particularly where they depict AIDS as a disease of the socially outcast have contritbuted to many misconceptions. Failure to emphasize that the means of transmission are limited, and that casual infection is impossible, arouses unnecessary fears. UNDP hopes in time to build an informed network of journalists concerned about AIDS issues.

Working to Change the Legal Climate

UNDP has begun t.o work with lawyers, policy-makers, and human rights activists in the region to create an ethical and legal environment which support rather than discriminates against people living with HIV. While the detention of HIV-positive individuals is an extreme case of the negative use of the law, there are other examples of discriminatory legal practice. Hospitals and laboratories have been required to report the names of all those testing HIV -positive, often leading to leaks of confidentiality and social rejection. Regulations which expose people to loss of jobs, household eviction, and victimization in ways that seem infinitely less endurable in the present than the prospect of sickness and death in the future support the process of denial, HIV's deadliest ally.

The repressive use of the law, by driving HIV underground, also obstructs the process of charting the epidemic. Where it restricts the advertisement of condoms or of safe sex messages, it inhibits action for prevention. Since the law reflects moral judgments made by society at large, it is important that it be used to provide a supportive policy framework. Policy-makers must be encouraged to use the law to prohibit discrimination and support the rights of people with HIV to privacy and aceess to services. The decriminalization of some activities, such as homosexuality and prostitution, may help the building of bridges to socially outcast groups in order to gain their co-operation in HIV prevention.

The law can also be used indirectly to lessen the vulnerability of certain groups exposed to HIV infection. Improvements in the status of women would enable them to protect their sexual health and their rights of inheritance to property; also to give them better access to decent, reasonably paid, jobs. In some countries, a review of the marriage code and the family code, particularly elements which do not afford sufficient protection to girls from early marriage, easy abandonment, and sexual exploitation, is needed in response to the threat which AIDS presents to women and family life.

UNDP is setting up an HIV legal network in the region to raise awareness about the need to integrate considerations about the law into HIV and AIDS policy, and to promote appropriate legal responses. This network will include policy-makers, lawyers, people living with HIV, and community-based organizations. The first step in this process is a Regional Consultation to be held in late 1992.

In Conclusion

The presence of AIDS in a country characterized by a poor standard of human development can set off a downward spiral of damage to hard-won gains in health and living standards. Existing social and economic deprivation produces an environment in which the spread of HIV occurs; and, in turn, the HIV epidemic intensifies deprivation among families already operating within perilously overstretched margins. Because AIDS cuts down people in the prime of life, the ramifications of HIV infection demand a special response from bodies at local, national, and regional levels, in the government, commercial, and non-governmental sectors.

THE HIV/AIDS EPIDEMIC AND ITS CONSEQUENCES

Phase I Spread of the virus	Phase II Illness and death	Phase III Survivors	Phase IV Social and economic impact	Phase V Long-term potential impact
		DISCRIPTION		
Initial spread is hidden but increasing numbers of people becoming infected	Spread of virus continues and infected people increasingly become ill and die.	Children, spouses elderly and others left without support	Depletion of the labour force and military; adverse impact on productive and social sectors, families, communities.	Possibility of social and political unrest, destitution, social disintegration, devastation of aspiration and economies
		POLICY CONTEXT		
Behaviour change: * Education * Prevention * Legislation Other preventive measures Surveillance	Attitudinal Change: * Living positively * Fear * Discrimination Confidentiality Income maintenance and housing Social and psychological support Home care and services Treatment Employment and education Legal rights Community management	Maintain in community Immediate assistance programmes Counselling and social support Education and health Income-generation Legal protection	Monitoring systems Sectoral strategies Personnel policies Education, training policies Strengthening of health/ social sectors Planning methodologies	Minimizing potential impact on individuals, communities and nations.

Countries of the Asian and Pacific Region will have to make the following critical choies:

- # The type of prevention policies adopted and the extent of resources directed to the epidemic in its early stages.
- # The extent to which community responses are integrated into and complemented by the governmental response.
- # The extent to which governments assist the infected, their families and carers, to remain an integral part of their Communities.
- # Whether, and at what stage, governments, the private sector and others begin to plan to minimize adverse social and economic impacts.

Upon the choices made will depend the degree of crisis posed by HIV and AIDS to human and economic development in Asia and the Pacific.

29

Facing the Challenges of HIV/AIDS/STDs: A Gender-based Response

1. Why Gender and HIV/AIDS/STDs?

"One of the most striking features of the response to the HIV epidemic to date is how few of the policies and programmes we have developed relate to women's life situations. The daily lives of women and the complex network of relationships and structures which shape them are well known to women and well documented. Despite this, our theories, research agendas, policies and programmes have not been grounded in and informed by these experiences."

Elizabeth Reid[1]

As the HIV/AIDS epidemic and sexually transmitted diseases (STDs) continue to advance worldwide, we are learning ever more about how they affect individuals, households, families, communities, organizations and nations The individual loss has been enormous, particularly in those countries and regions affected early on. AIDS is increasingly recognized in developing countries as a serious concern for socio-economic development as a whole. Its impact is seen in family and community structures and relationships and in sectors as varied as education, employment, health care, social welfare, agriculture and the judiciary.

Economic consequences are already apparent. In highly affected countries, the business sector is experiencing increased absenteeism as employees fall ill, care for the sick or attend funerals. Loss of experienced and skilled workers in the formal and informal sectors may lead to lower productivity, savings and investments. In subsistence and small-scale agriculture, loss of labour may result in changes in farming patterns and food shortages.

Strategies to prevent the spread of HIV have focused on the promotion of condom use, reduction of numbers of sexual partners and treatment of STDs[2]. Many of these responses, however, have failed to address social, economic and power relations between women and men, among men and among women. These relationships, together with physiological differences, determine to a great extent women's and men's risk of infection, their ability to protect themselves effectively and their respective share of the burdens of the epidemic:

— Women are physiologically more vulnerable to HIV infection than men. Young women are especially at risk and AIDS death rates are highest in women in their 20s.

— Stereotypes related to HIV/AIDS and STDs and their association with marginalized groups (e.g., sex workers) contribute to blaming women for the spread of HIV. Fear of stigmatization inhibits people from taking preventive measures and leads women and men to assess their own risks inadequately. Moreover, many ideas and expectations regarding male and female (sexual) behaviour neither encourage men to act responsibly and protect themselves and their partners from infection nor stimulate women to challenge notions of female inferiority and social structures which keep them vulnerable.

— Low social status and economic dependence prevent many women and young people (e.g., street-children) from controlling their own risk With little negotiating power, they are often unable to insist on safer sex; disproportionately poor, they may have little choice other than to barter sex for survival.

— As society's traditional care-givers, women carry the main psychosocial and physical burdens of AIDS care. Yet they have the least control over and access to the resources they need to cope effectively; few men share domestic responsibilities and family care with their partners.

Although the necessity of focusing on women's needs has been highlighted time and again, especially since 1990 when the theme of World AIDS Day was "Women and HIV/AIDS", women continue to bear the brunt of the epidemic and to be highly vulnerable to infection. Reducing their—and men's—risk of infection demands gender-based responses that focus on how the different social expectations, roles, status and economic power of men and women affect and are affected by the epidemic. This involves analysis of gender stereotypes, redefinition of male and female relationships and roles, promotion of cultural beliefs and values supporting mutually responsible behaviour and exploration of ways to reduce inequalities between women and men. A supportive environment can be created thereby, enabling women and men to undertake prevention and cope better with the epidemic.

Women and men both have much to gain from increased gender sensitivity in general development policy, planning and programmes and particularly by national AIDS/STD programmes, AIDS service organizations and related services. At all levels a gender-based focus on problems and solutions is urgently needed.

A gender-based response to HIV/AIDS and STDs focuses on how different social expectations, roles, status and economic power of men and women affect and are affected by the epidemic.

It analyses gender stereotypes and explores ways to reduce inequalities between women and men so that a supportive environment can be created, enabling both to undertake prevention and cope better with the epidemic.

This publication aims to provide policy-makers, planners and programme implementers with information and ideas to help them incorporate a gender-based approach to HIV/AIDS and STDs into their policies and programmes. It highlights the nature and scale of the epidemic, explores the concepts of gender and a gender-based approach and the ways HIV/AIDS and STDs affect and are affected by gender. Suggestions are made for approaches and strategies to address some of the problems.

It is hoped that the analysis, information, ideas and examples will help stimulate many more gender-sensitive initiatives to help us cope with HIV/AIDS and STDs more successfully.

2. How Extensive are HIV/AIDS and STDs?

At the end of 1994, a cumulative total of 1,025,073 AIDS cases (adults and children) worldwide had been reported to WHO. The actual number of AIDS cases is unknown because of under diagnosis, incomplete reporting and reporting delays. However, an estimated 4.5 million AIDS cases have occurred in adults and children since the beginning of the epidemic (Figure. 29.1).

An estimated 18 million adults (13-15 million alive) and 1.5 million children have been infected with HIV. Of the adults, 7-8 million are women (most of childbearing age, Figure 29.2). WHO forecasts that, by the year 2000, 30-40 million HIV infections will have occurred, 90 per cent in developing countries. Moreover, an estimated 5 million children under 10 years of age will be orphaned, losing one or both parents.

The proportion of women with HIV and AIDS has increased dramatically. By 1994, women represented 40 per cent of all new AIDS cases; up to 50 per cent of all new HIV infections were in women, mainly those aged 15-24 years.* Female vulnerability has

---

* *All figures are based on WHO reports unless otherwise indicated.*

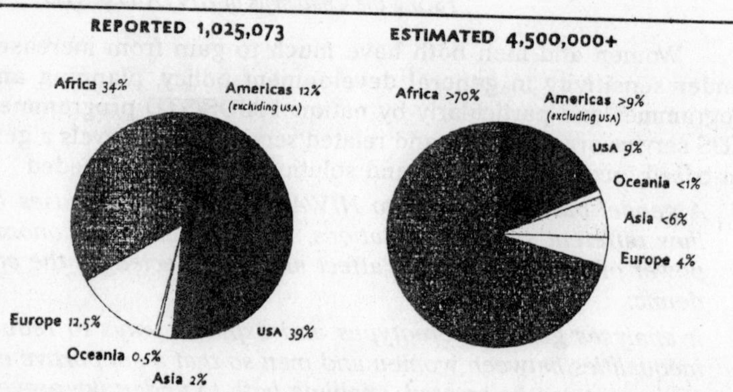

Figure 29.1. Total numbers of reported and estimated AIDS cases (adults and children) from the late 1970s/early 1980s until late 1994 *(Source: WHO/GPA)*

become increasingly clear in Africa and Asia. By the year 2000, an estimated I4 million women will have been infected with HIV and about 4 million will have died of AIDS.

HIV is transmitted predominantly through sexual intercourse (70-80 per cent of infections). Mother-to-child transmission and needle-sharing by drug users each account for 5-I0 per cent of all HIV infections, while needlestick accidents among health workers account for less than 0.01 per cent of resorted cases.

Higher proportions of young women than young men acquire HIV infection through sex. Their exposure to the virus at an earlier age, coupled with physiological factors, increases their risk. In countries with high HIV prevalence, the greatest numbers of reported AIDS cases occur among women aged I5-34 years and men aged 25-44 years (Figure 29.3).

HIV infection due to blood transfusion is more common in women than men.Women more often have blood transfusions because of anaemia and complications during pregnancy and childbirth. Perinatal transmission occurs during pregnancy, delivery or breast-feeding. The chance that a child of a seropositive woman will also be infected with HIV-I is 33 per cent overall, with transmission reported to be as high as 48 per cent in some developing countries. [3]

Regional Patterns

In regions where initially more men than women were infected, there is now a marked increase in infections transmitted through heterosexual intercourse. In Europe, 15.4 per cent of new infections in adults in I993 were due to heterosexual transmission. In France, heterosexual transmission increased from I9 per cent in

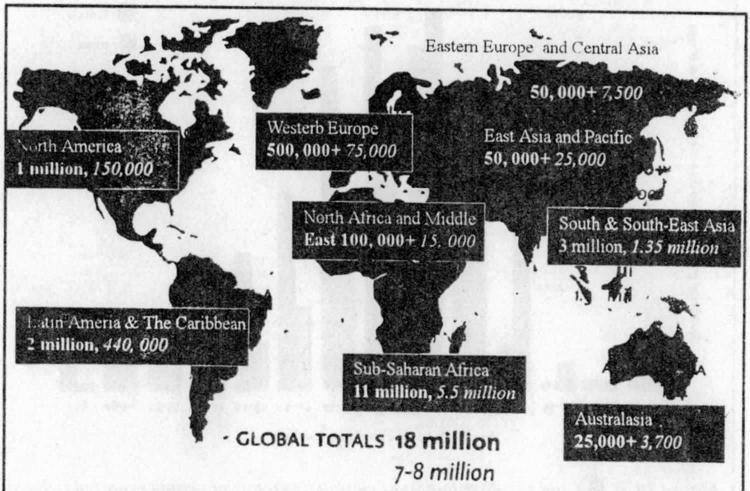

Eastern Europe and Central Asia
50,000+ 7,500
North America
1 million, 150,000
Westerb Europe
500,000+ 75,000
East Asia and Pacific
50,000+ 25,000
North Africa and Middle East 100,000+ 15,000
South & South-East Asia
3 million, 1.35 million
Latin Ameria & The Caribbean
2 million, 440,000
Sub-Saharan Africa
11 million, 5.5 million
Australasia
25,000+ 3,700
GLOBAL TOTALS 18 million
7-8 million

Figure 29.2. Estimated distribution by region of total HIV infections in adults (bold) and women (italics) from the late 1970s /early 1980s until late 1994.
(Source: WHO/GPA)

I991 to almost 25 per cent in I993. In I993 in the USA, AIDS cases in women were almost Is per cent higher than in I992; in nine major cities AIDS has become the leading cause of death among women of childbearing age.

In sub-Saharan Africa, HIV has been transmitted predominantly through heterosexual intercourse since the beginning of the epidemic. More than half of newly infected adults are female (11-12 women for every 10 men). The annual number of infections is still increasing. In Francistown, Botswana, for example, HIV prevalence in pregnant women rose from 8 per cent in 1991 to about 35 per cent by I993. In some countries, e.g., Cote d'Ivoire, Zaire and Uganda, AIDS has become the leading cause of adult death[4].

Seroprevalence rates in North Africa and the Middle East appear relatively low but are increasing. In Djibouti, for example, HIV prevalence has reached I4 per cent among men attending STD clinics and 4 per cent among women seeking antenatal care.

In Latin America and the Caribbean region, a shift from transmission through primarily homosexual intercourse to bisexual and heterosexual transmission as well as injecting drug use has taken place since the early I980. In Brazil, one woman was infected with HIV for I00 men in I 984; by I 994 this was one woman for four men.

Half of the newly infected adults in Asia are women. In a border town in Shan State, Myanmar, 6-I0 per cent of women registered at public maternal and child health centres were already seropositive in early I995 [5].

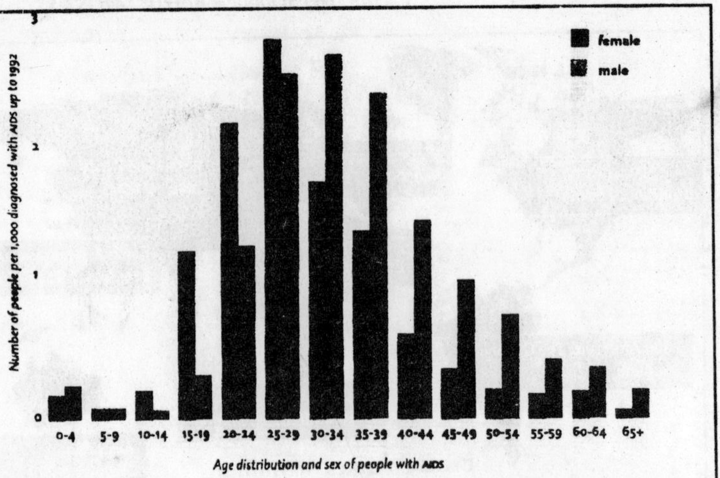

Figure 29.3. Age and sex distribution of cumulative totals of people reported to have AIDS (Source : "Young people first!", AIDS Action, 1994, 25, p. 2).

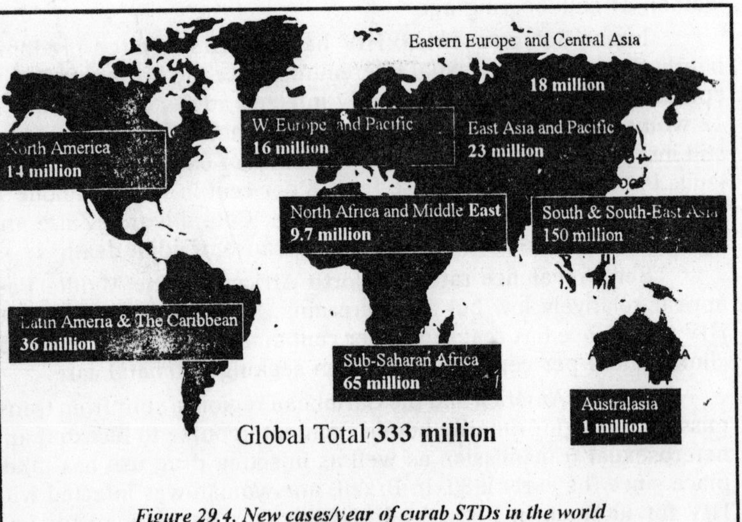

Figure 29.4. New cases/year of curab STDs in the world (Source: WHO/GPA)

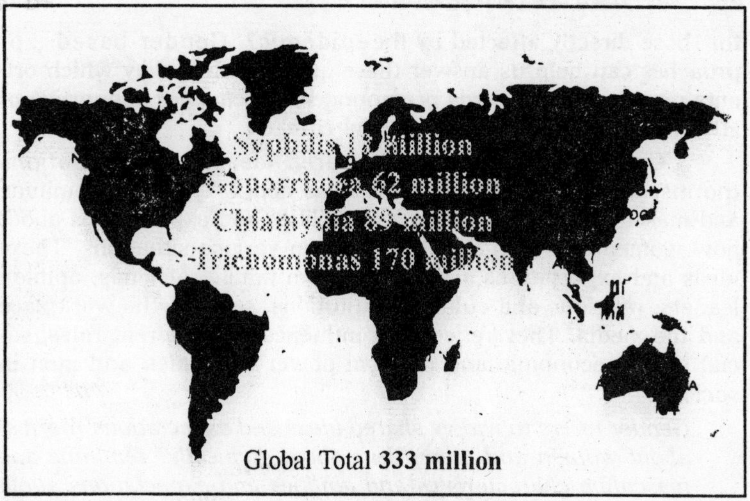

Figure 29.5. Estimated new cases/year of treatable syphilis, gonorrhoea, chlamydia and trichomonas (Source: WHO/GPA)

Sexually Transmitted Diseases

STD rates remain high in much of the world. Each year about 330 million new cases of STDs occur, of which more than 90 per cent are in developing countries (Figures. 29.4-29.5). Overall infection rates for STDs are higher in women than men. Ulcerative STDs, including syphilis and chancroid, and STDs causing inflammation, such as gonorrhoea and chlamydial infection, facilitate transmission of HIV in both women and men. Women, however, are disproportionately affected. As with HIV, women often acquire STDs at an earlier age than men. Gonorrhoea and syphilis are asymptomatic in 50-80 per cent of women against less than I0 per cent of men. In women, they often go untreated, especially in countries with inadequate STD programmes. The secondary health consequences of STDs are more serious for women as they may contribute to infertility, ectopic pregnancy, cervical cancer, premature delivery, stillbirth, low birth weight and neonatal infections. Ectopic pregnancy, cervical cancer and sepsis following pelvic inflammatory disease can be fatal.

3. What Does a Gender-based Response Involve?

What changes are needed to create an environment enabling women and men to protect themselves and each other? How can they collaborate equally in providing adequate care and support for those directly affected by the epidemic? Gender-based approaches can help us answer these questions in a way which orients programmes towards promoting social changes supportive of HIV/AIDS and STD prevention and care.

Gender refers to widely shared ideas and expectations (norms) about women and men: ideas about "typically" feminine and masculine *characteristics* and abilities and expectations about how women and men should behave in various situations. These ideas and expectations are learned from families, friends, opinion leaders, religious and cultural institutions, schools, the workplace and the media. They reflect and influence the different roles, social status, economic and political power of women and men in society.

> *Gender refers to widely shared ideas and expectations (norms) about women and men: ideas about "typically" feminine and masculine characteristcs and abilities and expectations about how women and men should behave in various situations. These ideas and expectations are learned from families, friends, opinion leaders, religious and cultural institutions, schools, the workplace and the media. They reflect and influence the different roles, social status, economic and political power of women and men in society.*

Status and power affect the individual's risk of infection and communities' abilities to cope with the epidemic. The low status and power of women and young people lead to their subordination and restrict their possibilities of taking control of their lives in relation to HIV/AIDS and STDs. Societal pressures also make it difficult for men to change their behaviours in this regard. Their sexual behaviour may be influenced by their relations with other men and women (e.g., fathers, sons, mothers, sisters, peers)[6].

Below, three examples show how gender is related to norms affecting HIV/AIDS and STD prevention and care. The examples are simplified. In-depth gender analysis would also consider other differences that interact with gender to create situations of dominance and subordination, such as age, class, ethnicity and religion[7].

Norms Concerning Parenthood

In most societies, women's primary role in life is to bear and nurture children. Although responsible fatherhood may be promoted, nen's main duty is seen to be earning a living and dealing with the broader society on behalf of the family.

Such norms have two broad implications in relation to HIV/AIDS and STDs. First, a false division is made between "reproductive" (women's) and "productive" (men's) roles[8]. The expectation that women must care for the children is extended to all household members needing support, e.g., the elderly, those who are ill with HIV/AIDS and/or orphaned children. Men are not usually expected to undertake care roles.

This supposed division does not correspond entirely to reality, however. Almost universally, women have always undertaken productive as well as reproductive work; it has simply been unpaid, unrewarded materially and unrecognized. In many African countries, for example, zell over half of the agricultural work is undertaken by women (68 per cent in Central African Republic and the Congo, 70 per cent in Gambia). Yet women do not gain equal access to educational opportunities or the paid labour market, both of which may contribute to social and economic indepenence and more self-assurance.

A second consequence is that childless women are not viewed as "fully adult" or may be considered deviant. Their social status is often low. If their childlessness is due to infertility, they may not know this or refuse to accept the diagnosis and try repeatedly (even with a variety of partners) to become pregnant. This of course implies that they have unprotected sex, thereby increasing their risk of exposure to HIV/STDs.

Moreover, when childless women express their opinions about community measures needed for HIV/STD prevention and care, their suggestions may not be fully respected or accepted by other community members. The voices of women who are mothers may also be given less credibility, because they are expected to confine themselves to household matters.

Sample statements reflecting the idea that women lure men into sex:

"Women should wear purdah [head-to-toe covering] to ensure that innocent men do not get unnecessarily excited by women's bodies and are not unconsciously forced into becoming rapists. If women do not want to fall prey to such men, they should take the necessary precautions instead of forever blaming men" (comment by a member of Malaysia's parliament during debates on the reform of rape laws[9].

"The child was sexually aggressive" (reason given by a Canadian judge for suspending the sentence of a man who had sexually assaulted a 3-year-old girl [9]).

"The female condom will increase immorality among women and single mothers. It is worse than the male condom, giving women the opportunity to do what they want. We are going to preach against these condoms-the church cannot condone their use"

(Parish priest in Kenya[10]).

Norms Concerning Sexuality

Among the numerous norms related to sex, many societies share ideas that women seduce men into having sex and that because male sexual needs are so strong, men cannot resist this. Such notions make men appear to be governed by their instincts, unable to control their behaviour and victims of female power. As a result, men are not expected to behave responsibly, while women's sexuality and behaviour are controlled. For example, in many countries, girls who become pregnant must leave school, while boys who father children can continue their education with no requirement to contribute to child care. To protect men from themselves, social rules may also deprive women of the freedom to move about freely and lead to situations in which women, instead of their attackers, are blamed for sexual abuse.

These ideas form an obstacle to HIV/STD prevention because they absolve men from taking responsibility for they sexual behaviour. They may also prevent women from taking measures to protect themselves. For example, women may be reluctant to buy and carry condoms because they will be accused of wanting to "entice" men into having sex. Women may be reluctant to report abuse because they fear this will affect their position in society: if it becomes known that a young girl has been sexually abused (the result, of a tial in some countries she will have difficulty marrying because both women and men see her as "spoiled".

Norms Concerning Power in Relationships

In many societies, men are expected to control women in all aspects of relationships. This involves desicion-making on when and whom a a girl/women will marry, when and how she will have sexual relations, when and how many children she will have, household expenditures, etc.

This type of male power is supported by tradition and social norms. Women learn, for example, that their first loyalty must be to their kin and families, causing them to act in ways that reinforce rather than challenge female subordination. Oftén, female family members enforce community norms saying, for instance, male relatives must assume authority over widows. In addition, men may impose their will on women, even resorting to violence to do so. Coupled with economic dependence on men, ideas and expectations concerning so-called "proper' male and female roles make it difficult or impossible far women to demand that men share responsibility for preventing sexual and perinatal transmission of HIV/STDs.

Gender analysis and gender-based programmes can help

women and men redefine their relationships in a mutually beneficial way. As women move into traditionally "male domains", men can be encouraged to begin sharing responsibilities in the "female domain". Some women already exert considerable power, if often in subtle ways. Their existing strengths should be recognized and their self-confidence and social skills expanded. Men can be helped to see how their privileged position and social roles orient them more towards relationships involving authority and competition and, perhaps, conflict than Collaboration. As the dynamics of male-female relationships change, communities will be able to benefit from the potential of all their members to minimize the impact of HIV/AIDS and STDs.

— "Right now I'm pregnant. It was an accident, I was planning to go to the clinic but my husband took away my card. He wanted more children so I became pregnant" (woman in Kenya [11]).

— " I told my husband that it was better to use condoms, the doctor said so. The doctor had also given me some to use at home. My husband became very angry and asked who gave me permission to bring those condoms home" (woman in Kenya [12]).

4. Why do HIV / AIDS/ STDs affect Women more?

Women's vulnerability to HIV/AIDS and STDs is partly determined by physiological factors. It further reflects their wider social, sexual and economic vulnerability. The central issue is inequality. Economic need, lack of job opportunities, poor access to education and training and cultural expectations of female submissiveness and male dominance combine to prevent women from actively making choices and decisions about their lives, particularly with regard to limiting sexual risks and protecting their and their families' health. For the same reasons, men are led to deny risk and avoid responsibility, not only for their partners but for themselves. For both sexes this situation needs to change.

Physiological Vulnerability

Women and Men

Researchers estimate that women's risk of HIV infection from unprotected sex is at least twice that of men. Semen, which has high concentrations of virus, remains in the vaginal canal a relatively long time. Women are more exposed through the extensive surface area of mucous membrane in the vagina and on the cervix through which the virus may pass. In men, the equivalent area is smaller, mainly the entrance to the urethra in a circumcised man plus, in an uncircumcised man, the delicate skin under the foreskin. Circumcision in males (not in females!) appears to have some protective value against STDs, including HIV. Men and women's risk of HIV escalates manyfold if STDs are present [13].

Young Women

Young women are at even greater risk than mature women (except for menopausal women in whom thinning of the vaginal mucosa increases susceptibility to infection). A teenager's vagina is not as well lined with protective cells as that of a mature woman. Her cervix may be more easily eroded, potentially enhancing risk of HIV infection. She also faces potential bleeding at first intercourse through tearing of the hymen. In cultures where sex with very young girls is condoned, sexual intercourse is especially likely to cause trauma. In some countries, girls as young as 12 may be married to men three times their age. In addition, girls aged 17 years or younger who have unprotected sex are at increased risk of developing cervical cancer. Sexually active young women may easily contract herpes simplex and human papilcomavirus infections.

All these factors make young women especially vulnerable at a time when their negotiating and economic power is last making them easier targets for sexual coercion and exploitation. This situation is worsened when more men, especially in high HIV-prevalence areas, seek out ever younger female partners in the belief that they are least likely to be infected. This is the most risky pattern of sexual partnership, as a group more likely to have HIV already (older men) transmits the virus to a group with low levels of infection (young girls).

Sexually Transmitted Diseases

Who estimates that about 330 million cases of treatable STDs exist worldwide at any time yet women may have these infections without realizing it some 50-80 per cent of STDs in women are asymptomatic or gounnoticed because they are internal. Women are much less likely than men to seek timely treatment for STDs for this reason. Stigma attached to STDs, especially for women, inaccessibility of clinics, lack of money and too many other responsibilities further prevent them from getting treatment. Negative attitudes of health workers towards women presenting with STDs may be another major deterrent to their seeking treatment or even contraceptive advice. This is true of teenage girls in South Africa, for example[14].

Shyamala, India: "From one end of the room, partitioned by a curtain, a voice, loud and haranguing, came through the silence. It was unmistakably the doctor's. 'Spread your legs!.......Tell me, where is it paining? Now tell me properly! Is it or isn't it paining? How are we supposed to understand anything if you won't talk? OK. Now you can go'...Suddenly the nurse's voice boomed: 'Everybody go and pass urine and come back! I quickly followed three other women towards the single toilet...Back in the waiting room, some men had appeared. Two seemed to have come with their wives and two others .....powere hospital orderlies. I noticed their eyes stray towards the gap in the curtain"[15].

Culture Practices

Certain cultural practices may exacerbate women's physiological risk of HIV infection, especially when HIV is widespread in the population. Many women actively support these practices because they enhance their social status and security with their partners. Examples:

— In some parts of the world, women use herbal and other agents in the vagina to cause dryness, heat and tightness. This practice is carried out because people believe men prefer "dry sex" (in which women feel like virgins) and because they think that female secretions are unclean. The substances used can cause inflammation and erosion of the vaginal mucosa, making it easier far HIV to enter.

— Excessive rubbing of the genitals during foreplay and intercourse, or "rough sex", can lead to sores in the mucous membrane.

— Anal intercourse carries higher risks of HIV transmission because of frequent lesions. Although H is often associated with homosexual contacts, heterosexual couples practise it to preserve virginity, to protect against pregnancy, far (usually male) sexual pleasure and in a search for sexual variety.

— Female genital mutilation (circumcision) is practised in various Countries. Infibulation fin which the labia minora and majora are cut away and the vulva is sewn shut leaving a pinhole opening for urination and menstruation) leads to extensive tearing and bleeding when sexual intercourse is attempted. it may also cause couples to practise riskier anal sex instead. The procedure itself could be risky if unsterilized instruments are used for several patients in succession. Less extreme circumcision, like removal of the clitoris hood, carries little risk during sex, but the procedure itself is potentially risky. Bleeding aver circumcision may lead to the need for blood transfusions with unscreened, possibly contaminated, blood.

Gender-Related Vulnerability and Obstacles to Prevention and Coping

Male Sexual Priority

Commonly, though not universally, male sexual needs are acknowledged to a greater extent than female needs. This may be reflected in the very terminology describing male sexual desire, genitals and partnerships compared with female equivalents. Many cultures use words to describe male sexual desire, genitals and partnerships compared with female equivalents. Many cultures use words to describe male sexuality in a positive way and female sexuality in a more negative and judgemental way. Many women and men define sex largely according to what they believe gives men pleasure, particularly penetration. Often women do not explore, let alone assert, their own preferences, because this is considered inappropriate.

"Everything is centred around the pleasure of the man," says a Zimbabwean women at a market. She sells herbs which, when put in the vagina, cause dryness and tightness. "So if these substances are harmful or even if discomfort is caused, it doesn't matter to the woman. She's doing what she thinks he wants. This is how we have been conditioned" [16].

The dominance of male needs and denial of female needs impedes open discussion between the sexes and limits people's chances of achieving mutually satisfying, respectful and safe forms of sexual behaviour. To curb HIV transmission, both partners should be able to express their worries about infection and use protective measures such as condoms out of respect and affection rather than as a sign of mistrust.

Sex within marriage,in particular, needs to be a source of mutual pleasure and bonding, rather than only a duty and a condition for procreation. However, it is within marriage or with regular partners that wonnen may have most difficult negotiating safer sex, such as condom use as this implies lack of trust and infidelity. But it is essential that they be able to do so, as most HIV-inicted women have been infected by their husband/regular partner.

Economic Vulner ability and Sexual Services

For women and men struggling with daily, concern about a disease that may kill[10] years hence is a luxury they can ill afford..Women's economic dependence makes them vulnerable and, for many, training and employment opportunities are few. If selling sex enables them to survive today, long term concerns remain out of focus. A Ghanaian woman engaged in sex work in Abidjan, Cote d'lvoire, commented, "I need to feed and clothe my children now. How can I worry about something that may not affect me for many years?"[17]

A ready market for sexual services exists almost worldwide and is a significant factor promoting the HIV epidemic. In some countries, it is reportedly the norm for young men's first sexual experiences to be with sex workers. Demand for sexual services is fuelled by cultural attitudes condoning or even encouraging male sexual freedom while repressing female sexuality. Migration, with its associated disruption of family life, partly promotes the demand for and supply of sexual services. Members of the armed forces away from home, displaced populations and affluent sex tourists from Europe, Japan, the Middle East, North America and the Pacific region further contribute to demand.

VULNERABILITY TO SEXUAL EXPLOITATION

Nhlungwane, South Africa: "A woman may go to look for employment all day and fail. On her way back home she might meet a man who wants to have sex with her. she will accept any amount of money in exchange for sex in order to purchase meals for herself and her children. She could get AIDS from that person". [8]

In Asia, daughters may be sold by the family to the sex industry because they need the income.

In Fiji, 8 out of 70 domestic workers reported that they are sexually abused by their employers. Female industrial workers are paid a pittance; some are also sexually abused by supervisors and employers. Because of these problems and increasing poverty, more of the women (often deserted wives) are engaging in sex work. As one sex worker said: "Why put up withyour boss demanding sex and receiving $ 30 a week when you can get more a day by selling your body?" [19].

At the same time, the boundaries of sex work are often blurred: payment and intimacy may range from a brief anonymous sex act for a specified fee through a gradation of casual and commercial interactions. In many societies, not only those with marked gender inequality, men entertain women or provide them with desired goods in return for sexual access on a one-off, short- or long-term basis. Sex may be demanded or bartered in the workplace to gain a job, promotion or trade permit. This is not usually considered sex work but is nonetheless related to economic need. Unfortunately, sex in these situations is often unsafe.

Control Over Sexual Relations within and out side Marriage

Marriage may be viewed as a social and economic commitment between individuals and families. Sexual access, procreation, childrearing and other services are universal to social expectations of marriage; romantic love and affection are not. Because of this, as well as lower social status and economic dependence, married women may be unable to challenge their husbands' extra-marital affairs or insist on condom use for themselves even when they know they are at risk. One philosophy professor used the Bible to justify this, arguing that women vowed to follow their husbands "in sickness and in health". in his view, this absolved husbands of the need to protect their wives; it did not apply the other way round.

Double standards—different sets of sexual rules for women and men—also may hold for other informal long- and short-term relationships. Various societal institutions may promote fidelity, on the one hand, yet also transmit the message that women should not question male unfaithfulness. Thus, heavy deep pressure may make it difficult for boys to resist experimenting with multiple premarital partners, while girls are expected to remain virgins until marriage or at least to remain faithful to one partner.

> *Havinei, Zimbabwe: [My husband] told me he'd been going with all sorts of women. He said that he couldn't see a woman passing by without falling in love with her. . . He always told me that I was lucky to be his wife. He said the ladies that he'd fallen in love with could fit into four or five buses, but he never took any of them as his wife. He told me to pray to God to say thanks for the husband that I'd been given"* [20],
>
> *Richard, Uganda: "After dropping out of school at age 17, I made friends with four boys who were prominent. We had quite a lot in common, only they engaged themselves in business and sexual life. We used to have evening walks from place to place, especially where there was entertainment and drinking. At such places, these boys could meet rnore than one sexual partner. They tried their best to persuade rne to do what they were doing, by sending me different girls so that we could exchange a word or two relating to sexual activity. I usually had fears and shyness. I didn't know how to start: what could she think of me and what could she say afterwards? How would I engage in actual physical intercourse?*
>
> *After all their pressures, the group was not happy with me at*

all. They felt that I didn't belong and started tc tease me with a lot of embarrassing questions and statements like: 'You will suffer from backache because of not releasing the semen. Richard, you seem to be impotent - were you castrated?' To sum it up, they deserted me on those grounds". [21],

A further potential source of risk is polygamy, usually meaning multiple wives rather than multiple husbands. If no partner has sex outside the group, this can be a safe system but if any one is infected, all may be at risk.

To curb the epidemic, marriage should be squarely acknowledged as a major risk factor for women in many societies. The simplistic message of lifelong monogamy is a poor one if one partner already has HIV infection and will not use condoms. It has been observed that some men who learn or fear they have HIV infection marry to ensure someone will care for them when they become sick [22].

Violence Against Women

Violence against women, especially rape, is a risk factor that is inadequately recognized or addressed. In South Africa, an estimated 370,000 women are raped every year; in the United States, the Department of Justice reports that a woman is raped every six minutes[23]. Ironically, marital violence is more tolerated by society than violence outside marriage, to the extent that rape within marriage is not a recognized offence in many parts of the world. The woman's word is usually given less credit than that of the rapist. It is also traumatic and difficult for women to report rape and secure a conviction; the extreme is reached in some Islamic countries where a male witness to the rape is required.

> *Young girls who may be raped by a male relative or who are married off as children are especially vulnerable to* HIV/STD *infection. At a maternity hospital in Lima, Peru, 90 per cent of the young mothers aged 12-16 years had been raped by their (step)fathers or another close family member. In Jamaka, 40 per cent of pregnant girls between 11 and 15 years of age reported that their first intercourse was forced". Meanwhile, in India, nearly 16 per cent of 133 middle and upper-class postgraduate students said they hadbeen sexually abused before the age of 12 years* [21].

Violence against women is sometimes socially condoned. Many would argue that widely distributed films and television portrayals of women as sex objects and victims of abuse reinforce the acceptability of violence against them. In some countries ritualized violence, including rape, is condoned in certain circumstances.

*In **Papua New Guinea**, various factors in tribal life combine to place women in situations of HIV/STD infection risk. Customs encourage strong male bonding mechanisms that are played out during frequent group sex events. Many men participate in having sex with one woman and several other men. Even though this is often against the woman's will, it is not considered rape in the legal sense or condemned*[24].

In the worst situations, physical and sexual violence against women are commonplace. Wars and armed conflicts, generally accompanied by widespread rape, now have the added risk of spreading HIV and STDs. The physical trauma of violent sex, often multiple rape, makes transmission particularly likely. Indeed, any coerced sex increases the likelihood of micro-lesions in the vaginal mucosae which may then be entry points for HIV.

Blame and Rejection

Despite the realities of infection patterns, gender stereotypes allow women to be blamed for spreading HIV/STDs. Men are often reported to be infected by sex workers or casual girlfriends, who may be castigated by men and women alike, while less blame tends to fall on men than women who have multiple partners. Indeed, in some African and Asian cultures, it is believed that men must regularly release semen to avoid ill hearth.

*Married women in Palembang, **Indonesia**, who knew little about AIDS, associated it with "loose women" rather than believing themselves to be at risk. They believed that AIDS was contracted through "sexual contact with the lower class of commercial sex workers" and that the high class had usually been protected from STDs. They also said that AIDS comes from "promiscuous women and multiple partners"*[25].

Although for both sexes alcohol consumption reduces a sense of responsibility and leads to risk taking, women are more likely to be criticized for this. Male drunkenness is widely tolerated, men being excused for giving way to "natural urges".

Men in some societies may boast about STDs because these show they are "real men" who have sexual relations. For a boy growing up this may be part of his initiation into manhood. But for a woman the story is different; she is more likely to be looked down on as loose or unclean. In much of southern Africa, for example, STDs are derogatorily termed "women's disease" and men blame women for their infections. A doctor's wife in Australia with pelvic inflammatory disease was told by her health worker that she should be ashamed of herself: "someone in your position coming in with a problem like this"[26].

If HIV infection is discovered first in a wife, perhaps because she is the first tested when a baby falls sick, she is readily blamed. Her husband may refuse to be tested or, if found positive, accuse her of infidelity to cover his own behaviour. She may equally be blamed by other relatives, regardless of whose infection was discovered first.

At the same time, the denial of women's sexuality and the social assumption that they must be "pure" make it hard for women to acknowledge any other sexual experiences they may have had even before marriage. To do so is to court divorce or blame, even from female relatives. This blocks women from assessing their own risk and discussing risk behaviours and situations with their partners. Women living with HIV (perhaps more so than men) are even expected to become sexually inactive.

BLAME AND REJECTION

Sylvia, The Netherlands: "I only dared tell my two sisters after a year. One thought I might be imagining it because I still looked healthy, didn't I? My other sister felt it was my fault. If I had lived well, with a complete family [including a husband], it wouldn't have happened to me. . . My ex-partner told others, too.. . Because people gossiped about me, the vice police started following me; they had heard I was whoring around and infecting everyone. Of course, they couldn't prove that" [27].

Reina, The Netherlands: "When a person is infected with HIV, that does not mean that sex disappears from her or his life, even though some people think those living with HIV/AIDS should never have sex again. Of course, none us of living with the virus wants to pass it on to others. . . we want to have sex for the same reasons you do: because we like it, to express love, to gain consolation or security. In that, we are like everyone else" [28].

Blame can also lead to institutionalized human rights violations, e.g., the compulsory screening of sex workers. Women carrying condoms may be charged by police as sex workers; thus even when they act to safeguard themselves, this may backfire.

Lack of Information

Many women have poor understanding of their own bodies, mechanisms of HIV/STD transmission and their level of risk in unprotected sex. Many men also lack adequate information about their own bodies and tend to have even less information about women's bodies and needs.

Addressing these gaps in information and understanding is difficult because many poor men, and even more women, have low level of education and literacy and have lime access to printed information on HIV/AIDS and STDs. Men are more often able to gain information from radio and television. Consequently women hear about HIV/STDs later and not infequently have little or incomplete information about transmission. This may prevent them from assessing adequately their own risks. A female merchant in Senegal commented: "I don't need condoms because I am not a prostitutes have a husband and children. It is rare that during my travels I fall to the advances of a man. When I do, it is with someone I trust. I only choose to have sexual relations with men who are clean and visibly healthy, polite, and capable of respecting me. These men know me, trust me and know that they don't need to use condoms with me."[29]

Communication

Poor communication between parents and children and between partners about relationships, male and female sexual needs and responsibilities exacerbates risk..Youth as well as adult can be taught to discuss sex-related issues (health, needs, relationship; ideally, this should become an accepted norm.

Communicating can be hard

Somchai, Thailand: "I want someone to talk to, but it is very difficult to open up. I cannot talk to my wife about this. she does not have much to say about it and rarely exchanges conversation with me. I don't really know how she feels or what she really thinks. She is a very good wife but we cannot be friends [30].

***Woman, South Pacific:** "I was aware my husband was having casual sex when not with me, but I was too ashamed to ask him to take precautions. I kept telling myself, next time. My advice to young mothers is, 'Don't ever wait for next time.' Now I have big regrets. I'm so lucky that I didn't have any more children after I was infected" [31].*

Family Stress

Women's traditional family roles are arduous. Rural women in many pans of the world are primarily responsible for subsistence agriculture and, in rural and urban areas, informal sector activities. Women usually undertake most household tasks, go through pregnancy, childbirth and lactation, and rear children. Large numbers of women are in fact household heads but lack sufficient authority, money and material resources, family and formal support to provide adequately for their children and themselves. AIDs-related stigmatization and the extra care burdens brought on by the disease worsen existing gender inequalities, increasing women's vulnerability and exploitation.

In an African country, when Janet's husband learned that she had HIV infection, he threw her out with their two small children. Janet's father had died of AIDS and her mother was sick but trying to look after Janet's seven younger siblings. The logical outcome was for Janet to return to her parents' home and help. Her mother has since died, leaving Janet to care for all nine children. None are in school, all are malnourished. They live in one room, a corner of which is partitioned off and rented out to provide a small income. This, and what the older girls can earn from selling sex, keeps the family alive. No help has been forthcoming from Janet's husband nor from other relatives on either side.

The impact of AIDS on the family may be devastating, with both parents and sometimes one or more children becoming ill and dying. Girls may be withdrawn from school to look after their families, thus increasing their economic and social vulnerability when they grow up. The elderly also take up an increasing care burden when they themselves may be frail.

"A nurse: "In many countries in Africa families admit they have had to disrupt the schooling of the girl children; first, because they need another pair of hands to help them in caring for the sick, and second, because the family resources are reduced and the little funds available go into meeting the basic survival needs of the family.... They seem to see this as one big disadvantage of the home-care programme activities".[32]

AIDS makes decision-making about child-bearing, abortion and breast-feeding much more difficult. Available services may or may not provide helpful advice or be sensitive to the stress women face around these and other sexual health issues. In fact, women and couples may face humiliation and misinformation in the very centres and at the hands of the so-called professionals supposed to help them.

Pung, Thailand: "It all happened with my first pregnancy when I had a blood test. The nurse asked me some questions and finally told me I was infected with the HIV virus.. . I brought my husband in for testing and he tested HIV-positive. . . I remember crying when both of us sat in front of the nurse. She asked us what we wanted to do with our unborn child. She suggested aborting the child and added that it would be free of charge. If I agreed to do so, I was also required to have a hysterectomy.

I talked to my husband and we both agreed to have an ultrasound to see if our child was healthy. The technician said the child was healthy and strong. Then she looked at my HIV status and suddenly replied: 'No, no you cannot keep the child'; her voice was so threatening. 'You must abort the child', she insisted.

My husband said it is probably better to abort the child, letting go now was better than losing it when the child grew and became as lovely as our dreams. I was not sure myself but was in a state of shock. I asked the nurse if I could have a sterilization that was reversible. She looked at me with surprise and asked if I still had hope for a cure. On the form there was only a hysterectomy so she wrote that I wished not to have a permanent sterilization operation.

I had my child aborted, with a special deal: abortion with sterilization — free of charge. But I still don't know what kind of sterilization I got. I am not sure if it is a reversible or permanent sterilization. I have no way of knowing what has been done to my own body"[33].

Home Care

In areas where the epidemic is already severe, particularly sub-Saharan Africa, hospitals cannot cope and much patient nursing is done at home Numerous home-care programmes have been developed by church and community groups or as hospital outreach programmes. Alns service organizations provide counselling, material and practical help, spiritual support nursing care and advice. Excellent work is performed by dedicated staff, yet coverage remains low, often under 10 per cent. Visits from support teams may be on a fixed and infrequent schedule, and cost-effectiveness and sustainability remain serious concerns. The extra burden inevitably falls on the family, in particular on women.

In other regions, such as Latin America, the Middle East and Asia, some hospitals, clinics and social services do not provide care because staff are still afraid to accept people with HIV/AIDS. Stigmatization and discrimination may also prevent families and community members from providing support.

The growing orientation towards home care may, in fact, worsen women's situation, particularly as men are often the first to become sick. The wife may have to nurse her husband while her own health deteriorates, but the main expenditures are for his care. There may be no appropriate care-givers to nurse her through her sickness. Rather than an excessive focus on home care, developing a continuum of care between hospitat clinic, local hospice and other community care is preferable, a strategy supported by WHO. This enables health workers at the local clinics, community health workers and neighbours to help when appropriate and when requested by the family.

ASPANE, in Mexico, helped Yolanda, 26 years old. She lived in a "house" of carton near garbage dump in a Mexico City suburb with her 3-year-old son and 5-year-old daughter. When her partner died of AIDS and her neighbours discovered that Yolanda was also HIV-positive, they tried to drive her away. Yolanda sought refuge with her mother-in-law, but her daughter was sexually abused by a brother-in-law in that household. In desperation, Yolanda turned for help to a charitable organisation for abandoned children. After proving that her children were HIV-negative, so that the organization would accept them, the Department of Social Welfare helped Yolanda to transfer custody of the children legally to the organization. They went there when she died.

Men need to be motivated to assume stronger care roles in the family, both for the sick and in general around child care. Health and welfare concerns cannot remain women's preserve. If this can be achieved, husbands may be less likely to desert women who are found to have HIV and will write wills or other wise provide for their families when they themselves are dying.

Legal and Human Rights

At present, women's rights in many countries are curtailed. They may have little right to land, to inherit property, even to keep their own children when their husbands die. AIDS throws these problems into stark relief because more women are being widowed at a young age and will themselves face an early death. Safeguarding their children's future may be a desperate worry for these women, yet they may lack the means to provide for them without extended family support. In some countries, women am traditionally inherited by the deceased husband's brother. Their economic and social survival may depend on their acquiescence.

On the other hand, after the death of, husband, women around the world may be disinherited by the husband's relatives, particularly if they blame the woman for his death.

At another level, marries women's confidentiality may be broken with relative impunity leading to violence or desertion if their husbands blame them for infection. Meanwhile, women may not be informed of their partners' HIV status. The right of partner notification versus strict confidentiality is being debated in many countries and different policies are being developed. For women the outcome is particularly crucial as infection often enters the family through the husband. Uninfected wives could, in theory, protect themselves but only if access to information is accompanied by the economic, social and legal means to take preventive action.

VIOLATIONS OF HUMAN RIGHTS

ASPANE in Mexico helps Rosa, who contracted HIV from her bisexual husband. He abandoned her and their four children when he learned that she, too, was HIV-positive. Rosa's in-laws blamed her for the HIV infection and consequently refused to offer her any help or information about her husband, who went into hiding for fear of being made legally responsible for child support.

Deborah in Uganda lost her husband to AIDS and is herself very sick. Her brother-in-law tried from the very beginning to inherit her, but she categorically refused so as not to infect him and his wife. He repeatedly told her he does not care that she has AIDS and is willing to take the risk of becoming infected. He harassed her for almost a year; when she held firm and refused, he cut off all financial support to her and he four children. Once she refused him, she was ostracized by the entire family and cannot rely on them for anything, even moral support. Now, he is trying to claim the land that his brother left jointly to them[34].

The rights of women living with HIV to bear children or seek an abortion are hotly debated. A British woman living with HIV was angered and upset by accusations that her choice to have a baby was selfish as the child risked infection or, if it lived, would certainly be orphaned fairly young[35]. In many developing countries a woman's status is highly dependent on motherhood; much more than in Britain it may be of great importance to an HIV-positive woman to have a child.

The issue of sex work also raises difficult legal and ethical problems. While soliciting remains illegal in most countries, sex workers remain vulnerable to abuse, are difficult to reach with HIV/STD prevention and support programmed and face increased stigma. Yet arrangements for sex work may involve minors, abduction and coercion; these aspects of the trade must be stopped. AIDS is giving rise to increased public outrage about these human rights violations.

"When life became difficult in her native village of Melamchi in the Nepali hills, Geeta moved to Kathmandu where she worked as a housemaid. When her cousin promised her a better job in a carpet factory in India, she jumped at the opportunity: 'I didn't realise that I was sold to a Nepali brothel keeper in India until the lady told me to engage in business. . . I wept and wept. I was shocked to be sold by my own relative. I went mad. They admitted me into a mental hospital. After a year, I was ultimately forced into prostitution. I never liked it—that was not what I had wanted. But you can't fight against luck and fate.'

Geeta was sent home with 200 Indian rupees (US$ 6.50) for her transport after she tested HIV-positive. Back in Melamchi, she found her mother had died and her father refused to take her back. Determined to begin a new life, she rented a liquor shop with her savings. The shop was successful until her HIV status became known in the village-then business collapsed and she was forced to close down". [36]

Another neglected area is the rights of homosexual women and men to social acceptance, child care, marriage and inheritance. Lesbian relationships are a preferred lifestyle for some women and generally carry a low risk of HIV infection. However, societal intolerance precludes many women from exploring this option even if they would like to. Male gay relationship are more common in some societies, but their very existence may be denied or condemned, leading gay men to marry and engage in bisexual contacts even if they prefer only to have sex with men. "Talk to any African government about homosexual issues and the spread of AIDS, and they simply tell you that homosexual activities only go on in the Western world," said Obi Zikora, president of Gentlement Alliance, in Nigeria [37]. "The stigma attached to homosexuality frightens away many who should be examined from going to doctors."

As with sex workers, legal rights for homosexuals and lesbians need to be strengthened and societal intolerance challenged if they are to cope better with HIV and AIDS and not be driven underground.

Structural Patterns

Economic policies widening the gap between rich and poor countries and rich and poor people within nations exacerbate the conditions for HIV/STD transmission. For example, economic structural adjustment programmes may have a negative impact on rural and urban poverty, national debt and trade relations. These policies hamper countries' capacity to provide social, educational and medical support to affected families and communities, especially if food subsidies are cut and social, welfare and health expenditures are reduced.

The epidemic has hardest the developing world and the poor inner cities of industrialized countries, which are least able to cope. Furthermore, poverty increasingly has a female face: UNDP estimates that 70 per cent of the world's poor are women. As prevention efforts are stepped up, communities' abilities to cope must also be strengthened. Only through improving coping capacity will fear and stigma around AIDS be reduced, allowing prevention strategies to really work.

Within this framework, empowering women and reducing gender inequalities are critical. The structural basis of gender inequality must be challenged by promoting personal attitude and behaviour change. Women must gain access to the education, training and employment they need to achieve sexual relations on equal terms and to control their risk of HIV/STDS. Cultural expectations that exonerate men from taking responsibility for health and welfare concerns must be transformed, along with the structural conditions of work, housing, migration, etc., that prevent this from becoming a reality.

> *Woman, Zimbabwe: "My husband passed away from AIDS when he was 35; he was ill for six months. He used to work as a general labourer in a big firm and only came home at weekends. We had eight children, but the last two both died. This leaves me with six children to feed. It is very hard. The two eldest have had to leave school to try and earn money, but I am trying to keep the youngest four in school.*
>
> *In the early stages of my husband's illness we could cope. It became difficult when he lost his job. We had to spend a lot of his savings on special food for him, and he lost his medical aid cover. I grow maize and try to make money selling crochet work, but it is not sufficient. I cannot get a proper job —in these days it is even more difficult as a woman because it is men who are expected to work.*
>
> *My husband's workplace helped with the funeral and will pay me a small pension for four years. But he had not worked there long so the amount is low. My husband's brother is supposed to take care of us. He knows our problems but did not help at all during my husband's illness nor after his death. Now he wants to marry me, but I think it is in order to take my husband's estate, not to help us. I am lucky because my husband left a letter instructing that his property was to remain with us and that I should not marry his brother in the traditional way. Fortunately, the headman and the other village elders support this decision because they know that this brother did not help us when my husband was alive. Otherwise it would be very hard for me to refuse. I have to think of my children. But by refusing to marry I lose any hope of help from him.*
>
> *If I die, the oldest children will have to take care of the young ones. I cannot trust my husband's brother, and I do not think*

his first wife would treat them well. My own two sisters cannot take the children because their husbands will not allow this. It is not traditional and they have their own families. The women take care of the children, but it is the husbands who must make the decision about this."

5. Can Women and Men reduce risks and share responsibilities?

The goal of our response to HIV/AIDS and STD is to decrease vulnerability to infection, reduce stigmatization and discrimination and curb the epidemic socio-economic impact. This will be best achieved through gender-based approaches promoting shared responsibility for prevention and care between women and men.

To ensure wider development and implementation of gender-sensitive strategies, collective action is required. Women's organizations and networks can help by reinforcing such strategies, sensitizing and mobilizing women and men, and making linkages to other gender-based initiatives in society. Collaboration and co-ordination between UN system agencies, governments and NGO networks may further serve to reinforce gender-sensitive responses.

Gender-sensitive strategies must address both short and longer-term needs and goals Short-term strategies focus on people immediate needs in specific communities, including obtaining basic information about HIV/AIDS and STD, gaining access to sexual health education, acquiring condoms and obtaining back-up support for home-based care.

Longer-terme strategies are directed at underlying cultural and social structures. They aim to promote mutual respect between men and women and equal access to all types of resources. The goals of longer terms strategies include, but are not limited to:

- changing ideas and social norms that keep women in an inferior social position
- achieving shared decision-making power between women and men at all levels: in relationships, community affairs, political and economic bodies, etc.
- creating structural changes to give women equal access to education, training and income-earning opportunities.
- reallocating work responsibilities so that women and men share them fairly
- encouraging legalization of traditional marriages or

unions where this would strengthen the rights of women to property, inheritance and children.

Governments and NGOs are now beginning to integrate a gender perspective in to their HIV/AIDS/STD programmes. Women living with HIV/AIDS are playing an increasingly important role in this process. Below, examples from programmes around the world show how a gender-based response is being developed. The examples are randomly grouped action areas. Gender-sensitive strategies must be developed simultaneously in all of them:

— creating a supportive and enabling environment
— research
— facilitating access to information and services
— changing the way we think and act
— sensitizing and mobilizing men
— combating discrimination
— developing gender-sensitive care and support
— living positively with HIV/AIDS.

A Supportive and Enabling Environment

The social environment must enable people to achieve effective prevention and care. Policy, legal and human rights, economic, social, cultural and educational structures are needed that benefit women to the same extent as men. If such structures are developed, then women and men will have a much better chance to change the social norms and values oppressing them in their daily lives. Although structural changes take time to achieve, strategies must be developed to address them at the same time as grassroots initiatives improve women's daily life situation.

Structural Measures

Decreasing women's economic dependence is an important step towards enabling them to reduce infection risks for themselves and their families. A credit scheme established by the Grameen Bank and Bangladesh Rural Advancement Committee (BRAC), for example, enables rural women to establish an independent income by offering them loans. The programme has enhanced women's autonomy and self-confidence and led to increased contraceptive use[38].

In addition to income-generating schemes, other structural measures are necessary. These include guaranteeing women:

— better access to schooling, vocational training and higher education

— equal access to employment and equal pay for equal work
— equitable access to social and health services
— legal and human rights protection equal to that of men
— better representation in political and economic bodies
— freedom from restrictive cultural expectations and practices.

Political and Community Support

Broad political and bureaucratic support is necessary if governments are to implement the measures outlined above. This can be facilitated if NAPS are made intersectoral, involving not only the health sector but also ministries and departments such as women's affairs, education, labour, justice, agriculture, defence and social affairs. By creating links among these sectors, the HIV/AIDS epidemic can illustrate why women must gain greater access to education, paid employment and social services. NAPS can further mobilize support for a gender-based response by formulating policies that provide various ministries and NGOs with a framework for action.

INCORPORATING GENDER AND WOMEN'S CONCERNS INTO NATIONAL RESPONSES

The first generation of National AIDS Programmes (NAPS) were gender neutral in their approach. Health education messages ignored gender disparities and roles in sexual and family relations. One and all were simply urged to "stick to one partner", avoid casual sex, reduce the number of sexual partners or use condoms.

As awareness gradually developed, NAPS started to address specific issues confronting women in relation to HIV/ AIDS. The initial approach was to "mobilize women" through women's NGOs as agents of health education and information. When concern arose about women's heightened vulnerability to HIV, interventions were developed to enable women to talk about sexual safety and condom use with their partners. This approach was criticized because it neglected men and the fact that men control the circumstances under which most women are exposed to risk or protected from infection.

Analysis of gender disparities and women's disadvantaged socio-economic status is now being incorporated into national HIV/AIDS policies. The challenge is to integrate gender considerations into all aspects of programme development. Botswana's National Information, Education and

Communication Strategy for HIV/AIDS Prevention places gender prominently among factors related HIV/STD spread. Guidelines for gender interventions for men and women are a key component for district programme planning. By determining how gender disparities affect women throughout their lifetime, interventions can be facilitated at community, school and workplace levels to ensure that girls do not grow into adults with increased vulnerability to HIV/STD infection.

Interventions also need to take account of women's responsibility for providing family and community care. Programmes developed by social welfare agencies, NGOS, employers, etc. should make provision for these responsibilities. Education and communication programmes should encourage sharing of domestic responsibilities and tasks between men and women.

Only when countries address gender disparities squarely in their economic political and social development strategies will incorporation of gender and women's concerns into HIV/AIDS programmes have a sustainable impact.

Tshidi Moeti, former Botswana NAP Manager

"The most critical decision of my life was to reveal to representatives of Caribbean media that I had tested positive for the AIDs virus. Coming face-to-face with a battery of journalists was a nerve-racking experience. I decided to impose this agony on myself in an effort to dispel some of the myths surrounding HIV-positive peoples. During my presentation, information that would usually be regarded by journalists as a 'juicy story' was instead treated as a moving commentary. On the admission of some of the journalists, my presence and commentary were edifying and represented their first opportunity to understand the plight of HIV-infected persons."

A Women living with HIV[39]

CREATING A SUPPORTIVE ENVIRONMENT

When sex workers in Calabar, Nigeria, wanted their customers to use condoms, they failed to get support from the people who influence their working conditions, such as hotel owners, managers and chairladies (head sex workers) . The Cross River State AIDS Programme (CRSAP) therefore approached them on the sex workers' behalf.

A special STD clinic was established to serve the women near their working sites. Collective actions were fostered to protect the sex workers' interests. The hotel managers and chairladies began backing the women's demand for higher fees and their right to refuse clients who wouldn't use condoms. The sex workers also were able to retain fees when clients attempted to renege on condom use. Harassment and extortion by security agents decreased, to.

The women reported more confidence in handling problems with clients, hotel owners and the police. They also organized a self-help group called Nka Iban Uko (Women of Courage), which focuses on skills training and services for their children[40].

Governmental and NGO programmes mobilizing communities to create conditions for effective prevention and care need expansion. Besides serving as a channel for information on HIV/AIDS and STDs, the media can mobilize public support for gender-sensitive programmes by highlighting the effects of the epidemic on women. Media workers may also be enlisted to help create a climate tolerant towards those affected by or responding to HIV/AIDS.

Policy-Making and Agenda-Setting

To ensure broad-based support, all agencies and government ministries must add HIV/AIDS and STDs to their action agendas. In this way, alliances for policy-related advocacy as well as new initiatives will arise at the national and community levels:

— After a national workshop in Malaysia where women were trained to organize HIV/AIDS awareness workshops, such meetings were held even in the most remote parts of the country. By linking women's umbrella organizations, duplication of effort was avoided and time and money saved [41].

— In England, regional seminars were organized on the theme "Women, AIDS and the Future" in collaboration with local women's organizations. Activities carried out by participants afterwards included: reporting on HIV/AIDS to local organizations; planning similar seminars in their area; talking with men, family, friends and colleagues about HIV/AIDS; writing advocacy letters to government ministers; holding study days/meetings with church groups; and writing articles for the press[42].

— The Society for Women and AIDS in Africa (SWAA) raises political awareness concerning gender in relation to HIV/AIDS and STDs and provides a voice for women in many parts of the continent. SWAA has national member organization in more than 20 countries.

Research

Biomedical studies-e.g., on opportunistic infections in women and ways to reduce perinatal transmission (including through breast-feeding)are increasing in scope but need expansion. More support is required for research on female-controlled methods to prevent HIV/STD infection, including the female condom. The current research priority is to develop microbicide, which appear to have great potential for acceptance. Other important topics for a gender-sensitive research agenda include:

- barriers to female control HIV/STD risks and ways to overcome them
- how young women and men define personal risk in relation to different types of relationship
- how men and women currently protect themselves against infection
- barriers to female and male STD treatment and how to improve access
- improving contact tracing for STDs
- the effects of HIV infection during various phases of a woman's life cycle (e.g., in relation to onset of menstruation and menopause)
- the appropriateness of counselling messages and methods in meeting women's and men's specific concerns
- partner notification, confidentiality and information sharing
- the division of labour concerning reproductive and productive tasks at the household and community levels and how these contribute to maintaining women in their current lower status and increase their burdens related to care.

NGOs and research institutes have not waited for international leader ship and donor funding to undertake studies in these areas. Research must be demystified so that more local organizations develop their own research agendas. Some of the most useful findings come from simple small-scale studies, especially when their results are linked directly to the implementing service agencies.

Exciting developments are taking place through participatory action research in which community members explore topics such as differences in knowledge and information sources for boys and girls, traditional communication channels used by women and men and inter generational family communication. The findings indicate how educational programmes can be better structured and channelled.

Dissemination of research results urgently needs expansion. This can be facilitated by linking researchers and NGOs. The International Center for Research on Women (USA) worked with Comprehensive Health for Women (SIPAM) and the Programme in Gender Studies of the National Autonomous University in Mexico to document and analyse their studies and programmes on women and AIDS. A forum held to discuss the results with NGOs, researchers and government institutions resulted in the formation of a permanent researcher NGO network[43].

Establishment of "inter-country" projects is another approach. For example, FEIM in Argentina and the Movimiento Paulina Luisi in Uruguay together planned action research and an intervention to increase gender awareness and prevention possibilities for poor and lower middle-class women[44]. They then compared their findings, identifying concerns that are country-specific and broader in scope.

Donor organizations can contribute to dissemination of research findings by funding the publication of research reports and researchers' participation in national and international meetings. Many UN agencies have distribution channels that might be expanded to include dissemination of studies carried out by governments and NGOS.

Facilitating Access to Information and Services

Information Dissemination

Printed materials can be improved by involving women and men in creating more appropriate messages and materials that address their specific concerns. Funding is also needed for translation of texts into local languages to allow greater access to printed information.

Including HIV/STD information in a variety of health programmes, such as mother and child health and family planning, reaches more people. The Guatemalan Association for the Prevention and Control of AIDS conducted educational sessions and small-group workshops on health and sexuality, self-esteem, partner communication and communication with adolescent children for women waiting at antenatal clinics [45]. Fears that discussions about HIV/STDs would cause the women to worry, increasing their stress levels during pregnancy, appeared unfounded. On the contrary, women reported that they felt relaxed and less apprehensive in talking about condoms, infidelity, STDs and AIDS with their partners. More than half of those interviewed postpartum said they shared written materials with their partners.

Information channels other than health services are also available. Traditional community counsellors, women and men's associations, church-based groups, sports and recreational clubs provide entry points for individual and group educational sessions. Other possibilities include labour and trade unions and groups participating in agricultural and small-enterprise projects. Training peer educators has proved particularly effective among women from various walks of life. NGOs have further explored ways to reach women whose mobility is restricted, e.g., girls living in slums and female prisoners.

REACHING OUT TO WOMEN

Both existing and new communication channels can be used to reach out to women and girls.

Traditional Associations

The Cheikh Anta Diop University in Senegal mobilized members of a well-respected women's association, the Dimba, to help organize community education sessions. Dimba membership is restricted to women who coped well with difficult circumstances, like infertility problems, repeated miscarriages and adopting orphans. They are influential because their members have thorough knowledge of women's and infants' illnesses. The University also worked with women ofthe Laobe ethnic group, who provide advice about reproductive health and sexuality. Laobe women are traders who make and sell products designed to enhance sexual pleasure; they were persuaded to sell condoms as an erotic product [29].

Adolescent Girls

World Vision designed a sex and family education programme for low-income adolescent girls in Bombay, India. The girls had little information about reproduction and almost none about HIV/STDs. They seemed trapped in a "culture of silence" that did not permit them to voice their opinions, feelings or concerns on any issue.

Parental and community support were essential to permit the girls to participate (e.g., providing child care for younger siblings). A community AIDS/STD awareness programme was therefore implemented, including meetings with mothers, teenage boys and young men, and a street play dramatizing women's status at different stages in life. The meetings stressed the value of educational interventions for the girls.

Topics discussed with the girls included: being a woman, female puberty, sexuality, sexual exploitation and harassment, health problems (with specific reference to HIV/STDs) and the development of an action plan to protect oneself against infection. The programme had to encourage the girls to talk. As the sessions progressed, they became more self-confident, freely voicing their opinions, suggestions and criticisms. The feedback was very positive, with the girls asking for more sessions[46].

Women Prisoners

"My partner used a condom because he saw the signs on my arms. That hurt me. Now I know something more about AIDS and I have changed my mind: I think that he did the right thing because both of us ran less risk." This comment came from a participant in the "Women, AIDS, Information" Project at the women's prison Le Nuove in Turin, Italy.

The 3-month project was initiated at the prisoners' request. The project team helped the women discuss HIV-testing, how to reduce infection risks and how to live with seropositive persons without fear or rejection. The women then developed a story that could be used as the basis for a video.

The intervention enabled the women to share their experiences as equals and realize they were capable of carrying out such a project. They began discussing the possibility of having relationships with other groups working on AIDS both inside and outside prison[47].

Reorientation of Services

NAPS, local governments and NGOS are reorienting services to better meet fee needs of women and men. They are providing information and condoms to men and women at sites they regularly visit (e.g., clubs, cafes, hairdressers). Clinics are being located where people live (e.g., STD clinics located in sex worker districts, mobile clinics). This enables people to acquire what they need without much effort.

- A programme in Haiti, which sells condoms in places where women feel comfortable buying them, aims to give women skills in negotiating social and cultural barriers to condom use. Product packaging is discreet, with advertising stressing women's right to control their sexuality [48].
- Government and NGOs in Calcutta, India, have increased female sex workers' access to STD services and health care for their children by opening a general health clinic in a local youth club. The clinic runs during the day and the club at night. Peer educators participate in outreach activities[49].
- The Filipino NGO Kabalikat provides comprehensive

services to female, male and youth sex workers by training peer educators, running a drop-in centre, offering short-term shelter and nutritional support and providing medical and residential care to those who need support[50]. In Colombia, PROFAMILIA runs male family planning clinics, emphasizing that family planning is a right. The men are offered general counselling, STD/HIV diagnosis, vasectomies and a free hotline. The programme has resulted in more early consultations related to STDs and increased condom use[51].

These types of programmes need to be replicated, along with increasing efforts to make the female condom and spermicides more accessible and affordable.

STD diagnosis and treatment are of special importance since STDs increase vulnerability to HIV. Because most STD diagnostic tests are too costly or require equipment unavailable at the primary health care level, WHO recommends syndromic management based on the identification of collections of STD signs and symptoms (syndromes). Any woman presenting with a particular syndrome is treated for all STD infections commonly associated with those symptoms.

To increase the accessibility and acceptability of STD services, stigmatization and the negative attitudes of staff must be reduced. Contact tracing procedures guaranteeing confidentiality also need further development.

Changing the Way we think and Act

Programmes can facilitate community exploration of how gender is related to prevention and care by addressing the following kinds of question: —Beliefs: how can people be assisted to re-examine ideas related to HIV/AIDS/STDs and sexuality which hinder prevention, e.g., men need to release semen to stay healthy, women must receive semen to promote an unborn baby's growth?

— *Relationships*: how are relationships defined, e.g., what kind of contact do the partners have in casual, regular and other types of relationship? What makes a relationship good? Who usually makes decisions in relationships? What circumstances in relationships increase or decrease risks of HIV/STD infection?

— *Sexuality*: why, with whom and in what circumstances do women and men engage in sex? What needs and desires do women and men have regarding sex and what do they understand of each other's needs? What types of sexual practices and needs are or are not considered normal and why? How do various aspects of sexuality affect risks of HIV/STD infection?

— *Power between women and men*: how should power relations between women and men be changed? How can women gain greater control over their lives and situations contributing to their risk of HIV/STD infection, e.g., condom use, types of sexual activity, extra-marital sex?

— *Care and support*: who provides what types of care and support to family members and needy people in the community? Why is caretaking divided between women and men in a particular way? What needs to be done to ensure that women and men both participate actively in providing care and support?

CREATING GENDER AWARENESS AND BUILDING SKILLS TO ACT ON IT

Around the world, communities are becoming more conscious of gender issues and acting to address them:

Women, Children, Citizenship and Health (MCCS), an NGO in Sao Paulo, Brazil, recruits women for sensitization workshops from mothers' clubs, unions, political parties, professional associations, community groups and feminist organizations. MCCS adapted its approach to safer sex when it was recognized that family planning programmes have emphasized use of "long-term" and "inexpensive" methods, such as sterilization and the pill. Barrier methods, such as condoms and spermicides, are frequently identifed as inefficient, inappropriate for lower-income groups and too complex for use by uneducated persons. MCCS encourages women to think about contraception in relation to HIV/STDs in the broader context of their overall health[52].

Julliet Awino, a widowed mother in Uganda, stars in "Strings Attached", a play portraying her personal experience with HIV/AIDS. It emphasizes practices that undermine women's role in society and the home, making them vulnerable to HIV transmission, such as: male pre- and extra-marital sexual activity, hostility from in-laws who blame wives for family problems, abandonment without rights and property if a woman refuses sexual "ritual cleansing" when she becomes a widow. The drama has contributed to an increase in people writing wills to regulate inheritances*[53].

In Kalabo, Zambia, women aware that girls in their area were especially vulnerable to HIV formed a committee to focus on communal attitudes towards sexuality and behaviours affect-

ing women. They organized seminars for more than 600 women, through churches, hospitals and health centres, to stimulate extensive community discussions about female sexuality and gender roles. As a result, the traditional initiation ceremony for girls was revised to include information on reproductive health and HIV/STDs [54].

In Mali, a primary health care project (SSP-Segou) and programme focused on improving women's status (PROFED) generated discussions on gender and sexual health among the general community and young women in particular during a needs assessment study. To break down barriers against discussing sexuality, they developed a drama with the villagers about a woman who has problems giving birth. It was acted out for the entire village, following an introduction by a male village leader concerned about women's situation. The audience became highly involved, worrying about the sick woman and giving advice to the husband. In this climate male and female researchers could address all kinds of topics from the perspective of both sexes. Some previously taboo subjects, like the negative consequences of female circumcision and sexual violence against women as a risk factor for HIV/AIDS, were dealt with publicly for the first time. The group discussions were geared towards analysing the villagers' problems and mobilizing them into action. The first step was to re-establish a village pharmacy [55].

Participatory group methodologies increase awareness and motivate adults and youth to devise solutions to the gender-based problems they identify. Skills building needs to be an important component of such approaches so that women and men learn how to talk about sex and relationships, resist pressure from peers and partners to engage in unwanted practices and stand up for their rights (e.g., resisting service providers' pressure to have an abortion or sterilization). The capacity to practise such skills is based on a sense of self-worth, a perception of one-self as capable and assertive. Examples of approaches that build self-esteem and gender awareness include:

— using drama and visual arts to help women "discover" their abilities and talents.
— role-play (e.g., to develop safer sex negotiation skills)
— vocational training and education (e.g., production skills, relating skills, managing skills)
— peer education programmes.

Ritual cleansing is a custom among some African cultures wherein the spouse of a deceased man or woman has sexual intercourse with a member of the spouse's family in order to allow the dead person's spirit to attain rest; it also ensures that the spirit will not bother the surviving spouse.

Changes in attitudes need to begin in childhood. Although parents are expected to play the primary role, in many societies talking about sexuality and related issues between parents and children is difficult. A study in Zimbabwe, for example, found that parent-child communication is severely limited, especially in the case of fathers, who are often absent, remote and moody.[56] Research in Mexico showed that adolescents want more communication about sex with their parents than they actually have. Obstacles included parental time/work constraints. not being able to reach agreement, lack of trust and knowledge and embarrassment.[57] Such studies indicate that parents want help to improve their ability to communicate, for instance, through NGO and church training activities for couples.

When questioned, many parents indicate they are willing for others to deliver prevention messages to their children as long as they are informed about the content. Media campaigns can help create a supportive environment for this. NGOs and schools can offer courses and activities for schoolchildren and out-of-school youth that explore gender relations, values, sexuality and related issues. Stressing the effects of positive as well as negative peer pressure is an important component of such programmes. As few teachers and youth workers have been trained to deal with such subjects, organizations such as UNICEF, WHO and UNESCO, as well as NGOS, are assisting governments to develop appropriate materials and training programmes for them. Training of youth peer educators has also shown promising results.

HELPING YOUNG PEOPLE

Two programmes in Asia and Africa are teaching young people the skills needed to insist on safer sex. One programme focuses on pre-marital abstinence and fidelity within marriage and the other on condom use.

In Africa, Aid for AIDS fosters the creation of positive self-images among boys and girls, emphasizing respect for girls. "It's great to be a girl" is an attitude crucial for boys and girls to absorb. The programme uses drama, role-play and discussions to teach young people how to resist peers who try to make them do things they don't want to do. The idea of positive peer pressure is promoted through Anti AIDS Clubs, in which friends help one another stand by mutually agreed behaviours, e.g.: 1. We will make friendships with lots of other boys and girls more important than "pairing off". 2. We will commit ourselves to avoid sex before marriage. 3. We will especially help and care for any of our friends who have HIV infection.

The University of Chiang Mai in Thailand developed special materials for young female factory workers. Research had shown that a lack of communication between women and men, reluctance to discuss condom use ("men's business") and misconceptions about moral goodness andAIDS (if someone looks and acts good, they are perceived as HIV-free) were major obstacles to prevention. Two booklets with discussion starters addressing these factors are used by female peer educators trained to facilitate group discussions and lead group activities.

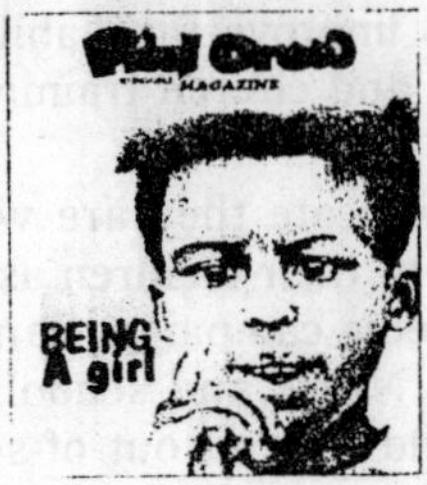

Care International in Kenya promotes respect for girls in a publication for schoolchildren

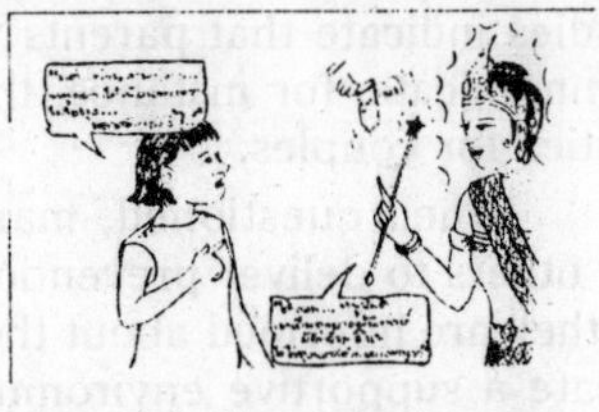

A Thai comic book uses humour to persuade young women to discuss condom use

A romantic illustrated novel shows the consequences of not discussing sexual behaviour. It tells the story of factory worker Lamyai, who falls in love with Tong Dee. Because he is good, she doesn't ask about his past. Despite warnings from a co-worker, they have unprotected sex. When Tong Dee enters military service to earn money for their marriage, he is tested and found HIV-positive; Lamyai also has the virus and, after working on for a few years, eventually dies.

To demonstrate what girls can say to negotiate condom use, a humorous comic book focuses on a young woman named Jon Di. Before she leaves to work at the factory, Jon Di prays to the Spirit of Good Health: "Please turn something near to me into a living thing —to be my friend—to protect me when I go to Chiang Mai." The Spirit does so, producing Brother Protector Condom, an invisible flying condom. The Spirit promises that if Jon Di and Brother Condom save five young women from AIDS, she will make Brother Condom into a real friend. Jon Di completes the assignment successfully, whereupon the Spirit changes Brother Condom into a young man with a condom head. After protest from Jon Di, the Spirit makes him a completely human companion.

DAVID CUNNINGHAM, Zimbabwe,
KATHLEEN CASH, BUPA ANASUCHATKUL and
WANTANA BUSAYAWONG, Thailand

ENLISTING INFLUENTIAL MEN

The Thai Health Project for Tribal People (HPTP) has trained

influential male community leaders as health educators for isolated hill tribe communities. The headmen, who also act as village counsellors, already have the respect, position and credibility necessary to promote new information. They are also experienced in talking to large groups.

The training seminars include practice teaching sessions. One headman, for example, used a picture of a young girl being sold into sex work to talk about the man who had taken her away and what happened to her once she was in town. HPTP teams visit the headmen several months after the seminars to ask about any problems they have using the materials and what is going well.

Knowledge changes are occurring in villages taught by the headmen. In one tribe, the initial survey showed that 85 per cent of the people had heard of AIDS, but none understood that it could be transmitted from mother to child. After teaching by the headman, 98 per cent of the villagers understood this.

Lori Rowe, Thailand

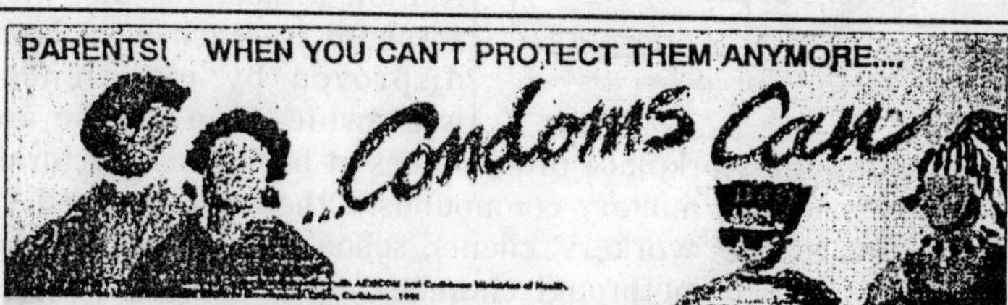

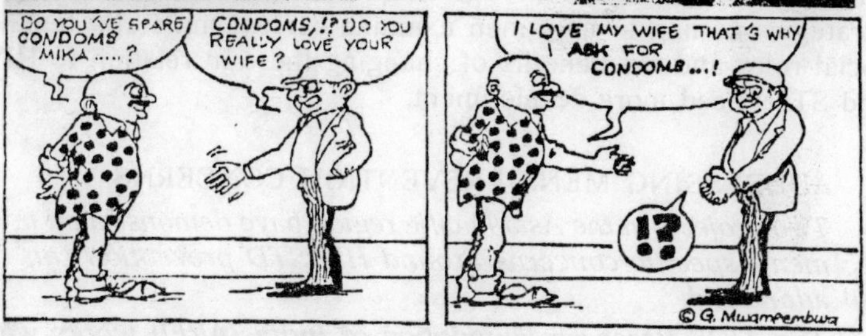

Sensitizing and Mobilizing Men

Men must be sensitized and mobilized to a greater extent for an effective response to HIV/AIDS and STDs. Since men occupy most positions of influence, their participation in advocating gender-sensitive policies and programmes is essential.

Some men are, ofcourse, already aware in this regard. Others, however, have not yet thought about the fact or placing women at a disadvantage. A Filipino NGO, HASIK, has developed a gender training programme for male staff invarious types of organization to address this.[58] Through games, exercises, song, dances and discussions, the men articulate their own ideas about why women are oppressed. Then they address how to change the institutions that determine gender roles, concluding with the formulation of action plans which help the men translate what they have learned into organizational professional goals and schemes.

The collaboration of village headmen, male religious authorities and businessmen in educational interventions and home- and community-based care is most important. They act as role models for the community and can set the example for acceptance of "new" ideas concerning men's and women's responsibilities in preventing HIV transmission and coping with AIDS

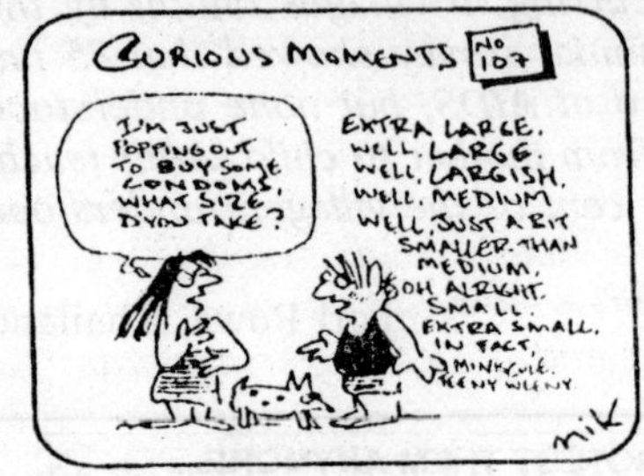
CURIOUS MOMENTS
NO 107
I'M JUST POPPING OUT TO BUY SOME CONDOMS, WHAT SIZE D'YOU TAKE?
EXTRA LARGE. WELL, LARGE. WELL, LARGISH. WELL, MEDIUM WELL, JUST A BIT SMALLER THAN MEDIUM. OH ALRIGHT. SMALL. EXTRA SMALL. IN FACT,
MIK

Beer coasters (mats) in Australia use humour to challenge male sexuality myths

Information and behavioural change programmes specifically targeting men and boys need replication. Objections that men are hard to-reach have been disproved by experiences worldwide. Men can be approached through workplace programmes at businesses, factories and settings such as military compounds. Others are targeted by interventions for sex workers' clients, school-based programmes and activities carried out through churches and recreational groups. Strategies aiming to help men examine current male and female social roles and the benefits of changing these in relation to HIV and STDs need more development.

ADDRESSING MENS PREVENTION CONCERNS

Two projects in the Asia/Pacific region have demonstrated how men's specific concerns around HIV/STD prevention can be addressed:

The AIDS Research Foundation of India (ARFI) works with sex-worker clients in Madras, emphasizing the health benefits of condom use. Truck drivers keep condoms in their trucks to fix radiator hose leaks. ARFI used this practice to start small groups talking about how "leaks during sex" can be fixed. Condoms are provided through transit-stop shops, where they are sold together with items men frequently buy. The truckers also receive key chains containing a compartment for a condom. Since most of the transit-stop teashops play music, a cas-

sette on safety (both on the road and at roadside, "It's all in the rubber", has been distributed with funds from a truck tyre manufacturing company.

Peer opinion leaders tell port/dock workers a story about a man who practices safer sex. To reinforce the message, posters on condom use are displayed in wine shops and barber shops, where the dock workers read the evening newspaper. Some men have been recruited as condom depot holders; a dispensary at the port provides free STD services. Short street plays reinforce the safer sex message. Since the programme started, condom sales have increased at the transitstop and port shops.[59]

The Heterosexual Men's Project in New South Wales, Australia, conducted focus-group discussions with building workers aged between 17-60 years to determine what was important to them in preventing HIV prevention. The groups comprised men from English- and non-English speaking backgrounds and included single, divorced, separated and single men, men in long-term relationships and fathers. Two issues highlighted by the workers were the role of alcohol in promoting unsafe behaviour and difficulties in communicating about sex with women.

Based on the men's suggestions, a campaign was designed using messages on beer coasters and toilet stickers, in pubs and clubs. The beer coasters used "themes" to demystify safe sex and challenge some male sexuality myths. The toilet stickers aimed to facilitate discussion of condom use between men and women by providing humorous ice breakers. Billboard, bus and magazine advertising messages addressed the link between STDs and HIV/AIDS.

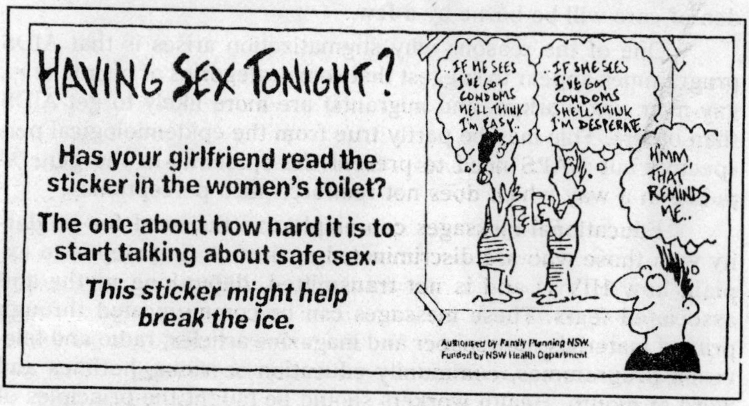

Evaluation showed that 50 per cent of the men familiar with the campaign saw it as personally relevant: 19 per cent of those who had read the beer coasters and stickers said they were

helpful in providing conversation starters on safe sex with their partners: 27 per cent said it led them to discuss this with their colleagues. Generally, the campaign messages were best recalled by men 18 to 24 years old, single men and condom users. Recommendations made for future campaigns included:

- *tailor messages to emphasize that condoms promote health rather than prevent disease*
- *employ humour to challenge aspects of male culture that do not support safer behaviour*
- *develop dynamic and flexible approaches to address men's sexual health needs in the context of changing life roles*
- *use medical centres, youth services and sexual health centres to provide information and resources*
- *use the media, particularly men's magazines, to support sexual health education*
- *locate future campaigns in venues where alcohol is consumed such as clubs and pubs [60].*

Combating Discrimination

Women and men living with HIV/AIDS, their families and people negatively associated with the epidemic (e.g., homosexuals, sex workers, street-children, migrants and foreigners) still face stigmatization and discrimination. Combating this is an important public health strategy. If people are to engage in safer sex, they must feel confident that they will not be abused or abandoned by their partners. If potential careproviders condemn those living with the virus, adequate care and support cannot be given and the burden of care will be borne by a few.

One of the reasons why stigmatization arises is that AIDS programmes appear to suggest that some categories of people (e.g., gay men, sex workers and migrants) are more likely to get AIDS than others. This may be partly true from the epidemiological perspective but NAPS need to present the epidemic to the general public in a way which does not reinforce such perceptions.

Educational messages can emphasize the need for solidarity with those who are discriminated against. A first step is to explain how HIV is and is not transmitted, debunking myths and associated fears. These messages can be communicated through printed materials, newspaper and magazine articles, radio and television programmes, community education sessions, hotlines and word of mouth. Health workers should be taught the principles of universal precautions that should apply to blood and body fluids from all patients, not only those they know or suspect to be HIV-infected.

Personalizing the epidemic also works well: when people tell their stories, they provide concrete examples rather than distant images of "AIDS victims" or "HIV carriers". The first woman to speak out publicly in the Philippines greatly increased the impact of the NAP campaigns, helping raise the general public's awareness in a positive way. Persons living with HIV are often in the forefront of actions to challenge discrimination. A woman working for a care agency in Canada, for example, sued her employer after she was dismissed because her serostatus became known She won her case, simultaneously giving other seropositive women encouragement to stand up for their nights. [61]

NGOs can play a useful "watchdog role" regarding human rights violations. The International Gay and Lesbian Human Rights Commission, for example, publishes an *Act or Alert* bulletin to publicize discrimination and stimulate responses to specific abuses. Amnesty International and many NGOS document discrimination cases so that these can be brought to the attention of the government and press. Lobbying for changes in discriminatory laws and the passage or endorsement of protective ones (e.g., the UN Convention for the Elimination of All Forms of Discrimination against Women) is another important action area. Many NGOs also publish HIV/AIDS rights charters and refer persons suffering discrimination to legal services so that they can pursue their rights.

Further work must be done to change customary and written laws so women have legal recourse in cases of abuse, loss of maintenance and discrimination over inheritance. Many women are unaware of their rights and don't know that they are legally protected against certain abuses. This knowledge gap is slowly being filled by lawyers' groups and NGOs worldwide through "legal literacy" programmes, making the law accessible to women and promoting their capacity to understand and assert their rights.[62]

PROMOTING LEGAL LITERACY

"Ugandan women have almost the same rights as men according to the law books, but in reality tradition rules", says Winnie Sekadde of FIDA, a legal aid organization for women in Uganda. "It means for example that they have no right to property and income."

The HIV/AIDS epidemic has presented FIDA with a growing number of cases regarding property and succession rights, although maintenance money is still the biggest issue. "Women get into trouble when their husbands die because of the gap between traditional customs and official laws. Women in rural areas are not aware of the written laws. Even if they are, the pressure to comply with tradition is enormous."

According to the traditional customs, when a woman marries, her father receives a bride price from her husband. She then belongs to her husband's clan. She must take care of his household and work his land; any earnings go to her husband. "Women are economically and socially completely dependent on their husbands," Sekadde says. "If a man dies, she loses everything to his clan, even the right to custody over her children."

According to written laws in Uganda, women have a right to their own income and a small inheritance. In practice, however, women almost never get this. The amount is divided if a man has more than one wife, which is common in Uganda. Other family members can also claim possessions. In case of doubt, judges may also fall back on customary law, often to the detriment of women. FIDA is therefore lobbying for a women-friendly law, with fewer opportunities for interpretation by judges.

Because not many women know about laws, FIDA educates them through village seminars, radio and television programmes and newspaper articles. FIDA has also formed a team to persuade villagers to write wills.

Cases relating to sexual abuse of children are increasing. Children are regarded as "safe partners" because generally they are notyet infected. Girls have been abused by grandfathers, uncles and teachers. To make pupils aware of these problems, FIDA performs education theatre at schools. [63]

Developing Gender-Sensitive Care and Support

A first step towards making care and support systems more sensitive to the specific needs of women and men is to re-evaluate policies and assess whether they are gender sensitive. Training programmes for care-providers and counsellors need adaptation so that, for example, they respect women's wishes and needs regarding pregnancy, breast-feeding, abortion and sterilization and deal with the potential negative consequences of testing women but not their partners for HIV.

Follow-up counselling and support for women and men living with HIV/AIDS requires expansion. Social and legal assistance must be available even when people cannot pay. Women's lack of money worsens their burden when they care for family members and yet lack care for themselves, especially if the husband dies first. Seropositive women especially need ways to generate an income despite suffering periodic bouts of illness: "When my husband died of AIDS, I found it difficult to make ends meet. I decided to grow tomatoes, but did not have enough money to start the project. When I had almost given up hope, I got into conversation with some women in my village who were in a similar situation as myself. One of them suggested we pool our resources to support one another. The plan worked out quite well. I am now able to take better care of myself and my family. Our group's plan also ended up being an inspiration to other women in the village" (Tanzania).[64]

LIGHTENING THE BURDEN OF CARE

Communities in sub-Saharan Africa recognize that as more households are affected by the epidemic, community life suffers unless affected women and children are supported in coping[65]*:*

In Rakai District, Uganda, men developed an income-generating project to help them support 26 children orphaned due to AIDS. They registered as an association and received training and a loan from the NGO World Vision for a bee-keeping project. In their first season, the association harvested nearly 25 litres of honey to raise funds needed to help them in their role of care-takers.

The University Teaching Hospital in Zambia used to test children suspected of being HIV-positive, then gave the test results only to mothers. Fathers who later learned their children were HIV-positive blamed the mothers and refused to be tested themselves. SWAA helped change this policy. Now, when children show clinical symptoms suggesting HIV infection, the parents are called in together for counselling and both parents and child are tested simultaneously. The test results are given to the parents together during additional counselling. This process has reduced blaming and tension between spouses.

Because much of the care and support for people affected by HIV/AIDS now falls on women's shoulders, a major task is to find ways of lessening women's extra workload. One way is to provide help with home-care nursing. In south Thailand, nurses are assisted by La Trobe University (Australia) in sharing skills with village women so that they can manage those sick with infectious diseases (including HIV/AIDS and STDs) more effectively and efficiently.[66]

Analysis of successful programmes is needed to determine what it is that motivates people (especially men) to volunteer their time, energy and resources to community- and home-based care and support.

In sights then need to be shared widely so that new initiatives can benefit from them and volunteer support can be maintained long term.

Living Positively with HIV/AIDS

Women and men around the world often feel isolated when they learn of their diagnosis. Women especially have difficulties in contacting peers in the same situation. Yet this provides great psychological benefits: "When the woman at the clinic said, 'Would you like to meet another woman with HIV?' and gave me her phone number, I couldn't wait to get home. . . As soon as I met her, it just changed my life. I realized I hadn't done anything wrong, I wasn't a criminal... We've formed a womens group . . . I can talk about problems that have happened. Not just to do with HIV... Just supporting each other, having good fun, having a laugh" (England).[67]

Associations of women living with HIV/AIDS are helping participants find ways to cope. They also give the epidemic a human—and female—face when their members speak out on how HIV/AIDS affects them In 1992, the International Community of Women Living with HIV/AIDS (ICW) was created at the International Conference on AIDS in Amsterdam. Since then, this coordinating body has provided women most directly affected by the epidemic with a voice at global and regional levels. Through a network of worldwide representatives, they provide policy input to UN agencies.

ICW has also inspired the formation of associations of seropositive women in many other countries. At the national and community levels, seropositive women are joining together to make the ideal of living positively with the virus a reality:

— The National Women and HIV Project in Canada created a coalition of Hlv-positive women by supporting regional networks and developing communication tools 168].

— The Argentine Network of Women Living with HIV/AIDS (ANW) gives women information about AIDS, helps access treatments and medications through state and private services and makes referrals to NGOs and governmental social services.[69]

— Many seropositive women who care for their households alone must also plan for their families' future, especially the children. Due to discrimination and frequent illness, their access to the labour market is also restricted. Women Touch in Sao Paulo, Brazil, helps provide them with work, an income and special protection.[70]

Such initiatives demonstrate that women and men living with HIV/AIDS are not the problem but part of the solution. To prove we truly care - not only in the sense of caring for but also caring about people living with HIV/AIDS—we must ensure that our response to the epidemic gives these women and also men a central role in policy and programme formulation, implementation and evaluation.

A PERSONAL TESTIMONY

"I became pregnant with my fourth child in 1988. My health deteriorated and I had persistent vaginal itching and abnormal pains. I complained during antenatal check-ups but didn't get proper treatment for my vaginal infection. They took my blood for an HIV-test without my consent.

After I delivered, they tested my child, too. Then the doctor just told me that they had taken our blood and the results for both of us were positive. When I broke the news to my husband, he left me that very same night, after calling me names and accusing me of being unfaithful and a prostitute. I later learned that he had already been tested and was HIV-positive but didn't have the courage to tell me.

I confided my HIV status to my sister, a nurse. Because of stigmatization and discrimination, she told me not to tell anyone else. I kept quiet but felt as if everybody knew that I was HIV-positive. I was so lonely, isolated and afraid of leaving my children without any information on AIDS. I spent most of my time crying and the loss of my child at five months made my condition worse. Fortunately, I didn't have to give up my job because it was my only source of support.

In 1992, I was invited to attend a conference organized by Dutch seropositive women. I accepted though I was afraid to talk about my status and had never been involved in AIDS activities. I went because I wanted to meet people who were also dying of AIDS. But I was wrong about that. The conference gave me self-confidence and courage to talk about my status to friends and family, including my children and co-workers.

Back home I began giving my personal testimony during workshops, seminars and on national radio. I introduced the idea of forming a support group for women whose husbands had died of AIDS because I saw many widows who were suffering from property-grabbing by the relatives of their deceased husbands. At first we met just to share our personal experiences, give each other moral and psychological support and break our isolation and fear.

Eventually, we established the National Association of People with HIV/AIDS in Malawi (NAPHAM) with the aim to promote health through self-care and support. We care for one another when one falls sick and are now trying to involve our families. Most of the women are poor housewives. NAPHAM therefore promotes self-reliance through income-generating

RESEARCHERS	YES	SOMEWHAT	NO
>Do you explore the implications of gender inequality in relation to HIV/AIDS and STDS?	☐	☐	☐
>Does your research focus on issues of special relevance to women and men:	☐	☐	☐
— Women controlling their risk	☐	☐	☐
— Women's scope for decision-making in different situations	☐	☐	☐
— Women's right to control fertility	☐	☐	☐
— Factors motivating men to share decision-making regarding fertility control	☐	☐	☐
— HIV transmission through breast-feeding	☐	☐	☐
— Female-controlled prevention methods	☐	☐	☐
— Factors motivating women and men to discuss mutual rsponsibility in relation to prevention	☐	☐	☐
— Factors facilitating women's and/or men's ability to undertake prevention			
— Women's and/or men's access to health services that address their specific concerns (including STD treatment)	☐	☐	☐
— Rape and violence	☐	☐	☐
— Sex work	☐	☐	☐
— Sexual practices facilitating HIV transmission	☐	☐	☐
— Female circumcision in relation to HIV/STDs	☐	☐	☐
— Female care roles and their impact on production and education	☐	☐	☐
— Factors motivating men to participate in domestic tasks and care	☐	☐	☐
— Inheritance rights	☐	☐	☐

>Do you explore which information channels are most appropriate for different age and gender groups?	☐	☐	☐
>Do you use these channels to communicate research findings and other information?	☐	☐	☐
>Have you researched barriers to women's participation in programme activities?	☐	☐	☐

POLICY-MAKERS, PROGRAMME DEVELOPERS AND IMPLEMENTERS

>Are all programme implementers able to address gender issues?	☐	☐	☐
>Are women's organizations involved in policy and programme development and decision-making processes?	☐	☐	☐
>Do women and men share programme goals?	☐	☐	☐
>Do your interventions combat violence against women and girls (active policy goals, educational programmes, legislation)?	☐	☐	☐
> Do your programmes consider differences in gender roles, access to resources and decision-making that affect women's and men's abilities to protect themselves?	☐	☐	☐
>Do your programmes consider differences in male and female life experiences ?	☐	☐	☐
>Do your programmes differentiate between male and female health needs throughout the life cycle?	☐	☐	☐
>Do your programmes call for gender-based sexual health education in school curricula?	☐	☐	☐
>Do your programmes encourage couples, parents and/or children to discuss sexual health?	☐	☐	☐
>Do your programmes address the need to motivate men to inform their wives if they are HIV-positive?	☐	☐	☐

	Yes	Somewhat	No
>Do your interventions aim to develop and strengthen men's concern and caring for their families?	☐	☐	☐
>Do your education and communication programmes encourage men to share domestic responsibilities and tasks?	☐	☐	☐
>Do your programmes encourage social welfare agencies, NGOs, employers, etc. to provide or make allowances for child and patient care?	☐	☐	☐
PROGRAMME ACTIVITIES			
>Do you organize activities at locations and times convenient to both women and men?	☐	☐	☐
>Do you provide child-care services during activities and meetings?	☐	☐	☐
>Do you create situations in which women and/or men can talk freely about their opinions, feelings and needs?	☐	☐	☐
>Do you try to ensure that men and women hear and respond to one another's concerns and needs in a constructive manner?	☐	☐	☐
PROMOTING SAFER SEX			
Do your programmes:			
>challenge double standards between men and women regarding a) teenage sexuality, b) casual sex, and c) sex outside marriage?	☐	☐	☐
>address difficulties in condom use from women's and men's perspectives?	☐	☐	☐
>teach both women and men how to use condoms?	☐	☐	☐

>promote easy access to condoms for women and men?	☐	☐	☐
>enhance women's and men's skills in negotiating safer sex?	☐	☐	☐
>enhance women's self-confidence?	☐	☐	☐
>address sexual abuse?	☐	☐	☐
>promote attitudes to relationships that meet women's and men's sexual needs?	☐	☐	☐

PROVIDING HEALTH AND CARE SERVICES

Do your programmes:

>ensure equal access by men and women, particularly for STD treatment?	☐	☐	☐
>make family planning services attractive and accessible to men?	☐	☐	☐
>encourage men to take on greater care roles in the family?	☐	☐	☐
>address inheritance laws and customs where these put women and children at a disadvantage?	☐	☐	☐
>address the different financial problems affecting women and men?	☐	☐	☐
>ensure that girls' care roles and lack of money do not exclude them from school?	☐	☐	☐
>include men as volunteers in providing community and home care services?	☐	☐	☐

activities. By making soap and raising chickens we are able to pay school fees for some of our members' children.

I know God is keeping me for a purpose which I yet have to fulfil. Today I am in the eighth year from the time I was diagnosed. I'm still living because I have a will to live and want to help those who are suffering as I did."

Winnie Chikafumbwa, Malawi

6. HOW GENDER SENSITIVE IS YOUR WORK?

The enormous cost and suffering caused by the HIV/AIDS epidemic is forcing serious re-evaluation of norms values and conditions related to genden. Such analysis may lead to fundamental improvements that can benefit misions of people—women, men and children—in societies around the world.

The following Checklist is designed to help policy implementers and programme planners assess the gender sensitivity of their HIV/AIDS and STD policies and programmes. First determine which areas pertain to your type of activities. Responses to the questions may then be answrere *"yes"*, *"somewhat"* and *"no"*.

References

1. Reid., E., Gender, knowledge and responsibility. In J. Mann et al., eds., *AIDs in the World*, Cambridge London: Harvard University Press, 1992, p. 657.
2. Heise, L. L. & C. Elias, Transforming AIDs prevention to meet women's needs a focus on developing countries. *Social Science and Medicine*, 1995, 40/7: 931-943.
3. Dabis, F. et al., Estimating the rate of mother to-child transmission of HIV Report of a workshop on methodological issues Ghent (Belgium), 17-20 February 1992 AIDS, 1993, 7:11391148.
4. De Cock, K. M. et al., The public health implications of AIDS research in Africa JAMA, 1994, 272:481.
5. Nyo Nyo, *National Programme for Training Urban and Rural Women on STD/HIV In Myanmar* WHO/GPA Meeting on Effective Approaches for the Prevention of HIV/AIDs in Women, Geneva, February 1995.
6 Reid, E., *Women's dreaming: women, sexuality and development.* Presentation at the Women's Studies Conference, Sydney, Australia, November 1994.
7 Thin, N., Women's status and rights. In: M. de Bruyn, ed., *Advancing women's statues women and men together? Critical reviews and a selected annotated bibliography.* Amsterdam:: KIT Press, 1995.
8 du Guerny, J. & E:. Sjoberg, Inter relationships between gender relations and the HIV/AIDS epidemic: some possible consideration for policies and programmes AIDS, 1993,7/8: 1027 - 1034.

9 Heise, L. L. et al., *Violence against women: the hidden health burden.* World Bank Discussion Paper No. 255. Washington, D.C.: IBRD/World Bank, 1994.

10 Muhindi, B., 'Immoral' female condom. World AIDs, July 1993, p. 3.

11 Marres, D., *AIDS and childbearing: an explorative study among Kenyan women* [Dutch] M.A Thesis. Maastricht: University of Limburg, 1992, p. 27.

12 Marres, p. 33.

13 Flummer, F. A. etal., *The effect of HIV infection on the clinical features and response to treatment of genital ulcer disease (GUD) due to chancroid.* Presentation at the VII International Conference on AIDS, Florence, June 1991

14 Karim, Q.A., personal communication, September 1994.

15 Nataraj, S., No way to treat a woman. *Populi,* November 1994, p. II.

16 PANOS quoted in *Sunday Mail* (Harare), 18 December 1994.

17 Personal communication, November 1994.

18 Karim, Q. A. et al., *Women and AIDS in Natal/KwaZulu, South Africa: determinants of the adoption of HIV protective behaviour.* Washington, D.C.:ICRW, 1994.

19 Soroptomists and SPC co-operate. *Pacific AIDs Alert Bulletin,* 1994, 9:8.

20 Lee, S., ed., *our voices, our lives: life stories of women living with HIV/AIDS in Zimbabwe* Harare: Body Positive, 1 994, p 59.

21 Seruunkuma, R., Living with HIV/AIDs :a personal testimony. *AIDs Health Promotion Exchange,* 1994, 3:7

22 Ray, S., personal observation, 1 995.

23 Armstrong, S., The last taboo. *World AIDs,* 1993, 29:6-9.

24 Jenkins, C., An epidemic with a future? *World AID,* 1993, 29: 2.

25 Surapaty, R.M. et al., *Knowledge about AIDs and husband-wife communication among married women in. Palembang, Indonesia* Presentation (PD 0132) at the X International Conference on AIDs,Yokohama, Japan, 1994.

26 Personal communication, November 1993.

27 Van den Berg, D. & M. Swenne, Eenzame strijd. *HIV Nieuws,* September-October 1993, pp.13-15.

28 Foppen, R., "Let's form a club of 'sexually-disabled' women". AIDS *Health Promotion Exchange,* 1994, 3: 12-13.

29 Niang, C.I., *Socio -cultural factors favouring HIV infection and the integration of traditional women's associations in AIDS prevention strategies in Kolda, Senegal* Washington, D.C: ICRW, 1994.

30 Apisuk, C. & N. Apisuk, eds., *Living with HIV.* Nontburi: NAAM-CHEWIT Project, 1994, p 6.

31 Berer, M.&S. Ray, *Women & AIDs, an international resource book.* London: Pandora 1993, p. 248.

32 Ngcongco, V.N., *Nursing, home care, and HIV.* X International Conference on AIDS, Yokohama, Japan,1994.

33 Apisuk & Apisuk, pp. 10-11.

34 Topouzis, D., *Uganda: the socio-economic impact of HIV/AIDS on rural families with an emphasis on youth.* TCP/UGA/2256 paper. Rome: FAO, 1994, p. 20.

35 Personal communication, London, March, 1994.

36 Sharma, J., Fighting against. *World AIDs,* March, 1994, p.h..

37 Africa's largest population begins AIDS campaign. *Herald* (Zimbabwe), 13 December 1991 .

38 Hashemi, S. *Credit programmes, women's empowerment and contraceptive use in rural Bangladesh.* WHO/GPA Meeting on Effective Approaches for the Prevention of HIV/AIDS in Women, Geneva, February 1995.

39 Fitzpatrick, L., Reflections from a workshop on the media and AIDS prevention: participation makes a difference. *AIDs Health Promotion Exchange,* 1991, 1: 13-15.

40 Esu-Williams, E.,Country Watch: Nigeria *AIDs Health Promotion Exchange,* 1992: 1: 13-14.

4 1 Shahabudin, S.H., HIV/AIDS awareness workshops for women. *Report of a Consultation on Women and HIV/AIDS,* Geneva: WHO/GPA, December 1993.

42 Dibb, L., Country Watch: England. *AIDs Health Promotion Exchange,* 1992, 3: 8-9.

43 Weiss, E. & M. Rehra, *Fostering collaboration between researchers and NGOS on women and AIDS,* Washington, D.C., 1994.

44 Bianco, M., personal communication, 1995.

45 Bezmalinovic, B. et al., *Guatemala City Women: empowering a vulnerable group to prevent HIV transmission.* Washington, D.C.: ICRW, 1994.

46 Bhende, A., *Evolving a model for AIDS prevention education among low-income adolescent girls in urban India.* Washington, D. C., ICRW, 1993.

47 Mazzola, E., Country Watch: Italy. *AIDS Health Promotion Exchange,* 1992, 3: 7-8.

48 Surena, Y., *Women's Protection Project: condom social marketing for women in Haiti.* WHO/GPA Meeting on Effective Approaches for the Prevention of HIV/AIDs in Women, Geneva, February 1995.

49 Dasgupta, P., personal communication, 1995.

50 Urban, M.T., personal communication, 1995.

5 1 Guttierez, A., *Man/Hombre/Homme: meeting male reproductive health care needs in Colombia.* WHO/GPA Meeting on Effective Approaches for the Prevention of HIV/AIDS in Women, Geneva, February 19

52 Kalckmann, S., personal communication, 1995.

53 Awino, J., Country Watch: Uganda. *AIDs Health Promotion Exchange.* 1992,3:6-7.

54 Blaauw., C., personal communication, 1994.

55 Prochaska, R., personal communication, 1995.

56 Wilson, D. et al., *Intergenerational communication within the family: implications for developing STD/HIV prevention strategies for adolescents in Zimbabwe.* Washington, D.C.: ICRW, 1994.

57 Givaudan, M. et al., *Strengthening intergenerational communication*

within the family: an AIDS prevention strategy for adolescents. Washington, D. C.: ICRW, 1994.

58 Constantino-David, K., A model of gender training for men. In: A. Rao et al., eds., *Reflections and learnings: gender trainers workshop report.* Amsterdam: Royal Tropical Institute, pp. 58-61.

59. Raman, S., Positive reinforcement to promote safer sex among clients *AIDs Health Promotion Exchange,* 1992, I:6-9.

60. Venables, S & J. Tulloch, *Your little head thinking instead of your big head. The Hetero sexual Men's Project.* Australia: Family Planning NSW, 1993.

61. Trudy, personal communication, 1995.

62. Schuler, M. & S. Kadirgamar-Rajasingham, eds., *Legal literacy: a tool for women's empowerment.* New York: PACT Communications, 1992.

63. Ars, B., Alice erfde alleen de ziekte van haar overleden man. *Internationale Samen werking,* February 1995, pp. 2, 3.

64 Msuya,W. et al., *Life first A practical guide for people with HIV/AIDs and their families* Mwanza: AMREF/Kuleana, 1993, p.69.

65 *Action for Children affected by AIDS: Programme Profile and lesson learned* Geneva: WHO/UNICEF, 1994.

66 Parsons, C., personal communication, 1995.

67 Richardson, A. & D. Bolle, *Wise before their time.* London: Fount Paperbacks, HarperCollins Publishers Limited, 1992, pp.77-78.

68 *Canadian women and AIDS projects and committees inventory.* Edmonton: Canadian AIDS Society - National Women and HIV Project, 1995.

69 Perez, P., Country Watch :Argentina. *AIDs Health promotion Exchange.* 1994, 3: 11-12.

70 Eugenia, personal communication, 1995.

INTERNATIONAL ENCYCLOPAEDIA OF AIDS-2

HIV/AIDS
ISSUES AND CHALLENGES
Part-II

Editor
Dr. Digumarti Bhaskara Rao
M.Sc. , M.A., M.A., M.Ed., Ph.D.
R. V. R. College of Education
Guntur–522 006
Andhra Pradesh. (INDIA)

2000
DISCOVERY PUBLISHING HOUSE
NEW DELHI-110 002

First Published-2000

ISBN 81-7141-524-5 (Set)

Published by:
DISCOVERY PUBLISHING HOUSE
4831/24, Ansari Road, Prahlad Street,
Darya Ganj, New Delhi-110 002 (*INDIA*)
Phone: 3279245
Fax: 91-11-3253475

Printed at:
Arora Offset Press
Laxmi Nagar, Delhi 110 092.

Preface

The HIV/AIDS is a new phenomenon in the human society. HIV destroys the immune system of human individuals, producing a defenselessness fatal state known as AIDS. The World Health Organisation has estimated that already one in every two hundred and fifty adults in the world is infected with Human Immunodeficiency Virus and according to WHO's projections a total of forty million men women and children worldwide will have been infected with HIV by the turn of this twentieth century. Visualising the devastating effects of the HIV/AIDS epidemic within our life times and beyond is difficult. Probably, no other disease in recent times has had the impact on human society generated by HIV/AIDS.

The HIV/AIDS epidemic has brought into focus many health related ethical, legal and human rights issues. This epidemic requires immediate and effective responses in new programming areas: attitudinal and behavioural changes, community-based care and support initiatives, and the maintenance of human development in the face of increasing rates of illness and deaths. At this point, education enters the scene as it can alter the HIV/AIDS situation since it brings change in the behaviour of the people.

This *International Encyclopaedia of AIDS* presents the worldwide information about HIV/AIDS, issues and challenges, reports and reviews, ethics laws and human rights, and educational activities and programmes to keep the policy makers, planners, professionals, activists, researchers, educationists, teachers and students well informed of the epidemic.

Dr. Digumarti Bhaskara Rao
26 January 1999
The Republic Day of India

Acknowledgements

I am thankful to the World Health Organisation and its associated offices for using their material namely School Health Education to prevent AIDS and STD: A Resource Package for Curriculum Planners-Handbook for Curriculum Planners. Student's Activities, Teachers' Guide, Global Programme on AIDS-HIV Prevention and Care: Teaching Modules for Nurses and Midwives, Global Programme on AIDS. Community HIV Prevention Handbook; STD care Management-workbooks 1-7, Facing the Challenge of HIV/AIDS STDs: A Gender-based Response; HIV/AIDS and STD surveillance Data Management and Use-Report, Bangkok, 1995; Carrying out HIV Sentinal Surveillance-A Guide for Programme Managers, AIDS Prevention and Care in the workplace: Enhancing the Role of Private Sector; HIV Testing Policies and Gidelines; Carrying out HIV Sentinel surveillance; AIDS Prevention; Understanding and Living with AIDS; AIDS: A Modern Epidemic; HIV/AIDS in South-East Asia: IXth meeting of the National Programme Managers, New Delhi, 1993; Information, Education and Communication: A Guide for AIDS Programme Managers, Handbook on AIDS Home Care; HIV/AIDS in South-East Asia: A Pictorial summary; etc.

I am thankful to the United Nations Development Programme, UNDP's HIV and Development Programme, and UNDP's Regional Projects on HIV and Development for using their material namely Economic Implications of AIDS in Asia; Socio Economic Implications of the Epidemic; NGOs Working with Sex workers; NGO Responses to HIV/AIDS in Asia-Case Studies; HIV in the Workplace: Dealing with the Issues-Role Plays, Development and the HIV Epidemic, Law Ethics and HIV; HIV Law and Law Reform; Issue Papers; Study Papers; Working Papers; etc.

I am thankful to the Health and Nutrition Centre, Republic of Philippines for using its material namely sourcebook on HIV/AIDS Prevention Education for Tertiary Educational Institutions.

I am thankful to the Curriculum Development Programme, Ministry of Education, Government of Thailand for using its material namely Institutional Modules for AIDS Education.

I am thankful to US Department of Health and Human Services: Whitman-Walker Clinic, Inc., USA; East-West Centre, USA; National AIDS Control Organisation, Government of India; Academy of Culture Communication Education Science and Service, Guntur, United Nations and its agencies for using their material.

I am grateful to Bhaskar Bhattacharji; V. Alexeev, Geeta Sethi, Elizabeth Reid, Mina Mauerstein-Bail, A. A. Trinidad, Palomi Cuchi. D. Pushpa Latha for their kind co-operation.

Dr. Digumarti Bhaskara Rao,
Secretary
ACCESS
D-43, S.V. N. Colony,
Guntur-522 006

Contents

30

Lost Souls

Ms. Elizabeth Reid
UNDP, New York

William James in *The Moral Philosopher and the Moral Life* explores the hypothesis a world in which millions can live full and happy lives on one simple condition: that a certain lost soul on the far-off edge of things should lead a life of lonely torment.

Except for this one person, people in this world lead lives of happiness, of unthreatened well-being. More than that, it is only because of the isolated torment of this lost soul that their happiness can exist and continue. The suffering of that one person creates the possibility of their serenity. Without this suffering, their utopia could not be.

James implicitly poses the question: could one accept happiness under such conditions?

It seems to me that two questions can be distinguished. Firstly, if faced with such a situation, could we accept happiness at this cost? Secondly, what would happen to us if we did if we were prepared to pay this price for happiness?

The second question is addressed by Ursula Le Guin in a short story entitled "The Ones Who Walk Away From Omelas" (*The Wind's Twelve Quarters*, Bantam Books, 1976). She describes the city of Omelas, bright-towered by a sparkling sea. The people are gifted, creative happy in their relationships and their work. But they all know one thing: the tenderness of the friendships, the wisdom of their scholars, the health of their children and even the abundance of their harvest wholly depend on one child's abominable misery.

This child lives in a windowless basement under one of their beautiful buildings. The child and the circumstances that it lives in are a sickening and a shocking sight. It has not always lived there. It can remember sunlight and its mother's voice.

All young people as they reach an age of maturity are told about the child and most go to see it. They feel disgust, anger, outrage, impotence. They would like to do something for to child, but if the child were brought out into the sunlight, out of that vile place, then their way of living, its lack of cares, its untrammelled joys would, in that moment, wither away. These are the terms: if the child is even spoken to, the world as they know it would cease to exist. The terms are absolute.

The children rage and brood. But then they begin to rationalism even if the child could be released, it is now too degraded and deprived to be able to know any real joy:

> "it has been afraid too long ever to be tree ot fear. Its habits are too uncouth for it lo respond to humane treatment. Indeed, after so long it would probably be wretched without walls about it to protect it, and darkness for its eyes, and its own excrement to sit in."

They begin to see, and accept, a terrible justice in reality. Just as we have: we accept poverty, extreme poverty, in our midst, for example. For us, it rarely has a human face.

But let us return to the first question, the one William James poses and the question that might allow us to understand better how such lost souls come about: could we accept happiness at such a price?

James acknowledges human frailty. An impulse would arise within us, he feels, to clutch at the happiness so offered. However, he argues, it would be immediately suppressed by the knowledge of how hideous would be its enjoyment when deliberately accepted as the fruit of such a bargain. In James world, there must be no lost souls to degrade us.

A similar fundamental moral dilemma faces the world with the coming of the HIVepidemic: would we accept the ability to continue our past way of life at such an inhuman cost, the cost of quarantining, isolating and rejecting those infected with HIV? Are we as morally decent as William James? Or would we find such a cost acceptable? Will the Lost Souls of the epidemic be those we push away from ourselves so that we can continue to live as we were living before this epidemic, those we reject, imprison, repudiate?

Our past way of life has its roots in a world that has fundamentally changed. The HIV virus is now in our midst. In a social setting, we cannot tell where it is, whom it has infected. Potentially therefore, each and every act of unprotected sexual intercourse can be an occasion for its further transmission.

There is a widespread reluctance to change, to act in the present in a way that is consistently protective. This should not cause much surprise. Sexual behaviour has consistently and throughout history been marked by a widespread refusal to take responsibility for these acts and a refusal in particular to take precautionary and protective measures. The consequences of this refusal have included unwanted pregnancies and the trauma of abortion or birth in such circumstances, widespread infertility, shame and significant morbidity, including that of sexual partners and children. To this list are now added all of the tragic consequences of HIV infection.

We know how to protect ourselves from HIV infection. However, the means to prevent the spread of HIV. unlike many other pathogens, depends not just on the impersonal application of technology but on human attributes, ultimately on both self-love and altruism. Changes are required not only to human behaviour, but to the very way that our society is structured and to our social values. The spread of the virus is much harder to slow down in conditions of social alienation, of poverty, even of wealth.

One change has occurred: the consequences of HIV infection are more feared than the consequences of other diseases that can be sexually transmitted. This fear could be a motivating force for each of us to make the required protective changes. Or it could reinforce the past refusal to accept responsibility for our conduct. In the latter case, the demand will be that the protection of the majority requires stringent measures to be taken against those infected. There will be pressure to shift the focus of HIV policy away from behaviour change in the whole community to identification, surveillance and isolating of those already infected. Emphasis will be placed, perhaps exclusively, on compulsory contact tracing, on the quarantining or sexual emasculation of those considered by the authorities to be unresponsive. In this way, the community's refusal to change its past ways of behaving, to act in a morally responsible way, will create our own lost souls, forced to pay the price for us all.

This has been recognised in national HIV policies in which one of the most important guiding principles has been that each person must take responsibility for preventing himself or herself from becoming infected sexually or through needle sharing. This responsibility cannot be thrust upon the infected and their cares. The nature of transmission and infection is such that each person in our community, not just the infected, must carry this responsibility. Those infected need the space and the support to learn how to live full and responsible lives knowing that they are infected; the whole community needs the knowledge, the means and the support to protect themselves .

The way a community responds to the HIV epidemic seems to be influenced by at least two factors. The first lies in the boundaries communities draw to define themselves: who is one of us and who is not. HIV policy responses to infection among drug users differ according to whether drug users are seen by the State or the community as enemies or as victims. New York and Edinburgh exemplify the first, and the HIV policy response has been a punitive mobilisation of the law rather than the setting in place of protective measures such as programmes for needle distribution and disposal. A similar distinction can be drawn between policy responses with regard to homosexuals, where the HIV policy alternatives have been either gross and culpable neglect along with calls for quarantining or tattooing or, alternatively, supportive measures which have assisted the gay community to develop an effective response.

Policy responses are more humane and supportive where those infected are accepted as an integral part of the community. There may be alienation, discrimination and stigma but nevertheless the community struggles to encompass and include the differences. Where the infected are ostracized, seen as enemies of the people, the policy responses mirror this perception. The implicit message is that the infected are expendable, their lives of little or no value to the community. The result is inevitably violation, violence and murder.

A second influencing factor seems to be leadership style. A recent study of eight us communities and their reactions to a HIV-infected school child in their midst (*Learning by Heart* David L, Kirp, Rutgers UP, 1989) shows that each community that responded with compassion and humanity had a leadership that created the conditions for arriving at a decision rather than imposing decisions on the community. Without this leadership, communities were adrift, reacting too often with bigotry, hatred and violence.

This leadership style has béen adopted in too few countries. Public statements by leaders, policy discussion papers and public hearings, discussions and debates are important means to significantly broaden community knowledge of these complex issues and to increase community participation in the processes of decision making.

Resistance to change is a human characteristic. But this tendency must be struggled against for the price of resisting change is now too high. To ensure that our response to the epidemic does not lead to the underpinning of our way of life by the torment of lost souls will require at least the following:

— that we continue to struggle to encompass and include everyone within the bounds of our community;
— that we continue with a participatory, inclusive and open style of leadership and decision making;
— that our protection and prevention policies continue to be directed at the whole community; and
— that we begin to conceptually explore and understand the high moral cost of doing otherwise.

The creation of lost souls can destroy the mogul-fabric of a society. There were some who walked away from Omelas. But they were few.

31

Towards an Ethical Response to the HIV Epidemic

Ms. Elizabeth Reid
UNDP, New York

Here in Africa, as elsewhere in the world, the HIV virus is not infiltrating a benign world.

The realities of which we are a part include:

— the brutal and seemingly senseless slaughter taking place in Rwanda, and which has taken place in Angola, Liberia and elsewhere;

— the purposeless disintegration of a once proud and homogenous nation state in Somalia which has parallels to Zaire:

— the degradation of life in the slums of Abijan, or Nairobi, or Lagos, or Soweto, and elsewhere;

— the pervasive corruption of the educated elite and the consequent rarity of a courageous and altruistic leadership;

— the swelling ranks of the disinherited: men without occupation, youth without education, the hungry, the landless, the lawless and the rootless;

— the increasing presence of eroded fields, discarded plastic bags, unpassable roads, crumbling makeshift shelters and disease; and

— the often base motives of the intervening powers, be they former colonial powers, other nation states, international organizations, the drug cartels or multinational corporations.

Another way of looking at these realities is to note that we are living in a world where increasingly:

— the concept of nation states, and so of national boundaries, are, in many instances, becoming irrelevant;

— the reach of national governments is shrinking and larger and larger tracts of land or expanses of dwellings are ungoverned and ungovernable by national authorities;

— legal systems are becoming marginalized or irrelevant and their place taken by military and paramilitary forces, vigilante groups, private security services, bandits and criminals, with the resulting summary executions, necklacing, roadblocks, ambushes, extortion and terror; and

— the delicate balance which must hold between the government, the military and the people for governance and participation to be possible is no longer in equilibrium.

These are not the only realities and, even where they hold sway, they may not be irreversible but they are realities very relevant to the HIV epidemic.

In the shanty towns and slums, wherever the military move, along the new drug routes in Africa and amongst the educated elites, the virus is spreading with a rapidity difficult to conceive. Its spread is directly linked to the economic, cultural, strategic and political conditions which are fueling widespread social and moral disintegration.

In turn, as it spreads, it itself is contributing to the creation of poverty, crime, alcoholism, economic disintegration, landlessness and hopelessness, with thc despair and deaths of those concerned. This is especially true where the epidemic remains wrapped in silence, where people live in fear that they might be infected but cannot find out, where sexual partners do not talk to each other and parents do not ensure that someone, be it they themselves or someone else, continues to talk to their children. Perhaps the most culpably silent are those to whom people turn as role models, for counsel or for leadership.

Furthermore, the response in Africa to date has been based on the concept of nation states. It has assumed an effective reach of centralized bureaucracies and formal institutions, including the law. There has been no acknowledgement of their limitations because the epidemic and its response has been seen as addressable from outside by technological interventions—a drug, a condom, a test kit. There has been little thought given to the limit of governmental action in attitudinal and behavioural change, in getting people to talk amongst themselves and to care for and about each other. Yet these latter lie at the heart of an effective response.

These issues are too important not to question their impact on the epidemic and not to accept that these realities are as relevant to our understanding of HIV as is a surveillance system or an anti-discrimination law. Those who have more chance of surviving this epidemic, whether adults, adolescents or children, may well live in slums or shanty towns. The difference between those communities which will survive and those that will not will lie in the values to which the community subscribes and, most importantly, those by which it strives to act.

A basic question thus becomes what sort of communities are those which have a chance of surviving and how can they be enabled to overcome all of the influences that are sapping and undermining their moral and social vitality? Just as people must want to create a community within a slum, within a village or of a nation in which they can live without fear and with hope for the future, with respect for each other and with the gift of life for their children, without crime, assault, filth and poverty, so too must people want to create a world within which we can co-exist peacefully with this virus, within which we do not pass it on, in the living of our lives from one to another.

Hence the work that UNDP has been associated with in the creation and stimulation of the African Network on Ethics, Law and HIV. The most notable thing about the epidemic, and the basis for hope for a future, lies in the remarkable fact that, somehow or other, this epidemic can bring out, not the worst, but the best in people: courage, compassion. concern for self and others. Hope for the future is grounded in the courage and behaviour of those most deeply affected, the people living with HIV and AIDS, many of whom are with us here today. Strikingly, these are not often those in whom their families and their nations have invested, the highly educated of this continent, nor are they usually those in whom the people have placed their trust, the politicians and leaders, religious, traditional or otherwise. They come, very often, from the same living conditions which drive others to crime or alcohol or violence. The courageous in this movement are mostly drawn from the villages, the slums, from lives marked by poverty or hardship, from humbler occupations and vocations. The vast majority of them will never attend a meeting on HIV except with their neighbours.

UNDP believes that this initiative will contributing significantly to ensuring that this courage and commitment to a better world for self and others is not lost. For people to continue to speak out and be engaged and for their individual actions to form the basis of a mass movement for social change, there must be an enabling and empowering ethical and legal environment. This will require a critical mass of courageous, informed and engaged people in each country who will speak out, advocate, lobby, advise, draft and defend to this end. These individuals could be more effective and supportive to each other when linked together into a national network. Thus a process was begun two years ago which has now resulted in national networks coming into existence in nine of the ten countries participitating in the process. The tenth country, South Africa, has established its networks independently and is now joining this regional effort.

By means of a Planning Meeting, held in Accra last October, and this Inter-Country Consultation, the process is now underway of linking these national networks into an African Network on Ethics, Law and HIV through which experiences can be exchanged, strategies discussed and shared to address common problems and a regional strategy developed. As resources allow, these networks will be expanded and more countries included.

This initiative, to be effective, must lead to a world where those most affected, those who live their daily lives within the confines of this epidemic, must be able to speak and act for the good of their societies, without recrimination, without retaliation, without repudiation. But it must also lead to a greater understanding of and impetus towards the kind of society in which people will be able to survive this epidemic and an identification of the value system or systems which will foster this. This, I have argued, cannot be done in isolation from the social and economic conditions which determine the pattern and speed of its spread.

Fortunately, I believe, although this must be tested in the crucible of reality, that the principles required to address this epidemic and those required to address the complex reality of the world on which it is feeding overlap.

There is a need, often overlooked, to distinguish two types of principles:

- those that must guide and shape the actions of those working to overcome this epidemic, and your presence here today bears witness to the fact that we all of us fall into that category; and
- those that will enable a community to survive through the tragedy in which we are already living and which is to come.

I will not attempt to give an exhaustive list of such principles but only an indicative one. Let me first start with the first type for they are less frequently discussed. These are the principles required to guide the actions of those working to assist others, as well as themselves, to respond to the epidemic, be they doctors, leaders, lawyers, researchers, development workers, counsellors, or whatever, those one might simply call the outsiders: those outside of a family, village or nation working with it.

The principle of being informed: each person engaged in or a part of the response to the epidemic needs actively in an ongoing manner to continue the quest to understand this epidemic in all its complexity and as it unfolds and changes. This principle is a prerequisite for the conceptual and programmatic flexibility demanded by the epidemic.

The principle of association: to work within this epidemic is to work in partnership with those living the virus. Those who do not know them as partners and confidants, who do not spend time in their company, should not represent them, speak for them, speak about them, attend conference on the subject, be employed as consultants, receive research grants or project financing, or head national programmes. If this principle is not respected, we run the risk of setting false priorities and designing irrelevant or infective programmes.

The principle of engagement: since each of us is affected, that is, there is no Them and Us within this epidemic, then each of us is and must be engaged, not just as actors, but active in our own interest and in the interests of those we love and care for. What we are facing can not be used as a situation of gain, nor as a situation of being employed, for the good of others or otherwise, nor as a situation of exploitation. To work, to be available, to volunteer, to spend one's time, to contribute one's talents is the engagement that this epidemic draws, and demands, from each person. Linked to this principle is the principle of language. It is equally important that the language used not divide the world into Them and Us, that it not strip those infected of their dignity nor define their identity as a human being in terms of their infection.

The principle of empowerment: this principle marks the manner in which we must work: as equals, in partnership, each bringing their own experience and skills to the partnership in a process of mutual capacity building. This is a difficult process. The experience of UNDP in working in partnership has led us to believe that one can only enter into true partnerships with people with similar value systems, in particular with those who are engaged. There may well be a diversity of beliefs, experiences, capacities, ways of thinking or working, disciplines and cultures; the critical value required for partnership is engagement. Furthermore, we have discovered that true partnership can only occur between or among equals, where all concerned are secure in their identities, their self-esteem and their place in the world.

Paradoxically, perhaps, it has often been easiest for UNDP to enter into partnership with those living with HIV and AIDS, those closest to them, and those working with them in the art of living. Perhaps it is because they have made the transition from knowing that they are infected to being able to take up their daily lives once more as someone living with the virus. This seems to create a will to live that they have to live and the determination that life be worth living which themselves produce the required self-esteem and security in their identity required for a partnership of mutual capacity building.

The principle of consensus-building: by its nature, this epidemic requires each person to face up to its realities. It is not a matter of some knowing and then providing direction to others and organizing them to carry out their directives. Rather, on the base of each couple, each family, each community, a process of consensus building must be catalysed so that all are involved in the discussions and in the decision making.

Turning briefly to those principles which will enable communities to survive and overcome this epidemic. These have been better mapped in the papers for this meeting and in the emerging discussion and literature on the nature of a community-based response, although there is still much work to do. These could include, as basic principles from which other more specific principles and directives for action can be derived, the following.

The principle of knowledge: that each person has the right to be able to determine their infection status in conditions of confidentiality and with counselling, and that this service must be voluntary, accessible and affordable. This principle is an essential prerequisite of the principle of openness, the imperative of this epidemic that the silence be shattered, the fear and the denital confronted and that each person be actively encouraged to talk about and decide upon this reality in all aspects of their life.

The principle of human dignity: that the essential human dignity of each person be respected in all aspects of their lives. This principle is ceaselessly and unrelentingly transgressed in the daily lives of women, a reality shared by the swelling ranks of the disinherited. Those most directly affected by this epidemic, who have been able to take up again their daily lives are now challenging us to honour it in principle and practice, to refind in our lives an unwavering commitment to mutual respect and trust as the basic values of human life.

The principle of protection: that all means of protecting themselves from infection or reinfection, both the technology, including condoms, and information, be available, affordable and accessible to each person who, reflecting on his or her life situation, sexuality, beliefs and values, has taken a decision to so protect themselves.

The principle of inclusion: that those most directly affected by the epidemic remain an integral part of their communities, with the right of access to all benefits available to others: education, training, employment, health and legal services, social support and benefits, sport, marriage etc. This principle is thus associated with the principle of non-discrimination and its behavioural imperatives against rejection, neglect, repudiation and stigmatization.

The principle of representation: that those most directly affected by the epidemic, living its realities in their daily lives, should participate in all discussions, activities and decision-making with respect to the epidemic.

The principle of compassion: this is the acknowledgement that each person is linked by relations of kinship, love, neighbourliness, empathy, dependency, respect or solidarity. To change and sustain the required changes, to be cared for, to be sheltered and provided for requires others. They cannot be achieved in isolation for they are not solitary or individual activities. Compassion is the ethical reflection of this interdependence.

The challenge facing this meeting lies in contributing to a process of better understanding the complex dynamics of the epidemic in its African setting, in reflecting on how one can create, catalyze and facilitate the building of consensus around the value systems or principles by which communities wish to live and nations to govern, and in adopting a set of principles, individually and collectively, which can guide our behaviour as activists in our struggle to bring about a world in which we wish to live and within which we can continue to live.

32

TB/HIV Connection: What Health Care Workers Should Know

US Department of Health
and Human Sciences
Atlanta Georgia 30333

Tuberculosis (TB) is seen with increasing frequency among persons infected with the human immunodeficiency virus (HIV), the virus that causes acquired immunodeficiency syndrome (AIDS). HIV infection is one of the strongest known risk factors for the progression of TB from infection to disease. However, of the diseases associated with HIV infection, TB is one of the few that is transmissible, treatable, and preventable.

Patients who have active. infectious TB pose a potential occupational hazard to health care workers (HCWs) if the disease is not promptly diagnosed and eftectively treated. This booklet presents information about diagnosing, managing, and preventing TB in persons with HIV infection and preventing and treating TB in health care workers.

TB AND HIV IN THE UNITED STATES

- An estimated 1.0 million persons in the United States are infected with HIV.
- An estimated 10 to 15 million persons in the United States are infected with *Mycobacterium tuberculosis,* the organism that causes TB.
- In 1990, approximately 5per cent of all AIDS patients also had TB. In some areas, as many as 58 per cent of persons with TB are HIV seropositive.

FACTS ABOUT HIV INFECTION

Mode of Transmission

HIV is not spread by casual contact. It is spread primarily through sexual contact or through sharing needles used to inject drugs. HIV can also be spread from pregnant women to their unborn children or from women to children through breast-feeding. In addition, HIV has been transmitted to persons who received HIV-infected blood products or transfusions of HIV-infected blood. Since July 1985, however, all blood donations have been tested for HIV infection, and those tound to contain HIV antibodies are discarded. Now the risk of infection from blood products or blood transfusions is very low. In a few instances, HIV has been transmitted to HCWs through unintentional needle-stick exposures to HIV-intected blood.

Pathogenesis

HIV is a retrovirus consisting of a central ribonucleic acid (RNA) surrounded by coats of virus-specific protein. In HIV-infected persons, the immune system recognizes the virus protein as foreign material and produces antibodies that are directed against this material. This is accomplished through complex mechanisms involving the white blood cells and the virus.

One important type of white blood cell is the lymphocyte, of which there are two types: B lymphocytes (B cells) and T lymphocytes (T cells). T cells include helper (CD4+) T cells and suppressor (CD8+) T cells. In persons infected with HIV, the total number of helper T cells is decreased because the virus infects the cells, reproduces within them, and then destroys them. As a result, immune defense mechanisms are impaired.

The helper (CD4+) T cell is the primary target for HIV infection because the virus is attracted to the CD4+ surface marker. Because the CD4+ T cell co-ordinates a number of immunologic functions, a loss of these cells leads to a progressive impairment of the immune response.[1] For example, low CD4+ counts are associated with anergy, the inability to mount a response to delayed-type hypersensitivity skin test antigens. Therefore, some HIV-infected persons with CD4+ counts of less than 200 who are cointected with M. tuberculosis may have a false-negative reaction to the tuberculin skin test..[2]

In addition as the number of CD4+ T cells decrease, the risk and severity of opportunistic diseases increases.[1] Some of the common opportunistic diseases experienced by persons infected with HIV are *Pneumocystis carinii* pneumonia, Kaposi's sarcoma, esophageal or bronchial candidiasis, extrapulmonary cryptococcosis, disseminated *Mycobacterium avium* complex, cytomegalovirus, HIV wasting syndrome, severe herpes simplex, toxoplasmosis of the brain, pulmonary TB, extrapulmonary TB, and other disseminated mycobacterial diseases.[3]

When people who are infected with HIV become ill with opportunistic diseases and infections, have CD4+ counts of less than 200, or have a CD4+ percentage of total lymphocytes of less than 14 per cent, they are generally said to have AIDS. As of January 1, 1993, pulmonary tuberculosis is an AIDS-defining disease in the expanded surveillance case definition for AIDS among adolescents and adults.[1]

High-Risk Behaviours for HIV Infection

Current or past behaviours that put persons at high risk for HIV infection include

injection drug use
sexual activity between men
sexual activity with someone who is infected with HIV
sexual activity with someone who has practiced any of the above behaviours.

Other factors which increase the risk for HIV infection include:

sexual activity with someone whose drug use or history of sexual behaviour is unknown (especially persons with multiple partners)
receipt of blood products or blood transfusions between 1978 and 1985.

FACTS ABOUT HIV-RELATED TB

Mode of Transmission

TB is a communicable disease caused by the bacterium *Mycobacterium tuberculosis,* often called the tubercle bacillus. It is spread from person to person through the inhalation of airborne particles containing *M. tuberculosis.* These particles, also called droplet nuclei, are produced when a person with infectious TB of the lung or larynx forcefully exhales, such as when coughing, sneezing, speaking, or singing. These infectious particles can remain suspended in the air and inhaled by someone sharing the same air. TB is transmitted in closed areas where ventilation is poor. The risk of transmission increases when susceptible persons share air for prolonged periods with a person who has untreated pulmonary

TB. Persons who have TB in extrapulmonary sites (not including laryngeal TB) are usually not considered infectious to other people. However, under unusual circumstances, TB has been transmitted to HCWs from patients with extrapulmonary TB.[4,5]

Pathogenesis

TB infection may occur when droplet nuclei are inhaled through the nose and mouth and then move down the trachea into the lungs and along the branches of the airways (the bronchi) until they reach the small air sacs of the lung (the alveoli). TB infection usually begins in the alveoli, where tubercle bacilli are initially able to multiply. During the first few weeks after infection, tubercle bacilli can spread from their initial location in the lungs (usually in the lower portions), to the lymph nodes in the center of the chest, and then to other parts of the body by way of the bloodstream. Tubercle bacilli can reach all areas of the body, but they often travel to the areas that are most susceptible to TB disease, such as the upper portions of the lungs, the kidneys, the brain and the bones. Within 2 to 10 weeks, the hody's immunologic response to the tubercle bacilli usually prevents the bacteria from multiplying and spreading more.

TB Infection and Disease

TB infection in a person who does not have active disease is not considered a case of TB. Persons with TB infection who do not have disease:

cannot infect others;
usually have a positive reaction to the tuberculin skin test;
usually have a negative chest radiograph and no clinical symptoms of TB;
have tubercle bacilli in their bodies. Although contained, these bacilli remain viable (and capable of producing active disease at any time.

TB disease does not develop in everyone who is infected. In the United States, about 90 per cent of infected persons remain infected for life and never develop symptoms of TB. But in about 5 per cent of infected persons, disease develops in the first or second year after infection. and in another 5 per cent it develops later in life (this varies with age and immunologic status). The risk that active TB will develop in a person coinfected with TB and HIV is about 86 per year. In contrast, the risk that it will develop in a person infected only with TB is 5 per cent to 10 per cent, during a lifetime.

Most cases of TB (approximately 85per cent) occur in the lungs (pulmonary TB). But disease may occur at any site in the body, such as the larynx the lymph nodes, the brain, the kidneys, or the bones (extrapulmonary TB). Extrapulmonary TB and unusual presentations of pulmonary TB are more common among HIV-infected persons than among persons not infected with HIV.

The signs and symptoms of TB vary according to the location of the disease. General signs and symptoms may include fatigue, feeling ill, loss of appetite, weight loss, fever, and night sweats. In addition to the general signs and symptoms, pulmonary TB usually causes cough, chest pain, coughing up sputum, and sometimes coughing up blood (hemoptysis); TB of the spine may cause pain in the back; and TB of the kidney may cause blood in the urine. Table 32.1 summarizes selected clinical characteristics of persons with TB infection, active pulmonary TB, or extrapulmonary TB.

The development of HIV-related TB disease can follow either of two courses. First, if a person who has latent TB infection becomes coinfected with HIV, active TB may develop as HIV weakens the person's immune system. Second, if a person who has preexisting HIV infection becomes infected with TB,TB infection may progress rapidly to disease .

TABLE 32.1
Selected Clinical Characteristics of Persons with Tuberculosis Infection, Active Pulmonary Tuberculosis, or Extrapulmonary Tuberculosis

	TB Infection	Active Pulmonary TB	Extra Pulmonary TB
Skin Test Result	usually positive	usually positive	usually positive
Signs and Symptoms	none	cough, hemoptysis, fever, night sweats, weight loss, fatigue, chest pain, and anorexia	depends on site in body affected general signs and symptoms: fever, night sweats, weight loss, fatigue, feeling ill, and loss of appetite
Infected	yes	yes	yes
Infectious	no	usually (before effective treatment)	usually not

Risk Factors for TB

Anyone who has shared airspace with a person who has infectious TB is at risk for TB. Some persons are considered to be at high risk for TB infection and disease because they are more likely than others to be exposed to someone with TB: foreign-born persons from areas with a high prevalence of TB; residents and employees of long-term care facilities and correctional facilities; and medically underserved populations, including the poor, the homeless, high-risk racial and ethnic minority groups, and injection drug users (IDUs). Other persons are at high risk for TB disease once they are infected with TB: immunocompromised persons (especially HIV-intected persons), persons with other medical risk factors (such as diabetes, end-stage renal disease, and being 10 per cent or more below ideal body weight), and IDUs.

Screening for TB Infection

The Mantoux tuberculin skin test is the recommended method of skin testing to determine whether a person is infected with *M. tuterculosis.* Multiple-puncture tests should not be used because the results are less reliable. The Mantoux skin test is performed by injecting 0.1 ml of 5 tuberculin units (TU) of purified protein derivative (PPD) intradermally, usually on the forearm. The patient's arm is examined 48 to 72 hours later for induration (palpable swelling) around the site of injection. The diameter of the indurated area across the forearm is measured. The area of erythema (redness) around the indurated area does not indicate infection with *M. tuberculosis* and should not be measured. A positive reaction to the tuberculin test usually means the patient has been infected with *M. tuberculosis.* For HIV-infected persons, a tuberculin skin test reaction of 5 or more millimeters of induration is considered positive.

All persons known to have or suspected of having HIV infection should be given a PPD tuberculin skin test. Persons coinfected with TB and HIV may have a false-negative skin test reaction because of anergy. Anergy is the inability to mount a delayed-type hypersensitivity (DTH) response to skin test antigens because of immunosuppression, which can be caused by certain medical conditions (e.g. HIV infection) or drugs. According to recent studies, HIV infection can depress tuberculin reactions even before the signs and symptoms of HIV infection develop.[2]

Testing for Anergy

Because persons with HIV infection are more likely to have

an anergic response to a tuberculin skin test, these persons should be evaluated for DTH anergy at the time of tuberculin testing. The likelihood of a false-negative skin test result increases as the CD4+ T-cell count decreases. For this reason, a previous positive skin test result should be considered evidence of TB infection, even if the current skin test result is negative.

For anergy testing, Mantoux tuberculin testing should be accompanied by Mantoux testing with two DTH antigens (i.e., *Candida,* mumps or tetanus toxoid). The reactions should be measured 48 to 72 hours after the test is administered. Induration of 3 or more millimeters to any of the antigens is considered evidence of DTH responsiveness; failure to respond to all of the antigens is considered anergy. In general, persons who respond to DTH antigens but who have a negative reaction to tuberculin are not considered infected with *M. tuberculosis.* HIV-infected persons who are anergic (and thus tuberculin skin test negative) and who are at increased risk for TB should be considered for preventive therapy. Anergic persons who are at increased risk for TB but who choose not to take preventive therapy should be informed about the signs and symptoms of TB and instructed to report promptly for medical evaluation if any of these develop.

Tuberculin Skin Test Reaction in Persons Vaccinated with BCG

Outside the United States, many countries use Bacille Calmette-Guerin (BCG) vaccination as part of their TB control activities, especially for infants. The size of tuberculin skin test reactions caused by BCG vaccination varies by the strain and the dose of the vaccine the age and the nutritional status at vaccination, the number of years since vaccination, and the frequency of tuberculin testing. Alter BCG vaccination, it is usually impossible to distinguish between a tuberculin skin test reaction caused by mycobacterial infection or by vaccination. However, BCG-induced tuberculin skin test reactivity wanes over time. Also, because BCG is used more often in countries where the prevalence of TB is high, BCG-vaccinated persons are more likely to have been exposed to TB. Therefore, these persons should be considered infected with *M. tuberculosis* if they have a positive reaction to 5 TU of PPD tuberculin. They also should be evaluated for TB disease and managed accordingly.

Preventive Therapy for TB Infection

Taken correctly by infected persons. preventive therapy can reduce the risk of TB by more than 90 per cent,. The recommended preventive therapy regimen is isoniazid (INH) at a dosage of 5 mg/kg daily for adults and 10 mg/kg daily for children to a maximum of 300 mg, for at least 6 continuous months for adults and 9 continuous months for children. For HIV-infected persons, preventive therapy is recommended for at least 12 months. Patients given preventive therapy should be monitored monthly for adherence to therapy and for drug side effects, especially the signs and symptoms of hepatitis.

Diagnosis of TB Disease

The key to diagnosing TB in HIV-intected persons is to suspect it for persons with signs or symptoms suggestive of the disease: coughing up sputum or blood, weight loss, fatigues night sweats, and fever.

Persons who have a positive skin test result and persons with TB symptoms (regardless of the skin test result) should be evaluated with a chest radiograph to rule out pulmonary TB. Health care workers must be aware that TB may present in unusual ways in HIV-infected persons. For example, it may cause infiltrates in any lung zone with no cavities, or it may cause mediastinal or hilar lymphadenopathy. Almost any abnormality on a chest radiograph may indicate TB. The radiograph may even appear entirely normal, while sputum or lung fluid specimens are culture positive for *M. tuberculosis.*

Patients who have abnormal chest radiographs should have sputum specimens collected for acid-fast bacilli (AFB) examination. For this examination the specimen is smeared onto a glass slide and stained with a fluorochrome stain or a conventional stain (e.g., Ziehl-Neelsen or Kinyoun). Laboratory personnel use the microscope to look for AFB on the smear. AFB are bacteria that remain stained even after they have been washed in an acid solution. Tubercle bacilli are one kind of AFB. Fluorochrome stains offer two advantages over conventional stains: they make the AFB easier to see, and they allow slides to be examined much more quickly.

Because AFB are not always tubercle bacilli, patients who have positive smears do not necessarily have TB. Furthermore, patients who have negative smears may have TB because negative smears do not rule out the possibility of TB. A culture result that is positive for M. *tuberculosis* is the only definitive proof of TB disease. Nevertheless, TB treatment should be started if the smear is tound to be positive before the culture results are known. Drug susceptibility testing is recommended for the first *M. tuberculosis* isolate for all patients, and it should be performed on additional isolates if culture results remain positive after the patient has received 3 months of therapy or if the patient does not seem to respond to therapy. Drug susceptibility results should be promptly reported to the hcalth care provider and the health department.

Contact Investigation

Contact investigation, one of the best ways to find persons who require treatment or preventive therapy for TB disease or infection, should begin as soon as a person is suspected of having TB. All new TB cases and suspected cases should be promptly reported to the health department by the health care provider. Early reporting is essential for the prompt evaluation of contacts of persons who have infectious TB. If a person's medical history and clinical findings suggest TB, health care workers should not wait for culture results before starting a contact investigation. Contact investigations are usually pertormed by the staff of health department TB control programmes, although hospital infection control officers and the staff of correctional and long-tenn care facilities may also conduct them.

Evaluations should be convenient for the contact. This may require that tuberculin testing and sputum collection be done in the field and that transportation to facilities be provided for radiographic and other examinations. The evaluation should proceed in an orderly manner, starting with persons who are most likely to have been infected, such as members of the patient's immediate family or others who have recently shared the same indoor environment with the source patient for prolonged periods. The highest priority should be given to rapidly examining close contacts who are children and persons who are HIV -infected because they are at high risk far active disease if infected with TB. For example, life-threatening TB meningitis or miliary TB can develop in newly infected children within weeks of infection unless preventive therapy is administered.

Close contacts of highly infectious persons, especially high-risk contacts (such as children and immunosuppressed persons), should be considered for preventive therapy even if their initial tuberculin skin test result is negative (less than S millimeters). A second skin test should be given 12 weeks after contact with the infectious person ended; if this result is also negative, preventive therapy may be stopped.

The HIV infection status of contacts alters the approach to both the investigation and the use of preventive therapy. Appropriate counseling and HIV testing for contacts whose HIV status is unknown is advisable. HIV-infected contacts should be considered fo preventive therapy, regardless of their tuberculin skin test results.

HIV Counseling and Testing

Counseling is an integral part of HIV antibody testing programmes. The primary purposes of counseling and testing are to help uninfected individuals initiate and sustain behavioural changes that reduce their risk of becoming infected and to help infected individuals avoid infecting others. Pre- and post-test HIV counseling are available from specially trained health care workers in some TB control programmes or from facilities that provide these services, e.g., HIV testing and counseling centers, sexually transmitted disease (STD) clinics, and some primary care clinics. HIV counseling must be client-centered—that is, tailored to the behaviours, circumstances, and special needs of the person being served.

All persons suspected of having active TB or persons with a confirmed diagnosis of active TB should be asked about behaviours that increase the risk for HIV infection. Knowing the HIV antibody status of these persons is essential because TB skin test interpretation, preventive therapy, and treatment regimens for HIV-seropositive patients are different from those for HIV-seronegative patients. Because not all persons who engage in behaviours that put them at high risk for HIV infection will admit to these behaviours during an interview, all TB patients should be urged to have an HIV antibody test.

The HIV antibody test is not a test for AIDS; rather, it is a blood test that detects antibodies made by the body in response to infection with HIV. Persons who have a positive HIV antibody test result are infected with HIV, and they can infect others. Persons who have a negative test result probably are not infected with the virus. However, there is a slight chance that an HIV-infected person can test negative for antibodies because antibodies usually do not develop until 6 to 12 weeks after infection. Persons who test negative for HIV can become infected in the tuture if they engage in any high-risk behaviours. Informed consent should be obtained from all persons tested.

Some states mandate the reporting of all persons infected with HIV. Health care workers who perform HIV testing should learn about the laws and reporting procedures in their areas. Centers for Disease Control and Prevention (CDC) guidelines for HIV counseling and testing have been published and are available through the CDC National AIDS Clearinghouse (1-800-458-5231).[6,7]

Treatment of TB Disease

TB is usually curable if it is diagnosed early and if effective treatment is instituted without delay. TB must be treated for a long

TABLE -32.2
REGIMEN OPTIONS FOR THE TREATMENT OF TB IN CHILDREN AND ADULTS

TB Without HIV Infection			TB With HIV Infection
Option 1	Option 2	Option 3	
Administer daily INH, RIF, and PZA for 8 weeks followed by 16 weeks of INH and RIF daily or 2-3 times/week*. In areas where the INH resistance rate is not documented to <4%, EMB or SM should be added to the initial regimen until susceptibility to INH and RIF Is demonstrated. Continue treatment for at least 6 months and 3 months beyond culture conversion. Consult a TB medical expert if the patient is symptomatic or smear or culture positive after 3 months.	Administer daily INH, RIF, PZA, and SM or EMB for 2 weeks followed by 2 times/week* administration of the same drugs for 6 weeks (by DoT§), and subsequently, 2 times/week administration of INH and RIF for 16 weeks (by DOT). Consult a TB medical expert if the patient is symptomatic or smear or culture positive after 3 months.	Treat by DOT, 3 times/week* with INH, RIF, PZA, and EMB or SM for 6 months.† Consult a TB medical expert if the patient is symptomatic or smear or culture positive after 3 months.	Options 1, 2, or 3 can be used, but treatment regimens should continue for a total of 9 months and at least 6 months beyond culture conversion.

* All regimens administered 2 times/week or 3 times/week should be monitored by DOT for the duration of therapy.

† The strongest evidence from clinical trials is the effectiveness of all four drugs administered for the full 6 months. There is weaker evidence that SM can be discontinued after 4 months if the isolate is susceptible to all drugs. The evidence for stopping PZA before the end of 6 months is equivocal for the 3 times/week regimen, and there is no evidence on the effectiveness of this regimen with EMB for less than the full 6 months.

§ DOT—Directly observed therapy.

TABLE -32.3
Dosage Recommendations for the Treatment of TB in Children* and Adults
Dosage

	Daily Dose		Twice-Weekly Dose		Thrice-Weekly Dose	
Drugs	Children	Adults	Children	Adults	Children	Adults
Isoniazid	10-20mg/kg Max. 300mg	5 mg/kg Max.300mg	20-40mg/kg Max. 900mg	15 mg/kg Max. 900mg	20-40mg/kg Max. 900mg	15 mg/kg Max. 900 mg
Rifampin	10-20 mg/ kg Max. 600 mg	10 mg/kg Max. 600 mg	10-20 mg/kg Max. 600 mg	10 mg/kg Max. 600 mg	10-20 mg/kg Max. 600 mg	10 mg/kg Max. 600 mg
Pyrazinamide	15-30 mg/kg Max. 2gm	15-30 mg/kg Max.2gm	50-70 mg/kg	50-70 mg/kg	50-70 mg/kg	50-70mg/kg
Ethambutol†	15-25 mg/kg Max. 2.5 gm	15-25 mg/kg Max. 2.5 gm	50 mg/kg	50 mg/kg	25-30 mg/kg	25-30 mg/kg
Streptomycin	20-40 mg/kg Max. 1gm	15 mg/kg Max. 1 gm	25-30 mg/kg	25-30 mg/kg	25-30 mg/kg	25-30 mg/kg

* Children $\leqslant$12 years of age.
† Ethambutol is generally not recommended for children whose visual acuity cannot be monitored (children <6 years of age). However, ethambutol should be considered for all children with organisms resistant to other drugs, if susceptibility to ethambutol has been demonstrated or susceptibility is likely.

time compared with most other infectious diseases. If treatment does not continue for a sufficient length of time (at least 6 months), enough tubercle bacilli may survive to make the patient ill and infectious again; also, ineffective treatment may foster the development of drug-resistant mycobacteria.

Because of the increase in drug-resistant TB, all TB patients should be given a fourdrug regimen of INH, rifampin (RIF), pyrazinamide (PZA), and ethambutol (EMB) or streptomycin (SM) until the drug susceptibility results are known. If the susceptibility results show no drug resistance, EMB or SM can be discontinued and the other drugs continued until PZA has been given for 2 months (initial phase). For HIV-negative persons, INH and RIF should then be continued for another 4 months (continuation phase), including at least 3 months of therapy after the culture results become negative. For HIV-positive persons, the continuation phase is 7 months; therapy should last a total of 9 months, including at least 6 months of therapy after the culture results become negative. In general, persons coinfected with TB and HIV respond well to TB treatment. Intermittent treatment regimens should be considered when giving daily therapy is impractical. Guidelines for the initial therapy of TB were updated and published in 1993.[8] Tables 32.2 and 32.3 (see pages 10 and 11) list regimen options and recommended dosages for the treatment of TB in adults and children.

Directly observed therapy (DOT) should be considered for all patients because of the difficulty in predicting which patients will adhere to a prescribed treatment regimen. DOT is the observation by a health care worker or other designated person of patients as they ingest anti-TB medications. The patient and provider should agree on an effective DOT routine that maintains the patient's Confidentiality and takes into account each patient's needs, living and employment conditions. and preferences. DOT can be arranged and administered in a variety of settings or locations, including TB clinics, community health centers, migrant clinics, homeless shelters, prisons or jails, nursing homes, schools, drug treatment centers, hospitals, HIV/AIDS clinics or living facilities, or occupational health clinics.

A variety of persons may administer DOT: physicians, nurses, health department personnel, health care aides, nursing home staff, correctional facility personnel, staff of community-based organizations, school nurses or teachers, staff of drug treatment centers, volunteers, social and welfare caseworkers, clergy, or other community leaders. Persons giving DOT who are not physicians or nurses should be supervised by a physician or a nurse. DOT can be given daily or intermittently (i.e., two or three times a week). Intermittent regimens are easier to implement than daily regimens, and they cost less. The use of incentives or enablers (such as transportation or car/bus fare to the DOT sites) may promote patient adherence to a DOT programme. When patients not receiving DOT demonstrate nonadherent behaviours (such as refusing pills or missing clinic appointments), the situation should be brought to the attention of the appropriate public health officials. These patients should be given DOT. Inadequate therapy is a major cause of multidrug-resistant TB.

Patients should be evaluated for and questioned about symptoms of drug toxicity at least once a month during therapy, even if no problems are apparent. Patients should be instructed to look for adverse reactions to the medications they are receiving. If symptoms suggestive of drug toxicity occur, appropriate laboratory testing and medical evaluation should be performed immediately. For patients treated with RIF who are also taking methadone, an increased methadone dosage may be necessary to avoid withdrawal symptoms caused by the interaction between the two drugs.[9]

The effectiveness of treatment can be evaluated by monitoring patients' sputum smear results. Also, sputum cultures should be obtained at least monthly until the results are negative. Appropriate consultation should be sought for patients whose smear or cut results do not convert to negative within 3 months. A positive sputum culture is the only definitive sign of treatment failure, and the persistence or reappearance of organisms in the smear should create a high index of suspicion.

As a general rule, regimens that are adequate for treating pulmonary TB in adults children are also effective for treating extrapulmonary disease. However, some experts recommend 9 months of therapy for patients with disseminated disease, miliary disease disease involving the bones or joints, or tuberculous lymphadenitis. Adjunctive therapies such as surgery and corticosteroids, may be used in some circumstances.

MULTIDRUG-RESISTANT TB

An extremely serious aspect of the TB problem in the United States is the recent increase in multidrug-resistant TB (MDR TB). From 1990 through late 1992, CDC investigated eight outbreaks of MDR TB in hospitals and correctional facilities in New York Florida and New Jersey. These outbreaks have included almost 300 cases virtually all due to organisms resistant to both INH and RIF Some cases were due to organisms resistant to at least seven antituberculosis drugs. Most of the patients in these outbreaks were infected with HIV. Mortality among patients with MDR TB in these outbreaks ranged from 72 per cent to 89 per cent and the median intervals between TB diagnosis and death ranged from 4 to 16 weeks. The transmission ol MDR TB to health care workers and prison guards was documented in these outbreaks.

Some persons are at high risk for drug-resistant TB: persons who have been recently exposed to drug-resistant TB especially it they are immunocompromised; TB patients who failed to take medications as prescribed; TB patients who were prescribed an ineffective treatment regimen; and persons previously treated for TB. Clinicians who are not familiar with the management of patients who have MDR TB or patients who have been exposed to MDR TB should seek expert consultation.

PREVENTION AND TREATMENT OF TB IN HEALTH CARE WORKERS

Health care facilities that provide care for patients at risk for TB should maintain active surveillance for TB among HCWs. All HCWs, including those with a history of BCG vaccination, should be given a Mantoux tuberculin skin test upon employment. For the initial tuberculin skin test, a two-step testing procedure is recommended. Two-step testing reduces the likelihood that a boosted skin test reaction will be interpreted as representing recent infection. If the reaction to the first tuberculin skin test is negative, a second test should be given 1 to 3 weeks later. If the reaction to this second test is positive, it probably represents a boosted reaction. Based on the second test result, the person should be classified as being TB infected or not and managed accordingly. HCWs known to have previous positive tuberculin test results or known to have completed adequate treatment or preventive therapy should be exempt from further screening unless they show symptoms suggestive of TB. HCWs should be educated about the signs and symptoms of TB and told to seek medical assistance promptly if these symptoms develop.

HCWs who have negative skin test results should be retested periodically to screen for new infection and disease. HCWs who may be exposed to patients with TB or who are involved in high-risk procedures (such as bronchoscopy) should be retested at least every 6 months. HCWs in other areas should be retested annually. Data on skin test conversions should be reviewed periodically to estimate the risk of acquiring new infection for each area of the facility. The frequency of retesting may be altered according to this analysis.

In addition to being screened periodically, HCWs should be evaluated for TB disease or infection if they have been exposed to a potentially infectious TB patient with whom recommended infection control procedures have not been taken. CDC has published guidelines for preventing the transmission of TB in health care settings.[10] HCWs who have been exposed to TB should be given a Mantoux tuberculin skin test as soon as possible after exposure. These HCWs should be managed in the same way as other contacts. If the initial skin test result is negative, the test should be repeated 12 weeks after the exposure ended. Exposed persons who have skin test reactions of 5 millimeters or greater or who have symptoms suggestive of TB should be evaluated with a chest radiograph. HIV infected HCWs may have a negative skin test result because of anergy. These persons should be given preventive therapy if they are likely to have been infected with TB after exposure. Persons known to have previous positive skin test reactions who have been exposed to an infectious patient do not require a repeat skin test or a chest radiograph unless they have symptoms suggestive of TB.

HCWs who have positive skin test results but who do not have active TB should be evaluated for their risk of HIV infection and considered for preventive therapy. If HIV infection is considered a possibility, counseling and HIV antibody testing should be strongly encouraged.

HCWs with pulmonary or laryngeal TB pose a risk to patients and to other employees while they are infectious. Therefore, they should be restricted from work until they begin receiving adequate treatment, they are no longer coughing, and they have three consecutive negative sputum smears. HCWs who are receiving preventive therapy for TB infection do not pose a risk to others, and they should be allowed to continue their usual work activities.

Remember! The key to preventing TB infection, disability from TB disease, and death is to consider the diagnosis of TB in high-risk groups, make the diagnosis as quickly as possible, and initiate effective, directly observed therapy for persons found to have TB.

References

1. Centers for Disease Control and Prevention. 1993 revised classification system for HIV infection and expanded surveillance case definition for AIDS among adolescents and adults. *MMWR.* 1992;41 (No.RR-17): 1-19.
2. Centers for Disease Control. Purified protein derivative (PPD)-tuberculin anergy and HIV infection: guidelines for anergy testing and management of anergic persons at risk of tuberculosis. *MMWR.* 1991 ;40(No. RR-5): 1-5.
3. Curran JW, Chamberland M. Epidemiology and prevention of AIDS and HIV infection. In: Mandell GL Douglas RG, Bennett JE. eds. *Principles and Practice of Infections Diseases* 3rd ed. New York, NY: Churchill Livingston; 1990:1029-1046.
4. Hutton MD, Stead WW, Cauthen GM, Bloch AB, Ewing WM. Nosocomial

transmission of tuberculosis associated with a draining abscess. *J Infest Dis.* 1990; 161:286-295.

5. Frampton MW. An outbreak of tuberculosis among hospital personnel caring for a patient with a skin ulcer. *Ann Intern Med.* 1992;117:312-313.
6. Centers for Disease Control and Prevention. Technical guidance on HIV counseling. *MMWR.* 1993;42(No. RR-2):8-17.
7. Centers for Disease Control. Public Health Service guidelines for counseling and antibody testing to prevent HIV infection and AIDS. *MMWR.* 1987;36(No. 31):509-515.
8. Centers for Disease Control and Prevention. Initial therapy for tuberculosis in the era of multidrug resistance: recommendations of the Advisory Council for the Elimination of Tuberculosis. *MMWR* 1993;42(No. RR-7):1-8.
9. Kreek MJ. Garfield JW, Gutjahr CL. Ginsti LM. Rif, ampin-induced methadone withdrawal. Engl. J Med 1976;294: 1104-6.
10. Centers for Disease Control. Guidelines for preventing the transmission of tuberculosis in health care settings, with special focus on HIV-related issues. *MMWR.* 1990;39(No. RR-17): 1-29.

33

HIV Testing Policies and Guidelines

WHO-Regional Office for South-East Asia
New Delhi, India

INTRODUCTION

The Acquired Immune Deficiency Syndrome (AIDS) was first recognized in the United States in 1981. The etiological agent, Human Immunodeficiency Virus (HIV), was isolated in 1984 and a laboratory test for HIV became commercially available the following year. This enabled health care workers to diagnose HIV infection, individuals to know whether or not they were HIV infected, and most importantly, medical science to understand HIV/AIDS better. The availability of these tests has also led to misconceptions regarding the role of HIV testing. These misconceptions were particularly witnessed worldwide during the early stages of the epidemic, and not unexpectedly are presently being noted in a number of countries in Asia. Many individuals, particularly health care workers, seem to believe that the spread of HIV can be controlled by identifying people with HIV infection, and testing of hospital patients or groups of people practising high risk behaviour are often advocated. This paper discusses some issues related to the use and appropriateness of HIV testing in the overall context of national AIDS control programmes.

PURPOSE OF HIV TESTING

Compared to any other type of disease, the issues related to the diagnosis of HIV infection are far more complex AIDS is invariably fatal and infection is lifelong. No drugs are available to cure AIDS or to render an HIV-infected person non-infectious. Since HIV is spread mainly through sexual contact, individuals known to be infected with HIV are unfortunately often stigmatized and discriminated against. Such a situation results from the lack of proper understanding regarding the mode of transmission, particularly the fact that HIV infection cannot be transmitted by casual social contact or through the respiratory route . Unlike other diseases, identification of people with HIV infection or AIDS, therefore, is neither rational nor appropriate.

HIV testing is recommended by the World Health Organization (WHO) only for selected purposes.[1] These include (1) screening of blood including blood products, and organs and tissues for transplantation; (2) epidemiological surveillance, particularly HIV sentinel surveillance using unlinked anonymous HIV testing methodology where all personal details of the person being tested are removed from the blood samples so that the results of HIV testing cannot be linked with the identity of the person—the specific purposes of testing in these situations are to ensure blood safety or to conduct epidemiological surveillance respectively; (3) diagnosis of symptomatic infection among those clinically suspected of having AIDS; and finally (4) early diagnosis of HIV infection among asymptomatic persons who would like to know their HIV status. In the latter two situations HIV testing is carried out with informed consent and with strict maintenance of confidentiality. No situation other than the four listed above warrant HIV testing, and there is no place in national AIDS prevention and control programmes for testing without informed consent. Experience shows that any kind of HIV testing without the full and informed consent of the person concerned is counter-productive as well as wasteful of resources.

PUBLIC HEALTH RATIONALE AGAINST MANDATORY TESTING

Public health rationale should always be kept in mind when testing of any population group including foreigners, refugees, hospital patients or individuals engaged in high risk behaviour is contemplated. The 45th World Health Assembly, to which all countries were signatory, noted that "there is no public health rationale for any measures that limit the rights of the individual, notably measures establishing mandatory screening".[2] Studies and public health experience have also shown that HIV testing carried out on a voluntary basis and with appropriate counselling is more likely to promote behaviour change than mandatory testing.[3] Furthermore, mandatory testing measures can be counter-productive because they tend to drive those at high risk of HIV infection "Underground, as a result of which such persons do not have access to education and counselling programmes". Such initiatives not only damage the credibility of the health services, but also create a false sense of security among the general public that all HIV-infected persons are known and that there is no need to take necessary precautions. From the cost point of view, testing is an expensive business, not only to National AIDS Programmes because of the high cost of HIV kits but also to individuals from the psychological point of view when the results of HIV testing are inadvertently disclosed and confidentiality is not always maintained. Additional details addressesing the question "Can mandatory HIV testing stop the AIDS epidemic?".

HIV TESTING IN HEALTH CARE SETTINGS

Many health care workers, however, seem to mistakenly believe in programmes of mandatory HIV testing or of testing without consent because of the fear of contracting HIV in the health care setting. Although there is a risk of HIV being transmitted in these settings, this risk is very small. For example, in the United States, more than 250,000 patients have so far been diagnosed as having AIDS, including 8,467 cases among health care workers of which only six (0.07 per cent) were due to occupational transmission[4]. While thousands of needle stick injuries occur every year, only 33 documented HIV infections have so far resulted from occupational injuries in the health care setting. In studies of health care workers who were exposed to HIV through needle stick injuries, the risk has been shown to be less than 0.4 per cent.[4,5] The risk of HIV transmission following mucous membrane or skin exposure to HIV infected blood, body fluids or tissues is even lower. Based on such data, testing of ambulatory or hospitalized patients for HIV on a routine basis for HIV has not been adopted as a general policy in the United States or other countries with prolonged experience of HIV/AIDS, and is not recommended by WHO. Rather, the application of universal precautions in infection control procedures is recommended as the best way to minimize HIV transmission in the health care setting.

In spite of this, there have been a number of situations where patients attending health facilities have been or are being tested for HIV. For example, many advocate testing in antenatal clinics on the notion that women may want to know whether they are infected in order to make a decision regarding having a baby. It has, however, been seen that such women, after having been provided counselling, are likely to participate in testing voluntarily. Moreover, routine testing of pregnant women may discourage many women from attending antenatal clinics because of the fear of being tested without their knowledge. Experience in other countries shows that relatively few women elect to have an abortion when they are properly informed and counselled (Kervin O'Reilly, personat Communication). Similarly, testing of patients attending hospital, particularly for surgery, cannot be justified.

Should patients with STDs be tested for HIV routinely? This issue has been much debated because of the close association between STD and AIDS. The consensus among the international scientific community is that all STD patients should be offered appropriate counselling and STD care without having to resort to mandatory HIV testing. If HIV testing is at all required and/or asked for, this can be provided through voluntary testing with appropriate pre- and post-test counselling. From the economics point of view, any requirements for HIV testing are likely to constitute additional burdens to STD control programmes as the cost of HIV tests would add to the already high costs of STD drugs.

Regarding the testing of blood donors, WHO advocates the concept of screening of donated blood rather than the testing of donors.[6] This in essence means that blood samples are subjected to antibody testing and those found positive are discarded without relating the test to the individual. However, if blood donors are to be tested for HIV and if they are to be notified of the results, they must know in advance that the blood is to be tested for HIV and they should give their informed consent to testing. This also entails provision of pre- and post-test counselling. There is, however, a danger that if blood banks offer facilities for HIV testing, many people, including those with high risk behaviour, may use these services to determine their HIV status thus compromising/endangering the safety of blood. In summary, the only roles that HIV testing can play in the health care setting are to assist in the diagnosis of HIV infection in patients with clinical signs compatible with AIDS and to offer voluntary testing services to people who wish to know their HIV status. In both the situations, the testing should be voluntary with provision of adequate pre- as well as post-test counselling.

VOLUNTARY TESTING AND COUNSELLING

Voluntary HIV testing always in conjunction with counselling has a place in national AIDS control programmes within the comprehensive range of measures for HIV/AIDS prevention, care and supports[7]. HIV testing, to be beneficial, should however be entirely voluntary and anonymous, with no possibility of breech of confidentiality. Voluntary HIV testing should be part of a comprehensive counselling programme which provides support services such as condoms and treatment for STDs. It should however be noted that counselling on its own is a valuable intervention even if HIV testing is not available or if the person decides not to be tested.

The current availability in the Asian region of HIV/AIDS counselling, of voluntary HIV testing and of HIV counselling and voluntary testing is limited, with the exception of Thailand. In countries where these services are not yet widely available, their introduction should proceed cautiously in order to ensure that confidentiality or anonymity is guaranteed and that the services are delivered in a manner most likely to result in benefits to the individual and to public health.

In conclusion, HIV testing has an important role to play in national AIDS control programmes. However, it should be carried out in a rational manner and without resort to coercive approaches. Mandatory testing or testing without informed consent is not only counter productive but also wasteful of scarce resources. The spread of HIV cannot be controlled by mandatory testing of hospital patients or high risk groups in the population; such efforts have failed everywhere they have been tried. HiV testing should be carried out only for those purposes which are specific objectives of National AIDS Control Programmes.

SOME QUESTIONS AND ANSWERS ON HIV TESTING POLICIES AND GUIDELINES

Can Mandatory HIV Testing Stop the AIDS Epidemic?

Forcing someone to undergo medical testing of any kind is an invasion of privacy and a violation of human rights. This is a fundamental reason why WHO and its member countries have taken a strong position against forced testing for HIV. But what about protecting the health of the public? The following Questions & Answers explain why compulsory HIV testing, far from protecting the public health, can actually endanger it. They have been contributed as the first of an occasional series by Suzanne Cherney, GPA's communications scientist, who encourages readers to suggest topics for exploration in future issues of Global AIDS news.

Q. Some people say that the reason AIDS continues to spread is that we aren't aggressive enough about finding out who is infected with the human immunodeficiency virus (HIV). Shouldn't we be testing everyone for HIV—if necessary, against their will?

A. If a person tests positive for HIV, it means that he or she has HIV infection and, scientists believe, will ultimately develop AIDS—a fatal disease for which there is at present no cure. But this can take 10 or even 15 years, and some people would prefer to live those healthy years without knowing their diagnosis. In addition, people with HIV infection or AIDS can suffer exclusion, discrimination and even persecution. *So testing for HIV is a very serious matter.*

People who are counselled about the personal and social implications of taking an HIV test can of course decide to be tested voluntarily. But forcing someone to undergo HIV testing is a highly coercive, intrusive measure.

Q. But why worry only about the infected people? Surely compulsory testing is justified in the case of a fatal epidemic disease?

A. There are a number of reasons why compulsory testing for HIV makes no sense. To begin with, *testing someone for HIV just gives you a diagnosis, and a diagnosis alone never stopped an epidemic.* Testing only helps if there are ways of breaking the chain of transmission. For example, when you test donated blood prior to transfusion and discard the infected blood, you are helping to prevent the spread of the virus. The testing of blood for transfusion, and of tissues or organs for transplantation, is the only area where testing needs to be compulsory.

Q. Testing has helped contain other infections diseases. Why not AIDS?

A. Because HIV is different. There is no drug available that can cure the infection or make the person uninfectious—that is, incapable of transmitting the virus to another person. And once a person is infected with HIV, it's for life. A person who tests positive for syphilis can be cured with a short course of antibiotics. A person diagnosed with tuberculosis can be made uninfectious with antibiotics. When someone tests positive for meningitis, the individuals in close contact with him or her can be treated and/or vaccinated. With HIV, there is no medical way to "test and treat" or "test and vaccinate" so as to break the chain of transmission.

Q. Yes, but people with HIV are nevertheless a danger to others. They could be isolated.

A. They don't need to be, because HIV infection is not "contagious" in the usual sense. Unlike tuberculosis, it doesn't spread through coughing. Unlike typhoid, it can't be transmitted through food or water. You can't catch HIV from swimming with an infected person, or sharing an office or home, or drinking from the same cup. So locking up infected people is not justified or practical. It's not even necessary isolate HIV-infected people when they're hospitalized.

We all have a responsibility to look after ourselves. And the fact that HIV spreads mainly through sexual intercourse means that uninfected people are not defenseless against the virus. They have ways of protecting themselves from HIV without locking up the infected individuals. They can abstain from sex, stay faithful to an uninfected partner, engage in sex without penetration, or else use a condom every time for sexual intercourse.

Q. **Still, if we could screen the whole population through compulsory testing and then isolate the infected people for life, it might stop the epidemic.**

A. Mass HIV testing sounds straightforward.. In practice, it's extremely costly, logistically unwieldy, incapable of identifying everyone who is infected, and fraught with problems that could be avoided by offering voluntary tests and guaranteeing the confidentiality of the test results.

Logistically, it's impossible to take blood samples from everyone, test them, and give everyone their results on the same day. So, even if the authorities managed to trace all infected people (clearly, many won't turn up voluntarily to find out their test results) and isolate them, this wouldn't prevent sexual contact between the uninfected and those who have yet to be tested.

And even if these logistic obstacles could somehow be eliminated, no mandatory testing programme can expect to identify all HIV-infected people. Individuals who think they might be infected can go to extremes to avoid testing and follow-up, given the serious consequences of a positive HIV test—especially when there is a threat of isolation.

Not all HIV-infected people will be identified even if they are tested. Most commercially available HIV tests work by detecting not the virus itself but antibodies to the virus which the person's immune system produces following infection with HIV. But it takes up to 12 weeks, or sometimes more, for those HIV antibodies to be produced and become detectable in a blood sample. This is the "window period" during which the infected person continues to test negative.

At best, an HIV test result is a "snapshot" of someone's infection status today. It's no guarantee that he or she won't become infected tomorrow, or next week or month —and how often can people be tested?

In any case, periodic testing of the entire population is prohibitively expensive in terms of staff time, transport of blood samples, and so on. (The actual HIV test kits account for only a fraction of the total costs). in many developing countries, testing the whole population just once would cost more than the government is able to spend on all health care in a year.

Q. Surely some countries have attempted to test everyone?

A. No. The financial and logistic impossibility of testing the whole population periodically has been recognized even by the few countries that have devoted most of their AIDS budget to testing. And most of these now realize that instead of mandatory testing—which failed to stop the epidemic—they should use their resources for preventive measures of proven effectiveness, such as informing the general public about HIV transmission, making condoms cheap and accessible, providing school-based education for young people, and ensuring blood safety.

Q. Even if you can't identify and trace all infected people, you could at least isolate the ones you find.

A. Apart from being a serious violation of human rights, lifetime isolation would be an unnecessary economic burden on the individuals' families and on society. In many places in Africa, and increasingly in Asia, 10 per cent or more of all young adults are infected. Isolation means forfeiting their economic productivity during the decade or so of good health that these young adults can expect. It means depriving their families of breadwinners and care-givers. And it means keeping thousands or even millions of fit individuals fed, clothed and looked after for years on end—at government expense.

Q. I am still concerned about all the healthy people walking around with HIV who don't even know they have the virus. Granted that isolation makes no sense and that there is no medical way of curing them or making them uninfectious. Compulsory testing would at least force them to find out their diagnosis and take precautions against transmitting the virus to others.

A. In other words, won't people who learn they are HIV-infected through compulsory testing simply avoid unsafe sex from then on? To begin with, not even voluntary counselling and testing achieves a uniformity "preventive" effect. When testing is purely voluntary, and people are presumably well motivated to protect themselves and their loved ones, the evidence shows that some infected people manage to change their sexual behaviour, others do not.*

* *(For example, helpful behaviour change (increased condom use) in couples who seek voluntary testing together and find out that just one of them is HIV infected).*

Is compulsory testing likely to be more effective than this in achieving behaviour change? On the contrary. First of all, someone who is forced to and out he or she is infected may have less interest in protecting others—or even in self-protection (safer sex protects both partners). But the main point is that a permanent, lifelong change in sexual behaviour isn't achieved automatically or quickly. The consistent use of condoms, for example, takes continuing motivation, will power, personal commitment. It takes the availability of inexpensive and readily accessible condoms. And for someone in a long-term relationship, it takes the full co-operation of the other partner. *The bottom line is that HIV prevention rests on the individual's willingness to avoid unsafe behaviour. Will power and motivation can't be coerced.* You don't gain people's voluntary co-operation by forcing them to be tested.

Q. True, but even if the infected person doesn't voluntarily adopt safer behaviour, at least other people can be warned...

A. Who? Medical test results are supposed to remain confidential. Imagine how suspicious we would be of doctors if they turned into law enforcement officers ! We'd stop seeking medical help for a whole range of problems if we thought our diagnoses would be handed out.

This doesn't mean that voluntary contact tracing is useless, though with HIV it's far less useful than for syphilis or gonorrhoea, where the sexual contact can be tested, treated and cured. But it's obvious that people infected with HIV will be less likely to volunteer information about their sex partners if they suspect that those individuals in turn may be forced into testing. Once again, making the test mandatory instead of voluntary makes it less rather than more effective.

Suppose an infected man refuses to use condoms or tell his wife about the infection. What will happen if the health care provider doesn't keep the diagnosis confidential but goes ahead and informs her? The wife might decide to leave the relationship, assuming she is economically able to do so. But while that might help her (if she is still uninfected), there are two reasons why it might endanger the public health. First, her rejected husband may well and new sex partners—and the epidemic will continue to spread. Or, if she is infected but doesn't know it, she might infect her new partners. Secondly, there is ample evidence that in places where test results aren't kept strictly confidential, people simply avoid HIV testing and continue to behaves though they were not infected. Helpful behaviour change that might have occurred as a result of voluntary counselling and testing is thus forfeited.

Q. In some places, couples have to get tested for syphilis before marrying. Why not for HIV?

A. Even with syphilis, a curable disease, experience from around the world shows that mandatory premarital screening has little or no impact on the public health. For HIV, mandatory testing makes even less sense. First, fear of a compulsory test will dissuade many couples from marrying where such a requirement exists—a disadvantage that voluntary test doesn't entail. Second, why pick the time of marriage? People often begin their sexual experimentation well before that. (indeed, if premarital sex were rate, testing before marriage would turn up virtually no positive HIV results!). And, most important sex with other partners can and does take place after marriage. For the many people whose mason risk of HIV is their partner's extramarital activity, a negative premarital test offers no protection—just an illusion of safety.

Q. But HIV can be transmitted from an infected woman to her fetus or newborn. Wouldn't it be helpful at least to insist on testing all pregnant women?

A. Once a woman is pregnant the fetus may well be infected already although there is no way to know this. At this stage the only possibilities for prevention are abortion, a decision not to breast-feed (although in many settings bottle-feeding may be more risky for the baby, or perhaps treatment with an antiviral drug around the time of delivery (this is still experimental). All these are major decision which cannot be forced on any woman but which she must take, if at all, voluntarily. Therefore, voluntary counselling and testing is what should be offered. Forced testing may also dissuade pregnant women from seeking medical care.

In any case, the best time for prevention is prior to pregnancy. Married or unmarried people need to be aware of all the implications of HIV infection before they decide whether to have children.

Q. Some employers test job applicants before hiring them. Does that make sense?

A. No. It won't protect the general public. And it won't protect the firm's employees because HIV infection is not "contagious" and doesn't spread at the workplace. The emphasis in any form should be on preventing infections among the existing workforce, which is always far larger than the number of new staff recruited each year. Some employers provide their workers with AIDS education, encouragement for condom use, and care for sexually transmitted diseases (STDs) such as syphilis and chancroid, which if left untreated greatly increase a person's susceptibility to HIV infection. They report a decrease in STD rates among their employees, which is good news on two counts. It means employees are less likely to get HIV and, for companies that offer or reimburse STD care, it means a decrease in company expenditure.

Q. I can see why forcing ordinary people to be tested is useless. What about restricting compulsory testing to high-risk groups?

A. At first sight this seems more practical than compulsory testing of the general population testing of the general population, but in fact it's got even more problems. To begin with, many such groups are hard to define, and even harder to locate. For example, men who have unprotected sex with prostitutes are clearly at high risk - but how do you identify them? And where do you draw the line? At those who seek out a sex worker twice a year? Or those who do so every payday? And what about their wives - are they a high-risk group to be tested? In many places, after all, most women with HIV have been infected by their one partner—their husband.

Q. One well defined group, at least, is drug users who inject their drugs. Isn't it true that they are at high risk of acquiring HIV?

A. Yes. If they don't use new or freshly sterilized equipment every time they inject, they can easily become infected—and pass the virus on to their sex partners. So the most urgent need is to reach them to clean their equipment carefully each time, never share it with anyone, or exchange their used syringes for sterile ones—and to encourage them to use condoms for sex. (Over the longer term, they need encouragement to switch from drug injecting to safer forms of drug use, or no drug use at all). These socalled "harm reduction" measures are clearly vital for the public health as well as for the users themselves.

The biggest hurdle for harm-reduction programmes is that drug users live on the margins of society. Almost everywhere, drug use is secretive or frankly illegal, and users are mistrustful of authorities. In many placres, health workers have to persuade the local police not to arrest drug users who come in for education, new syringes, bleach or condoms. Any threat of mandatory HIV testing would scare them away even more, doom the harm-reduction programmes to failure, and endanger the public health.

Q. **Shouldn't we at least insist that sex workers be HIV-negative?**

A. This is yet another idea that sounds fine in theory but works poorly in practice. Compulsory testing is as counterproductive for prostitutes as it is for drug users. Authorities need to work with prostitutes, not against them. They need to strengthen their ability to demand condom use by clients. (This is the standard harm-reduction measure for commercial sex work). if prostitutes are harassed an driven away by the threat of mandatory testing, they will be out of reach of effective harm-reduction programmes.

Prostitutes who can't escape testing and turn out to be HIV-positive may be fired (if they work in a brothel) or lose their registration. But this doesn't protect the public health. Infected individuals will simnly move on to another place. Where there is a systcm of registration, the infected sex workers will join the ranks of unofficial prostitutes, who generally have even less power to negotiate safer sex. Testing doesn't even protect the local clients. No matter how many "condom only" signs are posted, any brothel owner (or government official) who insists on testing sex workers - and lets the clients know that they are HIV-negative—is sending a clear message that if a client doesn't want to use a condom, he'll still be safe. Of course, the client may well be infected himself and infect the prostitute, who will then infect others who decide not to use a condom, and so on. Testing sex workers even as often as every 3 months still means that, because of the "window period", they can have HIV for nearly half a year—and infect many clients—before their infection is diagnosed.

Q. **You may well ask, why test the prostitutes and not their clients?**

A. From the standpoint of common decency, it's just as important to safeguard sex workers as sex work clients. From the standpoint of public health, protecting the prostitutes is even more important. Besides, there's something illogical about putting the responsibility for HIV prevention and safe sex on the sex worker. After all, in almost all cases, whether the prostitute is male or female, it's the client who has to wear the condom!

If condom use by men is the key, why not try to test STD patients systematically for HIV? After all, they're mostly men. And by coming down with a disease like syphilis or chancroid, they have proven that they are engaging in unsafe sex and are at risk of HIV.

There's no doubt that men (and women) with an STD are a very important "audience" indeed when it comes to HIV prevention. Attendance at a clinic or doctor's office provides the ideal opportunity for educating them about AIDS and condom promotion — just at the time they are confronted with evidence of their vulnerability to all STDs. But people with an STD need encouragement to seek care at the earliest possible sign of disease. Any threat of mandatory testing would frighten them away.

Q. So compulsory testing can't even help with people who engage in high-risk behaviour?

A. No. When it comes to drug injectors, sex workers and STD patients, mandatory HIV testing has nothing to recommend it—and multiple disadvantages as compared with voluntary testing. First, people are hard to track down for compulsory testing, and expensive to trace for follow-up. Then, what do you achieve? When you and infected individuals, you can't isolate them for life or enforce behaviour change. Indeed, voluntary testing is more likely to result in the adoption of safe behaviour.

Not only are the "benefits" of compulsory testing illusory, but the side effects are a positive danger to the public health. The main ones are driving vulnerable people away from harm-reduction and other prevention programmes, and encouraging a false sense of HIV-free security in the general population. Voluntary testing hasn't got these disadvantages. Hence, there's nothing to be gained for the public health, and much to be lost, by making HIV tests compulsory instead of voluntary and confidential .

Q. Aren't coercive measures ever necessary?

A. Yes. It is occasionally necessary to override people's individual rights in the interests of public health. For example, WHO recommended obligatory vaccination against smallpox until it was eradicated, and still endorses the need for mandatory vaccination against yellow fever for people travelling from zones where this disease is endemic. If one day a medicine is found that can make HIV-infected people noninfectious to others, WHO will re-examine its policy on HIV testing. For the moment, AIDS happens to be a disease for which coercive testing is not only pointless but harmful to the public health.

In the AIDS era, there is no way to sideline the infected people so that everyone else can go on living as before. Today, everyone has a responsibility to avoid unsafe behaviour.

References

1. WHO Global Programme on AIDS. Recommendations for the selection and use of HIV antibody tests, Weekly Epidemiological Record No. 20, 1992, p.145-149.
2. World Health Assembly Resolution 45.35, 14 May 1992
3. WHO Global Programme on AIDS. Global strategy for the prevention and control of AIDS, 1992 update. AIDS Series No.12.
4. Ciesielski C. et al. Occupationally acquired HIV infection - United States. 9th International Conference on AIDS, Berlin, 1993 (Abstract WS-c12-1).
5. Report of a WHO Consultation on the Prevention of Human immunodeficiency Virus and Hepatitis B virus transmission in the Health Care Setting, Geneva, 11-12 April 1991.
6. Gobal Blood Safety initiative. Consensus statement on screening of blood donations for infectious agents transmissible through blood transfusion, Geneva, 30 Jan.-1 Feb..1990. WHO/LBS/91.1.
7. WHO Global Programme on AIDS. Statement from the consultation on Testing and Counselling for HIV infection, Geneva, 16-18 November 1992. WHO/GPA/INF/93.2.

34

Universal Precautions for Prevention of Transmission of Human Immunodeficiency Virus, Hepatitis B Virus, and Other Bloodborne Pathogens in Health-Care Settings

INTRODUCTION

The purpose of this report is to clarify and supplement the CDC publication entitled "Recommendations for Prevention of HIV Transmission in Health-Care Settings"[1].

In 1983, CDC published a document entitled "Guideline for Isolation Precautions in Hospitals"[2] that contained a section entitled "Blood and Body Fluid Precautions." The recommendations in this section called for blood and body fluid precautions when a patient was known or suspected to be infected with bloodborne pathogens. In August 1987, CDC published a document entitled "Recommendations for Prevention of HIV Transmission in Health-Care Settings"[1]. In contrast to the 1983 document, the 1987 document recommended that blood and body fluid precautions be consistently used for all patients regardless of their bloodborne infection status. This extension of blood and body fluid precautions to *all* patients is referred to as "Universal Blood and Body Fluid Precautions" or "Universal Precautions." Under universal precautions, blood and certain body fluids of all patients are considered potentially infectious for human immunodeficiency virus (HIV), hepatitis B virus (HBV), and other bloodborne pathogens.

Universal precautions are intended to prevent parenteral, mucous membrane, and nonintact skin exposures of health-care workers to bloodborne pathogens. In addition, immunization with HBV vaccine is recommended as an important adjunct to universal precautions for health-care workers who have exposures to blood [3,4].

Since the recommendations for universal precautions were published in August 1987, CDC and the Food and Drug Administration (FDA) have received requests for clarification of the following issues: (1) body fluids to which universal precautions apply, (2) use of protective barriers, (3) use of gloves for phlebotomy, (4) selection of gloves for use while observing universal precautions, and (5) need for making changes in waste management programmes as a result of adopting universal precautions.

Body Fluids to Which Universal Precautions Apply

Universal precautions apply to blood and to other body fluids containing visible blood. Occupational transmission of HIV and HBV to health-care workers by blood is documented [4,5]. Blood is the single most important source of HIV, HBV, and other bloodborne pathogens in the occupational setting. Infection control efforts for HIV, HBV, and other bloodborne pathogens must focus on preventing exposures to blood as well as on delivery of HBV immunization.

Universal precautions also apply to semen and vaginal secretions. Although both of these fluids have been implicated in the sexual transmission of HIV and HBV, they have not been implicated in occupational transmission from patient to health-care worker. This observation is not unexpected, since exposure to semen in the usual health-care setting is limited, and the routine practice of wearing gloves for performing vaginal examinations protects health-care workers from exposure to potentially infectious vaginal secretions.

Universal precautions also apply to tissues and to the following fluids: cerebrospinal fluid (CSF), synovial fluid, pleural fluid, peritoneal fluid, pericardial fluid, and amniotic fluid. The risk of transmission of HIV and HBV from these fluids is unknown; epidemiologic studies in the health-care and community setting are currently inadequate to assess the potential risk to health-care workers from occupational exposures to them. However, HIV has been isolated from CSF, synovial, and amniotic fluid [6-8], and HBsAg has been detected in synovial fluid, amniotic fluid, and peritoneal fluid.[9-11] One case of HIV transmission was reported after a percutaneous exposure to bloody pleural fluid obtained by needle aspiration.[12] Whereas aseptic procedures used to obtain these fluids for diagnostic or therapeutic purposes protect health-care workers from skin exposures, they cannot prevent penetrating injuries due to contaminated needles or other sharp instruments.

Body Fluids to Which Universal Precautions Do Not Apply

Universal precautions do not apply to feces, nasal secretions, sputum, sweat, tears, urine, and vomitus unless they contain visible blood. The risk of transmission of HIV and HBV from these fluids and materials is extremely low or nonexistent. HIV has been isolated and HBsAg has been demonstrated in some of these fluids; however, epidemiologic studies in the health-care and community setting have not implicated these fluids or materials in the transmission of HIV and HBV infections.[13,14] Some of the above fluids and excretions represent a potential source for nosocomial and community-acquired infections with other pathogens, and recommendations for preventing the transmission of nonbloodborne pathogens have been published. [2]

Precautions for Other Body Fluids in Special Settings

Human breast milk has been implicated in perinatal transmission of HIV, and HBsAg has been found in the milk of mothers infected with HBV.[10,13] However, occupational exposure to human breast milk has not been implicated in the transmission of HIV nor HBV infection to health-care workers. Moreover, the health-care worker will not have the same type of intensive exposure to breast milk as the nursing neonate. Whereas universal precautions do not apply to human breast milk, gloves may be worn by health-care workers in situations where exposures to breast milk might be frequent, for example, in breast milk banking.

Saliva of some persons infected with HBV has been shown to contain HBV-DNA at concentrations 1/1,000 to 1/10,000 of that found in the infected person's serum.[15] HBsAg-positive saliva has been shown to be infectious when injected into experimental animals and in human bite exposures.[16,18] However, HBs Ag-positive saliva has not been shown to be infectious when applied to oral mucous membranes in experimental primate studies[18] or through contamination of musical instruments or cardiopulmonary resuscitation dummies used by HBV carriers [19.20]. Epidemiologic studies of nonsexual household contacts of HIV-infected patients, including several small series in which HIV transmission failed to occur after bites or after percutaneous inoculation or contamination of cuts and open wounds with saliva from HIV-infected patients, suggest that the potential for salivary transmission of HIV is remote. [5,13,14,21,22] One case report from Germany has suggested the possibility of transmission of HIV in a household setting from an infected child to a sibling through a human bite [23]. The bite did not break the skin or result in bleeding. Since the date of seroconversion to HIV was not known for either child in this case, evidence for the role of saliva in the transmission of virus is unclear. [23] Another case report suggested the possibility of transmission of HIV from husband to wife by contact with saliva during kissing. [24] However, follow-up studies did not confirm HIV infection in the wife [21].

Universal precautions do not apply to saliva. General infection control practices already in existence—including the use of gloves for digital examination of mucous membranes and endotracheal suctioning, and handwashing after exposure to saliva —should further minimize the minute risk, if any, for salivary transmission of HIV and HBV[1,25]. Gloves need not be worn when feeding patients and when wiping saliva from skin.

Special precautions, however, are recommended for dentistry[1]. Occupationally acquired infection with HBV in dental workers has been documented[4], and two possible cases of occupationally acquired HIV infection involving dentists have been reported [5,26]. During dental procedures, contamination of saliva with blood is predictable, trauma to health-care workers' hands is common, and blood spattering may occur. Infection control precautions for dentistry minimize the potential for nonintact skin and mucous membrane contact of dental health-care workers to blood-contaminated saliva of patients. In addition, the use of gloves for oral examinations and treatment in the dental setting may also protect the patient's oral mucous membranes from exposures to blood, which may occur from breaks in the skin of dental workers' hands.

Use of Protective Barriers

Protective barriers reduce the risk of exposure of the health-care worker's skin or mucous membranes to potentially infective materials. For universal precautions, protective barriers reduce the risk of exposure to blood, body fluids containing visible blood, and other fluids to which universal precautions apply. Examples of protective barriers include gloves, gowns, masks, and protective eyewear. Gloves should reduce the incidence of contamination of hands, but they cannot prevent penetrating injuries due to needles or other sharp instruments. Masks and protective eyewear or face shields should reduce the incidence of contamination of mucous membranes of the mouth, nose, and eyes.

Universal precautions are intended to supplement rather than replace recommendations for routine infection controt such as handwashing and using gloves to prevent gross microbial contamination of hands. [27] Because specifying the types of barriers needed for every possible clinical situation is impractical, some judgment mum be exercised.

The risk of nosocomial transmission of HIV, HBV, and other

bloodborne pathogens can be minimized if health-care workers use the following general guidelines:*

1 Take care to prevent injuries when using needles, scalpels, and other sharp instruments or devices when handling sharp instruments aher procedures; when deaning used instruments; and when disposing of used needles Do not recap used needles by hand; do not remove used needles from disposable syringes by hand; and do not bend, break, or otherwise manipulate used needles by hand Place used deposable syringes and needles, scalpel blades, and other sharp items in puncture-resistant containers for disposal Locate the puncture-resistant containers as close to the use area as is practical.

2 Use protective barriers to prevent exposure to blood, body fluids containing visible blood, and other fluids to which universal precautions apply. The type of protective barder(s) should be appropriate for the procedure being performed and the type of exposure anticipated.

3 Immediately and thoroughly wash hands and other skin surfaces that are contaminated with blood, body fluids containing visible blood, or other body fluids to which universal precautions apply.

Glove Use for Phlebotomy

Gloves should reduce the incidence of blood contamination of hands during phlebotomy (drawing blood samplesh, but they cannot prevent penetrating injuries caused by needles or other sharp instruments. The likelihood of hand contamination wdh blood containing HIV, HBV, or other bloodborne pathogens during phlebotomy depends on several factors: (1) the skill and technique of the health-care worker, (2) the frequency with which the health-care worker performs the procedure (other factors being equat the cumulative risk of blood exposure is higher for a health-care worker who performs more procedures (3) whether the procedure occursin a routine or emergency situation (where blood contact may be more likely and (4) the prevalence of infection with bloodborne pathogens in the patient population. The likelihood of infection after skin exposure to blood containing HIV or HBV will depend on the concentration of virus (viral concentration is much higher for hepatitis B than for HIV), the duration of contact the presence of skin lesions on the hands of the health-care worke and— for HBV—the immune status of the health-care worker. Although not accurately

† The August 1987 publication should be consulted for general information and specific recommendations not addressed in this update.

quantified, the risk of HIV infection following intact skin contact with infective blood is certainly much less than the 0.5 per cent risk following percutaneous needles tick exposures.[5] In universal precautions, all blood is assumed to be potentially infective for bloodborne pathogens, but in certain settings (e. g., volunteer blood-donation centers) the prevalence of infection with some bloodborne pathogens (e.g., HIV, HBV) is known to be very low Some institutions have relaxed recommendations for using gloves for phlebotomy procedures by skilled phlebotomists in settings where the prevalence of bloodborne pathogens is known to be very low.

Institutions that judge that routine gloving for all phlebotomies is not necessary should periodically reevaluate their policy. Gloves should always be available to health-care workers who wish to use them for phlebotomy. In addition, the following general guidelines apply:

1. Use gloves for performing phlebotomy when the health-care worker has cuts, scratches, or other breaks in his/her skin.
2. Use gloves in situations where the health-care worker judges that hand contamination with blood may occur for example, then performing phlebotomy on an uncooperative patient.
3. Use gloves for performing finger and/or heel sticks on infants and children.
4. Use gloves when persons are receiving training in phlebotomy.

Selection of Gloves

The Center for Devices and Radiological Health, FDA, has responsibility for regulating the medical glove industry. Medical gloves include those marketed as sterile surgical or nonsterile examination gloves made of vinyl or latex. General purpose utility ("rubber") gloves are also used in the health-care sewing, but they are not regulated by FDA since they are not promoted for medical use. There are no reported differences in barrier effectiveness between intact latex and intact vinyl used to manufacture gloves. Thus, the type of gloves selected should be appropriate for the task being performed.

The following general guidelines are recommended:

1. Use sterile gloves for procedures involving contact with normally sterile areas of the body.
2. Use examination gloves for procedures involving contact with mucous membranes, unless otherwise indicated, and for other patient care or diagnostic procedures that

do not require the use of sterile gloves.

3. Change gloves between patient contacts.
4. Do not wash or disinfect surgical or examination gloves for reuse. Washing with surfactant may cause "wicking" i.e., the enhanced penetration of squids through undetected holes in the glove. Disinfecting agents may cause deterioration.
5. Use general purpose untility gloves (e.g., rubber household gloves) for housekeeping chores involving potential blood contact and for instrument cleaning and decontamination procedures. Utility gloves may be decontaminated and reused but should be discarded if they are peeling, cracked, or discolored, or if they have punctures, tears, or other evidence of deterioration.

Waste Management

Universal precautions are not intended to change waste management programmes previously recommended by CDC for health-care settings.[1] Policies for defining, collecting, storing, decontaminating, and disposing of infective waste are generaly determined by institutions in accordance with state and local regulations. Information regarding waste management regulations in heakh-care settings may be obtained from state or local heath departments or agencies responsible for waste management.

Reported by: Center for Devices and Radiological Health, Food and Drug Administration, Hospital Infections Programme, AIDS Programme, and Hepatitis Br, Div of Viral Diseases, Center for Infectious Diseases, National Institute for Occupational Safety and Health, CDC.

Editorial Note: Implementation of universal precautions does not eliminate the need for other category- or disease-specific isolation precautions, such as enteric precautions for infectious diarrhea or isolation for pulmonary tuberculosis.[1,2] In addition to universal precautions, detailed precautions have been developed for the following procedures and/or settings in which prolonged or intensive exposures to blood occur: invasive procedures, dentistry, autopsies or morticians' services, dialysis, and the clinical laboratory. These detailed precautions are found in the August 21, 1987, "Recommendations for Prevention of HIV Transmission in Health-Care Settings".[1] In addition, specific precautions have been developed for research laboratories.[28]

References

1. Centers for Disease Control. Recommendations for prevention of HIV transmission in health-care settings. MMWR 1987;36(suppl no. 2S).
2. Garner JS, Simmons BP. Guideline for isolation precautions in hospitals. Infect Control 1983:4:245-325.
3. Immunization Practices Advisory Committee. Recommendations for protection against viral hepatitis. MMWR 1985;34:313-24,329—35.
4. Department of Labour, Department of Health and Human Services. Joint advisory notice: protection against occupational exposure to hepatitis B virus (HBV) and human immunodeficiency virus (HIV). Washington, DC:US Department of Labour, US Department of Health and Human Services, 1987.
5. Centers for Disease Control. Update: Acquired immunodeficiency syndrome and human immunodeficiency virus infection among health-care workers. MMWR 1988;37:229—34,239.
6. Hollander H. Levy JA. Neurologic abnormalities and recovery of human immunodeficiency virus from cerebrospinal fluid. Ann Intern Med 1987;106:692—5.
7. Wirthrington RH, Cornes P. Harris JRW, et al. Isolation of human immunodeficiency virus from synovial fluid of a patient with reactive arthritis. Br Med J 1987;294:484.
8. Mundy DC. Schinazi RF, Gerber AR, Nahmias AJ, Randall HW. Human immunodeficiency virus isolated from amniotic fluid. Lancet 1987;2:459-60.
9. Onion DK, Crumpacker CS, Gilliland BC. Arthritis of hepatitis associated with Australia antigen. Ann Intern Med 1971;75:29-33.
10. Lee AKY, Ip HMH, Wong VCW. Mechanisms of maternal-fetal transmission of hepatitis B virus. J Infect Dis 1978;138:668-71.
11. Bond WW, Petersen NJ, Gravelle CR, Favero MS. Hepatitis B virus in peritoneal dialysis fluid: A potential hazard. Dialysis and Transplantation 1982;11:592-600.
12. Oskenhendler E, Harzic M, Le Roux J-M, Rabian C, Clauvel JP. HIV infection with seroconversion after a superficiai needlestick injury to the finger [Letter]. N Engl J Med 1986;315:582.
13. Lifson AR. Do alternate modes for transmission of human immunodeficiency virus exist? A review. JAMA 1988;259:1353-6.
14. Friedland GH, Saltzman BR, Rogers MF, et al. Lack of transmission of HTLV-III/LAV infection to household contacts of patients with AIDS or AIDS-related complex with oral candidiasis. N Engl J Med 1986;314:344-9.
15. Jenison SA, Lemon SM. Baker LN, Newbold JE. Quantitative analysis of hepatitis B virus DNA in saliva and semen of chronically infected homosexual men. J Infect Dis 1987; 156: 299-306.
16. Cancio-Bello TP, de Medina M, Shorey J. Valledor MD, Schiff ER. An institutional outbreak of hepatitis B related to a human biting carrier. J Infect Dis 1982;146:652-6.
17. MacQuarrie MB, Forghani B. Wolochow DA. Hepatitis B transmitted by a human bite. JAMA 1974;230:723-4.

18. Scott RM, Snitbhan R. Bancroft WH, Alter HJ, Tingpalapong M. Experimental transmission of hepatitis B virus by semen and saliva. J Infect Dis 1980;142:67-71.
19. Glaser JB, Nadler JP. Hepatitis B virus in a cardiopulmonary resuscitation training course. Risk of transmission from a surface antigen-positive participant. Arch Intern Med 1985;145:1653—5.
20. Osterholm MT, Bravo ER, Crosson JT, et al. Lack of transmission of viral hepatitis type B after oral exposure to HBsAg-positive saliva. Br Med J 1979;2:1263-4.
21. Curran JW, Jaffe HW, Hardy AM, et al. Epidemiology of HIV infection and AIDS in the United States. Science 1988;239:610-6.
22. Jason JM, McDougal JS, Dixon G. et al. HTLV-III/LAV antibody and immune status of household contacts and sexual partners of persons with hemophilia. JAMA 1986;255:212-5.
23. Wahn V, Kramer HH, Voit T. Broster HT, Scrampical B. Scheid A. Horizontal transmission of HIV infection between two siblings [Letter]. Lancet 1986;2:694.
24. Salahuddin SZ, Groopman JE, Markham PD, et al. HTLV-III in symptom-free seronegative persons. Lancet 1984;2:1418-20.
25. Simmons BP, Wong ES. Guideline for prevention of nosocomial pneumonia. Atlanta: US Department of Health and Human Services, Public Health Service, Centers for Disease Control, 1982.
26. Klein RS, Phelan JA, Freeman K, et al. Low occupational risk of human immunodeficiency virus infection among dental professionals. N Engl J Med 1988;318:86-90.
27. Garner JS, Favero MS. Guideline for handwashing and hospital environmental control, 1985. Atlanta: US Department of Health and Human Services, Public Health Service, Centers for Disease Control, 1985; HHS publication no. 99-1117.
28. Centers for Disease Control. 1988 Agent summary statement for human immunodeficiency virus and report on laboratory-acquired infection with human immunodeficiency virus. MMWR 1988;37(suppl no. S4:1S-22S).

35

Preventing Transmission of Human Immunodeficiency Virus and Hepatitis B Virus to Patients During Exposure Prone Invasive Procedures

This document has been developed by the Centers for Disease Control (CDC) to update recommendations for prevention of transmission of human immunodeficiency virus (HIV) and hepatitis B virus (HBV) in the health-care setting. Current data suggest that the risk for such transmission from a health-care worker (HCW) to a patient during an invasive procedure is small; a precise assessment of the risk is not yet available. This document contains recommendations to provide guidance for prevention of HIV and HBV transmission during those invasive procedures that are considered exposure-prone.

INTRODUCTION

Recommendations have been made by the Centers for Disease Control (CDC) for the prevention of transmission of the human immunodeficiency virus (HIV) and the hepatitis B virus (HBV) in health-care settings.[1-6] These recommendations emphasize adherence to universal precautions that require that blood and other specified body fluids of all patients be handled as if they contain blood-borne pathogens.[1,2]

Previous guidelines contained precautions to be used during invasive procedures and recommendations for the management of HIV- and HBV-infected health-care workers (HCWs).[1] These guidelines did not include specific recommendations on testing HCWs for HIV or HBV infection, and they did not provide guidance on which invasive procedures may represent increased risk to the patient.

The recommendations outlined in this document are based on the following considerations:

- # Infected HCWs who adhere to universal precautions and who do not perform invasive procedures pose no risk for transmitting HIV or HBV to patients.
- # Infected HCWs who adhere to universal precautions and who perform certain exposure-prone procedures pose a small risk for transmitting HBV to patients.
- # HIV is transmitted much less readily than HBV.

In the interim, until further data are available, additional precautions are prudent to prevent HIV and HBV transmission during procedures that have been linked to HCW-to-patient HBV transmission or that are considered exposure-prone.

BACKGROUND

Infection-Control Practices

Previous recommendations have specified that infection-control programmes should incorporate principles of universal precautions (i.e., appropriate use of hand washing, protective barriers, and care in the use and disposal of needles and other sharp instruments) and should maintain these precautions rigorously in all health-care settings.[1,2,5] Proper application of these principles will assist in minimizing the risk of transmission of HIV or HBV from patient to HCW, HCW to patient, or patient to patient.

As part of standard infection-control practice, instruments and other reusable equipment used in performing invasive procedures should be appropriately disinfected and sterilized as follows:[7]

- # Equipment and devices that enter the patient's vascular system or other normally sterile areas of the body should be sterilized before being used for each patient.
- # Equipment and devices that touch intact mucous membranes but do not penetrate the patient's body surfaces should be sterilized when possible or undergo high-level disinfection if they cannot be sterilized before being used for each patient.
- # Equipment and devices that do not touch the patient or that only touch intact skin of the patient need only be cleaned with a detergent or as indicated by the manufacturer.

Compliance with universal precautions and recommendations for disinfection and sterilization of medical devices should be scrupulously monitored in all health-care settings.[1,7,8] Training of

HCWs in proper infection-control technique should begin in professional and vocational schools and continue as an ongoing process. Institutions should provide all HCWs with appropriate inservice education regarding infection control and safety and should establish procedures for monitoring compliance with infection-control policies.

All HCWs who might be exposed to blood in an occupational setting should receive hepatitis B vaccine, preferably during their period of professional training and before any occupational exposures could occur.[8,9]

Transmission of HBV During Invasive Procedures

Since the introduction of serologic testing for HBV infection in the early 1970s, there have been published reports of 20 clusters in which a total of over 300 patients were infected with HBV in association with treatment by an HBV-infected HCW. In 12 of these clusters, the implicated HCW did not routinely wear gloves; several HCWs also had skin lesions that may have facilitated HBV transmission.[10-22] These 12 clusters included nine linked to dentists or oral surgeons and one cluster each linked to a general practitioner, an inhalation therapist, and a cardiopulmonarybypass-pump technician. The clusters associated with the inhalation therapist and the cardiopulmonary-bypass-pump technician—and some of the other 10 clusters—could possibly have been prevented if current recommendations on universal precautions, including glove use, had been in effect. In the remaining eight clusters, transmission occurred despite glove use by the HCWs; five clusters were linked to obstetricians or gynecologists, and three were linked to cardiovascular surgeons.[6, 22-28] In addition, recent unpublished reports strongly suggest HBV transmission from three surgeons to patients in 1989 and 1990 during colorectal (CDC, unpublished data), abdominal, and cardiothoracic surgery.[29]

Seven of the HCWs who were linked to published clusters in the United States were allowed to perform invasive procedures following modification of invasive techniques (e.g., double gloving and restriction of certain high-risk procedures).[6,11-13,15,16,24] For five HCWs, no further transmission to patients was observed. In two instances involving an obstetrician/gynecologist and an oral surgeon, HBV was transmitted to patients after techniques were modified.[6,12]

Review of the 20 published studies indicates that a combination of risk factors accounted for transmission of HBV from HCWs to patients. Of the HCWs whose hepatitis B e antigen (HBeAg) status was determined (17 of 20), all were HBeAg positive. The presence of HBeAg in serum is associated with higher levels of circulating virus and therefore with greater infectivity of hepatitis-B-surface-antigen (HBsAg)-positive individuals; the risk of HBV transmission to an HCW after a percutaneous exposure to HBeAg-positive blood is approximately 30 per cent.[30-32] In addition, each report indicated that the potential existed for contamination of surgical wounds or traumatized tissue, either from a major break in standard infection-control practices (e.g., not wearing gloves during invasive procedures) or from unintentional injury to the infected HCW during invasive procedures (e.g., needle sticks incurred while manipulating needles without being able to see them during suturing.

Most reported clusters in the United States occurred before awareness increased of the risks of transmission of blood-borne pathogens in health-care settings and before emphasis was placed on the use of universal precautions and hepatitis B vaccine among HCWs. The limited number of reports of HBV transmission from HCWs to patients in recent years may reflect the adoption of universal precautions and increased use of HBV vaccine. However, the limited number of recent reports does not preclude the occurrence of undetected or unreported small clusters or individual instances of transmission; routine use of gloves does not prevent most injuries caused by sharp instruments and does not eliminate the potential for exposure of a patient to an HCW's blood and transmission of HBV.[6, 22-29]

Transmission of HIV During Invasive Procedures

The risk of HIV transmission to an HCW after percutaneous exposure to HIV-infected blood is considerably lower than the risk of HBV transmission after percutaneous exposure to HBeAg-positive blood (0.3 per cent versus approximately 30 per cent).[33-35] Thus, the risk of transmission of HIV from an infected HCW to a patient during an invasive procedure is likely to.be proportionately lower than the risk of HBV transmission from an HBeAg-positive HCW to a patient during the same procedure. As with HBV, the relative infectivity of HIV probably varies among individuals and over time for a single individual. Unlike HBV infection, however, there is currently no readily available laboratory test for increased HIV infectivity.

Investigation of a cluster of HIV infections among patients in the practice of one dentist with acquired immunodeficiency syndrome (AIDS) strongly suggested that HIV was transmitted to five of the approximately 850 patients evaluated through June 1991.[38] The investigation indicates that HIV transmission occurred during dental care, although the precise mechanisms of transmission have not been determined. In two other studies, when patients cared for by a general surgeon and a surgical resident who had AIDS were tested, all patients tested, 75 and 62, respectively, were negative for HIV infection.[39,40]. In a fourth study, 143 patients who had been treated by a dental student with HIV infection and were later tested were all negative for HIV infection.[41] In another investigation, HIV antibody testing was offered to all patients whose surgical procedures had been performed by a general surgeon within 7 years before the surgeon's diagnosis of AIDS; the date at which the surgeon became infected with HIV is unknown.[42] Of 1,340 surgical patients contacted, 616 (46 per cent) were tested for HIV. One patient, a known intravenous drug user, was HIV positive when tested but may already have been infected at the time of surgery. HIV test results for the 615 other surgical patients were negative (95 per cent confidence interval for risk of transmission per operation =0.0 per cent-0.5 per cent).

The limited number of participants and the differences in procedures associated with these five investigations limit the ability to generalize from them and to define precisely the risk of HIV transmission from HIV-infected HCWs to patients. A precise estimate of the risk of HIV transmission from infected HCWs to patients can be determined only after careful evaluation of a substantially larger number of patients whose exposure-prone procedures have been performed by HIV-infected HCWs.

Exposure-Prone Procedures

Despite adherence to the principles of universal precautions, certain invasive surgical and dental procedures have been implicated in the transmission of HBV from infected HCWs to patients, and should be considered exposure-prone. Reported examples include certain oral, cardiothoracic, colorectal (CDC, unpublished data), and obstetric/gynecologic procedures.[6, 12, 22-29]

Certain other invasive procedures should also be considered exposure-prone. In a prospective study CDC conducted in tour hospitals, one or more percutaneous injuries occurred among surgical personnel during 96 (6.9 per cent) of 1,382 operative procedures on the general surgery, gynecology, orthopedic, cardiac, and trauma services.[43] Percutaneous exposure of the patient to the HCW's blood may have occurred when the sharp object causing the injury recontacted the patient's open wound in 28 (32 per cent) of the 88 observed injuries to surgeons (range among surgical specialties=8 per cent=57 per cent; range among hospitals=24 per cent-42 per cent).

Characteristics of exposure-prone procedures include digital palpation of a needle tip in a body cavity or the simultaneous presence of the HCW's fingers and a needle or other sharp instrument or object in a poorly visualized or highly confined anatomic site. Performance of exposure-prone procedures presents a recognized risk of percutaneous injury to the HCW, and—if such an injury occurs—the HCW's blood is likely to contact the patient's body cavity, subcutaneous tissues, and/or mucous membranes.

Experience with HBV indicates that invasive procedures that do not have the above characteristics would be expected to pose substantially lower risk, if any, of transmission of HIV and other blood-borne pathogens from an infected HCW to patients.

RECOMMENDATIONS

Investigations of HIV and HBV transmission from HCWs to patients indicate that, when HCWs adhere to recommended infection-control procedures, the risk of transmitting HBV from an infected HCW to a patient is small, and the risk of transmitting HIV is likely to be even smaller. However, the likelihood of exposure of the patient to an HCW's blood is greater for certain procedures designated as exposure-prone. To minimize the risk of HIV or HBV transmission, the following measures are recommended:

- # All HCWs should adhere to universal precautions, including the appropriate use of hand washing, protective barriers, and care in the use and disposal of needles and other sharp instruments. HCWs who have exudative lesions or weeping dermatitis should refrain from all direct patient care and from handling patient-care equipment and devices used in performing invasive procedures until the condition resolves. HCWs should also comply with current guidelines for disinfection and sterilization of reusable devices used in invasive procedures.
- # Currently available data provide no basis for recommendations to restrict the practice of HCWs infected with HIV or HBV who perform invasive procedures not identified as exposure-prone, provided the infected HCWs practice recommended surgical or dental technique and comply with universal precautions and current recommendations for sterilization/disinfection.
- # Exposure-prone procedures should be identified by medical/surgical/dental organizations and institutions at which the procedures are performed.
- # HCWs who perform exposure-prone procedures should know their HIV antibody status. HCWs who perform exposure-prone procedures and who do not have serologic evidence of immunity to HBV from vaccination or from previous infection should know their HBsAg status

and, if that is positive, should also know their HBeAg status.

HCWs who are infected with HIV or HBV (and are HBeAg positive) should not perform exposure-prone procedures unless they have sought counsel from an expert review panel and been advised under what circumstances, if any, they may continue to perform these procedures.* Such circumstances would include notifying prospective patients of the HCW's seropositivity before they undergo exposure-prone invasive procedures.

Mandatory testing of HCWs for HIV antibody, HBsAg, or HBeAg is not recommended. The current assessment of the risk that infected HCWs will transmit HIV or HBV to patients during exposure-prone procedures does not support the diversion of resources that would be required to implement mandatory testing programmes. Compliance by HCWs with recommendations can be increased through education, training, and appropriate confidentiality safeguards.

HCWS WHOSE PRACTICES ARE MODIFIED BECAUSE OF HIV OR HBV STATUS

HCWs whose practices are modified because of their HIV or HBV infection status should, whenever possible, be provided opportunities to continue appropriate patient-care activities. Career counseling and job retraining should be encouraged to promote the continued use of the HCW's talents, knowledge, and skills. HCWs whose practices are modified because of HBV infection should be reevaluated periodically to determine whether their HBeAg status changes due to resolution of infection or as a result of treatment.[44]

NOTIFICATION OF PATIENTS AND F LOW-UP STUDIES

The public health benefit of nofficafon of pafents who have

*The review panel should include experts who represent a balanced perspective. Such experts might include all of the following: a) the HCW's personal physician(s), (b) an infectious disease specialist with expertise in the epidemiology of HIV and HBV transmission, (c) a health professional with expertise in the procedures performed by the HCW, and d) state or local public health official(s). if the HCW's practice is institutionally based, the expert review panel might also include a member of the infection-control committee, preferably a hospital epidemiologist. HCWs who perform exposure-prone procedures outside the hospital/institutional setting should seek advice from appropriate state and local public health officials regarding the review process. Panels must recognize the importance of confidentiality and the privacy rights of infected HCWs.

had exposure-prone procedures performed by HCWs infected with HIV or positive for HBeAg should be considered on a case-by-case basis taking into consideration an assessment of specfic risk, confidentialy issues, and available resources. Carefully designed and implemented follow-up studies are necessary to determine more precisely the risk of transmission during such procedures. Decisions regarding notification and follow-up studies should be made in consultation with state and local public health officials.

ADDITIONAL NEEDS

- # Clearer definition of the nature, frequency, and circumstances of blood contact between parents and HCWs during invasive procedures.
- # Development and evaluation of new devices, protective barriers, and techniques that may prevent such blood contact without adversely affecting the quality of parent care.
- # More information on the potential for HIV and HBV transmission through contaminated instruments.
- # Improvements in sterilization and disinfection techniques for certain reusable equipment and devices.
- # Identification of factors that may influence the likelihood of HIV or HBV transmission after exposure to HIV- or HBV-infected blood.

References

1. CDC. Recommendations for prevention of HIV transmission in health-care settings MMWR 1987; 36 (suppl.. no 25) 1-185
2. CDC . Update Universal precautions for prevention of transmission of human immunodeficiency virus, hepatitis B virus and other blood borne pathogens in health-care setlings. MMWR 1988;37 377-82,387-8
3. CDC. Heptitis Surveillance Report No. 48. Atlanta: U.S. Department of Health and Human Services, Public Health Service, 1982: 2-3.
4. CDC. CDC Guideline for Infection Control in Hospital Personnel Atlanta, Georgia: Public Health Service, 1983 24 pages (GPO# 6AR031 488305)
5. CDC. Guidelines for prevention of transmission of human immunodeficiency virus and hepatitis B virus to health-care and public-safety workers. MMWR 1989;38; (suppl. no. S-6): 1-37.
6. Lettau LA, Smith JD, Williams D, et al. Transmission of hepatise B with resultant restriction of surgical practice. Jama 1986; 255: 934-7.
7 CDC. Guidelines for the prevention and control of nosocomial infections guideline for handwashing and hospital environmental control Atlanta, Georgia Public Health Service, 1985: 20 pages (GPO# 544-436/24441).
8 Department of Labour, Occupational Safety and Health Administration.

Occupational exposure to bloodborne pathogens: proposed rule and notice of hearing Federal Register 1989;54. 23042-139

9 CDC.Protection against viral hepatitis: recommendations of the immunization practices advisory committee (ACIP) MMWR 1990 39:(no RR-2L)

10 Levin ML. Maddre; WC, Wands JR, Mendeloff Al. Hepatitis B transmission by dentists. JAMA 1974; 228 1139-40.

11 Rimland D, Parkin WE, Miller GB, Schrack WD. Hepatitis B outbreak traced to an oral surgeon. N Engl J Med 1977; 296: 953-8.

12. Goodwin D, Fannin SL, McCracken BB An oral-surgeon related hepatitis-B outbreak California Morbidity 1976 14.

13. Hadler SC Sorley DL, Acree KH, et al. An outbreak of hepatitis B in a dental practice. Ann Intern Med 1981 1981;95:133-8.

14. Reingold AL, Kane MA, Murphy BL, Checko P,. Francis DP, Maynard JE Transmission of hepatitis B by an oral surgeon J Infect Dis 1982;145:262-8.

15 Goodman RA, Ahtons JL, Finton RJ Hepaftis B transmission from dental personnel to patients unfinished business [Editorial. Ann Intern Med 1982;96:119.

16. Ahtons J. Goodman RA. Hepatitis B and dental personnel: transmission to patients and prevention issues J Am Dent Assoc 1983;106:219-22.

17. Shaw FE Jr, Barrett CL, Hamm R. et al. Lethal outbreak of hepatitis B in a dental practice JAMA 1986,255 3260-4.

18. CDC. Outbreak of hepatitis B associated with an oral surgeon, New Hampshire MMWR 1987;36:132-3.

19 Grob PJ, Moeschlin P. Risk to contacts of a medical practitioner carrying HBsAg [Letter] N Engl J Med 1975 293:197.

20 Grob PJ Bischof B. Naeff F. Cluster of hepatitis B transmitted by a physician Lancet 1981;2:1218-20.

21 Snydman DR, Hindman SH, Wineland MD, Bryan JA, Maynard JE Nosocomial viral hepatitis B. A cluster among staff with subsequent transmission to patients. Ann Intern Med 1976;85:573-7.

22. Coutinho RA, Albrecht-van Lent P. Stoutjesdijk L, et al Hepatitis B from doctors [Letter] Lancet 1982;1:345-6.

23. Anonymous Acuts hepatitis B associated with gynaecological surgery Lancet 1980;1:1-6.

24. Carl M, Blakey DL, Francis DP, Maynard JE. Interruption of hepatitis B transmission by modification of a gynaecologist's surgical technique. Lancet 1982;1:731-3.

25. Anonymous. Acute hepatitis B following gynaecological surgery. J Hosp Infect 1987;9:34-8.

26. Welch J. Webster M, Tilzey AJ, Noah ND, Banatvala JE. Hepatitis B infections after gynaecological surgery. Lancet 1989; 1 :205-7.

27. Haeram JW, Siebke JC, Ulstrup J. Geiram D, Helle I. HBsAg transmission from a cardiac surgeon incubating hepatitis B resulting in chronic antigenemia in four patients. Acta Med Scand 1981;210:389-92.

28. Flower AJE, Prentice M, Morgan G. et al. Hepatitis B infection following cardiothoracic surgery [Abstract].1990 International Symposium on Viral Hepatitis and Liver Diseases, Houston. 190;94.

29. Heptonstall J. Outbreaks of hepatitis B virus infection associated with infected surgical staff in the United Kingdom. Communicable Disease Reports 1991 (in press).
30. Alter HJ, Seef LB, Kaplan PM, et al. Type B hepatitis: the infectivity of blood positive for e antigen and DNA polymerase after accidental needlestick exposure. N Engl J Med 1976;295:909-13.
31. Seeff LB, Wright EC, Zimmerman HJ, et al. Type B hepatitis after needlestick exposure: prevention with hepatitis B immunoglobulin: final report of the Veterans Administration Co-operative Study. Ann Intern Med 1978;88:285-93.
32. Grady GF, Lee VA, Prince AM, et ai. Hepatitis B immune globulin for accidental exposures among medical personnel: final report of a multicenter controlled trial. J Infect Dis 1978;138:625-38.
33. Henderson DK, Fahey BJ, Willy M, et al. Risk for occupational transmission of human immunodeficiency virus type 1 (HIV-1) associated with ciinical exposures: a prospective evaluation. Ann Intern Med 1990;113:740-6.
34. Marcus R. CDC Co-operative Needlestick Study Group. Surveillance of health-care workers exposed to blood from patients infected with the human immunodeficiency virus. N Engl J Med 1988;319:1118-23.
35. Gerberding JL, Bryant-LeBlanc CE, Nelson K, et al. Risk of transmitting the human immunodeficiency virus, cytomegalovirus, and hepatitis B virus to health-care workers exposed to patients with AIDS and AIDS-related conditions. J Infect Dis 1987; 156:1 -8.
36. CDC. Possible transmission of human immunodeficiency virus to a patient during an invasive dental procedure. MMWR 1990;39:489-93.
37. CDC. Update: transmission of HIV infection during an invasive dental procedure - Florida. MMWR 1991; 40:21 -27,33.
38. CDC. Update: transmission of HIV infection during invasive dental procedures - Florida. MMWR 1991; 40: 377-81.
39. Porter JD, Cruikshank JG, Gentle PH, Robinson RG, Gill ON. Management of patients treated by a surgeon with HIV infection. [Letter] Lancet 1990;335:113-4.
40. Armstrong FP, Miner JC, Wolfe WH. Investigation of a health-care worker with symptomatic human immunodeficiency virus infection: an epidemiologic approach. Milit Med 1987;152:414-8.
41. Comer RW, Myers DR, Steadman CD, Carter MJ, Rissing JP, Tedesco FJ. Management considerations for an HIV positive dental student. J Dent Educ 1991;55:187-91.
42. Mishu B. Schaffner W. Horan JM, Wood LH, Hutcheson R. McNabb P. A surgeon with AIDS: lack of evidence of transmission to patients. JAMA 1990;264:467-70.
43. Tokars J. Bell D, Marcus R. et al. Percutaneous injuries during surgical procedures [Abstract]. Vll International Conference on AIDS. Vol 2. Florence, Italy, June 16-21, 1991:83.
44. Perrillo RP, Schiff ER, Davis GL, et al. A randomized, controlled trial of interferon alfa-2b alone and after prednisone withdrawal for the treatment of chronic hepatitis B. N Engl J Med 1990;323:295-301.

36

Prevention of HIV Transmission in Health-Care Settings

INTRODUCTION

Human immunodeficiency virus (HIV), the virus that causes acquired immunodeficiency syndrome (AIDS), is transmitted through sexual contact and exposure to infected blood or blood components and perinatally from mother to neonate. HIV has been isolated from blood, semen, vaginal secretions, saliva, tears, breast milk, cerebrospinal fluid, amniotic fluid, and urine and is likely to be isolated from other body fluids, secretions, and excretions. However, epidemiologic evidence has implicated only blood, semen, vaginal secretions, and possibly breast milk in transmission.

The increasing prevalence of HIV increases the risk that health-care workers will be exposed to blood from patients infected with HIV, especially when blood and bodyfluid precautions are not followed for all patients. Thus, this document emphasizes the need for health-care workers to consider all patients as potentially infected with HIV and/or other blood-borne pathogens and to adhere rigorously to infection-control precautions for minimizing the risk of exposure to blood and body fluids of all patients.

The recommendations contained in this document consolidate and update CDC recommendations published earlier for preventing HIV transmission in health-care settings: precautions for clinical and laboratory staffs [1] and precautions for health-care workers and allied professionals [2]; recommendations for preventing HIV transmission in the workplace [3] and during invasive procedures;[4] recommendations for preventing possible transmission of HIV from tears [5]; and recommendations for providing dialysis treatment for HIV-infected patients.[6] These recommendations also update portions of the "Guideline for Isolation Precautions in Hospitals" [7] and reemphasize some of the recommendations contained in

"Infection Control Practices for Dentistry".[8] The recommendations contained in this document have been developed for use in health-care settings and emphasize the need to treat blood and other body fluids from all patients as potentially infective. These same prudent precautions also should be taken in other settings in which persons may be exposed to blood or other body fluids.

DEFINITION OF HEALTH-CARE WORKERS

Health-care workers are defined as persons, including students and trainees, whose activities involve contact with patients or with blood or other body fluids from patients in a health-care setting.

HEALTH-CARE WORKERS WITH AIDS

As of July 10,1987, a total of 1,875 (5.8 per cent) of 32,395 adults with AIDS, who had been reported to the CDC national surveillance system and for whom occupational information was available, reported being employed in a health-care or clinical laboratory setting. In comparison, 6.8 million persons—representing 5.6 per cent of the U.S. labour force—were employed in health services. Of the health-care workers with AIDS, 95 per cent have been reported to exhibit high-risk behaviour; for the remaining 5 per cent, the means of HIV acquisition was undetermined. Health-care workers with AIDS were significantly more likely than other workers to have an undetermined risk (5 per cent versus 3 per cent, respectively). For both health-care workers and non-health-care workers with AIDS, the proportion with an undetermined risk has not increased since 1982.

AIDS patients initially reported as not belonging to recognized risk groups are investigated by state and local health departments to determine whether possible risk factors exist. Of all health-care workers with AIDS reported to CDC who were initially characterized as not having an identified risk and for whom follow-up information was available, 66 per cent have been reclassified because risk factors were identified or because the patient was found not to meet the surveillance case definition for AIDS. Of the 87 health-care workers currently categorized as having no identifiable risk, information is incomplete on 16 (18 per cent) because of death or refusal to be interviewed; 38 (44 per cent) are still being investigated. The remaining 33 (38 per cent) health-care workers were interviewed or had other follow-up information available. The occupations of these 33 were as follows: five physicians (15 per cent), three of whom were surgeons; one dentist (3 per cent); three nurses (9 per cent); nine nursing assistants (27 per cent);

seven housekeeping or maintenance workers (21 per cent); three clinical laboratory technicians (9 per cent); one therapist (3 per cent); and four others who did not have contact with patients (12 per cent). Although 15 of these 33 health-care workers reported parenteral and/or other non-needlestick exposure to blood or body fluids from patients in the 10 years preceding their diagnosis of AIDS, none of these exposures involved a patient with AIDS or known HIV infection.

RISK TO HEALTH-CARE WORKERS OF ACQUIRING HIV IN HEALTH-CARE SETTINGS

Health-care workers with documented percutaneous or mucous-membrane exposures to blood or body fluids of HIV-infected patients have been prospectively evaluated to determine the risk of infection after such exposures. As of June 30,1987, 883 health-care workers have been tested for antibody to HIV in an ongoing surveillance project conducted by CDC.[9] of these, 708 (80 per cent) had percutaneous exposures to blood, and 175 (20 per cent) had a mucous membrane or an open wound contaminated by blood or body fluid. Of 396 health-care workers, each of whom had only a convalescent-phase serum sample obtained and tested ⩾90 days post-exposure, one—for whom heterosexual transmission could not be ruled out—was seropositive for HIV antibody. For 425 additional health-care workers, both acute- and convalescent-phase serum samples were obtained and tested; none of 74 health-care workers with nonpercutaneous exposures seroconverted, and three (0.9 per cent) of 351 with percutaneous exposures seroconverted. None of these three health-care workers had other documented risk factors for infection.

Two other prospective studies to assess the risk of nosocomial acquisition of HIV infection for health-care workers are ongoing in the United States. As of April 30, 1987, 332 health-care workers with a total of 453 needlestick or mucous-membrane exposures to the blood or other body fluids of HIV-infected patients were tested for HIV antibody at the National Institutes of Health.[10] These exposed workers included 103 with needlestick injuries and 229 with mucous-membrane exposures; none had seroconverted. A similar study at the University of California of 129 health-care workers with documented needlestick injuries or mucous-membrane exposures to blood or other body fluids from patients with HIV infection has not identified any seroconversions.[11] Results of a prospective study in the United Kingdom identified no evidence of transmission among 150 health-care workers with parenteral or mucous-membrane exposures to blood or other body fluids, secretions, or excretions from patients with HIV infection.[12]

In addition to health-care workers enrolled in prospective studies, eight persons who provided care to infected patients and denied other risk factors have been reported to have acquired HIV infection. Three of these health-care workers had needlestick exposures to blood from infected patients.[13,15] Two were persons who provided nursing care to infected persons; although neither sustained a needlestick, both had extensive contact with blood or other body fluids, and neither observed recommended barrier precautions.[16,17] The other three were healthcare workers with non-needlestick exposures to blood from infected patients.[18] Although the exact route of transmission for these last three infections is not known, all three persons had direct contact of their skin with blood from infected patients, all had skin lesions that may have been contaminated by blood, and one also had a mucous-membrane exposure.

A total of 1,231 dentists and hygienists, many of whom practiced in areas with many AIDS cases, participated in a study to determine the prevalence of antibody to HIV; one dentist (0.1 per cent) had HIV antibody. Although no exposure to a known HIV-infected person could be documented, epidemiologic investigation did not identify any other risk factor for infection. The infected dentist, who also had a history of sustaining needlestick injuries and trauma to his hands, did not routinely wear gloves when providing dental care.[19]

PRECAUTIONS TO PREVENT TRANSMISSION OF HIV

Universal Precautions

Since medical history and examination cannot reliably identify all patients infected with HIV or other blood-borne pathogens, blood and body-fluid precautions should be consistently used for all patients. This approach, previously recommended by CDC [3,4], and referred to as "universal blood and body-fluid precautions" or "universal precautions," should be used in the care of all patients, especially including those in emergency-care settings in which the risk of blood exposure is increased and the infection status of the patient is usually unknown.[20]

1. All health-care workers should routinely use appropriate barrier precautions to prevent skin and mucous-membrane exposure when contact with blood or other body fluids of any patient is anticipated. Gloves should be worn for touching blood and body fluids, mucous membranes, or non-intact skin of all patients, for handling items or surfaces soiled with blood or body fluids, and for performing venipuncture and other vascular access

procedures. Gloves should be changed after contact with each patient. Masks and protective eyewear or face shields should be worn during procedures that are likely to generate droplets of blood or other body fluids to prevent exposure of mucous membranes of the mouth, nose, and eyes. Gowns or aprons should be worn during procedures that are likely to generate splashes of blood or other body fluids.

2. Hands and other skin surfaces should be washed immediately and thoroughly if contaminated with blood or other body fluids. Hands should be washed immediately after gloves are removed.
3. All health-care workers should take precautions to prevent injuries caused by needles, scalpels, and other sharp instruments or devices during procedures; when cleaning used instruments; during disposal of used needles; and when handling sharp instruments after procedures. To prevent needlestick injuries, needles should not be recapped, purposely bent or broken by hand, removed from disposable syringes, or otherwise manipulated by hand. After they are used, disposable syringes and needles, scalpel blades, and other sharp items should be placed in puncture-resistant containers for disposal; the punctureresistant containers should be located as close as practical to the use area. Large-bore reusable needles should be placed in a puncture-resistant container for transport to the reprocessing area.
4. Although saliva has not been implicated in HIV transmission, to minimize the need for emergency mouth-to-mouth resuscitation, mouthpieces, resuscitation bags, or other ventilation devices should be available for use in areas in which the need for resuscitation is predictable.
5. Health-care workers who have exudative lesions or weeping dermatitis should refrain from all direct patient care and from handling patient-care equipment until the condition resolves.
6. Pregnant health-care workers are not known to be at greater risk of contracting HIV infection than health-care workers who are not pregnant; however, if a health-care worker develops HIV infection during pregnancy, the infant is at risk of infection resulting from perinatal transmission. Because of this risk, pregnant health-care workers should be especially familiar with and strictly adhere to precautions to minimize the risk of HIV transmission.

Implementation of universal blood and body-fluid precautions for all patients eliminates the need for use of the isolation category of "Blood and Body Fluid Precautions" previously recommended by CDC [7] for patients known or suspected to be infected with blood-borne pathogens. Isolation precautions (e.g., enteric, "AFB" [7]) should be used as necessary if associated conditions, such as infectious diarrhea or tuberculosis, are diagnosed or suspected.

Precautions for Invasive Procedures

In this document, an invasive procedure is defined as surgical entry into tissues, cavities, or organs or repair of major traumatic injuries (1) in an operating or delivery room, emergency department, or outpatient setting, including both physicians' and dentists' offices; (2) cardiac catheterization and angiographic procedures; (3) a vaginal or cesarean delivery or other invasive obstetric procedure during which bleeding may occur; or (4) the manipulation, cutting, or removal of any oral or perioral tissues, including tooth structure, during which bleeding occurs or the potential for bleeding exists. The universal blood and body-fluid precautions listed above, combined with the precautions listed below, should be the minimum precautions for all such invasive procedures.

1. All health-care workers who participate in invasive procedures must routinely use appropriate barrier precautions to prevent skin and mucous-membrane contact with blood and other body fluids of all patients. Gloves and surgical masks must be worn for all invasive procedures. Protective eyewear or face shields should be worn for procedures that commonly result in the generation of droplets, smashing of blood or other body fluids, or the generation of bone chips. Gowns or aprons made of materials that provide an effective barrier should be worn during invasive procedures that are likely to result in the splashing of blood or other body fluids. All health-care workers who perform or assist in vaginal or cesarean deliveries should wear gloves and gowns when handling the placenta or the infant until blood and amniotic fluid have been removed from the infant's skin and should wear gloves during post-delivery care of the umbilical cord.
2. If a glove is torn or a needlestick or other injury occurs, the glove should be removed and a new glove used as promptly as patient safety permits; the needle or instrument involved in the incident should also be removed from the sterile field.

Precautions for Dentistry*

Blood, saliva, and gingival fluid from all dental patients should be considered infective. Special emphasis should be placed on the following precautions for preventing transmission of blood-borne pathogens in dental practice in both institutional and non-institutional settings.

1. In addition to wearing gloves for contact with oral mucous membranes of all patients, all dental workers should wear surgical masks and protective eyewear or chin-length plastic face shields during dental procedures in which splashing or spattering of blood, saliva, or gingival fluids is likely. Rubber dams, highspeed evacuation, and proper patient positioning, when appropriate, should be utilized to minimize generation of droplets and spatter.
2. Handpieces should be sterilized after use with each patient, since blood, saliva, or gingival fluid of patients may be aspirated into the handpiece or waterline. Handpieces that cannot be sterilized should at least be flushed, the outside surface cleaned and wiped with a suitable chemical germicide, and then rinsed. Handpieces should be flushed at the beginning of the day and after use with each patient. Manufacturers' recommendations should be followed for use and maintenance of waterlines and check valves and for flushing of handpieces. The same precautions should be used for ultrasonic scalers and air/water syringes.
3. Blood and saliva should be thoroughly and carefully cleaned from material that has been used in the mouth (e.g., impression materials, bite registration), especially before polishing and grinding intra-oral devices. Contaminated materials, impressions, and intra-oral devices should also be cleaned and disinfected before being handled in the dental laboratory and before they are placed in the patient's mouth. Because of the increasing variety of dental materials used intra-orally, dental workers should consult with manufacturers as to the stability of specific materials when using disinfection procedures.
4. Dental equipment and surfaces that are difficult to disinfect (e.g., light handles or X-ray-unit heads) and that may become contaminated should be wrapped with impervious-backed paper, aluminum foil, or clear plastic wrap. The coverings should be removed and discarded, and clean coverings should be put in place after use with each patient.

---

* General infection-control precautions are more specifically addressed in previous recommendations for infection-control practices for dentistry. [8]

Precautions for Autopsies or Morticians' Services

In addition to the universal blood and body-fluid precautions listed above, the following precautions should be used by persons performing postmortem procedures:

1. All persons performing or assisting in postmortem procedures should wear gloves, masks, protective eyewear, gowns, and waterproof aprons.
2. Instruments and surfaces contaminated during postmortem procedures should be decontaminated with an appropriate chemical germicide.

Precautions for Dialysis

Patients with end-stage renal disease who are undergoing maintenance dialysis and who have HIV infection can be dialyzed in hospital-based or free-standing dialysis units using conventional infection-control precautions.[21] Universal blood and body-fluid precautions should be used when dialyzing all patients.

Strategies for disinfecting the dialysis fluid pathways of the hemodialysis machine are targeted to control bacterial contamination and generally consist of using 500-750 parts per million (ppm) of sodium hypochlorite (household bleach) for 30-40 minutes or 1.5 per cent-2.0 per cent formaldehyde overnight. In addition, several chemical germicides formulated to disinfect dialysis machines are commercially available. None of these protocols or procedures need to be changed for dialyzing patients infected with HIV.

Patients infected with HIV can be dialyzed by either hemodialysis or peritoneal dialysis and do not need to be isolated from other patients. The type of dialysis treatment (i.e., hemodialysis or peritoneal dialysis) should be based on the needs of the patient. The dialyzer may be discarded after each use. Alternatively, centers that reuse dialyzers—i.e., a specific single-use dialyzer is issued to a specific patient, removed, cleaned, disinfected, and reused several times on the same patient only— may include HIV-infected patients in the dialyzer-reuse programme. An individual dialyzer must never be used on more than one patient.

Precautions for Laboratories †

Blood and other body fluids from all patients should be considered infective. To supplement the universal blood and body-fluid precautions listed above, the following precautions are recommended for health-care workers in clinical laboratories.

† Additional precautions for research and industrial laboratories are addressed elsewhere.[22,23]

1. All specimens of blood and body fluids should be put in a well-constructed container with a secure lid to prevent leaking during transport. Care should be taken when collecting each specimen to avoid contaminating the outside of the container and of the laboratory form accompanying the specimen.
2. All persons processing blood and body-fluid specimens (e.g., removing tops from vacuum tubes) should wear gloves. Masks and protective eyewear should be worn if mucous-membrane contact with blood or body fluids is anticipated. Gloves should be changed and hands washed after completion of specimen processing.
3. For routine procedures, such as histologic and pathologic studies or microbiologic culturing, a biological safety cabinet is not necessary. However, biological safety cabinets (Class I or II) should be used whenever procedures are conducted that have a high potential for generating droplets. These include activities such as blending, sonicating, and vigorous mixing.
4. Mechanical pipetting devices should be used for manipulating all liquids in the laboratory. Mouth pipetting must not be done.
5. Use of needles and syringes should be limited to situations in which there is no alternative, and the recommendations for preventing injuries with needles outlined under universal precautions should be followed.
6. Laboratory work surfaces should be decontaminated with an appropriate chemical germicide after a spill of blood or other body fluids and when work activities are completed.
7. Contaminated materials used in laboratory tests should be decontaminated before reprocessing or be placed in bags and disposed of in accordance with institutional policies for disposal of infective waste.[24]
8. Scientific equipment that has been contaminated with blood or other body fluids should be decontaminated and cleaned before being repaired in the laboratory or transported to the manufacturer.
9. All persons should wash their hands after completing laboratory activities and should remove protective clothing before leaving the laboratory.

Implementation of universal blood and body-fluid precautions for all patients eliminates the need for warning labels on specimens since blood and other body fluids from all patients should be considered infective.

ENVIRONMENTAL CONSIDERATIONS FOR HIV TRANSMISSION

No environmentally mediated mode of HIV transmission has been documented. Nevertheless, the precautions described below should be taken routinely in the care of all patients.

Sterilization and Disinfection

Standard sterilization and disinfection procedures for patient-care equipment currently recommended for use [25,26] in a variety of health-care settings—including hospitals, medical and dental clinics and offices, hemodialysis centers, emergency care facilities, and long-term nursing-care facilities—are adequate to sterilize or disinfect instruments, devices, or other items contaminated with blood or other body fluids from persons infected with bloodborne pathogens including HIV. [21,23]

Instruments or devices that enter sterile tissue or the vascular system of any patient or through which blood flows should be sterilized before reuse. Devices or items that contact intact mucous membranes should be sterilized or receive highlevel disinfection, a procedure that kills vegetative organisms and viruses but not necessarily large numbers of bacterial spores. Chemical germicides that are registered with the U.S. Environmental Protection Agency (EPA) as "sterilants" may be used either for sterilization or for high-level disinfection depending on contact rims.

Contact lenses used in trial fittings should be disinfected after each fitting by using a hydrogen peroxide contact lens disinfecting system or, if compatible, with heat (78 C-80 C [172.4 F-176.0 F] for 10 minutes.

Medical devices or instruments that require sterilization or disinfection should be thoroughly cleaned before being exposed to the germicide, and the manufacturers instructions for the use of the germicide should be followed. Further it is important that the manufacturer's specifications for compatibility of the medical device with chemical germicides be closely followed. Information on specific label claims of commercial germicides can be obtained by writing to the Disinfectants Branch, Office of Pesticides, Environmental Protection Agency, 401 M Street, SW, Washington, D.C. 20460.

Studies have shown that HIV is inactivated rapidly after being exposed to commonly used chemical germicides at concentrations that are much lower than used in practice.[27-30] Embalming fluids are similar to the types of chemical germicides that have been tested and found to completely inactivate HIV. In addition to commercially available chemical germicides, a solution of sodium hypochlorite (household bleach) prepared daily is an inexpensive and effective germicide. Concentrations ranging from approximately 500 ppm (1:100 dilution of household bleach) sodium hypochlorite to 5,000 ppm (1:10 dilution of household bleach) are effective depending on the amount of organic material (e.g., blood, mucus present on the surface to be cleaned and disinfected.. Commercially available chemical germicides may be more compatible with certain medical devices that might be corroded by repeated exposure to sodium hypochlorite, especially to the 1:10 dilution

Survival of HIV in the Environment

The most extensive study on the survival of HIV after drying involved greatly concentrated HIV samples, i.e., 10 million tissue-culture infectious doses per milliliter. This concentration is at least 100,000 times greater than that typically found in the blood or serum of patients with HIV infection. HIV was detectable by tissue-culture techniques 1-3 days after drying, but the rate of inactivation was rapid. Studies performed at CDC have also shown that drying HIV causes a rapid (within several hours) 1-2 log (90 per cent-99 per cent) reduction in HIV concentration. In tissue-culture fluid, cell-free HIV could be detected up to 15 days at room temperature, up to 11 days at 37 C (98.6 F), and up to 1 day if the HIV was cell-associated.

When considered in the context of environmental conditions in health-care faculties, these results do not require any changes in currency recommended sterilization, disinfection, or housekeeping strategies. When medical devices are contaminated with blood or other body fluids, existing recommendations include the cleaning of these instruments, followed by disinfection or sterilization, depending on the type of medical device. These protocols assume "worstcase" conditions of extreme virologic and micrological contamination, and whether viruses have been inactivated after drying plays no role in formulating these strategies. Consequently, no changes in published procedures for cleaning, disinfecting, or sterilizing need to be made.

Housekeeping

Environmental surfaces such as walls, floors, and other surfaces are not associated with transmission of infections to patients or health-care workers. Therefore, extraordinary attempts to disinfect or sterilize these environmental surfaces are not necessary. However, cleaning and removal of soil should be done routinely.

Cleaning schedules and methods vary according to the area of the hospital or institution, type of surface to be cleaned, and the amount and type of soil present. Horizontal surfaces (e.g., bedside tables and hard-surfaced flooring) in patient-care areas are usually cleaned on a regular basis, when soiling or spills occur, and when a patient is discharged. Cleaning of walls, blinds, and curtains is recommended only if they are visibly soiled. Disinfectant fogging is an unsatisfactory method of decontaminating air and surfaces and is not recommended.

Disinfectant-detergent formulations registered by EPA can be used for cleaning environmental surfaces, but the actual physical removal of micro-organisms by scrubbing is probably at least as important as any antimicrobial effect of the cleaning agent used. Therefore, cost, safely, and acceptability by housekeepers can be the main criteria for selecting any such registered agent. The manufacturers' instructions for appropriate use should be followed.

Cleaning and Decontaminating Spills of Blood or Other Body Fluids

Chemical germicides that are approved for use as "hospital disinfectants" and are tuberculocidal when used at recommended dilutions can be used to decontaminate spills of blood and other body fluids. Strategies for decontaminating spills of blood and other body fluids in a patient-care setting are different than for spills of cultures or other materials in clinical, public health, or research laboratories. In patient-care areas, visible material should first be removed and then the area should be decontaminated. With large spills of cultured or concentrated infectious agents in the laboratory, the contaminated areas should be flooded with a germicide before cleaning, then decontaminated with fresh germicidal chemical. In both settings, gloves should be worn during the cleaning and decontaminating procedures.

Laundry

Although soiled linen has been identified as a source of large numbers of certain pathogenic micro-organisms, the risk of actual disease transmission is negligible. Rather than rigid procedures and specifications, hygienic and common-sense storage and processing of clean and soiled linen are recommended .[26] Soiled linen should be handled as little as possible and with minimum agitation to prevent gross microbial contamination of the air and of persons handling the linen. All soiled linen should be bagged at the location where it was used; it should not be sorted or rinsed in patient-care areas. Linen soiled with blood or body fluids should be placed and transported in bags that prevent leakage. If hot water is used, linen should be washed with detergent in water at least 71 C

(160 F.) for 25 minutes. If low-temperature (≤ 70 C [158 F.]) laundry cycles are used, chemicals suitable for low-temperature washing at proper use concentration should be used.

Infective Waste

There is no epidemiologic evidence to suggest that most hospital waste is any more infective than residential waste. Moreover, there is no epidemiologic evidence that hospital waste has caused disease in the community as a result of improper disposal. Therefore, identifying wastes for which special precautions are indicated is largely a matter of judgment about the relative risk of disease transmission. The most practical approach to the management of infective waste is to identify those wastes with the potential for causing infection during handling and disposal and for which some special precautions appear prudent. Hospital wastes for which special precautions appear prudent include microbiology laboratory waste, pathology waste, and blood specimens or blood products. While any item that has had contact with blood, exudates, or secretions may be potentially infective, it is not usually considered practical or necessary to treat all such waste as infective.[23,26] Infective waste, in general, should either be incinerated or should be autoclaved before disposal in a sanitary landfill. Bulk blood, suctioned fluids, excretions, and secretions may be carefully poured down a drain connected to a sanitary sewer. Sanitary sewers may also be used to dispose of other infectious wastes capable of being ground and flushed into the sewer.

Implementation of Recommended Precautions

Employers of health-care workers should ensure that policies exist for:

1. Initial orientation and continuing education and training of all health-care workers—including students and trainees—on the epidemiology, modes of transmission, and prevention of HIV and other blood-borne infections and the need for routine use of universal blood and body-fluid precautions for all patients.
2. Provision of equipment and supplies necessary to minimize the risk of infection with HIV and other blood-borne pathogens.
3. Monitoring adherence to recommended protective measures. When monitoring reveals a failure to follow recommended precautions, counseling, education, and/or re-training should be provided, and, if necessary, appropriate disciplinary action should be considered.

Professional associations and labour organizations, through continuing education efforts, should emphasize the need for health-care workers to follow recommended precautions.

Serologic Testing for HIV Infection

Background

A person is identified as infected with HIV when a sequence of tests, starting with repeated enzyme immunoassays (EIA) and including a Western blot or similar, more specific assay, are repeatedly reactive. Persons infected with HIV usually develop antibody against the virus within 6-12 weeks after infection.

The sensitivity of the currently licensed EIA tests is at least 99 per cent when they are performed under optimal laboratory conditions on serum specimens from persons infected for $\geq$ 12 weeks. Optimal laboratory conditions include the use of reliable reagents, provision of continuing education of personnel, quality control of procedures, and participation in performance-evaluation programmes. Given this performance, the probability of a false-negative test is remote except during the first several weeks after infection, before detectable antibody is present. The proportion of infected persons with a false-negative test attributed to absence of antibody in the early stages of infection is dependent on both the incidence and prevalence of HIV infection in a population (Table 36.1).

The specificity of the currently licensed EIA tests is approximately 99 per cent when repeatedly reactive tests are considered. Repeat testing of initially reactive specimens by EIA is required to reduce the likelihood of laboratory error. To increase further the specificity of serologic tests, laboratories must use a supplemental test, most often the Western blot, to validate repeatedly reactive EIA results. Under optimal laboratory conditions, the sensitivity of the Western blot test is comparable to or greater than that of a repeatedly reactive EIA, and the Western blot is highly specific when strict criteria are used to interpret the test results. The testing sequence of a repeatedly reactive EIA and a positive Western blot test is highly predictive of HIV infection, even in a population with a low prevalence of infection (Table 36.2). If the Western blot test result is indeterminant, the testina sequence is considered equivocal for HIV infection.

When this occurs, the Western blot test should be repeated on the same serum sample, and, if still indeterminant, the testing sequence should be repeated on a sample collected 3-6 months later. Use of other supplemental tests may aid in interpreting of results on samples that are persistently indeterminant by Western blot.

TABLE -36.1.
Estimated Annual Number of Patients Infected with HIV not Detected by HIV-Antibody Testing in a Hypothetical Hospital with 10,000 Admissions/year*

Beginning pre valence of HIV Infection	Annual incidence of HIV Infection	Approximate number of HIV-infected patients	Approximate number of HIV-infected patients not detected
5.0%	1.0%	550	17-18
5.0%	0.5%	525	11-12
1.0%	0.2%	110	3 4
1.0%	0.1%	105	2-3
0.1%	0.02%	11	0-1
0.1%	0.01%	11	0-1

* The estimates are based on the following assumptions: (1) the sensitivity of the screening test is 99 per cent (i.e., 99 per cent of HIV-infected persons with antibody will be detected), (2) persons infected with HIV will not develop detectable antibody (seroconvert) until 6 weeks (1.5 months) after infection; (3) new infections occur at an equal rate throughout the year; (4) calculations of the number of HIV-infected persons in the patient population are based on the mid-year prevalence, which is the beginning prevalence plus half the annual incidence of infections.

TABLE -36.2.
Predictive Value of Positive HIV-Antibody Tests in Hypothetical Populations with Different Prevalences of Infection

	Prevalence of infection	Predictive value of positive test
Repeatedly reactive enzyme immunoassay (EIA)†	0.2%	28.41%
	2.0%	80.16%
	20.0%	98.02%
Repeatedly reactive EIA followed by positive Western blot (WB)§	0.2%	99.75%
	2.0%	99.97%
	20.0%	99.99%

* Proportion of persons with positive test results who are actually infected with HIV.
† Assumes EIA sensitivity of 99.0% and specificity of 99.5%.
§ Assumes WB sensitivity of 99.0% and specificity of 99.9%.

Testing of Patients

Previous CDC recommendations have emphasized the value of HIV serologic testing of patients for: (1) management of parenteral or mucous-membrane exposures of health-care workers, (2) patient diagnosis and management, and (3) counseling and serologic testing to prevent and control HIV transmission in the community. In addition, more recent recommendations have stated that hospitals, in conjunction with state and local health departments, should periodically determine the prevalence of HIV infection among patients from age groups at highest risk of infection.[32]

Adherence to universal blood and body-fluid precautions recommended for the care of all patients will minimize the risk of transmission of HIV and other blood-borne pathogens from patients to health-care workers. The utility of routine HIV serologic testing of patients as an adjunct to universal precautions is unknown. Results of such testing may not be available in emergency or outpatient settings. In addition, some recently infected patients will not have detectable antibody to HIV (Table 36.1).

Personnel in some hospitals have advocated serologic testing of patients in settings in which exposure of health-care workers to large amounts of patients' blood may be anticipated. Specific patients for whom serologic testing has been advocated include those undergoing major operative procedures and those undergoing treatment in critical-care units, especially if they have conditions involving uncontrolled bleeding. Decisions regarding the need to establish testing programmes for patients should be made by physicians or individual institutions. In addition, when deemed appropriate, testing of individual patients may be performed on agreement between the patient and the physician providing care.

In addition to the universal precautions recommended for all patients, certain additional precautions for the care of HIV-infected patients undergoing major surgical operations have been proposed by personnel in some hospitals. For example, surgical procedures on an HIV-infected patient might be altered so that hand-to-hand passing of sharp instruments would be eliminated; stapling instruments rather than hand-suturing equipment might be used to perform tissue approximation; electrocautery devices rather than scalpels might be used as cutting instruments; and, even though uncomfortable, gowns that totally prevent seepage of blood onto the skin of members of the operative team might be worn. While such modifications might further minimize the risk of HIV infection for members of the operative team, some of these techniques could result in prolongation of operative time and could potentially have an adverse effect on the patient.

Testing programmes, if developed, should include the following principles:

- # Obtaining consent for testing.
- # Informing patients of test results, and providing counseling for seropositive patients by properly trained persons.

- # Assuring that confidentiality safeguards are in place to limit knowledge of test results to those directly involved in the care of infected patients or as required by law.
- # Assuring that identification of infected patients will not result in denial of needed care or provision of suboptimal care.
- # Evaluating prospectively, (1) the efficacy of the programme in reducing the incidence of parenteral, mucous-membrane, or significant cutaneous exposures of health-care workers to the blood or other body fluids of HIV-infected patients and (2) the effect of modified procedures on patients.

Testing of Health-Care Workers

Although transmission of HIV from infected health-care workers to patients has not been reported, transmission during invasive procedures remains a possibility. Transmission of hepatitis B virus (HBV)—a blood-borne agent with a considerably greater potential for nosocomial spread—from health-care workers to patients has been documented. Such transmission has occurred in situations (e.g., oral and gynecologic surgery) in which health-care workers, when tested, had very high concentrations of HBV in their blood (at least 100 million infectious virus particles per milliliter, a concentration much higher than occurs with HIV infection), and the health-care workers sustained a puncture wound while performing invasive procedures or had exudative or weeping lesions or microlacerations that allowed virus to contaminate instruments or open wounds of patients.[33,34]

The hepatitis B experience indicates that only those health-care workers who perform certain types of invasive procedures have transmitted HBV to patients. Adherence to recommendations in this document will minimize the risk of transmission of HIV and other blood-borne pathogens from health-care workers to patients during invasive procedures. Since transmission of HIV from infected health-care workers performing invasive procedures to their patients has not been reported and would be expected to occur only very rarely, if at all, the utility of routine testing of such health-care workers to prevent transmission of HIV cannot be assessed. If consideration is given to developing a serologic testing programme for health-care workers who perform invasive procedures, the frequency of testing, as well as the issues of consent, confidentiality, and consequences of test results—as previously outlined for testing programmes for patients—must be addressed.

Management of Infected Health-Care Workers

Health-care workers with impaired immune systems resulting from HIV infection or other causes are at increased risk of acquiring or experiencing serious complications of infectious disease. Of particular concern is the risk of severe infection following exposure to patients with infectious diseases that are easily transmitted if appropriate precautions are not taken (e.g., measles, varicella). Any health-care worker with an impaired immune system should be counseled about the potential risk associated with taking care of patients with any transmissible infection and should continue to follow existing recommendations for infection control to minimize risk of exposure to other infectious agents.[7,35] Recommendations of the Immunization Practices Advisory Committee (ACIP) and institutional policies concerning requirements for vaccinating health-care workers with live-virus vaccines (e.g., measles, rubella) should also be considered.

The question of whether workers infected with HIV—especially those who perform invasive procedures—can adequately and safely be allowed to perform patient-care duties or whether their work assignments should be changed must be determined on an individual basis. These decisions should be made by the health-care worker's personal physician(s) in conjunction with the medical directors and personnel health service staff of the employing institution or hospital.

Management of Exposures

If a health-care worker has a parenteral (e.g., needlestick or cut) or mucousmembrane (e.g., splash to the eye or mouth) exposure to blood or other body fluids or has a cutaneous exposure involving large amounts of blood or prolonged contact with blood—especially when the exposed skin is chapped, abraded, or afflicted with dermatitis—the source patient should be informed of the incident and tested for serologic evidence of HIV infection after consent is obtained. Policies should be developed for testing source patients in situations in which consent cannot be obtained (e.g., an unconscious patient).

If the source patient has AIDS, is positive for HIV antibody, or refuses the test, the health-care worker should be counseled regarding the risk of infection and evaluated clinically and serologically for evidence of HIV infection as soon as possible after the exposure. The health-care worker should be advised to report and seek medical evaluation for any acute febrile illness that occurs within 12 weeks after the exposure. Such an illness--particularly one characterized by fever, rash, or lymphadenopathy— may be indicative of recent HIV infection. Seronegative health-care workers should be retested 6 weeks post-exposure and on a periodic basis thereafter (e.g., 12 weeks and 6 months after exposure) to determine whether transmission has occurred. During this follow-up period—especially the first 6-12 weeks after exposure, when most infected persons are expected to seroconvert—exposed health-care workers should follow U.S. Public Health Service (PHS) recommendations for preventing transmission of HIV. [36,37]

No further follow-up of a health-care worker exposed to infection as described above is necessary if the source patient is seronegative unless the source patient is at high risk of HIV infection. In the latter case, a subsequent specimen (e.g., 12 weeks following exposure) may be obtained from the health-care worker for antibody testing. If the source patient cannot be identified, decisions regarding appropriate follow-up should be individualized. Serologic testing should be available to a health-care workers who are concerned that they may have been infected with HIV.

If a patient has a parenteral or mucous-membrane exposure to blood or other body fluid of a health-care worker, the patient should be informed of the incident, and the same procedure outlined above for management of exposures should be followed for both the source health-care worker and the exposed patient.

References

1. CDC. Acquired immunodeficiency syndrome (AIDS): Precautions for clinical and laboratory staffs. MMWR 1982;31:577-80.
2. CDC. Acquired immunodeficiency syndrome (Aids) Precautions for health-care workers and allied professionals. MMWA 1983;32:450-1.
3. CDC. Recommendations for preventing transmission of infection with human T-lymphotropic virus type III,/ lymphadenopathy-associated virus in the workplace. MMWA 1985;34:681-6, 691-5.
4. CDC. Recommendations for preventing transmission of infection with human T-lymphotropic virus type III/ lymphadenopathy-associated virus during Invasive procedures. MMWR 1986;35:221-3.
5. CDC. Recommendations for preventing possible transmission of human T-lymphotropic virus type III, /lymphadenopathy-associated virus from tears. MMWR 1985;34:533-4.
6. CDC. Recommendations for providing dialysis treatment to patients infected with human T-lymphotropic virus type III/lymphadenopathy-associated virus infection. MMWR 1986;35:376-8, 383.
7. Garner JS, Simmons BP. Guideline for isolation precautions in hospitals. Infect Control 1983;4 (suppl) :245-325.
8. CDC. Recommended infection control practices for dentists MMWR 1986;35:237-42.
9. McCray E, The Co-operative Needlestick Surveillance Group. Occupational risk of the acquired immunodeficiency syndrome among health care workers. N Engl J Med 1986;314:1127-32.

10. Henderson DK, Saah AJ, Zak BJ, at al Risk of nosocomial infection with human T-cell Iymphotropic virus type III/ymphadenopathy-associated virus in a large cohort of intensively exposed health care workers. Ann Intern Med 1986; 104:W-7.
11. Gerberding JL, Bryant--LeBlanc CE, Nelson K, et al Risk of transmitting the human immunodeficiency virus, cytomegalovirus, and hepatitis B virus to health care workers exposed to patients with AIDS and AIDS-related conditions. J Infect Dis 1987;156:1-8.
12. McEvoy M, Poner K, Mortimer P. Simmons N. Shanson D. Prospective study of clinical, laboratory, and concillory staff with accidental exposures to blood or other body fiuids from patients infected with HIV. Bo Med J 1987;29:1595-7.
13. Anonymous. Needlestick transmission of HTLV-III from a patient infected in Africa. Lancet 1984;2:1376-7.
14. Oksenhendler E, Haizic M, he, Le Roux JM, Rabian C, Clauvel JP. HIV infection with seroconversion after a superficial needlesfick injury to the finger. N Engl. J Med 1986;315:582.
15. Neisson-Vernant C, Arfi S., Mathez D, Leibowdch J. Monplaisir N. Needlestick HIV seroconversion in a nurse. Lancet 1986;2:814.
16. Grint P. McEvoy M. Two associated cases of the acquired immune deficiency syndrome (AIDS). PHLS Commun Dis Rep 1985;42:4.
17. CDC. Apparent transmission of human T-lymphotropic virus type III/lymphadenopathy associated virus from a child to a mother providing health care. MMWR 1986;35:76-9.
18. CDC. Update: Human immunodeficiency virus infections in health-care workers exposed to blood of infected patients. MMWR 1987;36:285-9.
19. Kline RS, Phelan J. Friedland GH, et al Low occupational risk for HIV infection for dental professionals [Abstracts] fin: Abstracts from the III International Conference on AIDS, 1-5 June 1985. Washington, DC: 155.
20. Baker JL, Kelen GD, Sivenson KT, Quinn TC. Unsuspected human immunodeficiency virus in critically ill emergency patients. JAMA 1987;257:Z609-11.
21. Favero My. Dialysis-associated diseases and their control in: Bennett JV, Brachman PS, eds. Hospital infections. Boston: Little, Brown and Company, 1985:Z 67-84.
22. Richardson JH, Barkley WE, eds. Biosafety in microbiological and biomedical laboratories, 1984. Washington, DC: US Department of Health and Human Services, Public Health Service. HHS publication no. (CDC) 84-8395.
23. CDC. Human T-lymphotropic virus type III/lymphadenopathy-associated virus: Agent summary statement. MMWR 1986,35:540-2, 547-9.
24. Environmental Protection Agency. EPA guide for infectious waste management. Washington, DC : U.S. Environmental Protection Agency, May 1986 (Publication no. EPA/530-SW-86-014).
25. Favero MS. Sterilization, disinfection, arid antisepsis in the hospital. In: Manual of clinical microbiology. 4th ed. Washington, DC: American Society for Microbiology, 1985:129-37.

26. Garner JS, Favero MS. Guideline for handwashing and hospital environmental control, 1985. Atlanta: Public Health Service, Centers for Disease Control, 1985. HHS publication no. 99-1117.
27. Spire B. Montagnier L, Barre-Sinoussi F. Chermann JC. Inactivation of lymphadenopathy associated virus by chemical disinfectants. Lancet 1984;2:899-901.
28. Martin LS, McDougal JS, Loskoski SL. Disinfection and inactivation of the human T lymphotropic virus type III/lymphadenopathy-associated virus. J Infect Dis 1985; 152:400-3.
29. McDougal JS, Martin LS, Cort SP, et al. Thermal inactivation of the acquired immunodeficiency syndrome virus-III/lymphadenopathy-associated virus, with special reference to antihemophilic factor. J Clin Invest 1985;76:875-7.
30. Spire B. Barre-Sinoussi,,F, Doront D, Montagnier L, Chermann JC. Inactivation of lymphadenopathy-associated virus by heat, gamma rays, and ultraviolet light. Lancet 1985;1:188-9.
31. Resnik L, Veren K, Salahuddin SZ, Tondreau S. Markham PD. Stability and inactivation of HTLV-III/LAV under clinical and laboratory environments. JAMA 1986;255:1887-91.
32. CDC. Public Health Service (PHS) guidelines for counseling and antibody testing to prevent HIV infection and AIDS. MMWR 1987,3:509-15..
33. Kane MA, Lenau LA. Transmission of HBV from dental personnel to patients. J Am Dent Assoc 1985;110:634-6.
34. Lettau LA, Smith JD, Williams D, et. al. Transmission of hepatitis B with resultant restriction of surgical practice. JAMA 1986;255:934-7.
35. Williams WW. Guideline for infection control in hospital personnel. Infect Control 1983,4 (supply) :326-49.
36. CDC. Prevention of acquired immune deficiency syndrome (AIDS): Report of inter-agency recommendations. MMWR 1983;32:101-3.
37. CDC. Provisional Public Health Service inter-agency recommendations for screening donated blood and plasma for antibody to the virus causing acquired immunodeficiency syndrome. MMWR 1985;34:1-5.

37

HIV in the Workplace: Dealing with the Issues

Joyce Leyones and
Jenny Huddart
UNDP, New York

INTRODUCTION

Vinod, a skilled mechanic, has recently disclosed he is infected with HIV to his fellow worker and good friend Jyoti. He now sits isolated in the cafeteria.

Teresita, a beloved teacher in a rural community, has been dismissed from her job because of her HIV positive status.

What is obvious in these scenarios is that education about, and an understanding of, HIV has not taken place. Discrimination and dismissal will not remove the threat of HIV infection nor help to create a congenial workplace environment. The only protection we have against the spread of HIV is education. Clear, concise and medically correct facts help to reduce the fear and anxiety commonly associated with HIV and to prevent any loss in worker productivity which may result from these far too common responses.

Why is an Understanding of the Implications of HIV Important to the Workplace?

"Today there are 2.3 billion economically active people in the world. The workplace environment plays a central role in the lives of people everywhere. A consideration of HIV/ AIDS and the workplace will strengthen the capacity to deal effectively with the problem of HIV/AIDS at the local, national and international levels." (Statement from the Consultation on AIDS and the Workplace, WHO/ILO Geneva, June 1988).

HIV is a nondiscriminatory virus, affecting people of all cultures, religions and races. The most common route of transmission is unprotected sexual activity. This fact makes men and women in their most productive and sexually active years, those between 18-45 years of age, the most vulnerable group for becoming infected. The largest organized target audience of the vulnerable age group is found in the workplace where employers have a lot to lose if employees become infected with the virus.

Because of its infection pattern, unlike other epidemics, HIV directly affects the social and economic environment of the workplace. Due to the fear and stigma currently surrounding the virus, HIV can cause interpersonal, social and discriminatory problems within the workplace.

It can also affect the company's productivity when in later stages of the infection, increased absenteeism, loss of skilled labour, and costs of retraining or hiring new workers begin to take their toll.

One vital factor which distinguishes HIV from other diseases is that it can remain dormant in an individual for many years before the onset of illness. During this time, the individual can lead a healthy and productive life; this has psychological and economic implications for the worker as well as for the employer. Each can continue to receive the full benefits of the working relationship.

Another significant point about this virus, unlike other viruses, is that infection can be prevented by changes in personal behaviour. To lessen the impact of HIV on the workplace, it is important to develop a comprehensive HIV/ AIDS programme which includes workplace policies to ensure humane treatment of those who are HIV positive, prepares managers to answer questions and confrontations related to HIV, and teaches workers how the infection is transmitted and what they can do to prevent it. All employees should be supplied with the facts and support needed to practice the preventive behaviour which will reduce their vulnerability to infection and their fear of those infected. Some employers will also want to consider offering additional health services.

The Purpose of the Role Plays

Statistics have shown us that information alone is important but not enough to make people adopt the changes in behaviour necessary to protect themselves from HIV infection. This should not come as a surprise, for example, advertising campaigns against smoking do not stop smokers. Often a more personal experience is necessary to convince people to change their behaviour. The media have been successful in using well known characters to tell stories about living with HIV; community members with HIV have been able to convey the message. To reach a large audience, videos, films and slide shows have also been effective.

Another technique, which has great value in helping individuals to personalize issues, is to give them an opportunity to explore the predicament by involving them as participants in a simulation experience. Keeping this in mind, these role plays, based on reports of actual situations, have been developed to help managers confront and discuss the issues related to HIV in the workplace.

The role plays assist participants to:

1. Explore the issues surrounding HIV/AIDS in the workplace;
2. Identify the potential contributions of NGOs in assisting the business sector to address the issues of HIV/AIDS in the workplace;
3 Practice skills in developing co-operative strategies for dealing with HIV/AIDS in the workplace.

Before implementing these role plays, a basic understanding of HIV and AIDS is needed, including how the infection is (and is not) transmitted and its progression from infection to AIDS-related symptoms.

BACKGROUND

Basic Facts

What is AIDS?

Acquired Immunodeficiency Syndrome, AIDS is the result of infection with the Human Immunodeficiency Virus (HIV). The virus is transmitted primarily through sexual intercourse, although infection can also occur through the transmission of infected blood and blood products. Slowly, the virus disables the immune system which is the body's primary line of defense against disease. As the body's immune system breaks down, it becomes more vulnerable to a host of opportunistic infections which leave a person susceptible to pneumonia, tuberculosis, oral lesions and occasionally rare forms of cancer—diseases which rarely affect healthy immune systems. The symptoms and signs of HIV related illnesses are complex, vary greatly and can include persistent diarrhea, weight loss, oral and skin lesions, and loss of appetite. It is impossible to tell from looking at a person or by hearing his symptoms whether or not he is infected with the virus. It is important to note that these symptoms are commonly associated with many other diseases. Diagnosis of HIV infection can only be made through a blood test .

We know a great deal more about HIV now than we did when it was first identified in 1985. We know how it is transmitted, how the body reacts to it and most importantly, we know how to protect ourselves. We still do not know how to cure it and there is no definitive answer as to the origin of the virus. This gap in our knowledge has no bearing on the development of a workplace programme to control its transmission. The knowledge we do have clearly shows that casual contact, such as in the workplace setting, does not put a person at risk of infection.

HOW IS HIV TRANSMITTED?

There are only three ways the virus can be transmitted.

1. By having unprotected sexual intercourse with a person who has the virus. This accounts for approximately 80 per cent of the worldwide transmission of the virus; the percentage in developing countries is even greater.
2. By being injected with contaminated blood, blood products or unsterile equipment; 35 per cent of the worldwide transmissions occur in this manner. Five to ten per cent of global infections are due to the reuse of contaminated needles by intravenous drug users.
3. By an infected mother passing the virus onto her child through pregnancy or breastfeeding; this comprises 5-10 per cent of the entire transmission figure.

HOW IS HIV NOT TRANSMITTED?

The virus cannot be transmitted:

1. Through the air, by sneezing, coughing, or breathing
2. Through casual physical contact, such as touching, hugging or kissing
3. Through water, as in swimming pools
4. Through sharing utensils or food or the same telephone
5. Through toilets
6. Through mosquitoes

HOW CAN HIV TRANSMISSION BE PREVENTED?

1. By practicing safer sex: keeping to one partner whose sexual history is known to you; practicing non-penetrative sex or using a high quality latex condom for every act of sexual intercourse.
2. By always using clean, sterilized needles and avoiding unnecessary skin piercing.
3. By never sharing injecting drug equipment.
4. By receiving blood transfusions only when necessary and only with properly screened blood.

ISSUES

What are the Issues that HIV Brings into the Workplace?

As HIV enters the workplace, government agencies, companies and labour unions are all struggling to develop strategies to respond to the issues it raises. What follows is a discussion of these issues; relevant policy statements of the United Nations are included as a guide to help others determine their own response. (The complete UN HIV/AIDS Personnel Policy can be found in the p. No. 483).

1. DENIAL: A common misconception is that HIV is someone else's problem. It is a disease of selected groups commonly referred to as "high risk" groups, i.e., promiscuous people, intravenous drug users, foreigners.

This ignores the evidence that the greatest single mode of transmission of HIV is unprotected heterosexual intercourse. The virus does not put groups at risk. People practicing unsafe behaviour put themselves at risk.

Statistics demonstrate that the virus is already spreading at an alarming rate in Asia. By the year 2000, the number of the new cases in Asia is expected to surpass that of Africa, the overwhelming majority of them, men and women in their most economically productive years.

Continued beliefs that HIV only affects a selected population is a dangerous practice, allowing large sectors of society to feel protected from the epidemic thus blocking the understanding of the necessity to develop effective intervention strategies.

2. FEAR: Ten years into the epidemic and still the most common response to the subject of AIDS is fear Misinformation, misconceptions and dread of the unknown heighten the anxiety felt by those who have their first encounter with a person with AIDS, or someone known to have HIV.

   Fear is best handled by allowing people to express openly their concerns. Acknowledgment of their feelings and discussion about them helps to dissipate the fear.

3. DISCRIMINATION: Fear often leads to discrimination against people who have HIV Loss of jobs, friends, homes are not uncommon occurrences. Mistaken beliefs that casual contacts can spread the virus have led to the isolation and loss of dignity and respect to which people infected with the virus often become subject.

Presenting medically correct facts and discussing the

misconceptions that cause fear will reduce the discrimination that results from it.

4. CONFIDENTIALITY: A person's medical history is confidential Revelation of items such as a person's HIV status can lead to the consequences of his/her being stigmatized and subjected to discrimination.

HIV is still associated with discrimination and stigma due to misconceptions of how the virus is transmitted. Cases of people losing their jobs, homes and families have occurred after disclosure that they are infected with the HIV virus. The medical facts regarding transmission of the virus clearly prove that ordinary workplace behaviour and interaction does not lead to the spread of infection. To reduce disruption in the workplace and protect the infected individual, privacy about his/her status is required.

> United Nations Policy states "Confidentiality regarding all medical information, including HIV/AIDS status, must be maintained "

5. SCREENING: To attempt to create an HIV free environment business may consider screening or pretesting potential employees to determine their HIV status as a condition of employment.

The practice of eliminating HIV positive people from the workforce has no justification as a public health measure nor is it considered fair employment practice. Furthermore due to the "window period" or amount of time it takes between becoming infected and having antibodies to the virus form in the blood, screening would not even reveal all individuals who are HIV+. Even if the employer believed that screening would reduce the number of infected people who gain entrance into the workplace, pre-employment testing certainly does not prevent an employee from practicing behaviours that will expose him or her to infection after employment.

> UN Policy states: "There will be no screening of candidates for recruitment".

6. TESTING: Testing of employees has also been used as a means to eliminate workers who contract HIV while employed

Testing for HIV is not 100 per cent accurate; the "window period" makes the exact date upon which antibodies will appear in the blood undeterminable. Estimates range from 6 weeks to 6 months; however, researchers have found that some individuals take longer, sometimes years, to develop antibodies. Testing is an expensive prospect which must be repeated every 3-6 months if its objective is to identify all cases of HIV. In many countries, legal regulations limit the type of testing that can be required.

Testing should not be done unless a person is fully aware of the meaning and consequences of the test results and has provided his or her consent. An interview with a trained counsellor should give the individual interested in being tested an opportunity to express his concerns and to ask questions about the test. It is important to assure the individual that confidentiality is guaranteed. Counselling is essential both before testing and upon receipt of test results.

> UN Policy states: "Voluntary testing with pre-and post-counselling and assured confidentiality should be made available to all UN staff members and their families".

7. POLICY: Issues related to sick leave, increased inability to perform the same strenuous job, health insurance needs, retirement rules, and policies on hiring and dismissal will all need to be reviewed."

Policies should reflect the medical facts, confirm basic human rights, and ensure workplace harmony. In many instances, HIV can be added to the policy in existence on serious illnesses. In all cases, the policy should be endorsed by top management and understood at all levels.

A person's job not only provides him or her with daily subsistence but helps to define a person's life. Most people who have discovered themselves to be HIV+ are fully capable of carrying out their job responsibilities and find comfort in continuing their daily employment.

Under what circumstances should an HIV+ individual be dismissed or deemed ineligible for employment? Facts show that a person infected with HIV does not present a risk of infection for others in daily casual contact. Facts also show that once a person is infected, s/he can lead a healthy, active and productive life for an average of 7-10 years. If this person is capable of performing in his or her job, there is no medical justification for dismissal.

When related illnesses cause a person with HIV to need special attention, such as longer sick leave or a less strenuous job, businesses should accommodate the situation following the same policies as are applied to other illnesses.

> UN Policy states: (a) The only medical criteria for recruitment is fitness to work . (b) HIV infection or AIDS should not, of itself, be considered as a basis for termination of employment. (c) If fitness to work is impaired by HIV-related illness, reasonable alternative working arrangements should be made. (d) UN staff members should enjoy health and social protection in the same manner as other UN employees suffering from serious illness."

8. RESPONSIBILITY: Having a healthy and productive workforce is essential to the workplace. Preventive services such as condom promotion and counsellin.g referrals can be offered to ensure the personal health of workers Companies that provide health care should consider offering services for counselling and treatment of sexually transmitted diseases.

The simplest way to help employees protect themselves against infection is to provide accurate and up-to-date information. Messages on the need to have medical check ups for STD (Sexually Transmitted Disease) control are also important. The vulnerability to HIV increases when an STD is present.

After education, the best defense we have against HIV is the use of high quality condoms. Condoms act as a barrier preventing the virus from passing through, thereby reducing the risk of transmission. Having condoms available at the workplace for distribution or purchase is an innovative way of helping to ensure safer behaviour.

In the absence of a cure, counselling for individuals who have HIV or who suspect they might be infected takes on new significance. People need to express their frustration and anger. Often a linkup with a local health center or NGO can set up a referral system for pre- and post-test counselling, as well as, for illness related help.

Established links with hospitals or health care centers in which blood is known to be screened for the HIV virus can be a life saving matter.

> UN Policy: (a) UN Staff and their families should be provided with sufficient, updated information to enable them to protect themselves from HIV infection and to cope with the presence of AIDS. (b) All UN staff members and their families should be made aware of where safe blood may be obtained. (c) All UN staff members and their families should have access to condoms."

How can these Issues Best be Addressed?

The disruption in the workplace caused by the fear of HIV can be minimized by providing an HIV education and support system to all employees and by establishing HIV related personnel policies well in advance of any problems. However, only a comprehensive educational programme supported by top management will encourage employees to comply.

Successful workplace education programmes have approached executives first to help them develop an understanding of the basic facts regarding HIV. This knowledge can then be used to develop appropriate policy measures that will maintain a high level of worker productivity, ensure the rights and dignity of all, clarify legal issues, and create an atmosphere conducive to caring for and promoting the health of all workers.

Next, managers must understand and support the policy developed by their company and be knowledgeable enough about HIV/AIDS to respond to the concerns of their subordinates. They must be informed about their obligations once an employee becomes ill. They also need to know how to handle fearful workers and potential crisis situations.

Finally, a workplace education programme meeting the needs of all workers must be developed. Each programme must be tailored to the particular audience and company. Union representatives or worker spokespersons can be involved in the design of the educational programme. Logistical decisions regarding who, where, how and when this programme should be undertaken must be determined both to meet the objectives of the programme and to create the minimum disruption in the workplace.

Methods of Addressing the Issues

The first step in addressing the issues is acknowledging the need for an HIV/AIDS education programme. This needs to be followed up by contacts with professional groups who can assist in the development of that programme. In some countries, local health departments or National AIDS Committees may have material to assist in this process. The WHO has several publications that may be relevant. In other countries, local non-government agencies may be your strongest ally.

As the epidemic spreads at an increasing rate, many NGOs have realized the importance of developing preventive programmes. Many have targeted the workplace as an appropriate setting for their efforts. Training modules, videos, peer training programmes, and written materials have been developed to assist in comprehensive workplace intervention programmes. A business/NGO collaboration is a strong deterrent to the spread of HIV.

An NGO, after providing basic education about the medical facts and societal realities of HIV, can help management prepare workplace policies that will guide the company's response to questions and concerns about HIV. An NGO can also be asked to prepare management to deal with HIV related issues that are likely to arise in the workplace. Then, in conjunction with management, it can draw up the most effective and efficient method of providing training to line workers. If necessary, the NGO can offer ongoing support in the form of pre and post-test counselling, individual sessions or training of trainers; others can offer legal guidance, support for condom distribution, family counselling or education and an opportunity to allow people openly to discuss sexuality.

What Else can be Done?

As the worker actually begins to display signs of illness, accommodations may be worked out. Shorter work weeks, being able to work at home, more rest periods, a reduced work load, a restructuring of the job, relocation to a less demanding position have all been methods of dealing with an increased inability to perform the normal assignment.

How Else Can Business Contribute?

To increase the understanding of HIV in society and to reach other workplaces, the following suggestions are provided:

1. Share your company's experience with other companies. Personal experience works in helping others follow the lead. Use the media, Chambers of Commerce or newsletters.
2. Produce a video on AIDS in the Workplace for your company's educational programmeme. Share it with other firms.
3. Become an advocate for AIDS in the workplace legislation.
4. Host an AIDS in the Workplace Conference.
5. Volunteer to work for AIDS organizations and encourage employees to do the same.
6. Contributions from business to the non government community can include printing of brochures, photocopying of leaflets, providing space for meetings.
7. Start a resource library of AIDS information.
8. Raise funds for research or care facilities.
9. Provide HIV/AIDS information for the worker's family. Organize a meeting for spouses. Produce simple material for presentation to their children.
10. Provide informed speakers for schools and community groups.

I. GLOSSARY

AIDS.: Acquired Immune Deficiency Syndrome (AIDS) is the last stage of the virus known as HIV. The body's immune system has been seriously damaged, leaving it vulnerable to infections that can ultimately result in death.

ANTIBODY: A protein produced in the blood to fight infection.

AT RISK: Practicing behaviours which could lead to becoming infected with HIV, e.g., engaging in unprotected sex, sharing of unsterilized injecting equipment.

HIV: Human Immunodeficiency Virus (HIV) is the virus that causes AIDS.

HIV-: Having been tested for HIV antibodies in the blood and discovering that none exist.

HIV+: This signifies the status of one who has been found to have, through blood screening, antibodies to HIV in the blood. It indicates that one is infected with HIV and can infect others but it does not indicate a person has AIDS. It can also be referred to as being seropositive.

HIV TESTING: Screening the blood for HIV antibodies. The two most common tests are the ELISA and Western Blot.

NGO: Non Government Organization usually performing a service.

SAFER SEX: Engaging in sexual intercourse with the protection of a condom; having fewer sexual partners, keeping to one sexual partner whose sexual history is known to you.

SERONEGATIVE: see HIV

SEROPOSITIVE: See HIV+

STD: Sexually Transmitted Disease whose presence increases the possibility of HIV receptivity. HIV is predominately a sexually transmitted infection.

WINDOW PERIOD: The time between infection and the appearance of HIV antibodies in the blood system. This can vary greatly in length. It is also why mandatory testing is not an effective devise to determine the HIV status of individuals.

II. *UN HIV/AIDS*

Personnel Policy

A. Information, Education and Other Preventive Health Measures

(i) UN Staff and their families should be provided with sufficient, updated information to enable them to protect themselves from HIV infection and to cope with the presence of AIDS.

To this end all UN bodies are encouraged to develop and implement an active staff education strategy for HIV/AIDS utilizing inter alia, the handbook on AIDS for UN employees and their families produced by WHO and identifying in the field local sources experienced by HIV/ AIDS counselling, to provide confidential follow up. The staff of the UN Medical Service should be fully involved in such staff education programmes. They should receive any additional professional education that they may be required; and all pertinent information material on HIV and ADDS, supplied and updated by WHO, should be available through them at all duty stations

(ii) All UN staff members and their families should be made aware of where safe blood may be obtained.

To accomplish this task, the WHO Global Blood Safety Initiative, in co-operation with the UN Medical Service, should establish and regularly update a list of reliable and operational blood transfusion centres for circulation to UN headquarters, regional offices and duty stations. The UN Medical Services should also make efforts to ensure that blood transfusions are performed only when absolutely necessary.

(iii) UN Resident Co-ordinators must exercise their responsibility to adopt measures to reduce the frequency of motor vehicle accidents, not only because of their attendant high mortality and morbidity, but because they present a particular risk for HIV infection in those localities lacking safe blood supplies.

UN Resident Co-ordinators are, therefore, encouraged to consider the following measures for reinforcement or for general adoption if not already applied; and to circulate them to all personnel at the duty station together with instructions on the use of public transport.

* the fitting of and compulsory use of seat belts in all UN vehicles;
* proper training in off-road use of 4-wheel drives;
* prohibition against the personal use of vehicles when an official driver is available;
* compulsory use of helmets for all riders of motorbikes;
* organization of first-aid training sessions; and
* equipping UN vehicles with first-aid kits containing macromolecular solutions (plasma expanders).

(iv) All UN staff members and their families should have access to disposable syringes and needles.

The UN Medical Service should provide disposable syringes and needles to staff on duty travel to areas where there is no guarantee of the proper sterilization of such materials. They should be accompanied by a certificate in all UN official languages explaining the reasons why they are being carried. Regional offices and other duty stations should stock disposable injection material for the use of UN staff and their families. This stock should be available at UN dispensaries, where such exist, or at the WHO duty station in the country.

(v) All UN staff members and their families should have access to condoms.

Condoms should be available through UNFPA and/or WHO at those duty stations where there is not a reliable and consistent supply of high quality condoms from the private sector. Access should be free, simple and discreet.

B. Voluntary Testing, Counselling and Confidentialily

Voluntary testing with pre- and postcounselling and assured confidentiality should be made available to all UN staff members and their families.

Adequate and confidential facilities for voluntary and confirmatory testing and counselling should be made available locally to UN staff members and their families, with UN bodies acting in close collaboration with the UN Medical Service and WHO. Specific procedures must be developed by UN bodies to maintain confidentiality with respect to negative as well as positive results from an HIV test, including whether such a test has been taken. Only the person tested has the right to release information concerning his/her HIV status.

C. Terms of Appointment and Service

Pre-recruitment and Employment Prospects

(i) The only medical criterion for recruitment is fitness to work.

(ii) HIV infection does not, in itself, constitute a lack of fitness to work.

(iii) There will be no HIV screening of candidates for recruitment.

(iv) AIDS will be treated as any other medical condition in considering medical classification.

(v) HIV testing with the specific and informed consent of the candidate may be requited if AIDS is clinically suspected.

(vi) Nothing in the pre-employment examination should be considered as obliging any candidate to declare his or her HIV status.

(vii) For any assignment in a country which requires HIV testing for residence, this requirement must appear in the vacancy notice.

Continuity of Employment

(i) HIV infection or AIDS should not, of itself, be considered as a basis for termination of employment.

(ii) If fitness to work is impaired by HIV-related illness, reasonable alternative working arrangements should be made.

(iii) UN staff members with AIDS should enjoy health and social protection in the same manner as other UN employees suffering from serious illness.

(a) HIV/AIDS screening, whether direct (HIV testing), indirect (assessment of risk behaviours) or asking questions about tests already taken, should not be required.

(b) Confidentiality regarding all medical information, including HIV/AIDS status, must be maintained.

(c) There should be no obligation on the part of the employee to inform the employer regarding his or her HIV/AIDS status.

(d) Persons in the workplace affected by, or perceived to be affected by HIV/AIDS, must be protected from stigmatization and discrimination by co-workers, unions, employers or clients.

(e) HIV-infected employees and those with AIDS should not be discriminated against, including access to and receipt of benefits from statutory social security programmes and occupationally related schemes.

The administrative, personnel and financial implications of these principles under terms of appointment and service should be monitored and periodically reviewed.

D. Health Insurance Benefits Programmes

(i) Health insurance coverage should be available for all UN employees regardless of HIV status.

There should be no pre- or post-employment testing for HIV infection.

(ii) Health insurance premiums for UN employees should not be affected by HIV status.

No testing for HIV infection should be permitted with respect to any health insurance scheme.

III. RESPONDING TO AIDS: TEN PRINCIPLES FOR THE WORKPLACE

1. People with AIDS or HIV (Human Immunodeficiency Virus) infection are entitled to the same rights and opportunities as people with other serious or life threatening illnesses.
2. Employment policies must, at a minimum, comply with federal, state and local laws and regulations.
3. Employment policies should be based on the scientific and epidemiological evidence that people with AIDS or HIV infection do not pose a risk of transmission of the virus to coworkers through ordinary workplace contact.
4. The highest levels of management and union leadership should unequivocally endorse non discriminatory employment policies and education programmes about AIDS.
5. Employers and unions should communicate their support of these policies to workers in simple, clear and unambiguous terms.
6. Employers should provide employees with sensitive, accurate and up-to date education about risk reduction in their personal lives.
7. Employers have a duty to protect the confidentiality of employees' medical information.
8. To prevent work disruption and rejection by coworkers of an employee with AIDS or HIV infection, employers and unions should undertake education for all employees before such an incident occurs and as needed thereafter.
9. Employers should not require HIV screening as part of general pre-employment or workplace physical examinations.
10. In those special occupational settings where there may be a potential risk of exposure to HIV (for example, in health care, where workers may be exposed to blood or blood products), employers should provide specific, ongoing education and training, as well as the necessary equipment, to reinforce appropriate infection control procedures and ensure that they are implemented.

CITIZENS COMMISSION ON AIDS

February 1988

References

AIDS Education in the Workplace, An Education Guide for Managers produced by The San Francisco AIDS Foundation, 333 Valencia Street, Fourth Floor, P. O. Box 6182, San Francisco, California 94101-6182, USA.

Statement from the Consultation on AIDS and the Workplace, World Health Organization in association with International Labour Organization, Geneva, June 1988.

38

AIDS Prevention and Care in the Workplace:

Enhancing the Role of the Private Sector

Report of a Regional Work Shop,
New Delhi, 12-13 January, 1995

BACKGROUND

In South-East Asia, the human immunodeficiency virus (HIV), which causes acquired immunodeficiency syndrome (AIDS), is spreading as fast as it did in Africa a decade ago. Asia with its large population may soon surpass Africa in terms of both the total numbers of people infected and the number of new infections each year. WHO estimates that while there are over 18 million adults and 1.5 million children infected with HIV, this global figure will more than double, to between 30 and 40 million infections, by the year 2000. In South-East Asia, the epidemic's spread will be even more dramatic. The 2 million HIV infections now estimated in this region are projected to increase five-fold, to over 10 million by the year 2000.

HIV infection and AIDS do not only seriously affect health and life expectancy; if left unchecked, the epidemic will also greatly undermine the social and economic development of Asian countries. The epidemic will force national resources to be diverted from economic development to the health care of people with AIDS. This set-back for the business sector will be further accentuated by the loss of productivity when workers are forced to stay home either because they are sick themselves or because they need to take care of sick relatives. With industry facing a loss of skilled workers, the indirect costs of training or retraining new workers will be high. Moreover, the epidemic may even reduce consumer markets as increasing amounts of personal income will be spent on hospital bills and treatment for AIDS-related health problems. The need to check the epidemic is, therefore, urgent.

Unfortunately, there is no cure in sight, nor is a vaccine likely to be available in the foreseeable future. Only preventive measures can check the epidemic and these must, therefore, be implemented rapidly. This demands that each sector of society understands the implications of HIV infection and AIDS and responds to the challenge. The private sector in general, and business leaders in particular, represent a crucial component in this response. Apart from the self-interest involved, this sector could also play an effective leadership role in the fight against AIDS. Provision of education and information to the labour force, condom promotion, provision of access for the treatment of sexually transmitted diseases, institution of policies to stop discrimination and stigmatization are important contributions the private sector can make to reduce both the health and socio-economic impact of AIDS in the Region.

In order to discuss the role of the private sector, the South-East Asia Regional Office of the World Health Organization (WHO/SEARO) organized a regional workshop in New Delhi in January 1995. The specific objectives of the meeting were:

(1) To review the existing role of the private sector in HIV/AIDS prevention and care world wide in general and in the South-East Asia Region in particular;

(2) To identify and recommend strategies for developing or further strengthening HIV/AIDS prevention and care in business and other private sector workplaces, in the context of national AIDS programmes, and

(3) To develop guidelines, where possible, for the implementation of such policies and programmes at country level during 1995.

The meeting was opened by Dr. Samlee Plianbangchang, Acting Regional Director of WHO's South-East Asia Region, on behalf of Dr. Uton Muchtar Rafei, Regional Director. Expressing concern at the spread of HIV/AIDS in SEAR countries, particularly among people in their most productive years of life, Dr. Samlee. urged the private sector to actively participate in the national response by developing workplace policies and services. For the technical sessions of the workshop, Mr. P.R. Dasgupta from India was nominated as chairman, Dr. Supanya Lamsam from Thailand as co-chairman and Dr. Nyoman Suesan from Indonesia as rapporteur. For the list of participants and the programme of the workshop.

HIV AND AIDS IN SOUTH-EAST ASIA AND ITS IMPACT ON HEALTH

In the South-East Asia Region of WHO, HIV infection was first reported in 1984 from Thailand, but in most other countries in the Region the infection was not reported until 1986 and even later. However, it has now spread extremely rapidly and all the countries of the Region except DPR Korea have reported HIV infection. WHO estimates that currently there are more than two million HIV-infected people in South-East Asia (see Figure 38.1).

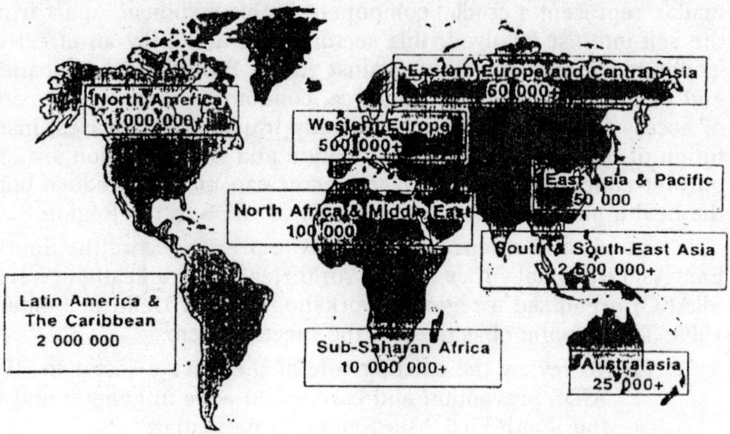

Figure 38.1. Estimated distribution of total adult HIV infections until mid-1994

The annual incidence of AIDS cases shows a steep rise in South-East Asia (see Figure 38.2). As of 1 October 1994, a total of 14,625 cases of AIDS have been reported in this region, Thailand and India contributing the largest numbers, viz. 13,246 and 905 respectively and thus accounting for almost 95 per cent of the total cases reported. The number reported each year is also increasing rapidly. In Thailand it increased from 82 in 1992 to 730 in 1992 and to 2092 in 1993. Of the cases reported in Thailand in 1994, nearly 80 per cent occurred in people between 20-44 years. Of these, 75 per cent occurred among 20-39-year olds, the most productive years of life. (see Figure 38.3).

Sentinel surveillance data and those from other studies indicate a rapid increase in HIV prevalence among individuals with risk-associated behaviour. For example, between 1985 and 1987, injecting drug users (IDUs) in Bangkok accounted for less than 1 per cent of the local HIV prevalence. This percentage dramatically increased to 40 by 1988 and appears to have stabilized at this level. In Manipur, India, HIV prevalence among IDUs is 54 per cent and in Myanmar a study indicates that in certain parts of the country it was as high as 71 per cent-in 1990-1991. Among female sex

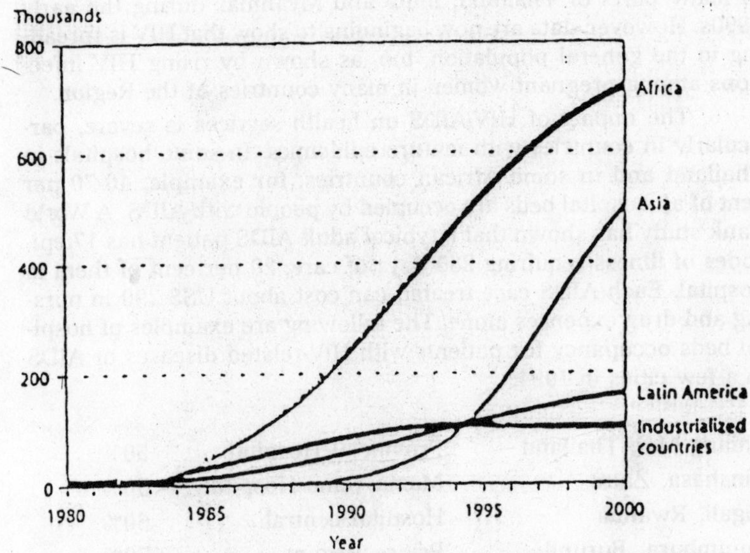

Figure 38.2. Estimated and projected annual AIDS incidences by "macro" region- 1980-2000

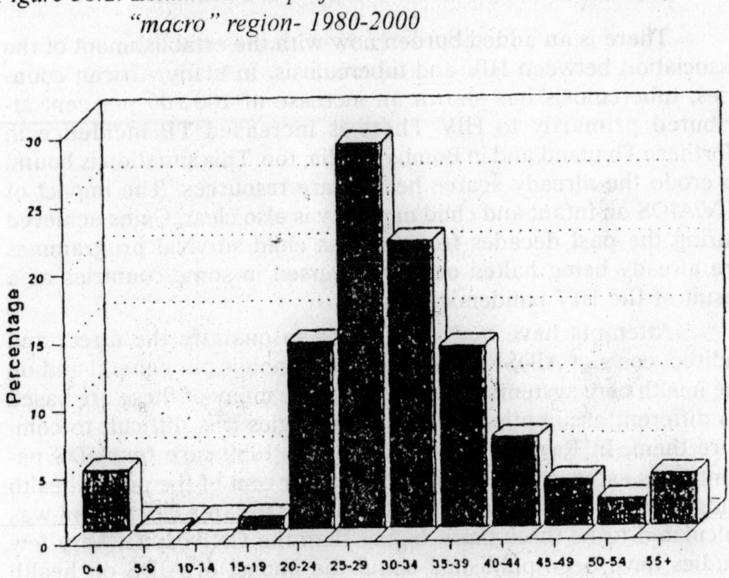

Figure 38.3. Reported AIDS cases by age, 1994

workers remarkable increases in HIV infection have also occurred in many parts of Thailand, India and Myanmar during the early 1990s. However, data are now beginning to show that HIV is spreading in the general population, too, as shown by rising HIV infections among pregnant women in many countries of the Region.

The impact of HIV/AIDS on health services is severe, particularly in countries with mature epidemics. In some hospitals in Thailand and in some African countries, for example, 40-70 per cent of all hospital beds are occupied by people with AIDS. A World Bank study has shown that a typical adult AIDS patient has 17 episodes of illness requiring 280 days of care, 20 per cent of them in hospital. Each AIDS case treated can cost about US$ 290 in nursing and drug expenses alone. The following are examples of hospital beds occupancy for patients with HIV-related diseases or AIDS in a few cities in 1994:

Chiang Mai, Thailand	Provincial Hospital	50%
Kinshasa, Zaire	Mama Yemo Hospital	50%
Kigali, Rwanda	Hospital central	60%
Bujumbura, Burundi	Prince Regent	70%

There is an added burden now with the establishment of the association between HIV and tuberculosis. In many African countries, tuberculosis has shown an increase of 100-200 per cent attributed primarily to HIV. There is increased TB incidence in Northern Thailand and in Bombay, India, too. This situation is bound to erode the already scarce health care resources. The impact of HIV/AIDS on infant and child mortality is also clear. Gains achieved during the past decades from various child survival programmes are already being halted or even reversed in some countries as a result of the HIV pandemic.

Attempts have now been made to quantify the direct and indirect costs of AIDS on the national economies in general and on the health care systems in particular. Since many of these are based on different assumptions and methodologies it is difficult to compare them. In Rawanda, for example, in 1989 care for AIDS patients was estimated to absorb about 5 per cent of the public health budget. In Kenya, the cost of a 60-day stay for an AIDS patient was calculated to be three times higher than the GNP/capita. Very few studies have been published about the impact of AIDS on health care personnel. "In the mid-80s, a study found that 6.4 per cent of the 2,384 hospital workers in Mama Yemo Hospital in Kinshasa, Zaire, were infected". Another study carried out in southern Zambia found that "the mortality rate among nurses in two hospitals had risen from 0.5 in 1980 to 2.7 per cent in 1991, presumably due to AIDS". Other studies are under way in eastern and southern Africa which will help in comparing the situation in different countries. The preliminary results seem to indicate the same trend. Apart from the rising financial costs that will be incurred, the attrition rates among these highly skilled and highly technical personnel will far exceed the training capacity of the countries concerned.

THE SOCIO-ECONOMIC IMPACT OF AIDS

Even though there is lack of well-planned social and behavioural research studies, it is clear that HIV primarily affects people during the most productive years of life, leading to premature death. Many of them are not only the mainstay of their families but that of the workforce as well. AIDS has a serious socio-economic impact. Virtually every adult who dies of AIDS leaves behind dependent family members. It is estimated that, by the year 2000 close to five million children would lose their mothers or both parents due to AIDS. Thus, in economic terms the indirect costs due to loss of productivity far exceed the health care costs. In Thailand, it is estimated that the health care cost for an AIDS patient is US$ 1500, as compared to the indirect cost to the economy of US$ 22, 000 in case of death. By the year 2000, the overall cost to Thailand and India on account of AIDS has been estimated at US$ 9 and 11 billion respectively. (see **Figure** 38.4). In addition, AIDS would have a negative impact on foreign investments and labour remittances from abroad.

Studies in Rawanda, Swaziland, Zaire and Zimbabwe point out that AIDS affects primarily people in the higher socio-economic bracket, those who represent the skilled workers, supervisors and managers of all important sectors of the economies of African countries. To replace them, a younger and less experienced labour and management workforce would have to be recruited. The consequences of this situation will vary according to the economic sector involved. In the mining industry in Zambia, for example, "the result is not necessarily a sudden collapse in output; rather there will be a steady but noticeable increase in breakdowns, accidents, delays and misjudgments, and output will suffer".

In every major company in countries with high prevalence rates of HIV and AIDS, there is anecdotal evidence to support this situation. A comment often made by company managers in Cote d'lvoire, Ghana, Kenya, Zambia and Zimbabwe is that in recent years they have noticed that death rates among staff are sometimes more than twice or three times higher than the rates observed over the previous years. These examples are drawn from sectors as diverse as the mining industry, banking, petroleum, insurance and transport, large commercial farms and agro-industries. Presumably,

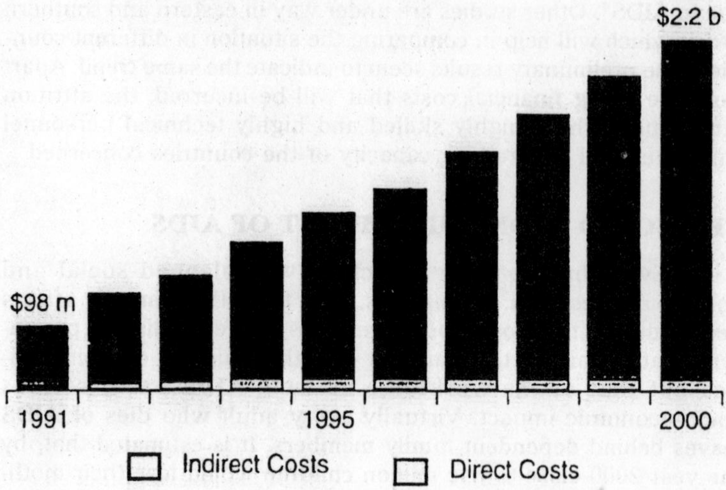

Figure 38.4. Estimated Direct and Indirect Costs, Thailand

the increases are related to the consequences of HIV and AIDS. One vivid example of the impact of HIV/AIDS on the private sector comes from Zambia. In 1987, of 12,204 employees in 33 businesses, 2.5 out of every 1000 employees died of AIDS. This figure increased to 18.3 in 1993—an eight-fold increase in annual employee deaths due to AIDS!

In the productive sector, an immediate consequence of HIV-related diseases and AIDS is the high level of absenteeism. A study carried out in Kenya substantiates this (see Fig. 38.5). As workers become increasingly afflicted with AIDS-related illness, their overall health conditions worsen and they take a longer time away from work to seek treatment. Even healthy workers are not spared because many, especially women, will also take time off to attend to the health needs of those family members who are infected and need care. A few companies have documented the high number of days their staff are away from work to attend funerals of family members and co-workers. As one interviewee in a study carried out in Uganda put it, death has become so common that if one wants to attend funerals one could easily end up losing a month's work

Another example of the socio-economic impact of the HIV pandemic comes from Nakambala sugar estate (NSE), Zambia. AIDS has resulted in 50 per cent of all the man-hours lost in the estate. If diarrhoeal diseases often associated with HIV are added as well, the figure rises to 60 per cent. Even when they return to work, infected workers often cannot perform their duties satisfactorily. Estimated numbers of AIDS deaths and medical releases due

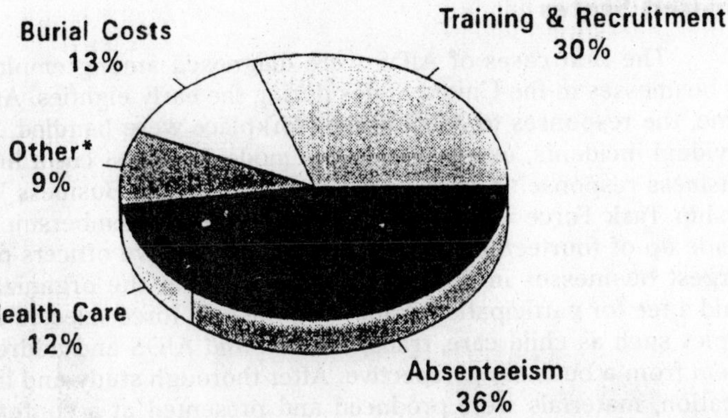

*Other includes labor turnover, funeral attendance, and productivity losses due to the inexperience of new workers
Sources: AIDS captions March 1995

Figure 38.5: AIDS-related costs to Kanyan business

to HIV/AIDS could well increase to 70 per cent during the year 1995/96.

As in many other African communities, healthy employees also absent themselves from work to care for sick relatives and to attend funerals. Absenteeism due to tuberculosis has also increased.

The social impact is considerable. HIV/AIDS-affected families in caring for the sick have to meet increasing medical expenses. Following death, the family loses not only the income, but also entitlement for housing 6 months after death. Those in seasonal employment are even more vulnerable because they do not get the full range of benefits. The number of orphans in the surrounding villages of Nakambala is also on the rise.

EXAMPLES OF PRIVATE SECTOR RESPONSE AND EXPERIENCES

The contribution of the private sector and the business community as equal partners in the national, regional and global efforts is crucial for the prevention and care of HIV/AIDS. Business and government leaders need to work together to set up AIDS programmes in the workplace. These programmes include AIDS education to prevent new infections among employees and their dependents. Programmes should also ensure that people with HIV infection and AIDS are treated fairly, humanely and without discrimination. A number of countries have put in place an HIV/AIDS programme in the workplace. Some examples are as follows:

United States

The first cases of AIDS were diagnosed among employees of businesses in the United States during the early eighties. At that time, the responses to AIDS in the workplace were handled as individual incidents, usually in a crisis mode. The first co-ordinated business response to AIDS began in 1985 with the Business Leadership Task Force (BLTF) in San Francisco. Its membership was made up of fourteen presidents and chief executive officers of the largest businesses in the city. Each member of the organization paid a fee for participation. Each year, the task force selected a few topics such as child care, transportation and AIDS and addressed them from a business perspective. After thorough study and investigation, materials were produced and presented at a conference for effectiv involvement of the private sector in public sector issues.

The conference, "An Epidemic of Fear: AIDS In The Workplace, held in March 1986, discussed the question of how employers should deal with AIDS in the workplace in a businesslike, consistent, cost-effective and compassionate way. The conference as well as the package or materials developed by BLTF and distributed to the members was the first attempt in the United States to address the impact of AIDS on business and set an early standard for a comprehensive business response to AIDS. Since then, other regions in the United States have also developed similar collaborative programmes. An example is the New England Corporate Consortium for AIDS Education, which produces timely and useful materials on AIDS at the workplace. Many big and small business houses are members of this consortium, which also organizes an annual conference on "WORLD AIDS DAY" to encourage and help the employers in New England to address AIDS issues in responsible, ethical and cost-effective ways. In 1986, the Surgeon-General of the United States urged that worksites should have a plan in operation for education of the workforce and care for patients with AIDS even before the first such case appeared at the worksite. Employees with AIDS should be treated like any other worker with a chronic illness.

Another significant response to the AIDS epidemic from business leaders in the United States was the founding, in 1987, of the National Leadership Coalition on AIDS, a non-profit charitable organization which brings together the collective resources of the private sector. The Coalition has grown steadily and now has a membership of more than 200 business houses. In the late 1980s, the US Congress provided funding for the Center for Disease Control (CDC) Atlanta, and the American Red Cross to develop comprehensive AIDS education and prevention activities for the workplace. Programmes designed by and for business underscore the principle that AIDS should be treated like any other life-threatening illness. Their AIDS policies thus are modelled on the policies existing for other life-threatening illnesses.

Employers of workers who have a higher risk of on-the job infection (hospitals, police departments, fire departments and emergency workers) have also developed specific infection control procedures and begun to use the concept of "universal precautions" to minimize the possibility of the spread of infection on the job, for all illnesses including AIDS.

Smaller businesses and some major industries such as airlines and restaurants have, however, only now begun to address AIDS and, for the most part, did not respond well initially.

The legal framework in the United States covering people with HIV/AIDS in the workplace is found in the federal law of 1990 pertaining to disabilities. This law took effect in July 1992 and is applicable to every business enterprise having more than 25 employees. In July 1993, all businesses with more than 15 employees were included. In addition to the federal law, at least 36 of the 50 states in the US provide state protection against discrimination in the workplace to people with disabilities.

Private sector standards as expressed by ten principles for the workplace developed by the Citizens Commission on AIDS for New York City/Northern New Jersey Region are also supported by the World Health Organization, the International Labour Organisation and major multinational corporations as well as by international business groups in Europe, North America, South America and Asia.

Africa

The business community in certain African countries, particularly those in sub-Saharan Africa which are hardest hit by the AIDS pandemic, have now begun to take an active interest in AIDS prevention and control. In a tripartite workshop on the role of the organized sector in reproductive health and AIDS prevention, held in 1994, the business community realized some important facts, viz. that AIDS leads to the loss of output and productivity, there is drain on the family income on account of caring for the sick and funerals; the cost to industry includes high cost of training, retraining and replacement of the workforce; possible increase in wage cost due to labour shortages and loss of consumer markets which will have a direct impact on several industrial sectors and an indirect impact on tourism and other service industries. Studies conducted in a bank in Zambia confirm these concerns. In June 1992, among 1800 staff, 40 deaths had already taken place and it is projected that by 1995 about 140 will die of AIDS. A snap check carried out on staff absentees on 17 July 1991 showed that 10 employees were on leave to attend funerals and 53 were on sick leave. Death claims on the state insurance corporation had increased from 200 in 1986 to nearly 800 in 1991. Many businesses have now started including AIDS in the workplace programmes. Although the involvement of the private sector in Africa is still at an early stage, it is nevertheless gathering momentum.

One example of the private sector in Africa actively engaged in AIDS prevention and control is that of the Debswana Diamond Company (Pty) Ltd., Botswana. The AIDS programme is implemented as a part of their occupational health programme, with the objective of raising the level of awareness among employees on HIV/AIDS through formal lectures, drama, distribution of literature and through briefing by people living with HIV/AIDS. The programme also aims to establish counselling and care support services through training the company hospital nurses as AIDS counsellors and using the existing professional counsellors working in the employee assistance programme.

Nepal

General Paper Industries, based in Kathmandu, which contributes 10 per cent of its annual export value for various community development activities, has organized camps to bring basic health services and simple AIDS awareness information to four remote mountainous villages in Nepal.

The HIV/AIDS awareness efforts received a boost in early 1993 when the company sponsored a half-page advertisement in the *Gorkhapatra* daily with the message "Use condoms to protect yourself against AIDS".

The first target population chosen for AIDS awareness were truck drivers who ply along the national transport route and are among the country's largest mobile groups. By educating drivers it was also possible to disseminate AIDS messages to distant parts of the country. Drivers are given prevention packages when they queue up to complete the required traffic registration at the Nagdhunga traffic police post. Each package contains two condoms, a simple brochure describing HIV transmission and its prevention, and a match box with the message *"Use Condoms to Protect yourself against Aids"* inscribed on it. The industry also organizes competitions among the transport workers and awards attractive prizes tc the best five suggestions on how to improve the AIDS education messages.

India

Since 1991, many small businesses in different parts of India have got involved in creating AIDS awareness. Attempts have been made by the private sector and nongovernmental organizations to provide condoms to long distance transport workers, and collaboration between agencies involved in such programmes is being strengthened.

Numerous corporate sector organizations, such as the Confederation of Indian Industry (CII) and the West Bengal Chamber of Commerce and Industry, have begun collaborating with the National AIDS Control Organization (NACO) for the integration of HIV/AIDS/STD prevention and control activities into health care, educational and other social sector activities already being carried out under the auspices of the corporate sector. A strategic plan is currently being developed by the West Bengal Chamber of Commerce to reach all member industries. The CII has prepared a proposal for initiating AIDS activities in the workplace and many other industries have expressed interest in initiating similar activities. As stated in a folder brought out by CII recently, it is committed to programmes related to AIDS and the workplace and states that "it is essential to plan. If you wait until you have a crisis in your hands, it may be too late to take effective and appropriate action". in partnership with ILO and WHO, a pilot programme is being planned to develop approaches and materials for the industrial sector, and the Indian Tobacco Company is discussing a possible partnership with NACO and the West Bengal State AIDS Cell to provide management assistance for intervention projects in the redlight areas of Calcutta.

The Shriram Industrial Enterprises Limited (SIEL) has also been active in HIV/AIDS prevention. In 1993 an AIDS sensitization programme organized by the company was attended by the top management of industries. SIEL now plans to hold national and regional seminars and workshops on AIDS in conjunction with NACO and WHO. Activities related to AIDS prevention will be carried out along with those on STD control and drug and alcohol abuse. SIEL also holds regular "AIDS Awareness Weeks" in its factories along with workshops and discussions at different managerial levels. Posters and banners are displayed and other educational materials distributed. A major activity in AIDS awareness was carried out through the Annual Marathon which was covered well by the media. The company is now in the process of formulating a programme of AIDS education and counselling and a workplace policy in consultation with the labour unions.

Deepam Educational Society for Health (DESH) based in Madras has been able to educate more than 200,000 employees about AIDS through the involvement of management associations and trade unions. The Society has conducted interactive programmes with many agencies such as the Southern Railway, large industrial houses like Ashok Leyland Ltd., Addison & Co. Ltd., Dock Labour Board, Binny Ltd., and the Madras Port Trust in Madras, India Cements in Salem and Cuddapah, and Larsen & Toubro Ltd. and Cable Corporation in Bombay. Workshops have also been organized for the benefit of employees of the Small Industries Service Institute. Through the Central Board of Workers Education worker-teachers representing various organizations have been trained. These training sessions have been well received, with requests for repeat workshops. More importantly, the programmes seem to have brought about a positive attitudinal change. The motto of DESH is to promote the fact that "the HIV/AIDS epidemic is everyone's concem", and to develop policies which will prepare the organizations to deal with the epidemic responsibly and knowledgeably and in a businesslike way.

Thailand

Until 1993, the response to AIDS in Thailand was mainly from the governmental and international agencies and nongovernmental organizations. There was no co-ordinated response from the private sector. A survey of the business community in 1992-93 revealed that while many were concerned about AIDS, particularly its impact on productivity, office morale and on health, few had done anything about it and many did not know where to go for education and information.

The Thai Business Coalition on AIDS (TBCA) was subsequently formed in 1993 as a non-profit organization of the private sector, for providing leadership through and beyond the AIDS epidemic. The need forAIDS education and information in the workplace and the establishment of workplace policies were supported by the Government, international agencies, universities and NGOs. The main role of TBCA is to develop leadership, promote education and information and co-ordinate the activities of the private sector. The present membership consists mostly of multinational companies and many large and medium Thai industries. Members of TBCA benefit through briefings given to key managers, in-house training and publication of a newsletter and manuals on workplace policies.

TBCA assists businesses in providing AIDS education to the workforce and in the development of a workplace policy. The Coalition expects to have 150 new corporate members by 1995-1996, and plans to provide 300 copies of workplace manuals and train about 30,000 employees and managers. The activities have so far received extensive media coverage and donations from NGOs and other agencies. Among its ten-point workplace principles are (i) combating discrimination against employees with HIV infection, (ii) maintenance of confidentiality, and (iii) providing workplace education and health care to all employees irrespective of their HIV status.

The several problems yet to be overcome include lack of adequate seed money, reluctance of local firms to join the Coalition and insufficient local training. However, given the many opportunities such as wide exposure and co-operation from the public sector, the coalition is expected to develop into a good model of the private sector's response in Asia. TBCA's future plan includes activities related to advocacy, co-ordinating training resources, undertaking community-based projects and developing regional branches.

PRIVATE SECTOR AND AIDS: A MODEL FOR HIV/AIDS PREVENTION AND CARE

Role of Private Sector

The impact of the AIDS epidemic is increasingly being felt by businesses across Asia. AIDS is fast becoming an obstacle to economic development, and the epidemic is forcing us to re-examine the role of the private sector in disease prevention and health promotion. The workplace is an appropriate and important setting for AIDS prevention because most people spend a significant part of their time at work. Thus, AIDS is an important private sector concern, and AIDS prevention makes good business sense.

An effective workplace AIDS prevention and care programme consists of a comprehensive and co-ordinated set of components, such as:

- # Policy development and practices that are clearly defined, understood, and consistently followed, and
- # Implementation of a workplace AIDS programme.

Policy Development and Practice

Policy is the foundation of a workplace AIDS prevention programme. An AIDS policy defines a company's position and its practices as they relate to employees with AIDS. Policies set standards of behaviour expected of all employees as well as standards for communication about AIDS. Policies help employees to know where to go for assistance and instruct supervisors and managers on how to manage AIDS in their work groups. Businesses that have successfully addressed HIV/AIDS suggest that it is useful to have a written policy stating the company's position and procedures that tell managers and employees about what is expected of them. A policy does not provide an entire HIV/AIDS prevention programme, it is the foundation, the first step, upon which a strong prevention programme can be built.

In June 1988, a group of experts representing governments, trade unions, business, public health, medicine, the legal profession and educators agreed on a joint WHO and ILO declaration on AIDS and the workplace which incorporated the following principles:

1. HIV/AIDS screening as part of an assessment of fitness to work is unnecessary and should not be required.
2. For persons already in employment, HIV/AIDS screening, whether direct (HIV testing), indirect (assessment of risk behaviour) or asking questions about tests already taken, should not be required.
3. Confidentiality regarding all medical information including HIV/AIDS must be maintained.
4. There should be no obligation on the employee to inform the employer of his or her HIV/AIDS status.
5. Persons in the workplace infected, or perceived to be infected, by HIV/AIDS must be protected from stigmatization and discrimination by co-workers, unions, employers or clients. Information and education are essential to maintain the climate of mutual understanding necessary to ensure this protection.
6. Employees and their families should have access to information and educational programmes on HIV/AIDS as well as to relevant counselling and appropriate referral.
7. HIV-infected employees should not be discriminated against; this means that they should have unreserved access to and receipt of standard social security and occupationally related benefits.
8. HIV infection by itself is not associated with any limitation on fitness to work. If fitness to work is impaired by HIV-related illness, reasonable working arrangements should be made.
9. HIV infection is not a ground for termination of employment. As with many other illnesses, persons with HIV-related illnesses should be able to work as long as they are medically fit for available and appropriate work.
10. In any situation requiring first aid in the workplace,

precautions should be taken to reduce the risk of the transmission of blood-borne infections, including hepatitis B, and standard precautions will be equally effective against HIV transmission.

Most businesses find that developing an HIV/AIDS policy takes less time than expected and is an interesting, informative and valuable experience. They also find that management and worker responses are surprisingly favourable. The biggest benefit is the knowledge that they are prepared to deal effectively with a serious problem and reduce the health and socio-economic impact of the epidemic significantly.

Successful HIV/AIDS policies used by businesses around the world share a number of the following basic principles.

1. People with HIV/AIDS are entitled to the same rights, benefits and opportunities as people with other serious or life-threatening illnesses.
2. Employment practices must, at a minimum, comply with national, regional and local laws and regulations.
3. Employment policies should be based on the scientific and epidemiological evidence that people with HIV/AIDS do not pose a risk of transmission of the virus to co-workers through ordinary workplace contact.
4. The highest levels of management and union leadership should unequivocally endorse nondiscriminatory employment policies and educational programmes related to the prevention and care of HIV/AIDS.
5. Employers and union leaders should communicate their support of these policies to workers in simple, clear and unambiguous terms.
6. Employers should provide employees with sensitive, accurate and up-to-date education about risk reduction in their personal lives.
7. Employers have a duty to protect the confidentiality of medical information in respect of all their employees.
8. To prevent work disruption and rejection by co-workers of an HIV/AIDS employee, employers and unions should undertake education for all employees before such an incident thereafter as needed.
9. Employers should not require HIV screening as part of pre-employment or general workplace physical examinations.
10. In special occupational settings where there may be a potential risk of exposure to HIV (working with blood or blood products). employers should provide specific. on-

going education and training, as well as the necessary equipment, to reinforce appropriate infection control procedures and ensure that they are implemented.

Implementation of Workplace AIDS Programmes

A comprehensive and on-going HIV/AIDS education and prevention programme must aim at bringing about changes in behaviour that will reduce the spread of AIDS through:

Formal and informal education
Condom distribution
Diagnosis and treatment of sexually transmitted diseases (STD).
Care, counselling and support services for workers and their families.

Formal and Informal Education

HIV/AIDS education includes a variety of approaches to address a broad range of issues. No matter what forms or approaches are used, there are specific core issues that should always be included as part of the educational programme. These are:

the company's policy or position on HIV/AIDS and procedures for handling HIV/AIDS-related problems or concerns
How HIV/AIDS is and is not transmitted
how to prevent the spread of HIV
how to respond to a co-worker with HIV/AIDS
benefits available to workers and family members with HIV/AIDS
confidentiality and privacy requirements
where to go for help and for additional information.

Use of Peers as Educators

Peer education is universally considered the most effective way to provide workers with HIV/AIDS education to initiate prevention activities focusing on behavioural change. Peer education will, however, need specific training and support, to be able to function effectively.

Peer educator training requires between two and five days of specialized instruction to develop in the trainees the necessary skills for education and prevention activities.

Some organizations may decide that instead of peer education, individuals or a small group of people should be responsible for conducting the company's formal and informal HIV/AIDS education and prevention activities. In any case, it is essential that the people identified as HIV/AIDS educators receive adequate training—even doctors who may not be equipped to deal with issues such as those related to sex, sexuality, condom use and behavioural change.

Trade unions also have a major role to play in educating their members on AIDS prevention.

Condom Distribution, Establishing System(s) that Maximize Condom use for AIDS Prevention

Condom distribution is a necessary part of an effective workplace HIV/AIDS prevention programme. Workers must be educated on how to use condoms correctly and simultaneously must also have easy access to them through an effective distribution system. Condoms will also prevent other sexually transmitted diseases (STDs).

Diagnosis and Treatment of Sexually Transmitted Diseases

Sexually transmitted diseases (STDs) are common among workers and contribute not only to absenteeism and medica care costs but also to the increased possibility of HIV transmission during sexual intercourse. HIV/AIDS education and prevention activities must, therefore, include learning and discussions among workers about STDs and their relationship to the transmission of HIV/AIDS as well as the provision of STD diagnosis and treatment services using, where appropriate, the syndrome approach. According to some studies, the cost of diagnosis and treatment for a worker with an STD is less than one day's wages whereas the costs of absenteeism and the resulting impact on productivity, medical costs, and other expenses can be many times the cost of diagnosis and treatment. It thus makes it cost effective to provide STD diagnosis and treatment as a support service to HIV/AIDS education and prevention activities. I many situations, provision of STD treatment services may not be possible for the company. However, it is the company's responsibility to ensur that employees are informed where these services are available and how they can access them. STD diagnosis and treatment should also include counselling services for workers and their families.

Care, Counselling and Support Services for Workers and their Families

Care includes counselling and support services for concerned

Workers and those diagnosed with HIV (following voluntary testing and counselling services), for workers who have AIDS and for their families. Care is an important part of a comprehensive workplace AIDS programme. Counselling and support are important both for the physical and mental welfare of workers and their families. Such services also increase the probability of sustained behavioural change and will help prevent the transmission of HIV.

Provision of comprehensive care services irrespective of the HIV status makes the other prevention activities concrete and real in the lives of workers and their families, because they provide personal and individual reinforcement for behavioural change, outside of the formal and informal group activities offered at work. Without the reinforcement of these services, HIV/AIDS education and prevention activities remain merely educational exercises without real-life application and are unlikely to bring about sustained behavioural change or reduce the transmission of HIV/AIDS.

CONCLUSIONS AND RECOMMENDATIONS

The private sector plays a significant and essential role in HIV/AIDS prevention and has the potential for impacting necessary behavioural change as no other sector in society can. Clear, straightforward, factual policies prepare businesses to deal with HIV/AIDS smoothly, responsibly and cost-effectively. HIV/AIDS education and prevention activities and services assist workers and their families to prevent the spread of HIV/AIDS and businesses derive the benefits of reduced costs, stable productivity, and a healthier workforce.

A comprehensive HIV/AIDS education and prevention programme must be developed which would include policy, education and prevention activities for workers, and accompanying support services. A responsible, assertive stand on HIV/AIDS can place a company among the ranks of business leaders in Asia, and around the world, who are collaborating successfully in confronting the HIV/AIDS epidemic.

The workshop deliberated in groups and, after discussions in the plenary, made the following recommendations·

1. In view of the fact that HIV/AIDS largely affects people in the most economically productive years of their lives, it is imperative that AIDS prevention and care activities are initiated at the workplace.
2. As the private sector has a crucial role to play in the provision of STD/HIV/AIDS education and prevention services to its employees, its resources must be harnessed to develop appropriate AIDS prevention and control

programmes in the workplace that will adequately respond to the unique national and local needs and situations prevalent in the respective countries.

3. The role of the private sector must fit into the overall national plan of action co-ordinated by the national AIDS programme of the respective countries. It is, therefore, important that the precise role the private sector can play in HIV prevention and care be defined by all parties, including the private sector itself.
4. In order to encourage and facilitate the participation of the private sector, information with respect to HIV/STD/AIDS, especially the projected national and/or sectoral impact (economic and otherwise) of the pandemic, be provided to the private sector in a business context.
5. To initiate an HIV/STD/AIDS education and prevention programme, it is necessary for the private sector to identify and involve key industrial leaders and workers' representatives in the planning, development and/or implementation of such programmes in the workplace.
6. To facilitate a partnership between the private sector and the national AIDS programme, the latter should initiate the establishment of a forum for regular exchange of information, experience and activities related to the private sector's response to HIV/STD/AIDS at regional, national and local levels.
7. Since policy is the foundation of a workplace AIDS prevention programme, a national policy for a workplace response to HIV/STD/AIDS should be developed through collaboration between the national programme and the corporate and workers' representatives as appropriate to each country.
8. In order to be cost-effective, HIV/STD/AIDS prevention and care programmes for the workplace should be developed, implemented and monitored utilizing existing structures through the development adaptation of manuals and appropriate training within existing human resources development programmes and through networking with relevant NGOs or community groups. In this process the skills, capacities and resources of the private sector should be utilized to the maximum extent.
9. In order to suport and sustain HIV/STD/AIDS prevention and care programmes in the workplace, mechanisms must be established for generating funds through the private sector.
10. To foster the private sector's response to the AIDS pan-

demic, a network should be established for the exchange of experiences between all industries and other businesses involved in HIV/STD/AIDS prevention and care activities, within and among countries.

SUMMARY

The human immunodeficiency virus (HIV), which causes AIDS, has now spread to all continents of the world. In Asia, HIV appeared later than in other parts of the world but is now spreading at a pace reminiscent of the situation in Africa about 10 years ago. Asia last year reported the biggest increase in the number of HIV infections, the cumulative infections todate being more than 2.5 million. More and more people are expected to be infected each year and soon there will be more Asians infected with HIV annually than those in Africa. The end of the pandemic is nowhere in sight. If left unchecked, it is estimated that between 30 and 40 million people worldwide will be infected by HIV by the year 2000, and of these, 8 to 10 million will be in Asia. The AIDS pandemic has, in addition, brought with it the resurgence of tuberculosis, which already accounts for over 1.5 million deaths annually in Asia. The devastating effect of this deadly combination has already been seen in Africa, where the incidence of tuberculosis has doubled and even tripled in many countries over the last five years.

As the dimension of HIV/AIDS increases, the workplace assumes very great importance. In 1994, about 2.3 billion people in the world were associated with the workplace either in the public sector or in the private sector. When AIDS affects, it is not only the breadwinners who die, but they leave behind families, old parents, children and spouses. AIDS therefore affects not only individuals and families but also communities in which businesses are located. AIDS particularly affects the private sector or businesses in profound and costly ways—in terms of illnesses and disabilities thereby causing decrease in productivity as workers remain absent due to illnesses or are away to care for sick families. In economic terms, the indirect costs due to loss of productivity far outweigh the health care costs. In Thailand, for example, a well-documented study estimates the health care cost for an AIDS patient at US$ 1,500, as compared to the indirect cost to the economy of US$ 22,000 in case of death. By the year 2000, the overall costs to Thailand and India on account of AIDS have been estimated at US$ 9 and 11 billion respectively.

The prevention and control of HIV infections and AIDS require the broadest possible commitment to supporting community-based initiatives to encourage young people to adopt and maintain protective social norms and practices. The contribution of the private sector and the business community as equal partners in national, regional and global efforts is crucial in this regard. To effectively meet the challenge posed by AIDS, business and government leadership must work together. In all countries, governments, through their national programmes, have taken initiatives to prevent HIV infection and to provide care and social support to those affected by HIV/AIDS and their families.

Besides supporting the national AIDS programmes in their work, what can individual businesses and the private sector do to prevent the spread of HIV/AIDS? To begin with, businesses can establish and urgently begin to implement workplace policies and programmes. The two main components of such programmes are: first, to ensure that people with HIV infection and AIDS are treated fairly, humanely and without discrimination; and second, to set up AIDS education programmes in the workplace with the objective of preventing new infections among employees and their dependents. The adoption of a corporate policy on AIDS, highlighting provision of education and information to employees and their families on a regular basis irrespective of their HIV status; strengthening facilities for the treatment of sexually transmitted diseases; ensuring accessibility to condoms and promoting 'no' to pre-employment HIV screening must be the goal of each business or industry. Advocacy by the management and fellow workers is an important component of a workplace policy against HIV-related discrimination. The private sector can also play a major advocacy role in helping to shape the national response to the AIDS epidemic. For example, the Thai Business Coalition on AIDS subscribes to its famous "Ten Principles". These principles recognize the need for businesses to treat people with AIDS in the same way as people with any other serious condition; to have non-discriminatory employment practices; and to protect the confidentiality of employees' medical and insurance information. They also include a policy on AIDS prevention by stating that AIDS education is to be provided to all staff. Provision of care and support is also included in the workplace initiatives.

To enhance implementation of these policies by the private sector, much advocacy and support is needed from the government sector. Orientation of, and group educational activities for, executives and trade union leaders will go a long way in evoking an early response. While educational and information programmes at the workplace are the responsibility of the private sector, technical and material support can be obtained from the national AIDS programme. Moreover, as each private enterprise may not have facilities for treatment of STDs, the management should have information about the nearest place where such facilities are available. The same is true with respect to availability of condoms. In some situations, some seed money will have to be provided to the private sector for conducting group educational activities and promoting peer education, but ultimately contributions must come from within the private sector itself. Press coverage of the AIDS control activities of the private sector will not only strengthen such activities but will also encourage many other private enterprises to join in this effort.

In the long term, continued dialogue with the management is needed to convince them that any delay in their responding to the pandemic will have grave consequences and that investing early in AIDS prevention does indeed make sound business sense!

39

Guidelines for Prevention of Transmission of Human Immunodeficiency Virus and Hepatitis B Virus to Health-Care and Public-Safety Workers

I. INTRODUCTION

A. Background

This document is a response to recently enacted legislation, Public Law 100-607, The Health Omnibus Programmes Extension Act of 1988, Title II, Programmes with Respect to Acquired Immune Deficiency Syndrome ("AIDS Amendments of 1988"). Subtitle E, General Provisions, Section 253(a) of Title II specifies that "the Secretary of Health and Human Services, acting through the Director of the Centers for Disease Control, shall develop, issue, and disseminate guidelines to all health workers, public safety workers (including emergency response employees) in the United States concerning

1. methods to reduce the risk in the workplace of becoming infected with the etiologic agent for acquired immune deficiency syndrome; and
2. circumstances under which exposure to such etiologic agent may occur."

It is further noted that "The Secretary [of Health and Human Services] shall transmit the guidelines issued under subsection (a) to the Secretary of Labour for use by the Secretary of Labour in the development of standards to be issued under the Occupational Safety and Health Act of 1970," and that "the Secretary, acting through the Director of the Centers for Disease Control, shall develop a model curriculum for emergency response employees with respect to the prevention of exposure to the etiologic agent for acquired immune deficiency syndrome during the process of responding to emergencies."

Following development of these guidelines and curriculum, "[t]he Secretary shall.

(a) transmit to State public health officers copies of the guidelines and the model curriculum developed under paragraph (1) with the request that such officers disseminate such copies as appropriate throughout the State; and

(b) make such copies available to the public."

B. Purpose and Organization of Document

The purpose of this document is to provide an overview of the modes of transmission of human immunodeficiency virus (HIV) in the workplace, an assessment of the risk of transmission under various assumptions, principles underlying the control of risk, and specific risk-control recommendations for employers and workers. This document also includes information on medical management of persons who have sustained an exposure at the workplace to these viruses (e.g., an emergency medical technicians who incur a needle-stick injury while performing professional duties). These guidelines are intended for we by a technically informed audience. As noted above, a separate model curriculum based on the principles and practices discussed in this document is being developed for use in training workers and will contain less technical wording.

Information concerning the protection of workers against acquisition of the human immunodeficiency virus (HIV) while performing job duties, the virus that causes AIDS, is presented here. Information on hepatitis B virus (HBV) is also presented in this document on the basis of the following assumptions:

the modes of transmission for hepatitis B virus (HBV) are similar to those of HIV,

the potential for HBV transmission in the occupational setting is greater than for HIV,

there is a larger body of experience relating to controlling transmission of HBV in the workplace, and

general practices to prevent the transmission of HBV will also minimize the risk of transmission of HIV.

Blood-borne transmission of other pathogens not specifically addressed here will be interrupted by adherence to the precautions noted below. It is important to note that the implementation of control measures for HIV and HBV does not obviate the need for continued adherence to general infection-control principles and general hygiene measures (e.g., hand washing) for preventing transmission of other infectious diseases to both worker and client. General guidelines for control of these diseases have been published.[1,2,3]

This document was developed primarily to provide guidelines for fire-service personnel, emergency medical technicians, paramedics (see section IV), and law-enforcement and correctional-facility personnel (see sectionV). Throughout the report, paramedics and emergency medical technicians are called "emergency medical workers" and fire-service, law-enforcement, and correctional-facility personnel, "public-safety workers." Previously issued guidelines address the needs of hospital-, laboratory-, and clinic-based health-care workers.[4,5] A condensation of general guidelines for protection of workers from transmission of blood-borne pathogens, derived from the Joint Advisory Notice of the Departments of Labour and Health and Human Services [6], is provided in section.[III]

C. Modes and Risk of Virus Transmission in the Workplace

Although the potential for HBV transmission in the workplace setting is greater than for HIV, the modes of transmission for these two viruses are similar. Both have been transmitted in occupational settings only by percutaneous inoculation or contact with an open wound, nonintact (e.g., chapped, abraded, weeping, or dermatitic) skin, or mucous membranes to blood, blood-contaminated body fluids, or concentrated virus. Blood is the single most important source of HIV and HBV in the workplace setting. Protection measures against HIV and HBV for workers should focus primarily on preventing these types of exposures to blood as well as on delivery of HBV vaccination.

The risk of hepatitis B infection following a parenteral (i.e., needle stick or cut) exposure to blood is directly proportional to the probability that the blood contains hepatitis B surface antigen (HBsAg), the immunity status of the recipient, and on the efficiency of transmission[7]. The probability of the source of the blood being HBsAg positive varies from 1 to 3 per thousand in the general population to 5 per cent-15 per cent in groups at high risk for HBV infection, such as immigrants from areas of high endemicity (China and Southeast Asia, sub-Saharan Africa, most Pacific islands, and the Amazon Basin); clients in institutions for the mentally retarded; intravenous drug users; homosexually active males; and household (sexual and non-sexual) contacts of HBV carriers. Of persons who have not had prior hepatitis B vaccination or postexposure prophylaxis, 6 per cent-30 per cent of persons who receive a needle-stick exposure from an HBsAg-positive individual will become infected[7].

The risk of infection with HIV following one needle-stick exposure to blood from a patient known to be infected with HIV is approximately 0.5 per cent.[4,5] This rate of transmission is considerably lower than that for HBV, probably as a result of the significantly lower concentrations of virus in the blood of HIV-infected persons. Table 39.1 off presents theoretical data concerning the likelihood of infection given repeated needlestick injuries involving patients whose HIV serostatus is unknown. Though inadequately quantified, the risk from exposure of nonintact skin or mucous membranes is likely to be far less than that from percutaneous inoculation.

Table 39.1.
The Risk of HIV Infection Following Needlestick Injury: Hypothetical Model

Prevalence of HIV Infection	Probability of Infection given Needlestick Injury with Blood Containing H1V	Problility of Infection given Random Needlestick (Unknown Serostatus)	Probabihty of Infection Given 10 Random Needlesticks	Probability of Infection Given 100 Random Needlesticks
(A)	(B)	A * B = (C)	$1-(1-C)^{10}$	$1-(1-C)^{100}$
0.0001	0.001	0.0000001	0.000001	0.00001
0.0001	0.005	0.0000005	0.000005	0.00005
0.001	0.001	0.000001	0.00001	0.0001
0.001	0.005	0.000005	0.00005	0.0005
0.01	0.001	0.00001	0.0001	0.001
0.01*	0.005	0.00005	0.0005	0.005
0.05	0.001	0.00005	0.0005	0.005
0.05	0.005	0.00025	0.0025	0.025

* For example, if the prevalence of infection in the population is 0.01 (i.e., 1 per 100) and the risk of a seroconversion following a needlestick with blood known to contain HIV is 0.005 (i.e., 1 in 200), then the probability of HIV infection given a random needlestick is 0.00005 (i.e., 5 in 100,000). If an individual sustains 10 needlestick injuries, the probability of acquiring HIV infection is 0.0005 (i.e., 1 in 2,000); if the individual sustains 100 needlestick injuries, the probability of acquiring HIV infection is 0.005 (i.e., 1 in 200).

D. Transmission of Hepatitis B Virus to Workers

1. Health-care workers

In 1987, the CDC estimated the total number of HBV infections in the United States to be 300,000 per year, with approximately 75,000 (25 per cent) of infected persons developing acute hepatitis. Of these infected individuals, 18,000-30,000 (6 per cent-10 per cent) will become HBV carriers, at risk of developing chronic liver disease (chronic active hepatitis, cirrhosis, and primary liver cancer), and infectious to others.

CDC has estimated that 12,000 health-care workers whose jobs entail exposure to blood become infected with HBV each year, that 500-600 of them are hospitalized as a result of that infection, and that 700-1,200 of those infected become HBV carriers. Of the infected workers,approximately 250 will die (12-15 from fulminant hepatitis,170-200 from cirrhosis, and 40-50 from liver cancer) . Studies indicate that 10 per cent-30 per cent of health-care or dental workers show serologic evidence of past or present HBV infection.

2. Emergency medical and public-safety workers

Emergency medical workers have an increased risk for hepatitis B infection.[8,9,10] The degree of risk correlates with the frequency and extent of blood exposure during the conduct of work activities. A few studies are available concerning risk of HBV infection for other groups of public-safety workers (law-enforcement personnel and correctional-facility workers), but reports that have been published do not document any increased risk for HBV infection.[11,12,13] Nevertheless, in occupational settings in which workers may be routinely exposed to blood or other body fluids as described below, an increased risk for occupational acquisition of HBV infection must be assumed to be present.

3. Vaccination for hepatitis B virus

A safe and effective vaccine to prevent hepatitis B has been available since 1982. Vaccination has been recommended for health-care workers regularly exposed to blood and other body fluids potentially contaminated with HBV. [7,14,15] In 1987, the Department of Health and Human Services and the Department of Labour stated that hepatitis B vaccine should be provided to all such workers at no charge to the worker. [6]

Available vaccines stimulate active immunity against HBV infection and provide over 90 per cent protection against hepatitis B for 7 or more years following vaccination.[7] Hepatitis B vaccines also are 70-88 per cent effective when given within 1 week after

HBV exposure. Hepatitis B immune globulin (HBIG), a preparation of immunoglobulin with high levels of antibody to HBV (anti-HBs), provides temporary passive protection following exposure to HBV. Combination treatment with hepatitis B vaccine and HBIG is over 90 per cent effective in preventing hepatitis B following a documented exposure.[7]

E. Transmission of Human Immunodeficiency Virus to Workers

1. Health-care workers with AIDS

As of September 19, 1988, a total of 3,182 (5.1 per cent) of 61,929 adults with AIDS, who had been reported to the CDC national surveillance system and for whom occupational information was available, reported being employed in a health-care setting. Of the health-care workers with AIDS, 95 per cent reported high-risk behaviour; for the remaining 5 per cent (169 workers), the means of HIV acquisition was undetermined.

Of these 169 health-care workers with AIDS with undetermined risk, information is incomplete for 28 (17 per cent) because of death or refusal to be interviewed; 97 (57 per cent) are still being investigated. The remaining 44 (26 per cent) health-care workers were interviewed directly or had other follow-up information available. The occupations of these 44 were nine nursing assistants (20 per cent); eight physicians (18 per cent), four of whom were surgeons; eight housekeeping or maintenance workers (18 per cent); six nurses (14per cent); four clinical laboratory technicians (9 per cent); two respiratory therapists (5 per cent) ; one dentist (2 per cent); one paramedic (2 per cent); one embalmer (2 per cent); and four others who did not have contact with patients (9 per cent). Eighteen of these 44 health-care workers reported parenteral and/or other non-needle-stick exposure to blood or other body fluids from patients in the 10 years preceding their diagnosis of AIDS. None of these exposures involved a patient with AIDS or known HIV infection, and HIV seroconversion of the health-care worker was not documented following a specific exposure.

2. Human immunodeficiency virus transmission in the workplace

As of July 31,1988,1,201 health-care workers had been enrolled and tested for HIV antibodyinongoing CDC surveillance of health-care workers exposed vianeedle stick or splashes to skin or mucous membranes to blood from patients known to be HIV-infected.[16] Of 860 workers who had received needle-stick injuries or cuts with sharp objects (i.e., parenteral exposures) and whose serum had been tested for HIV antibody at least 180 days after exposure, 4 were positive, yielding a seroprevalence rate of 0.47 per cent. Three of these individuals experienced an acute retroviral syndrome associated with documented seroconversion. Investigation revealed no non-occupational risk factors for these three workers. Serum collected within 30 days of exposure was not available from the fourth person. This worker had an HIV-seropositive sexual partner, and heterosexual acquisition of infection cannot be excluded. None of the 103 workers who had contamination of mucous membranes or nonintact skin and whose serum had been tested at least 180 days after exposure developed serologic evidence of HIV infection.

Two other ongoing prospective studies assess the risk of nosocomial acquisition of HIV infection among health-care workers in the United States. As of April 1988, the National Institutes of Health had tested 983 health-care workers, 137 with documented needle-stick injuries and 345 health-care workers who had sustained mucousmembrane exposures to blood or other body fluids of HIV-infected patients; none had seroconverted[17] (one health-care worker who subsequently experienced an occupational HIV seroconversion has since been reported from NIH).[18] As of March 15, 1988, a similar study at the University of California of 212 health-care workers with 625 documented accidental parenteral exposures involving HIV-infected patients had identified one seroconversion following a needle stick.[19] Prospective studies in the United Kingdom and Canada show no evidence of HIV transmission among 220 health-care workers with parenteral, mucous-membrane, or cutaneous exposures.[20,21]

In addition to the health-care workers enrolled in these longitudinal surveillance studies, case histories have been published in the scientific literature for 19 HIV infected health-care workers (13 with documented seroconversion and 6 without documented sero conversion). None of these workers reported non-occupational risk factors (see Tabler 39.2).

3. Emergency medical service and public-safety workers

In addition to the one paramedic with undetermined risk discussed above, three public-safety workers (law-enforcement officers) are classified in the undetermined risk group. Follow-up investigations of these workers could not determine conclusively if HIV infection was acquired during the performance of job duties.

Table 39.2
HIV-Infected Health-Care Workers with no Reported Non-occupational Risk Factors and for whom Case Histories have been Published in the Scientific Literature

Cases with Documented Seroconversion

Case	Occupation	Country	Type of Exposure	Source
1. *	NS†	United States	Needlestick	AIDS patient
2.	NS	United States	Needlestick	AIDS patient
3.	NS	United States	Needlestick	AIDS patient
4.	NS	United States	2 Needlesticks	AIDS patient, HIV-infected patient
5.	NS	United States	Needlestick	AIDS patient
6.	Nurse	England	Needlestick	AIDS patient
7.	Nurse	France	Needlestick	HIV-infected patient
8.	Nurse	Martinique	Needlestick	AIDS patient
9.	Research lab worker	United States	Cut with sharp object	Concentrated virus
10.	Home health-care worker	United States	Cutaneous#	AIDS patient
11.	NS	United States	Nonintact skin	AIDS patient
12.	Phlebotomist	United States	Mucous-membrane	HIV-infected patient
13.	Technologist	United States	Nonintact skin	HIV-infected patient
14.	NS	United States	Needlestick	AIDS patient
15.	Nurse	Italy	Mucous membrane	HIV-infected patient
16.	Nurse	France	Needlestick	AIDS patient
17.	Navy medic	United States	Needlestick	AIDS patient
18.	Clinical lab worker	United States	Cut with sharp object	AIDS patient
19.	NS	United States	Puncture wound	AIDS patient
20.	NS	United States	2 Needlesticks	2 AIDS patients
21.	Research lab worker	United States	Nonintact skin	Concentrated virus
22.	Home health-care provider	England.	Nonintact skin	AIDS patient
23.	Dentist	United States	Multiple needle-sticks	Unknown
24..*	Technician	Mexico	Multiple needle-sticks and mucous-membrane	Unknown
25.	Lab worker	United States	Needlestick, puncture wound	Unknown

#AIDS case.

{Cont.}.......

† Not specified.
# Motherwho provided nursing care for her child with HIV infection; extensive contact with the child's blood and body secretion and excretions occurred; the mother did not wear gloves and often did not wash her hands immediately after exposure.

II. PRINCIPLES OF INFECTION CONTROL AND THEIR APPLICATION TO EMERGENCY AND PUBLIC SAFETY WORKERS

A. General Infection Control

Within the health-care setting, general infection control procedures have been developed to minimize the risk of patient acquisition of infection from contact with contaminated devices, objects, or surfaces or of transmission of an infectious agent from health-care workers to patients.[1,2,3] Such procedures also protect workers from the risk of becoming infected. General infection-control procedures are designed to prevent transmission of a wide range of microbiological agents and to provide a wide margin of safety in the varied situations encountered in the health-care environment.

General infection-control principles are applicable to other work environments where workers contact other individuals and where transmission of infectious agents may occur. The modes of transmission noted in the hospital and medical office environment are observed in the work situations of emergency and public-safety workers, as well. Therefore, the principles of infection control developed for hospital and other health-care settings are also applicable to these work situations. Use of general infection control measures, as adapted to the work environments of emergency and public-safety workers, is important to protect both workers and individuals with whom they work from a variety of infectious agents, not just HIV and HBV.

Because emergency and public-safety workers work in environments that provide inherently unpredictable risks of exposures, general infection-control procedures should be adapted to these work situations. Exposures are unpredictable, and protective measures may often be used in situations that do not appear to present risk. Emergency and public-safety workers perform their duties in the community under extremely variable conditions; thus, control measures that are simple and uniform across all situations have the greatest likelihood of worker compliance. Administrative procedures to ensure compliance also can be more readily developed than when procedures are complex and highly variable.

B. Universal Blood and Body Fluid Precautions to Prevent Occupational HIV and HBV Transmission

In 1985, CDC developed the strategy of "universal blood and body fluid precautions" to address concerns regarding transmission of HIV in the health-care setting.[4] The concept, now referred to simply as universal precautions stresses that all patients should be assumed to be infectious for HIV and other blood-borne pathogens. In the hospital and other health-care setting, universal precautions" should be followed when workers are exposed to blood, certain other body fluids (amniotic fluid, pericardial fluid, peritoneal fluid, pleural fluid, synovial fluid, cerebrospinal fluid, semen, and vaginal secretions), or any body fluid visibly contaminated with blood. Since HIV and HBV transmission has not been documented from exposure to other body fluids (feces, nasal secretions, sputum, sweat, tears, urine, and vomitus), "universal precautions" do not apply to these fluids. Universal precautions also do not apply to saliva, except in the dental setting, where saliva is likely to be contaminated with blood.[7]

For the purpose of this document, human "exposure" is defined as contact with blood or other body fluids to which universal precautions apply through percutaneous inoculation or contact with an open wound, nonintact skin, or mucous membrane during the performance of normal job duties. An "exposed worker" is defined, for the purposes of this document, as an individual exposed, as described above, while performing normal job duties.

The unpredictable and emergent nature of exposures encountered by emergency and public-safety workers may make differentiation between hazardous body fluids and those which are not hazardous very difficult and often impossible. For example, poor lighting may limit the worker s ability to detect visible blood in vomitus or feces. Therefore, when emergency medical and public-safety workers encounter body fluids under uncontrolled, emergency circumstances in which differentiation between fluid types is difficulty if not impossible, they should treat all body fluids as potentially hazardous.

The application of the principles of universal precautions to the situations encountered by these workers results in the development of guidelines (listed below) for work practices, use of personal protective equipment, and other protective measures. To minimize the risks of acquiring HIV and HBV during performance of job duties, emergency and public-safety workers should be protected from exposure to blood and other body fluids as circumstances dictate. Protection can be achieved through adherence to workpractices designed to minimize or eliminate exposure and through use of personal protective equipment (i.e., gloves, masks, and protective clothing), whichprovide a barrier between the worker and the exposure source. In some situations, redesign of selected aspects of the job through equipment modifications or environmental control can further reduce risk. These approaches to primary prevention should be used together to achieve maximal reduction of the risk of exposure.

If exposure of an individual worker occurs, medical management, consisting of collection of pertinent medical and occupational history, provision of treatment, and counseling regarding future work and personal behaviours, may reduce risk of developing disease as a result of the exposure episode.[22] Following episodic (or continuous) exposure, decontamination and disinfection of the work environment, devices, equipment, and clothing or other forms of personal protective equipment can reduce subsequent risk of exposures. Proper disposal of contaminated waste has similar benefits.

III. EMPLOYER RESPONSIBILITIES

A. General

Detailed recommendations for employer responsibilities in protecting workers from acquisition of blood-borne diseases in the workplace have been published in the Department of Labour and Department of Health and Human Services Joint Advisory Notice and are summarized here.[6] In developing programmes to protect workers, employers should follow a series of steps: (1) classification of work activity, (2) development of standard operating procedures, (3) provision of training and education, (4) development of procedures to ensure and monitor compliance, and (5) workplace redesign. As a first step, every employer should classify work activities into one of three categories of potential exposure (see Table 39.3). Employers should make protective equipment available to all workers when they are engaged in Category I or II activities. Employers should ensure that the appropriate protective equipment is used by workers when they perform Category I activities.

As a second step, employers should establish a detailed work practices programme that includes standard operating procedures (SOPs) for all activities having the potential for exposure. Once these SOPs are developed, an initial and periodic worker education programme to assure familiarity with work practices should be provided to potentially exposed workers. No worker should engage in such tasks or activities before receiving training pertaining to the SOPs, work practices, and protective equipment required for that task. Examples of personal protective equipment for the pre hospital setting (defined as a setting where delivery of emergency health care takes place away from a hospital or other health-care setting) are provided in Table 39.4. (A curriculum for such training programmes is being developed in conjunction with these guidelines and should be consulted for further information concerning such training programmes.

Table 39.3
Summary of Task Categorization and Implications for Personal Protective Equipment

Joint Advisory Notice Category[1]	Nature of Task/Activity	Personal protective equipment should be: Available?	Worn?
I.	Directcontact with blood or other body fluids to which universal precautions apply	Yes	Yes
II.	Activity performed without blood exposure but exposure may occur in emergency	Yes	No
III.	Task/activity does not entail predictable or unpredictable exposure to blood	No	No

[1] U.S. Department of Labour, U.S. Department of Health and Human Services. Joint advisory notice: protection against occupational exposure to hepatitis B virus (HBV) and human immunodeficiency virus (HIV). Washington, DC: US Department of Labour, US Department of Health and Human Services, 1987.

To facilitate and monitor compliance with SOPs, administrative procedures should be developed and records kept as described in the Joint Advisory Notice.[6] Employers should monitor the workplace to ensure that required work practices are observed and that protective clothing and equipment are provided and properly used. The employer should maintain records documenting the administrative procedures used to classify job activities and copies of all SOPs for tasks or activities involving predictable or unpredictable exposure to blood or other body fluids to which universal precautions apply. In addition, training records, indicating the dates of training sessions, the content of those training sessions along with the names of all persons conducting the training, and the names of all those receiving training should also be maintained.

Whenever possible, the employer should identify devices and other approaches to modifying the work environment which will reduce exposure risk. Such approaches are desirable, since they don't require individual worker action or management activity. For example, jails and correctional facilities should have classification procedures that require the segregation of offenders who indicate through their actions or words that they intend to attack correctional-facility staff with the intent of transmitting HIV or HBV.

Table 39.4
Examples of Recommended Personal Protective Equipment for Worker Protection Against HIV and HBV Transmission in Prehospital[1] Settings

Task or Activity	Disposable Gloves	Gown	Mask	Protective Eyewear
Bleeding control with spurting blood	Yes	Yes	Yes	Yes
Bleeding control with minimal bleeding	Yes	No	No	No
Emergency child birth	Yes	Yes	Yes if splashing is likely	Yes if splashing is likely
Blood drawing	At certain times[4]	No	No	No
Starting an intravenous (IV) line	Yes	No	No	No
Endotracheal intubation esophageal obturator use	Yes	No	No unless splashing is likely	No unless splashing is likely
Oral/nasal suctioning manually cleaning airway	Yes[5]	No	No, unless splashing is likely	No, unless splashing is likely
Handling and cleaning instruments with microbial contamination	Yes	No, unless soiling is likely	No	No
Measuring blood pressure	No	No	No	No
Measuring temperature	No	No	No	No
Giving an injection	No	No	No	No

[1] The examples provided in this table are based on application of universal precautions Universal precautions are intended to supplement rather than replace recom

{Cont.}.........

mendations for routine infection control, such as handwashing and using gloves to prevent gross microbial contamination of hands (e g, contact with urine or feces)

[2] Defined as setting where delivery of emergency health are takes place away from a hospital or other health-care facility.

[3] Refers to protective masks to prevent exposure of mucous membranes to blood or other potentially contaminated body fluids. The use of resuscitation devices, some of which are also referred to as "masks".

[4] For clarification see A, and B.

[5] While not clearly necessary to prevent HIV or HBV transmission unless blood is present, gloves are recommended to prevent transmission of other agents (e.g., Her per simplex).

B. Medical

In addition to the general responsibilities noted above, the employer has the specific responsibility to make available to the worker a programme of medical management. This programme is designed to provide for the reduction of risk of infection by HBV and for counseling workers concerning issues regarding HIV and HBV. These services should be provided by a licensed health professional. All phases of medical management and counseling should ensure that the confidentiality of the worker's and client's medical data is protected.

1. Hepatitis B vaccination

All workers whose jobs involve participation in tasks or activities with exposure to blood or other body fluids to which universal precautions apply (as defined above) should be vaccinated with hepatitis B vaccine.

2. Management of percutaneous exposure to blood and other infectious body fluids

Once an exposure has occurred (as defined above a blood sample should be drawn after consent is obtained from the individual from whom exposur eoccurred and tested for hepatitis B surface antigen (HBsAg) and antibody to human immunodeficiency virus (HIV antibody). Local laws regarding consent for testing source individuals should be followed. Policies should be available for testing source individuals in situations where consent cannot be obtained (e.g., an unconscious patient). Testing of the source individual should be done at a location where appropriate pretest counseling is available; posttest counseling and referral for treatment should be provided. It is extremely important that all individuals who seek consultation for any HIV-related concerns receive counseling as outlined in the "Public Health Service Guidelines for Counseling and Antibody Testing to Prevent HIV Infection and AIDS". [22]

(a) Hepatitis B virus postexposure management

For an exposure to a source individual found to be positive for HBsAg, the worker who has not previously been given hepatitis B vaccine should receive the vaccine series. A single dose of hepatitis B immune globulin (HBIG) is also recommended, if this can be given within 7 days of exposure. For exposures from an HBsAg-positive source to workers who have previously received vaccine, the exposed worker should be tested for antibody to hepatitis B surface antigen (anti-HBs), and given one dose of vaccine and one dose of HBIG if the antibody level in the worker's blood sample is inadequate (i.e. <10 SRU by RIA, negative by EIA).[7]

If the source individual is negative for HBsAg and the worker has not been vaccinated, this opportunity should be taken to provide hepatitis B vaccination.

If the source individual refuses testing or he/she cannot be identified, the unvaccinated worker should receive the hepatitis B vaccine series. HBIG administration should be considered on an individual basis when the source individual is known or suspected to be at high risk of HBV infection. Management and treatment, if any, of previously vaccinated workers who receive an exposure from a source who refuses testing or is not identifiable should be individualized.[7]

(b) Human immunodeficiency virus postexposure management

For any exposure to a source individual who has AIDS, who is found to be positive for HIV infection,[4] or who refuses testing, the worker should be counseled regarding the risk of infection and evaluated clinically and serologically for evidence of HIV infection as soon as possible after the exposure. In view of the evolving nature of HIV post exposure management, the health care provider should be well informed of current PHS guidelines on this subject. The worker should be advised to report and seek medical evaluation for any acute febrile illness that occurs within 12 weeks after the exposure. Such an illness, particularly one characterized by fever, rash, or lymphadenopathy, may be indicative of recent HIV infection. Following the initial test at the time of exposure, seronegative workers shoul be retested

6 weeks, 12 weeks, and 6 months after exposure to determine whether transmission has occurred. During this follow-up period (especially the first 6-12 weeks after exposure, when most infected persons are expected to seroconvert), exposed workers should follow U.S. Public Health Service (PHS) recommendations for preventing transmission of HIV. [22] These include refraining from blood donation and using appropriate protection during sexual intercourse. [23] During all phases of follow-up, it is vital that worker confidentiality be protected.

If the source individual was tested and found to be seronegative, baseline testing of the exposed worker with follow-up testing 12 weeks later may be performed if desired by the worker or recommended by the health-care provider.

If the source individual cannot be identified, decisions regarding appropriate follow-up should be individualized. Serologic testing should be made available by the employer to ahl workers who may be concerned they have been infected with HIV through an occupational exposure as defined above.

3. Management of Human Bites

On occasion, police and correctional-facility officers are intentionally bitten by suspects or prisoners. When such bites occur, routine medical and surgical therapy (including an assessment of tetanus vaccination status) should be implemented as soon as possible, since such bites frequently result in infection with organisms other than HIV and HBV. Victims of bites should be evaluated as described above exposure to blood or other infection body fluids.

Saliva of some persons infected with HBV has been shown to contain HBV-DNA at concentrations 1/1,000 to 1/10,000 of that found in the infected person's serum. [5,24] HBsAg-positive saliva has been shown to be infectious when injected into experimental animals and in human bite exposures.[25-27] However, HBsAg-positive saliva has not been shown to be infectious when applied to oral mucous membranes in experimental primate studies [27] or through contamination of musical instruments or cardiopulmonary resuscitation dummies used by HBV carriers. [28,29] Epidemiologic studies of nonsexual household contacts of HIV-infected patients, including several small series in which HIV transmission failed to occur after bites or after percutaneous inoculation or contamination of cuts and open wounds with saliva from HIV-infected patients, suggest that the potential for salivary transmission of HIV is remote.[5,30-33] One case report from Germany has suggested the possibility of transmission of HIV in a household setting from an infected child to a sibling through a human bite.[34] The bite did not break the skin or result in bleeding. Since the date of seroconversion to HIV was not known for either child in this case, evidence for the role of saliva in the transmission of virus is unclear.[34]

4. Documentation of Exposure and Reporting

As part of the confidential medical record, the circumstances of exposure should be recorded. Relevant information includes the activity in which the worker was engaged at the time of exposure, the extent to which appropriate work practices and protective equipment were used, and a description of the source of exposure.

Employers have a responsibility under various federal and state laws and regulations to report occupational illnesses and injuries. Existing programmes in the National Institute for Occupational Safety and Health (NIOSH), Department of Health and Human Services; the Bureau of Labour Statistics, Department of Labour (DoL); and the Occupational safety and Health Administration (DOL) receive such information for the purposes of surveillance and other objectives. Cases of infectious disease, including AIDS and HBV infection, are reported to the Centers for Disease Control through State health departments.

5. Management of HBV- or HIV-infected workers

Transmission of HBV from health-care workers to patients has been documented. Such transmission has occurred during certain types of invasive procedures (e.g., oral and gynecologic surgery) in which health-care workers, when tested, had very high concentrations of HBV in their blood (at least 100 million infectious virus particles per milliliter, a concentration much higher than occurs with HIV infection), and the health-care workers sustained a puncture wound while performing invasive procedures or had exudative or weeping lesions or microlacerations that allowed virus to contaminate instruments or open wounds of patients. [35,36] A worker who is HBsAg positive and who has transmitted hepatitis B virus to another individual during the performance of his or her job duties should be excluded from the performance of those job duties which place other individuals at risk for acquisition of hepatitis B infection.

Workers with impaired immune systems resulting from HIV infection or other causes are at increased risk of acquiring or experiencing serious complications of infectious disease. Of particular concern is the risk of severe infection following exposure to other persons with infectious diseases that are easily transmitted if appropriate precautions are not taken (e.g., measles, varicella). Any worker with an impaired immune system should be counseled about the potential risk associated with providing health care to persons with any transmissible infection and should continue to follow existing recommendations for infection control to minimize risk of exposure to other infectious agents.[2,3] Recommendations of the Immunization Practices Advisory Committee (ACIP) and institutional policies concerning requirements for vaccinating workers with live-virus vaccines (e.g., measles, rubella) should also be considered.

The question of whether workers infected with HIV can adequately and safely be allowed to perform patient-care duties or whether their work assignments should be changed must be determined on an individual basis. These decisions should be made by the worker's personal physician(s) in conjunction with the employer's medical advisors.

C. Disinfection, Decontamination, and Disposal

As described in Section I.C. (4), the only documented occupational risks of HIV and HBV infection are associated with parenteral (including open wound) and mucous membrane exposure to blood and other potentially infectious body fluids. Nevertheless, the precautions described below should be routinely followed.

1. Needle and sharps disposal

All workers should take precautions to prevent injuries caused by needles, scalpel blades, andother sharp instruments or devices during procedures; when cleaning used instruments; during disposal of used needles; and when handling sharp instruments after procedures. To prevent needle-stick injuries, needles should not be recapped, purposely bent or broken by hand, removed from disposable syringes, or otherwise manipulated by hand. After they are used, disposable syringes and needles, scalpel blades, and other sharp items should be placed in puncture-resistant containers for disposal; the puncture-resistant containers should be located as close as practical to the use area (e.g., in the ambulance or, if sharps are carried to the scene of victim assistance from the ambulance, a small puncture—resistant container should be carried to the scene, as well). Reusable needles should be left on the syringe body and should be placed in a puncture-resistant container for transport to the reprocessing area.

2. Hand washing

Hands and other skin surfaces should be washed immediately and thoroughly if contaminated with blood, other body fluids to which universal precautions apply, or potentially contaminated articles. Hands should always be washed after gloves are removed, even if the gloves appear to be intact. Hand washing should be completed using the appropriate facilities, such as utility or restroom sinks. Waterless antiseptic hand cleanser should be provided on responding units to use when hand-washing facilities are not available. When hand-washing facilities are available, wash hands with warm water and soap. When hand-washing facilities are not available, use a waterless antiseptic hand cleanser. The manufacturer's recommendations for the product should be followed.

3. Cleaning, disinfecting, and sterilizing

Table 39.5 presents the methods and applications for cleaning, disinfecting, and sterilizing equipment and surfaces in the prehospital setting. These methods also apply to housekeeping and other cleaning tasks. Previously issued guidelines for health-care workers contain more detailed descriptions.[4]

4. Cleaning and decontaminating spills of blood

All spills of blood and blood-contaminated fluids should be promptly cleaned up using an EPA-approved germicide or a 1:100 solution of household bleach in the following manner while wearing gloves. Visible material should first be removed with disposable towels or other appropriate means that will ensure against direct contact with blood. If splashing is anticipated, protective eyewear should be worn along with an impervious gown or apron which provides an effective barrier to splashes. The area should then be decontaminated with an appropriate germicide. Hands should be washed following removal of gloves. Soiled cleaning equipment shouldbe cleaned and decontaminated or placed in an appropriate container and disposed of according to agency policy. Plastic bags should be available for removal of contaminated items from the site of the spill.

Shoes and boots can become contaminated with blood in certain instances. Where there is massive blood contamination on floors, the use of disposable impervious shoe coverings should be considered. Protective gloves should be worn to remove contaminated shoe coverings. The coverings and gloves should be disposed of in plastic bags. A plastic bag should be included in the crime scene kit or the car which is to be used for the disposal of contaminated items. Extra plastic bags should be stored in the police cruiser or emergency vehicle.

5. Laundry

Although soiled linen may be contaminated with pathogenic micro organisms, the risk of actual disease transmission is negligible. Rather than rigid procedures and specifications, hygienic storage and processing of clean and soiled linen are recommended. Laundry facilities and/or services should be made routinely available by the employer. Soiled linen should be handled as little as possible and with minimum agitation to prevent gross microbial contamination of the air and of persons handling the linen. All soiled linen should be bagged at the location where it was used. Linen soiled with blood should be placed and transported in bags that prevent leakage. Normal laundry cycles should be used according to the washer and detergent manufacturers' recommendations.

6. Decontamination and laundering of protective clothing

Protective work clothing contaminated with blood or other body fluids to which universal precautions apply should be placed and transported in bags or containers that prevent leakage. Personnel involved in the bagging, transport, and laundering of contaminated clothing should wear gloves. Protective clothing and station and work uniforms should be washed and dried according to the manufacturer's instructions. Boots and leather goods may be brush-scrubbed with soap and hot water to remove contamination.

7. Infective waste

The selection of procedures for disposal of infective waste is determined by the relative risk of disease transmission and application of local regulations, which vary widely. In all cases, local regulations should be consulted prior to disposal procedures and followed. Infective waste, in general, should either be incinerated or should be decontaminated before disposal in a sanitary landfill. Bulk blood, suctioned fluids, excretions and secretiond may be carefully poured down a drain connected to a sanitary sewer, where permitted sanitary sewers may also be used to dispose of other infectious wastes capable of being ground and ushed into the sewer, where permited sharp items should be placed in puncture-proof containers and other blood-contaminated items should be placed in leak-proof plastic bags for transport to an appropriate disposal location.

Prior to the removal of protective equipment, personnel remainingon the scene after the patient has been cared for should carefully search for and remove contaminated materials Debris should be disposed of as noted above.

IV. FIRE AND EMERGENCY MEDICAL SERVICES

The guidelines that appear in this section apply to fire and emergency medical services. This includes structural fire fighters, paramedics, emergency medical technicians, and advanced life support personnel. Fire fighters often provide emergency medical services and therefore encounter the exposures common to paramedics and emergency medical technicians. Job duties are often performed in uncontrolled environments, which, due to a lack of time and other factors, do not allow for application of acomplex decision-making process to the emergency at hand.

The general principles presented here have been developed from existing principles of occupational safety and health in conjunction with data from studies of health-care workers in hospital settings. The basic premise is that workers must be protected from exposure to blood and other potentially infectious body fluids in the course of their work activities. There is a paucity of data concerning the risks these worker groups face, however, which complicates development of control principles. Thus, the guidelines presented below are based on principles of prudent public health practice.

Fire and emergency medical service personnel are engaged in delivery of medical care in the prehospital setting. The following guidelines are intended to assist these personnel in making decisions concerning use of personal protective equipment and resuscitation equipment, as well as for decontamination, disinfection, and disposal procedures.

A. Personal Protective Equipment

Appropriate personal protective equipment should be made available routinely by the employer to reduce the risk of exposure as defined above. For many situations, the chance that the rescuer will be exposed to blood and other body fluids to which universal precautions apply can be determined in advance. Therefore, if the chances of being exposed to blood is high (e.g., CPR, IV insertion, trauma, delivering babies), the worker should put on protective attire before beginning patient care. Table 39.4) sets forth examples of recommendations for personal protective equipment inthe prehospital setting; the list is not intended to be all-inclusive.

1. Gloves

Disposable gloves should be a standard component of emergency response equipment, and should be donned by all personnel prior to initiating any emergency patient care tasks involving exposure to blood or other body fluids to which universal precautions apply. Extra pairs should always be available. Considerations in the choice of disposable gloves should include dexterity, durability, fit, and the task being performed. Thus, there is no single type or thickness of glove appropriate for protection in all situations. For situations where large amounts of blood are likely to be encountered, it is important that gloves fit tightly at the wrist to prevent blood contamination of hands around the cuff. For multiple trauma victims, gloves should be changed between patient contacts, if the emergency situation allows.

Greater personal protective equipment measures are indicated for situations where broken glass and sharp edges are likely to be encountered, such as extricating a person from an automobile wreck. Structural fire-fighting gloves that meet the Federal OSHA requirements for fire-fighters gloves (as contained in 29 CFR 1910.156 or National Fire Protection Association Standard 1973, Gloves for Structural Fire Fighters) should be worn in any situation where sharp or rough surfaces are likely to be encountered.[37]

While wearing gloves, avoid handling personal items, such as combs and pens, that could become soiled or contaminated. Gloves that have become contaminated with blood or other body fluids to which universal precautions apply should be removed as soon as possible, taking care to avoid skin contact with the exterior surface. Contaminated gloves should be placed and transported in bags that prevent leakage and should be disposed of or, in the case of reusable gloves, cleaned and disinfected properly.

2. Masks, eyewear, and gowns

Masks, eyewear, and gowns should be present on all emergency vehicles that respond or potentially respond to medical emergencies or victim rescues. These protective barriers should be used in accordance with the level of exposure encountered. Minor lacerations or small amounts of blood do not merit the same extent of barrier use as required for exsanguinating victims or massive arterial bleeding. Management of the patient who is not bleeding, and who has no bloody body fluids present, should not routinely require use of barrier precautions. Masks and eyewear (e.g., safety glasses) should be worn together, or a faceshield should be used by all personnel prior to any situation where splashes of blood or other body fluids to which universal precautions apply are likely to occur. Gowns or aprons should be worn to protect clothing from splashes with blood. If large splashes or quantities of blood are present or anticipated, impervious gowns or aprons should be worn. An extra change of work clothing should be available at all times.

3. Resuscitation Equipment

No transmission of HBV or HIV infection during mouth-to-mouth resuscitation has been documented. However, because of the risk of salivary transmission of other infectious diseases (e.g., herpes simplex and Neisseria meaningitidis)and the theoretical risk of HIV and HBV transmission during artificial ventilation of trauma victims, disposable air way equipment or resuscitation bags should be used. Disposable resuscitation equipment and devices should be used once and disposed of or, if reusable, thoroughly cleaned and disinfected after each use according to the manufacturer's recommendations.

Mechanical respiratory assist devices (e.g., bag-valve masks, oxygen demand valve resuscitators) should be available on all emergency vehicles and to all emergency response personnel that respond or potentially respond to medical emergencies or victim rescues.

Pocket mouth-to-mouth resuscitation masks designed to isolate emergency response personnel (i.e.,double lumen systems) from contact with victims' blood and blood contaminated saliva, respiratory secretions, and vomitus should be provided to all personnel who provide or potentially provide emergency treatment.

V. LAW-ENFORCEMENT AND CORRECTIONAL-FACLLLTY OFFICERS

Law-enforcement and correctional-facility officers may face the risk of exposure to blood during the conduct of their duties. For example, at the crime scene or during processing of suspects, law-enforcement officers may encounter blood-contaminated hypodermic needles or weapons, or be called upon to assist with body removal. Correctional-facility officers may similarly be required to search prisoners or their cells for hypodermic needles or weapons, or subdue violent and combative inmates.

The following section presents information for reducing the risk of acquiring HIV and HBV infection by law-enforcement and correctional-facility officers as a consequence of carrying out their duties. However, there is an extremely diverse range of potential situations which may occur in the control of persons with unpredictable, violent, or psychotic behaviour. Therefore, informed judgment of the individual officer is paramount when unusual circumstances or events arise. These recommendations should serve as an adjunct to rational decision making in those situations where specific guidelines do not exist, particularly where immediate action is required to preserve life or prevent significant injury.

The following guidelines are arranged into three sections: a section addressing concerns shared by both law-enforcement and correctional-facility officers, and two sections dealing separately with law-enforcement officers and correctional-facility officers, respectively. Table 39.4 contains selected examples of personal protective equipment that may be employed by law-enforcement and correctional-facility officers.

A. Law-Enforcement and Correctional-Facilities Considerations

1. Fights and assaults

Law-enforcement and correctional-facility officers are exposed to a range of assaultive and disruptive behaviour through which they may potentially become exposed to blood or other body fluids containing blood. Behaviours of particular concern are biting, attacks resulting in blood exposure, and attacks with sharp objects. Such behaviours may occur in a range of law-enforcement situations including arrests, routine interrogations, domestic disputes and lockup operations, as well as incorrectional-facility activities. Hand-to-hand combat may result in bleeding and may thus incur a greater chance for blood-to-blood exposure, which increases the chances for blood-borne disease transmission.

Whenever the possibility for exposure to blood or blood-contaminated body fluids exists, the appropriate protection should be worn, if feasible under the circumstances. In all cases, extreme caution must be used in dealing with the suspect or prisoner if there is any indication of assaultive or combative behaviour. When blood is present and a suspect or an inmate is combative or threatening lo staff, gloves should always be put on as soon as conditions permit. In case of blood contamination of clothing, an extra change of clothing should be available at all times.

2. Cardiopulmonary resuscitation

Law-enforcement and correctional personnel are also concern about infection with HIV and HBV through administration of cardiopulmonary resuscitation (CUR). Although there have been no documented cases of HIV transmission through this mechanism, the possibility of transmission of other infectious diseases exists.

Therefore, agencies should make protective masks or airways available to officers and provide training in their proper use. Devices with one-way valves to prevent the patients' saliva or vomitus from entering the caregiver's mouth are preferable.

B. Law-Enforcement Considerations

1. Searches and evidence handling

Criminal justice personnel have potential risks of acquiring HBV or HIV infection through exposures which occur during searches and evidence handling. Penetrating injuries are known to occur, and puncture wounds or needle sticks in particular pose a hazard during searches of persons, vehicles, or cells, and during evidence handling. The following precautionary measures will help to reduce the risk of infection:

An officer should use great caution in searching the clothing of suspects. Individual discretion, based on the circumstances at hand, should determine if a suspect or prisoner should empty his own pockets or if the officer should use his own skills in determining the contents of a suspect's clothing.

A safe distance should always be maintained between the officer and the suspect.

Wear protective gloves if exposure to blood is likely to be encountered.

Wear protective gloves for all body cavity searches.

If cotton gloves are to be worn when working with evidence of potential latent fingerprint value at the crime scene, they can be worn over protective disposable gloves when exposure to blood may occur.

Always carry a flashlight, even during daylight shifts, to search hidden areas. Whenever possible, use long-handled mirrors and flashlights to search such areas (e.g., under car seats).

If searching a purse, carefully empty contents directly from purse, by turning it upside down over a table.

Use puncture-proof containers to store sharp instruments and clearly marked plastic bags to store other possibly contaminated items.

To avoid tearing gloves, use evidence tape instead of metal staples to seal evidence.

Local procedures for evidence handling should be followed. In general, items should be air dried before sealing in plastic.

Not all types of gloves are suitable for conducting searches. Vinyl or latex rubber gloves provide little protection against sharp instruments, and they are not puncture proof. There is a direct trade-off between level of protection and manipulability. In other words, the thicker the gloves, the more protection they provide, but the less effective they are in locating objects. Thus, there is no single type or thickness of glove appropriate for protection in all situations. Officers should select the type and thickness of glove which provides the best balance of protection and search efficiency.

Officers and crime scene technicians may confront unusual hazards, especially when the crime scene involves violent behaviour, such as a homicide where large amounts of blood are present. Protective gloves should be available and worn in this setting. In addition, for very large spills, consideration should be given to other protective clothing, such as overalls, aprons, boots, or protective shoe covers. They should be changed if torn or soiled, and always removed prior to leaving the scene. While wearing gloves, avoid handling personal items, such as combs and pens, that could become soiled or contaminated.

Face masks and eye protection or a face shield are required for laboratory and evidence technicians whose jobs which entail potential exposures to blood via a splash to the face, mouth, nose, or eyes.

Airborne particles of dried blood may be generated when a stain is scraped. It is recommended that protective masks and eyewear or face shields be worn by laboratory or evidence technicians when removing the blood stain for laboratory analyses.

While processing the crime scene, personnel should be alert for the presence of sharp objects such as hypodermic needles, knives, razors, broken glass, nails,or othersharp objects.

2. Handling deceased persons and body removal

For detectives investigators evidence technicians all other who may have to touch or remove a body, the response should be the same as for situations requiring CPR or first aid: wear gloves and cover all cuts and abrasions to create a barrier and carefully wash all exposed areas after any contact with blood. The precautions to be used with blood and deceased persons should also be used when handling amputated limbs, hands, or other body parts. Such procedures should be followed after contact with the blood of anyone, regardless of whether they are known or suspected to be infected with HIV or HBV.

3. Autopsies

Protective masks and eyewear (or face shields), laboratory coats, gloves, and waterproof aprons should be worn when performing or at tending all autopsies. All autopsy material should be considered infectious for both HIV and HBV. Onlookers with an opportunity for exposure to blood splashes should be similarly protected. Instruments and surfaces contaminated during postmortem procedures should be decontaminated with an appropriate chemical germicide.[4] Many laboratories have more detailed standard operating procedures for conducting autopsies; where available, these should be followed. More detailed recommendations for health-care workers in this setting have been published. [4]

4. Forensic laboratories

Blood from all individuals should be considered infective. To supplement other worksite precautions, the following precautions are recommended for workers in forensic laboratories.

a. All specimens of blood should be put in a well-constructed, appropriately labelled container with a secure lid to prevent leaking during transport. Care should be taken when collecting each specimen to avoid contaminating the outside of the container and of the laboratory form accompanying the specimen.
b. All persons processing blood specimens should wear gloves. Masks and protective eyewear or face shields should be worn if mucous-membrane contact with blood is anticipated (e.g., removing tops from vacuum tubes). Hands should be washed after completion of specimen processing.
c. For routine procedures,such as histologic and pathologic studies ormicrobiological culturing, a biological safety cabinet is not necessary. However, biological safety cabinets (Class I or II) should be used whenever procedures are conducted that have a high potential for generating droplets. These include activities such as blending, sonicating, and vigorous mixing.
d. Mechanical pipetting devices should be used for manipulating all liquids in the laboratory. Mouth pipetting must not be done.
e. use of needles and syringes should be limited to situations in which there is no alternative, and the recommendations for preventing injuries with needles outlined under universal precautions should be followed.

f. Laboratory work surfaces should be cleaned of visible materials and then decontaminated with an appropriate chemical germicide after a spill of blood, semen, or blood-contaminated body fiuid and when work activities are completed.

g. Contaminated materials used in laboratory tests should be decontaminated before reprocessing or be placed in bags and disposed of in accordance with institutional and local regulatory policies for disposal of infective waste.

h. Scientific equipment that has been contaminated with blood should be cleaned and then decontaminated before being repaired in the laboratory or transported to the manufacturer.

i. All persons should wash their hands after completing laboratory activities and should remove protective clothing before leaving the laboratory.

j. Area posting of warning signs should be considered to remind employees of continuing hazard of infectious disease transmission in the laboratory setting.

C. Correctional-Facility Considerations

1. Searches

Penetrating injuries are known to occur in the correctional-facility setting, and puncture wounds or needle sticks in particular pose a hazard during searches of prisoners or their cells. The following precautionary measures will help to reduce the risk of infection.

A correctional-facility officer should use great caution in searching the clothing of prisoners. Individual discretion, based on the circumstances at hand, should determine if a prisoner should empty his own pockets or if the officer should use his own skills in determining the contents of a prisoner's clothing.

A safe distance should always be maintained between the officer and the prisoner.

Always carry a flashlight, even during daylight shifts, to search hidden areas. Whenever possible, use long-handled mirrors and flashlights to search such areas (e.g., under commodes, bunks, and in vents in jail cells).

Wear protective gloves if exposure to blood is likely to be encountered.

Wear protective gloves for all body cavity searches.

Table- 39. 5

Reprocessing Methods for Equipment Used in the Prehospital[1] Health-Care Setting

Sterilization:	Destroys	All form of microbial life including high numbers of bacterial spores.
	Methods:	Steam under pressure (autoclave), gas (ethylene oxide), dry heat, or immersion in EPA-approved chemical "sterilant" for prolonged period of time, e.g., 6-10 hours or according to manufacturers' instructions. Note: liquid chemical "sterilants" should be used only on those instruments that are impossible to sterilize or disinfect with heat.
	Use:	For those instrumetns or devices that pen etrate skin or contact normally sterile ar eas of the body, e.g., scalpels, needles, etc. Disposable invasive equipment eliminates the need to reprocess these types of items. When indicated, however, arrangements should be made with a health-care facility for reprocessing of reusable invasive instruments.
High-Level Disinfection:	Destroys:	All forms of microbial life except high numbers of bacterial spores.
	Methods:	Hot water pasteurization (80-100 C, 30 minutes) or exposure to an EPA-registered "sterilant" chemicals above, except for as hort exposure time (10-45 minutes or as directed by the manufacturer).
	Use:	For reusable instruments or devices that come into contact with mucous membranes (e.g., laryngoscope blades, endotracheal tubes, etc.).
Intermediate-Level	Destroys:	*Mycobacterium tuberculosis*, vegetative bacteria, most viruses, and most fungi, but does not kill bacterial spores.
	Methods:	EPA-registered "hospital disinfectant" chemical germicides that have a label claim for tuberculocidal activity; commer cially available hard-surface germicides or solutions containing at least 500 ppm free available chlorine (a 1: 100 dilution of com mon household bleach-approximately ¼ cup bleach per gallon of tap water).
	Use:	For those surfaces that come into contact only with intact skin, e.g., stethoscopes, blood pressure cuffs, splints, etc. and have been visibly contaminated with blood or bloody body fluids. Surfaces must be precleaned of visible material before the

{Cont.}.....

		germicidal chemical is applied for disin fection.
Low-Level Disinfection:	Destroys:	Most bacteria, some viruses, some fungi, but not *Mycobacterium tuberculosis* or bacterial spores.
	Methods:	EPA-registered "hospital disinfectants" (no label claim for tuberculocidal activity).
	Use:	These agents are excellent cleaners and can be used for routine housekeeping or removal of soiling in the absence of visible blood contamination.
Low-Level Disinfection:		Environmental surfaces which have become soiled should be cleaned and disinfected using any cleaner or disinfectant-agent which is intended for environmental use. Such surfaces include floors, woodwork, ambulance seats, countertops, etc.
IMPORTANT:	To assure the effectiveness of any sterilization or disinfection process, equipment and instruments must first be thoroughly cleaned of all visible soil.	

[1] Defined as setting where delivery of emergency health-care takes place prior to arrival at hospital or other health-care facility.

Not all types of gloves are suitable for conducting searches. Vinyl or latex rubber gloves can provide little if any, protection against sharp instruments and they are not puncture-proof. There is a direct tradc-off bctwccn lcvcl of protcction and manipulability. In other words, the thicker the gloves, the more protection they provide, but the less effective they are in locating objects. Thus, there is no single type or thickness of glove appropriate for protection in all situations. Officers should select the type and thickness of glove which provides the best balance of protection and search efficiency.

2. Decontamination and Disposal

Prisoners mayspit at officers and throw feces; sometimes these substances have been purposefully contaminated with blood. Although there are no documented cases of HIV or HBV transmission in this manner and transmission by this route would not be expected to occur, other diseases could be transmitted. These materials should be removed with a paper towel after donning gloves, and the area then decontaminated with an appropriate germicide. Following clean-up, soiled towels and gloves should be disposed of properly.

References

1. Garner JS, Favero MS. Guideline for handwashing and hospital environmental control, 1985. Atlanta: Public Health Service, Centers for Disease Control, 1985. HHS publication no. 99-1117.
2. Garner JS, Simmons BP. Guideline for isolation precautions in hospitals. Infect Control 1983; 4 (suppl):245—325.
3. Williams WW. Guideline for infection control in hospital personnel. Infect Control 1983; 4(suppl):326-49.
4. Centers for Disease Control. Recommendations for prevention of HIV transmission in health-care settings. MMWR 1987; 36 (suppl 2S).
5. Centers for Disease Control. Update: Universal precautions for prevention of transmission of human immunodeficiency virus, hepatitis B virus, and other bloodborne pathogens in health-care settings. MMWR 1988; 37:377-382,387-88.
6. U.S. Department of Labour, U.S. Department of Health and Human Services. Joint Advisory Notice: protection against occupational exposure to hepatitis B virus (HBV and human immunodeficiency virus HIV). Federal Register 1987; 52:41818-24.
7. Centers for Disease Control. Recommendations for protection against viral hepatitis. MMWR 1985; 34:313-324,329-335.
8. Kunches L M, Craven DE, Werner BG, Jacobs LM. Hepatitis B exposure in emergency medical personnel: prevalence of serologic markers and need for immunization. Amer J Med 1983; 75:269-272.
9. Pepe PE, Hollinger FB, Troisi CL, Heiberg D. Viral hepatitis risk in urban emergency medical services personnel. Annals Emergency Med 1986; 15(4):454 457.
10. Valenzuela TD, Hook EW, Copass MK, Corey L. Occupational exposure to hepatitis B in paramedics. Arch Intern Med 1985; 145:1976-1977.
11. Morgan-Capner P. Hudson P. Hepatitis B markers in Lancashire police officers. Epidemiol Inf 1988; 100:145-151.
12. Peterkin M, Crawford RJ. Hepatitis B vaccine for police forces [Letter]? Lancet 1986; 2: 1458-59.
13. Radvan GH, Hewson EG, Berenger S. Brookman DJ. The Newcastle hepatitis B outbreak: observations on cause, management, and prevention. Med J Australia 1986; 144:461-464.
14. Centers for Disease Control. Inactivated hepatitis B virus vaccine. MMWR 1982; 26:317-322, 327-328.
15. Centers for Disease Control. Update on hepatitis B prevention. MMWR 1987; 36:353-360, 366.
16. Marcus R. and the CDC Co-operative Needlestick Surveillance Group. Surveillance of health care workers exposed to blood from patients infected with the human immunodeficiency virus. N Engl. J Med 1988; 319:1118-23.
17. Henderson DK, Fahey BJ, Saah AJ, Schmitt JM, Lane HC. Longitudinal assessment of risk for occupational/nosocomial transmission of human immunodeficiency virus, type 1 in health care workers. Abstract #634; presented at the 1988 ICAAC Conference, New Orleans.

18. Barnes DM. Health workers and AIDS: Questions persist. Science 1988; 241:161-2.
19. Gerberding JL, Littell CG, Chambers HF, Moss AR, Carlson J. Drew W. Levy J. Sande MA. Risk of occupational HIV transmission in intensively exposed health-care workers: Follow-up. Abstract #343; presented at the 1988 ICAAC Conference, New Orleans.
20. Health and Welfare Canada. National surveillance programme on occupational exposures to HIV among health-care workers in Canada. Canada Dis Weekly Rep 1987; 13-37: 163-6.
21. McEvoy M, Porter K,Mortimer P. Simmons N. Shanson D. Prospective study of clinical, laboratory, and ancillary staff with accidental exposures to blood or body fluids from patients infected with HIV. Br Med J 1987; 294: 1595-7.
22. Centers for Disease Control. Public Health Service guidelines for counseling and antibody testing to prevent HIV infection and AIDS. MMWR 1987; 36:; 509-515.
23. Centers for Disease Control. Additional recommendations to reduce sexual and drug abuse-related transmission of human T-lymphotropic virus type III/lymphadenopathy associated virus. MMWR 1986; 35:152-55.
24. Jenison SA, Lemon SM, Baker LN, Newbold JE. Quantitative analysis of hepatitis B virus DNA in saliva and semen of chronically infected homosexual men. J Infect Dis 1987; 156:299-306.
25. Cancio-Bello TP, de Medina M, Shorey J. Valledor MD, Schiff ER. An institutional outbreak of hepatitis B related to a human biting carrier. J Infect Dis 1982; 146:652-6.
26. MacQuarrie MB, Forghani B. Wolochow DA. Hepatitis B transmitted by a human bite. JAMA 1974; 230:723-4.
27. Scott RM, Snitbhan R. Bancroft WH, Alter HJ, Tingpalapong M. Experimental transmission of hepatitis B virus by semen and saliva. J Infect Dis 1980; 142:67-71.
28. Glaser JB, Nadler JP. Hepatitis B virus in a cardiopulmonary resuscitation training course: Risk of transmission from a surface antigen-positive participant. Arch Intern Med 1985; 145:1653-5.
29. Osterholm MT, Bravo ER, Crosson JT, et al. Lack of transmission of viral hepatitis type B after oral exposure to HBsAg-positive saliva. Br Med J 1979; 2:1263-4.
30. Lifson AR. Do alternate modes for transmission of human immunodeficiency virus exist? A review. JAMA1988;259:1353-6.
31. Friedland GH, Saltzman BR, Rogers MF, et al. Lack of transmission of HTLV-III/LAV infection to household contacts of patients with AIDS or AIDS-related complex with oral candidiasis. N Engl J Med 1986; 314:344-9.
32. Curran JW, Jaffe HW, Hardy AM, et al. Epidemiology of HIV infection and AIDS in the United States. Science 1988; 239:610-6.
33. Jason JM, McDougal JS, Dixon G. et al. HTLV-III/LAV antibody and immune status of household contacts and sexual partners of persons with hemophilia. JAMA 1986; 255:212-5.

34. Wahn V, Kramer HH, Voit T. Bruster HT, Scrampical B. Scheid A. Horizontal transmission of HIV infection between two siblings [Letter]. Lancet 1986; 2:694.
35. Kane MA, Lettau LA. Transmission of HBV from dental personnel to patients. J Am Dent Assoc 1985; 110:634-6.
36. Lettau LA, Smith JD, Williams D, et al. Transmission of hepatitis B virus with resultant restriction of surgical practice. JAMA 1986; 255:934-7.
37. International Association of Fire Fighters. Guidelines to prevent transmission of communicable disease during emergency care for fire fighters, paramedics, and emergency medical technicians. International Association of Fire Fighters, New York City, New York, 1988.

40

Information, Education and Communication

1. INTRODUCTION

The pandemic of Acquired Immuno-deficiency Syndrome (AIDS) poses a unique challenge to public health planners and programme developers. With no cure in sight, we are forced to look closely at behavioural patterns and how to alter them to prevent AIDS. Since AIDS is primarily a sexually transmitted disease (STD), it is important that policy-makers, communicators and public health professionals examine the sexual behaviour patterns of the communities they are serving and develop strategies aimed at behavioural change.

Information, education and communication (IEC) plays a crucial role in bringing about this change. IEC is seen as an essential component of an AIDS prevention and care programme. However, IEC alone is not enough; it must be supported by health and social services and should be planned for in the context of the overall programme objectives and activities. One of the necessary conditions for effective implementation is the understanding of (and commitment to) the IEC framework among the key personnel in each country. Promoting this may need specific steps, including:

- — Involvement of such key persons in the finalization of an overall strategy.
- — Workshops that help to disseminate and clarify the strategy.

Implementation of IEC efforts in relation to HIV/AIDS requires an appropriate organizational set-up in each country and this must take place in close collaboration with other services. There are advantages in having an integrated IEC organization for all activities in the health sector. However, in such a case it is essential to have a nodal person—or even a small group—for focusing specifically on the IEC activities for HIV/AIDS. Implementation should be done in the context of the totality of the problem and the overall framework of the strategy. Thus, a 'total system' or holistic approach is essential. Not only does each of the elements—including planning, research, message design, production, dissemination, monitoring and evaluation—need attention, but the relationship between each, as also the overall process, must be addressed.

A concerted effort, through a well-planned and effectively implemented IEC strategy, should create the necessary conditions for bringing about favourable behavioural changes. It is only through this that the preventive steps will succeed and help in combating the spread of HIV/AIDS.

1.1 What is IEC ?

IEC is a broad term comprising a range of approaches, activities and outputs. Although the most visible component of IEC is frequently the materials produced and used, such as posters hanging on clinic walls, materials are only one component. Effective IEC makes use of a full range of approaches and activities.

Approaches may range from the use of mass media to inform or establish positive norms among the general population to the use of targeted interpersonal communication to help those at particular risk evaluate their own behaviour and develop new personal skills. IEC activities may include designing and providing training in communication skills, carrying out research on audiences to determine what information is needed and the most effective way of delivering it, as well as designing and producing the materials to support activities.

Overall, IEC must be integrated with all existing HIV/AIDS prevention and care programmes as well as with on-going training services. For example, promotion of condom use or STD treatment among individuals with high-risk behaviour will be effective only if condoms are also made accessible and STD treatment services are available and non-stigmatizing.

Similarly a positive social environment without discrimination and stigmatization will facilitate behavioural change.

1.2 How can this Guide Help?

This document provides guidelines for national AIDS programme managers on how to set priorities and systematically plan and implement IEC activities as part of AIDS prevention and care programmes. It describes steps for the planning, implementation and evaluation of IEC activities. To reinforce the step-wise approach, a specific example of IEC activities addressed to young people has been included in the text.

2. HIV/AIDS BURDEN IN THE SOUTH-EAST ASIA REGION

In the South-East Asia Region, HIV infection was first reported in 1984 in Thailand. In most other countries, HIV infection was not diagnosed until 1986 or later. Since then, however, HIV infection has spread rapidly. WHO estimates that, as of early 1995, there are more than 2 million HIV-infected people in the Region. Three-fourths of reported AIDS cases from the Region have acquired the infection through sexual intercourse and more than 80 per cent are in the age group of 15-49 years.

In view of the fact that heterosexual contact is the predominant mode of HIV transmission in the Region, the rates of sexually transmitted diseases are high and that there is considerable unprotected sexual activity, continued transmission of HIV in the general population appears inevitable unless effective measures are taken immediately. Furthermore, WHO estimates that while the annual number of HIV infections may peak in Africa by the mid-1990s, infections in Asia will continue to increase well into the early years of the next century. By the year 2000, it is probable that the cumulative number of infections in Asia will rise by 8-10 million and that the annual numbers will fat exceed those in sub-Saharan Africa (Figure-40.1).

The greatest tragedy, besides medical and health care costs, will be the loss of thousands of lives, particularly those of young adults in their most productive years and infants born to HIV-infected mothers, which will directly affect child survival rates.

3. THE ROLE OF IEC IN HIV/AIDS PREVENTION

All countries in the Region now have national AIDS prevention and care programmes and are organizing efforts to combat the spread of HIV which include IEC, condom programming, providing STD services, and ensuring blood safety.

The general goal of IEC is to promote and support appropriate changes in behaviour, especially among populations with high-risk behaviour. While cultural differences are likely to require different styles of presentation of material between countries and between different target groups, the desired behaviours or behavioural changes will be similar (or even the same):

- Postponement of first sexual encounter;
- Decrease in multiple-partner sex;
- Increase in condom use;
- Increased use of health services to treat STDs; and
- Increased use of clean syringes by injecting drug users.

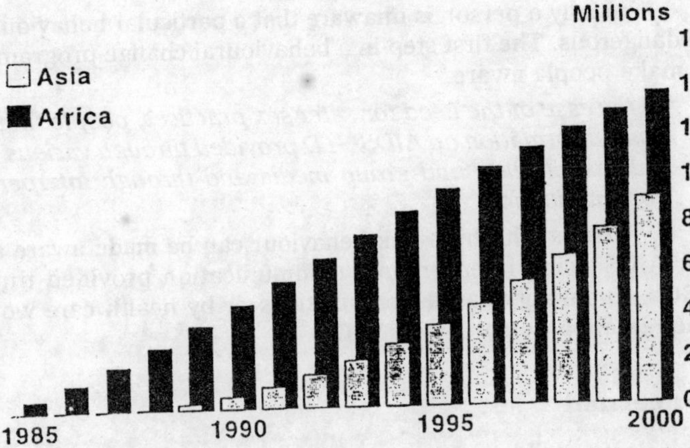

Figure 40.1. Estimated and projected cumutative adult HIV infections in Asia and Africa

3.1 Process of Behavioural Change: A Continuum

Bringing about a behavioural change is, however, a difficult process. The task is further complicated by the sensitive and personal nature of the issues, dealing as they largely do with sex and sexuality. A variety of approaches and messages will be needed to promote movement of individuals and populations along the continuum of behavioural change. The "adoption of safer sex" example below illustrates the various stages of the behavioural change model shown in Figure 40.2.

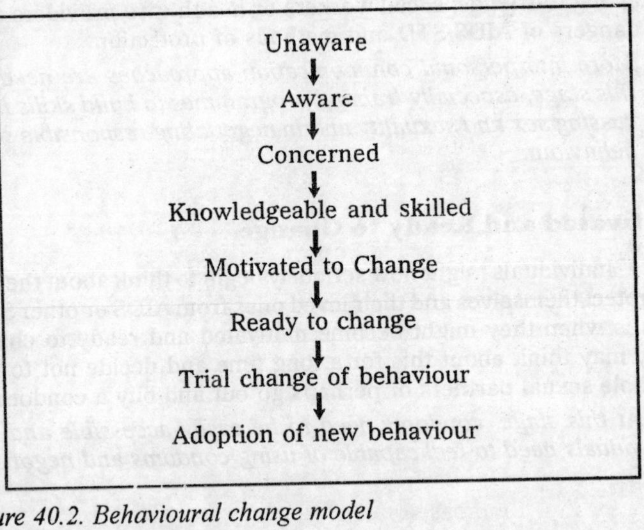

Figure 40.2. Behavioural change model

Unaware- aware

Initially a person is unaware that a particular behaviour may be dangerous. The first step in a behavioural change programme is to make people aware.

In the case of the need for safer sex practices, people first need basic information on AIDS/STD provided through various channels using mass and group media and through interpersonal communication.

Persons with high-risk behaviour can be made aware about HIV/AIDS using interpersonal communication provided through NGOs, community-based organizations or by health care workers when treating persons with STD.

Concerned

It is possible to be aware without being concerned. Information must be given is such a way that the audience feels it applies to them, i.e., the audience becomes concerned, and people are motivated to evaluate their own behaviour.

Mass media approaches aimed at the general population are less likely to be effective in creating concern and overcoming denial, particularly among those at greatest risk. Targeted communication and interpersonal approaches are therefore more useful.

Knowledgeable and Skilled

Once concerned, individuals may acquire more knowledge by talking to friends, social workers or health care providers about the dangers of AIDS/STD and methods of protection.

More interpersonal communication approaches are needed at this stage, especially training programmes to build skills in discussing sex and sexuality and in negotiating responsible sexual behaviour.

Motivated and Ready to Change

Individuals might now seriously begin to think about the need to protect themselves and their loved ones from AIDS or other STDs. This is when they might become motivated and ready to change. They may think about this for a long time and decide not to have multiple sexual partners or perhaps go out and buy a condom.

At this stage, condoms need to be easily accessible and individuals need to feel capable of using condoms and negotiating safer sex. Mass and targeted media can help provide a supportive environment by showing role models and promoting a positive view of safer sexual behaviour. Positive messages from peers are particularly effective.

Trial Change of Behaviour

At a later stage individuals are in a situation where a sexual encounter could take place and they have access to a condom. They could then decide to try the new behaviour.

The results of any trial will be evaluated. If the experience has been too difficult or embarrassing, due to lack of experience and skills, then they may not try again for a long time. Therefore, skills to *negotiate condom use, and to use condoms correctly, are essential.*

Adoption of New Behaviour

Finally, the individual decides to remain faithful to one faithful partner or regularly uses condoms as a source of protection from AIDS/STD.

Assuming the new behaviour continues to be evaluated as largely positive, sustained behavioural change could take place at this stage. Continuous messages of support and access to condoms are still essential.

Programmes must ensure that overall and individual stages of behavioural change are taken into consideration when IEC approaches and activities are being planned and implemented.

3.2 The Role of IEC in STD/AIDS Prevention and Control

(1) *Public education and targeted interventions:* education of the general population can best be carried out through the mass media. Additionally, while use of the mass media can be a most useful way to educate the population at large, experience indicates that more individualized, interpersonal channels of communication are needed, particularly for individuals engaged in high-risk behaviour. Efforts through the mass media may result in generating awareness and creating a positive environment, but interpersonal communication is a must for behavioural change. For this to occur, IEC efforts must be continuous.

Moreover, the mass media often do not reach those segments of a population which are most in need of information. Women, poorer communities, and those who operate on the fringes of society often have limited access to mass media. Traditional channels for communication, such as folk media including street theatres, are particularly effective in rural areas and urban slums. Other channels which also need to be explored include women's organizations and existing community networks. It is important to choose the right channel of communication for each target audience.

(2) *Advocacy:* IEC has an important role in advocacy. Policy and decision-makers have to be persuaded to take steps and/or initiate policies and services that will limit the spread of HIV infection and influence legislation. They must be made aware of the present magnitude and the frightening potential of HIV/AIDS, the consequent economic loss and the load on health services. Similarly, IEC efforts must also be directed to teachers, health and health-related workers and other intermediaries or 'influencers'. Equally important, through education programmes related to how HIV is not transmitted, IEC can assist in limiting discrimination and stigma and in promoting community acceptance of people with HIV or AIDS.

(3) *Support for various components of an AIDS Prevention and Control Programme:* IEC campaigns can promote seeking of quality STD services, which of course must be made available. IEC can also support efforts to promote voluntary blood donation and the implementation of universal precautions in health care settings.

4. LESSONS LEARNT FROM IEC PROGRAMME EXPERIENCES

Countries in South-East Asia can benefit from the experiences gained within as well as outside the Region. Learning from others allows programme managers to initiate more effective strategies and communication approaches to assist behavioural change. Such lessons illustrate the importance of selecting appropriate communication approaches, of targeting education and of integrating IEC with health and social services.

4.1 Using Appropriate Communication Approaches

Some examples of lessons learned about communication approaches early on in the AIDS pandemic in many countries include the following:

In many countries, including the U.K. and Australia, fear campaigns were initiated with the reasoning that people would be shocked into behavioural change. However, studies showed contrary results, since individuals at low risk became irrationally concerned and those at high risk turned away from the messages. Such approaches may provide short-term improvement but do not lead to sustained behavioural change.

Fear campaigns do not work and are not effective in bringing about behavioural change

Denial of the AIDS epidemic is a stage most countries have gone through. A slogan such as 'Do not have sex with foreigners' blames others. This slogan claims that only foreigners have AIDS and that AIDS does not exist in the home country. Denial is extremely dangerous as it allows individuals and policy-makers to lay the blame elsewhere and to block and unnecessarily delay needed action.

Denial or blame campaigns inhibit necessary action

In the United States, policy-makers initially believed that AIDS was a disease of gay men only and they ignored all the signs and evidence that AIDS was a sexually transmitted disease of the entire population. In India, and in some other South-East Asian countries, blame in many quarters is being placed on sex workers and drug users, when the HIV virus can already be found in many other pockets of society, for example, in clients who infect sex workers.

Moral messages may turn away the very people you want to reach or deny lifesaving information to those in need

AIDS education necessitates talking about sexual behaviour and methods of protection from HIV through sexual intercourse. To date, the only known method, barring abstinence, is condom use. However, in many countries, governments and religious organizations have prohibited the promotion of condom use with the argument that it would promote promiscuity. This has led to disastrous results in some countries. Studies have conclusively demonstrated that education on sex and methods of contraception in schools do not lead to an increase in sexual activity among youth; only to an increase in the use of contraceptive methods. In some cases, such education has instead led to an increase in the postponement of initiating sexual activity.

4.2 Designing Appropriate Audience Communications

Messages and delivery channels must be tailored for the specific target group. Consideration needs to be given to cultural acceptability, literacy levels, preferred sources of information, and available infrastructures. Communication must be gender sensitive and should be delivered through a variety of channels, packaged in different forms.

The development of messages should take place after rapid assessment of the current knowledge, attitudes, behaviour and practices (KABP) in relation to sexuality and AIDS/STDs. Population KABP studies have been found to be expensive, time-consuming and laborious. Qualitative methods have instead been found to be more useful.

Keeping all these issues in mind, guidelines which can assist in avoiding some of the mistakes of the past indicate that messages should:

— be consistent and accurate and disseminated in a continuous manner.
— be positive and aim to help people protect themselves and help those already infected to live productive and socially beneficial lives.
— be action oriented, so leading individuals to actions such as calling for more information, buying condoms, or using clean needles.
— be linked to service delivery. For example, information and counselling centres must be available to help people gain knowledge about the spread of infection and methods of prevention, and to counsel those in need. If condoms are being promoted, affordable condoms must be available in the area. STD treatment services should also be made easily accessible.
— offer options. For example, when dealing with difficult-to-change behaviour patterns such as drug use, it is helpful and more effective to provide the individual with options for action. For example 'Your chances of getting AIDS are high if you inject drugs, so don't inject: if you can't avoid injecting, don't share needles; if you can't avoid sharing, at least clean the needles before sharing'. Such behaviour options also apply to sexual transmission. For example: 'Your chances of contracting HIV/STDs increase if you have multiple sexual partners; so abstain from sex or stick to one uninfected partner; or practise safer sex such as condom use for every sexual encounter in situations of risk.'

4.3 Targeting AIDS Education

Another important lesson learned is the need to prioritize programme activities. Not everyone is at equal risk of contracting HIV. Identifiable groups of people who are engaged in behaviours which facilitate the spread of HIV can be targeted for priority prevention activities. These behaviours include having multiple sexual partners and sharing injecting equipment. People with a high prevalence of other sexually transmitted diseases also need to be targeted.

The groups at high risk may differ from city to city and area to area. It is important for each national or district-level programme to evaluate the risk determinants and identify the populations that may be at high risk of infection so that appropriate strategies to reach such populations can be developed on a priority basis.

Groups of individuals who share common high-risk behaviour might include, among others, commercial sex workers and their clients; injecting drug users; people with STDs; migrant workers; transportation workers—especially truck drivers; street children; and the military. Other general groups, such as women who have limited access to information and services or youth, also need special emphasis.

Targeted interventions among these populations, given the current epidemiological situation in the Region, will have the greatest impact on limiting the further spread of HIV.

4.4 IEC as a Part of an Integrated Intervention Package

Experience shows that IEC alone will not have a significant impact on the spread of HIV infection unless it is complemented by making available health and other services which address factors contributing to vulnerability to STD and HIV infection. Such an integrated approach among truck drivers, for example, would necessitate AIDS education in an interpersonal manner, the availability of condoms, STD services in a non-stigmatizing setting and possibly counselling services. For women, besides IEC, such an approach would entail the provision of STD services within MCH/FP and primary health care facilities along with the mobilization of women's organizations and counselling services. IEC should lead to action, and the means to facilitate that action must be in place and easily accessible.

No single organization can carry out all these activities. AIDS prevention and control activities need to draw on the wide range of multisectoral expertise and skills required for intervention development and implementation. This means close collaboration between government services and NGOs working with particular groups. If such programmes do not exist, it is essential that these be initiated urgently.

5. STEPS IN IEC PLANNING, IMPLEMENTATION AND EVALUATION

Effective IEC programmes are based within the overall context of the programme goals and can be developed following a systematic assessment of the target audiences and with their participation. The steps which need to be taken for the development of an effective IEC programme are as follows:

— Planning;
— Preparatory Activities and Materials Development;
— Dissemination and Utilization, and
— Monitoring and Evaluation.

A framework for IEC is presented in Figure 40.3.

5.1 Planning

First, the current situation must be reviewed. This will include a thorough assessment of the programme's IEC needs and existing IEC activities, identification of target audiences, formulation of achievable objectives, and identification of activities to be carried out as well as potential partners for implementation.

5.1.1 Situational Analysis

(a) The first step of a situational analysis is examination and analysis of existing national policies, especially those relating to Health, Education and Communication, and laws which can impact on AIDS/STD prevention efforts. For example, a national policy against condom promotion would need to be revised in the light of the AIDS pandemic. The organizational structure and manpower available for AIDS prevention should be analysed, while communication and outreach networks, both within the government as well as among NGOs, should be assessed for use in AIDS educational activities.

(b) Another task in situational analysis is examination of existing epidemiological, cultural and behavioural data and exploration of the existing situation from a number of points of view, including: past/present preventive actions and their effectiveness; the extent of spread of HIV in different groups and areas; assessment of vulnerable populations; and any information relating to particular groups of interest such as demographic data, social structure, the status of women and literacy levels. Every effort must be made to fully utilize existing data from studies in various fields, particularly including those in

Figure 40.3 IEC Framework

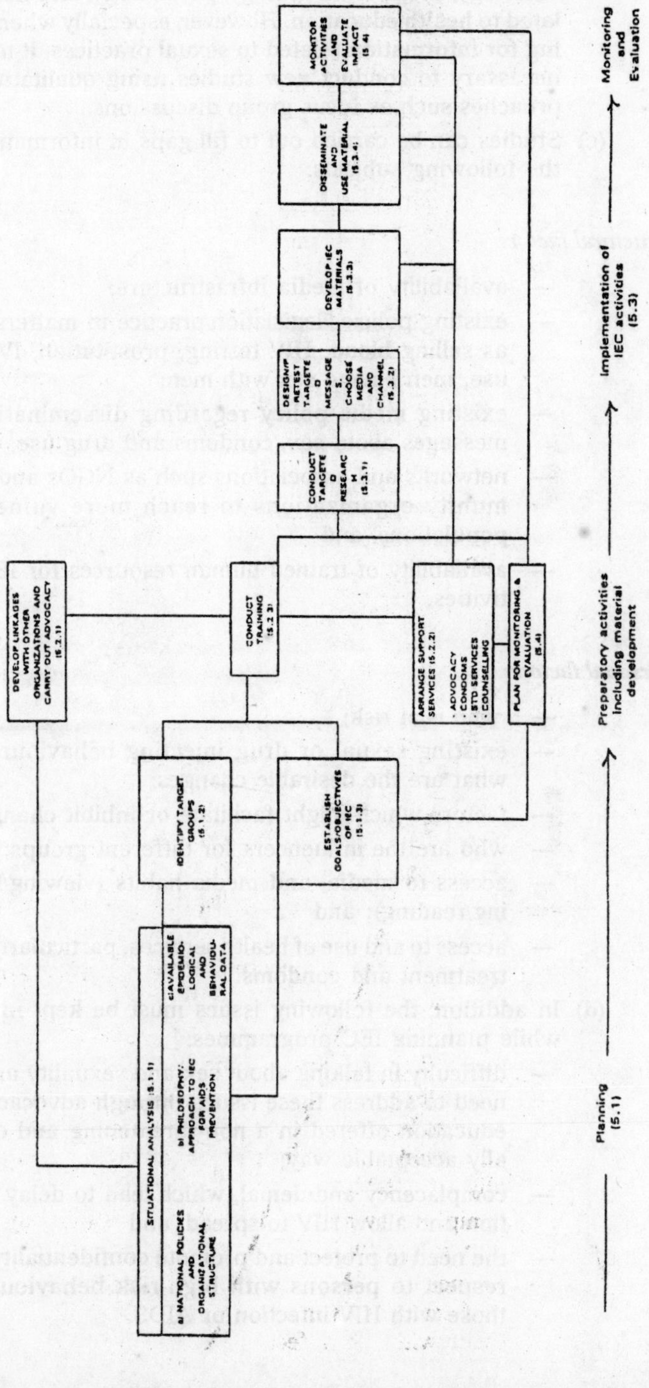

sociology, social anthropology, psychology, and fields related to health education. However, especially when looking for information related to sexual practices, it may be necessary to conduct new studies using qualitative approaches such as focus group discussions.

(c) Studies can be carried out to fill gaps in information on the following subjects:

Structural factors:

- availability of media infrastructure;
- existing policies/legislation/practice in matters such as selling blood, HIV testing, prostitution, IV drug use, men having sex with men;
- existing media policy regarding dissemination of messages about sex, condoms and drug use;
- networks and associations such as NGOs and community organizations to reach more vulnerable populations, and
- availability of trained human resources for IEC activities.

Personal factors:

- who is at risk;
- existing sexual or drug injecting behaviours and what are the desirable changes;
- factors which might facilitate or inhibit changes;
- who are the influencers for different groups;
- access to media, and media habits (viewing/listening/reading); and
- access to and use of health services, particularly STD treatment and condoms.

(d) In addition, the following issues must be kept in mind while planning IEC programmes:

- difficulty in talking about sex and sexuality and the need to address these issues through advocacy and education offered in a non-threatening and culturally acceptable way;
- complacency and denial, which lead to delay in action and allow HIV to spread; and
- the need to protect and promote confidentiality with respect to persons with high-risk behaviour and those with HIV infection or AIDS.

5.1.2 Identify Targets Groups

Identification and prioritization of target groups for the overall IEC programme is of great importance. In the absence of specific targeting, IEC messages tend to be very general, non-focused and, while they may provide information, they do not foster either change or action. Setting priorities is also necessary since resources are inevitably limited and their optimal use requires a clear understanding about which groups are to be the focus of attention.

Target groups for intervention should be identified according to criteria such as risk behaviour, population size, potential for contributing to spread of infection and accessibility. In South-East Asia, populations at high risk or vulnerable to HIV infection might include:

— adolescents and youth, especially street children;
— women in the reproductive age group (15-45 years); and
— known populations with a high prevalence of risk behaviour such as sex workers and their clients, injecting drug users, truck drivers and migrant populations.

5.1.3 Establish Goals, Objectives and Targets

IEC programme goals for each target group should describe the desired behavioural changes, while the specific objectives for each target group should be stated in measurable terms. This means that it will be possible to observe and measure progress towards meeting the objectives. For example, 'Within 12 months, 50 per cent of injecting drug users in one urban slum will stop sharing the injection equipment'; and, for IEC,' Within 12 months, 80 per cent of injecting drug users will be reached with accurate information on safer injecting practices'.

Realistic targets must be set taking into consideration the characteristics and situation of the target groups involved, the extent of communication infrastructure and the access that various groups have to information and services (e.g., radio and TV ownership/access in the case of education for the general population, or the presence of an NGO in the case of a population with high-risk behaviour); and the support services available.

Overall programme objectives for most of the target groups would include:

— decrease in number of sexual partners;
— increase in safe injecting practices (for injecting drug users);
— increase safer sex practices including condom use;
— enhance negotiating skills on sexual decisions;

— increase STD treatment-seeking behaviour;
— increase in health care-seeking behaviour (especially for women).
— reduction in STD rates.

5.2 Preparatory Activities

Essential preparatory activities include developing linkages, establishing co-ordination for essential services and ensuring availability of trained manpower.

5.2.1 Develop Linkages

Linkages for implementation of IEC activities within the government may be with the ministries of education, youth, women and child welfare, tourism, information and broadcasting, and transportation. Integration with MCH/FP programmes is an important strategy to reach women and should be a major priority. Collaboration with various ministries is also needed for advocacy to establish the sound policies needed for planning and implementation of effective IEC programmes.

NGOs are also important. While conducting the assessment and looking closer at identified vulnerable groups and high-risk behaviour groups, nongovernmental partners for implementing integrated programmes can be identified. Governments cannot do this work alone as they do not often have the close contact with vulnerable/high-risk populations that NGOs or community-based organizations may have. The national programme must provide technical and material support to NGOs in these activities.

5.2.2 Arrange Support Services

Planning in advance for provision of health services and supplies is essential for facilitating behavioural change and in generating an impact (effect) of IEC programmes. This includes physical inputs such as availability of condoms, bleach or needles, and also services such as counselling. Also included are allied health services such as the provision of STD clinics and primary health care facilities which are prepared to manage STDs. The services and availability of inputs will influence the objectives and targets set for the overall programme and for specific groups.

5.2.3 Conduct Training

Effective implementation of the IEC strategy requires that manpower needs are reviewed to ensure that personnel involved in implementation have the requisite knowledge and skills. Training is vital for ensuring that personnel have the ability to carry out programme activities as required. Development of appropriate training materials should be part of the total material development for IEC and training in communication skills needs to be emphasized. Long-term measures could include the incorporation of an HIV/AIDS IEC component into the curricula of basic training programmes for health and health-related workers, or workers in other sectors who will be providing STD/AIDS information. Short-term measures could include the promotion of inservice training and ensuring that all existing training materials dealing with AIDS/STD give consistent, correct information. The categories for training where special attention needs to be devoted are:

— Health and health-related workers
— Teachers
— NGO workers/volunteers, and
— Leaders or peers from high-risk populations and vulnerable groups.

5.3 Materials Development

Suitable partners should be identified to assist in materials development. This is especially important if ministries of health do not have the in-house capacity for development of IEC materials appropriate to meeting the needs of the programme. As a general strategy, it is suggested that the actual development of materials be contracted out to appropriate professionals, if available. The demands of targeting materials to produce sexual behaviour change may require skills beyond what is normally available.

When developing communication tools for a programme, it is important to call in communication professionals, if available, for every step in the process.

In this case, the manager's responsibility is to ensure that the contracting agency carries out all important steps. The following steps are essential:

5.3.1 Conduct Targeted Behavioural Research

Rapid research among specific target groups is needed for information during the development of appropriate communication strategies and tools. This entails a series of rapid qualitative studies to test relevant concepts and areas of perceived threat and needs of the targeted group. For example, one group may feel that AIDS is only spread by visiting sex workers and they may feel safe even though they habitually have multiple partners. They may use condoms with some partners and not with others.

Understanding behaviours and beliefs is essential for formulating effective, targeted IEC. This research, carried out when specific communication strategies and tools are being developed, will identify keys to behavioural change and help developers to tailor communication messages and materials to meet the needs of the identified population.

Maintaining confidentiality is essential; care must be taken to ensure that the research does not lead to the stigmatization or marginalization of any group.

5.3.2 Design Messages, Choose Media and Channels

Data and inputs from target groups can be used to determine the messages, and the medium and channels needed for conveying them (such as radio, TV, posters, interpersonal approaches, traditional media,) to each segment of the audience. This is the culmination of the conceptualization, analysis and planning exercise. Targeted IEC research, including an analysis of existing data, and a knowledge of the target group, plays an important role in selecting and defining the message, format, presentation, medium, etc., for each identified target group. At the design stage, the exact types of media, the channels for communication and the style should be determined. A balance between passive (e.g. posters, print or video) and interactive media must be created. In many cases, folk media such as puppetry, drama and story telling, can be used quite effectively to support interpersonal communication and should be actively considered as part of the overall IEC plan.

5.3.3 Develop IEC Materials

Development of draft materials is based on decisions about messages, media and channels to be used for delivery to each target group. Materials may consist of radio/TV spots, booklets, posters, handouts or hoardings, but these are not all. IEC also involves tools for use in interpersonal communication. It must be kept in mind that materials are a support tool for activities which lead to the achievement of goals and objectives. IEC materials alone will not produce behavioural change.

Pretesting of materials is one of the most important steps in materials development. Pretesting allows the evaluation of messages and materials with regard to acceptability and potential impact before large amounts of resources are used in production and distribution. Although it adds to the cost and time of producing materials, it prevents wastage of resources by ensuring that materials are effective.

Once draft materials are developed, they are carefully reviewed with groups selected from the specific target audience. For example, a TV spot providing general information on AIDS should be tested with samples from the general public using a rough story board or outline of the pictures and text, before even beginning to film the spot. This process should continue once the rough film has been shot. In this way, planners can be assured that, as much as possible, the spot will convey the information desired as effectively as possible. Pretesting should take place with every material from TV spots to more specific outreach materials being developed for non-literate audiences. Pretesting is cost-effective in the long run.

A summary of the steps to be followed in materials development is shown below:

MATERIALS DESIGN STEPS

Design prototype material
↓
Pretest
↓
Revise material
↓
Pretest again and produce

Setting up a resource centre where all materials (communication products) related to HIV/AIDS/STD are available would also be very helpful and cost-effective. These materials can be used as they are, if appropriate, or adapted and used as prototypes for new materials.

Cost and cost-effectiveness of materials. Determining affordability and cost effectiveness is important, as resources are always scarce. Cost-effectiveness of materials (in terms of development, production and dissemination costs as compared to their reach and effectiveness) is, therefore, an important consideration. In this context, it would be well to judiciously and selectively use expensive media such as film and TV. The glamour of these media often results in an overemphasis on their use, even though the cost of production and dissemination is extremely high. On the other hand, traditional media (including puppetry, traditional theatre and songs) and interpersonal communication tools (such as flip-charts and flash cards) are often neglected, though they are generally very cost-effective. Special efforts must, therefore, be made to use traditional media wherever they are more suitable.

What will it Cost?

Each step in the IEC development process can be reviewed to identify items and activities that will have to be contracted for. Items that are important to include in overall costing are:

— costs of targeted behavioural research
— costs of development of prototype or draft materials
— costs of pretesting
— costs associated with each type of medium: availability of in-house capacity for any aspects of production, the quality desired
— costs of producing sufficient copies for intended use
— costs of distribution or dissemination—whether it be freight or postal charges, trucking or buying air time on radio or TV
— costs of storage. Materials produced in quantities will require dry, secure storage space
— costs of reprints and revisions. All materials have a 'lifet' and will need replacement and updating.

5.3.4 Disseminate and Utilize Materials

Planning effective ways to make sure that materials reach their target audiences is as important as producing effective materials. It is often the case that good quality materials never reach those who need them or who could most effectively use them. Planning a distribution strategy and setting up a distribution network at the beginning is important.

Using materials to support IEC activities, through mass media or for interpersonal communication requires knowing how to use them effectively. Ideally, users will become familiar with different types of materials and methods for using them during communication training. At the very least, instructions and suggestions for use must be supplied along with the materials.

5.4 Monitoring and Evaluation

Monitoring and evaluation provide inputs for guiding and improving programme implementation, for appropriate redefinition or fine-tuning of messages and materials, for reworking objectives/goals and for the overall IEC approach.

Monitoring and evaluation must be built into the overall programme process. Monitoring and evaluation are essential parts of the overall IEC programme and must be planned for from the beginning. Monitoring and evaluation are, however, different.

Monitoring is a continuous activity, and provides immediate feedback so that timely corrective action can be taken. Evaluation, on the other hand, is carried out at regular intervals to assess programme effectiveness and impact.

5.4.1 Monitoring

Monitoring can be defined as the ongoing process of collecting and analysing information about implementation of the programme. It involves regular checking to see whether programme activities are being carried out as planned so that problems can be discussed and dealt with. It allows managers to follow the progress of planned activities, identify problems, give feedback to staff and solve problems before they cause delays.

Monitoring can answer questions such as:

— Have relevant health care workers and others received training?
— Are the appropriate services in place?
— Have the IEC materials been distributed to those they are intended for?
— Are the IEC materials being utilized?

(a) What to Monitor

Deciding what to monitor can begin by preparing a list of programme and activity targets and indicators as well as important tasks, performances and outputs.

A task is one of a set of actions required to carry out an activity. Examples are 'identify partners for work with vulnerable populations' or 'identify organizations for materials development'. Performance refers to how well a task is carried out. The quality is assessed by comparing current practice with established standards of performance. Examples are 'training health workers to give appropriate health education sessions on STD' or 'advising women at antenatal clinics on the risks of HIV infection and pregnancy'. Output refers to the quantity of items used to carry out activities or to the quantified result of carrying out a task. Examples are numbers of brochures printed or distributed, numbers of personnel trained, and numbers of condoms distributed.

(b) Adoption of Monitoring Methods, and Development and Adoption of Appropriate Tools for Monitoring

Programme activities can be monitored through checklists

of observations to be made during supervisory visits, regular checking of workplans, and use of reporting forms. Some monitoring methods for collecting data to measure indicators/progress are outlined below.

— Routine reports are reports of certain information submitted on a regular basis by all or most reporting sites in an area. Useful periodic records and reports that can be reviewed for monitoring IEC activities might include those on dissemination of print materials, training sessions held with NGOs and community organizations, advocacy meetings, new partners identified to reach vulnerable populations, and number of TV spots aired.

— Supervisory visits/reports are reports of visits by supervisors to oversee tasks and performances of workers, identify problems and help solve performance and output problems. Supervisory, activities may include observation, exit interviews, record reviews, or other ways of monitoring performance and output. When supervisory visits are carried out with appropriate checklists, the information gathered can be very useful for monitoring the programme. Regular supervisory visits are difficult to achieve, and transportation costs arc difficult to sustain. However, frequent supportive supervision is an indispensable monitoring method.

(c) Use of Monitoring Results

It is important to use what is learned from monitoring as feedback to the programme so that necessary corrective actions can be taken. Feedback should be quick and action oriented and aimed at making immediate changes to improve effectiveness. It will in particular, provide key inputs to modify the messages and media used to reach specific target groups and to make improvements/changes in services. Feedback assumes even greater importance in the context of the proposed strategy, since it has been suggested that implementation begin immediately, without waiting for the results of detailed research or large-scale surveys. Thus, IEC messages/products will be based on existing data/studies, which may not be fully adequate. Needed corrections and adjustments will have to be based on monitoring efforts which feed back into the redesign of the programme.

A system based on a short, quick and reliable feedback mechanism is essential. Such feedback will cover, with regard to IEC material, aspects such as target group interest in the material, comprehension of it, reaction to the format, language and characters used (if any), and visual appeal (where relevant).

5.4.2 Evaluation

Evaluation is the process of collecting and analysing information at regular intervals about the effectiveness and impact of either particular parts of the programme or the programme as a whole. A variety of different evaluation methods is possible depending on programme needs. Regardless of method, planning for evaluation, including development of programme indicators and planning for information collection, should take place at the beginning of the programmer to ensure that essential data will be available when needed.

Impact is measured against the programme objectives. Baseline data will be needed, and methods for collecting the information need to be spelled out so that the amount of change can be assessed.

At a given point in time, evaluation can answer such quantifiable, impact-related questions as:

— Are access to condoms and information on correct use-increasing?

— What proportion of health workers are providing health education?

— What proportion of prostitutes report the correct and consistent use of condoms?

— What proportion of the general population can cite at least two acceptable ways to protect themselves from HIV infection?

— What proportion of women who have been advised on the risks or HIV infection and pregnancy at antenatal clinics can cite two risk factors for HIV infection?

— What proportion of the general population who are sexually active can report that they are practising safer sex?

— Has the incidence of STDs declined?

Collection of appropriate baseline data is essential if an evaluation of impact is to take place

Evaluation can also be designed to help a programme manager understand why a programme is where it is. Did certain types of activities have bigger impacts than others? What types of problems occurred? How can such problems be solved or prevented in the future? Periodic programme reviews provide more qualitative or descriptive information on the status of the programme.

Evaluation should include not only the impact on the target audience, but must also cover an evaluation of other activities, such as training and/or utilization of services.

Some evaluation methods are outlined below:

Community surveys, such as the general population survey:

These are usually regionally (and sometimes nationally) focused investigations. They can be conducted as household surveys, which collect information from a representative sample of a population and are conducted by trained interviewers who go to the dwellings in a selected geographic area for face-to-face interviews, or targeted population surveys, which collect information about a population of particular interest, and are carried out in locations where these populations can be found.

Comprehensive programme reviews: These are carried out primarily for management purposes. They assess the relevance and adequacy of the national plan and existing policies including those related to IEC. They assess adequacy and appropriateness of the structure of the national AIDS programme, progress toward targets, and the efficiency of prevention and control activities. The objective of a review is to identify achievements and problem areas, including recommendations for solutions. Reviews also assess the adequacy of management information systems. Reviews are done at regular intervals; internal reviews are done by country staff every year and external reviews are done every two to three years by staff outside the programme.

Accumulation of monitoring results: This is a collection of monitoring data gathered over time that is judged valid and useful for evaluating certain components of programme activities that require repeated assessment.

Special studies and surveys: These are studies that assist in understanding specific operational issues. For example, a pilot study of a prevention strategy such as 'Use of peer educators for HIV prevention in prostitute populations' will eventually assist managers in deciding whether or not to expand the approach to a national scale. HIV or STD surveillance in antenatal clinics help the national AIDS programme to better understand trends in disease prevalence.

Depending on the methods selected, evaluation will provide an in-depth, integrated feedback, covering a longer time-scale and at a broader level than that provided by monitoring. It svill indicate the extent of success in meeting the behavioural objectives/goals of IEC, and provide inputs for changes or modifications in these, and possibly even the overall approach/philosophy of IEC.

6. IEC FOR SPECIFIC TARGET AUDIENCES - YOUTH AS AN EXAMPLE

This section illustrates the use of the IEC planning and implementation process with one target group: young persons - adolescents and youth—from 10 to 24 years of age. This group will need to be divided into segments due to the wide range of developmental stages and cultural norms.

6.1 PLANNING

6. 1.1 Situational Analysis

(1) National policy and organizational structure

In the case of youth it is important to know what policies are in place for: the health of youth of each segment, including children in school, condom use and sex education in schools. In light of the AIDS pandemic, the need for advocacy to change policies should also be assessed. An analysis should take place on how best to utilize the government structures for Youth and AIDS.

(2) Philosophy/approach to IEC for youth

At the central level a decision needs to be made on how to approach the topic of Youth and AIDS. This will entail a decision on sex education or life-style education in schools; how to handle discussion on condoms; and other issues. It is necessary to strike a delicate balance between the promotion of traditional values and a practical programme to meet the needs of young people who may already be sexually active.

(3) Examining existing data

The factors that need to be examined as part of the situational analysis have already been discussed. It is on the basis of such an analysis that one can identify youth as a priority target group. The situational analysis will also provide details that will help to further identify the target group and how to reach them, involvement with youth/sports or other organizations and key 'influencers' (e.g. teachers). Existing research reports may indicate the habits, preferences and effectiveness of different media, etc. for this target group. All this data will be crucial in:

— Further/finer stratification of the target group;
— Developing suitable messages;
— Ensuring participation and involvement of youth in the process (message design) and-where possible—in developing communication tools;
— Identifying and using peers as communicators;
— Identifying suitable media and means of reaching the

target group (including through influencers);

— Development of appropriate school curricula on AIDS; and

— Development of co-curricular activities for AIDS.

6.1.2 Target Group Identification

Youth, both male and female, can be further segmented in most countries as follows:

— Youth in school (urban and rural);

— Youth out of school in the urban setting;

— Youth out of school in the rural setting;

— Street youth or street children; and

— University students.

Each group has different levels of literacy and may have different behaviour patterns as well as information and service needs. It is also important to target parents and teachers.

The role of teachers and parents in informing and educating youth must be explored thoroughly. Often a well intentioned programme will fail because the important role of teachers and parents has been ignored.

6.1.3 Goals/Objectives/Targets/Indicators

For the specific target audience, it is now necessary to define the behavioural goals on the basis of the philosophy or approach and the situational analysis. In this, one also has to take note of the communication infrastructure that is available and the access that the target group has to various channels of communication such as mass media, print media and interpersonal channels.

For this target group (youth), the desired behavioural goals may be stated as follows:

— Delay sexual initiation (relevant for adolescents and younger people);

— Provide safer intimacy options;

— Reduce the number of sexual partners;

— Increase condom use;

— Discuss sexual matters openly;

— Actively seek information on sexual matters and seek counselling;

— Seek STD services; and

— Develop 'enabling skills' to promote healthy lifestyles.

In the Region as a whole, these would be the primary goals, since almost all the HIV infection is sexually transmitted. However, in certain parts of some countries (e.g. India, Thailand, Myanmar), injecting drug use is also a major problem. In such areas, the behavioural goals will have to emphasize sterilization and non-sharing of needles and other injecting equipment, while simultaneously attempting to reduce drug injecting itself. These messages should be integrated into promoting and supporting a positive life-style.

As noted in the previous section, the goals and objectives should be quantified or expressed in measurable terms as far as possible, and targets set. These will differ from country to country, depending upon the situation prevailing there. Specific indicators should be developed and a system to collect the appropriate information designed.

6.2. PREPARATORY ACTIVITIES AND MATERIALS DEVELOPMENT

6.2.1 Linkages with Existing Organizational Structure and other Organizations

Close and active collaboration with other agencies and programmes is vital for the success of any IEC strategy. In the case of youth, collaboration should be established with educational authorities and institutions (ministry of education, schools/colleges, universities, etc.) and with youth organizations (Ministry of Youth Services, scouts/guides and social service organizations, student bodies, etc.). Links should also be sought with youth cubs and sports organizations.

NGOs and voluntary organizations can play important roles because of the commitment and dedication of those involved. Also, they are generally able to establish a better rapport with young people and high-risk behaviour groups than official agencies, while their ability to reach out-of-school youth and street children is particularly high. The entertainment industry is geared largely to attracting young people. They would, therefore, be appropriate partners for many IEC activities.

In addition, strong linkages must obviously be established with other relevant health programmes) especially with STD and family planning services, for condom distribution.

6.2.2 Services

Services play an important role in supporting behavioural

change and facilitating the adoption of appropriate safe/preventive practices and behaviour.

For this target group the services include:

— Counselling, which is of special relevance for this age group;
— Condom distribution;
— STD/health services; and
— Information service ('hotline' through telephones, or a 'post box') providing relevant information on an anonymous basis.

6.2.3 Training

The categories to which special attention needs to be devoted for training in youthrelated activities include teachers, health workers, NGO workers and volunteers, youth leaders and peer groups.

6.2.4 Targeted Behavioural Research

IEC research can play a major role in designing the right messages. Such research will indicate the target audience's current level of knowledge including any misconceptions. Focusing IEC research on youth will help to find keys to overcoming the perceived invulnerability of youth - the 'it can't happen to me' syndrome.

6.2.5 Design of Targeted Messages and Media

The basic or core messages are:

— Delay sexual activity;
— Single sex partner (mutual faithfulness);
— Avoid penetrative sex; and
— Use latex condoms.

Some specific messages for this target group (youth and adolescents) would be:

— How HIV is transmitted and also how it is not;
— How to protect oneself and one's sexual partner from HIV;
— Seeking appropriate treatment for STDs;
— The STD and HIV relationship, i.e. recognition of how STD increases the risk of HIV;
— Proper condom use;

— Hazards of drug use, particularly injecting;
— Existence of support/counselling services and where to go for these; and
— Knowledge about human sexuality (development, behaviour, relationships), especially for adolescents.

The choice of medium for each message will depend upon the extent of access that the target group has to the medium. The situational analysis and IEC research should provide crucial data on this. In general, however, one may list the general products which might be appropriate for a general youth population:

— Broadcast media—especially targeted youth programming: audio and video cassettes;
— Books (including textbooks), magazines, newspapers;
— Films/movies;
— Street theatre, especially for street children and college students;
— NGOs and voluntary agencies; not necessarily those working on AIDS, but many others who are basically working with youth in areas such as health, women, development and water supply;
— Entertainment shows and sports—these are a very effective way of reaching urban youth;
— Exhibitions;
— Peer group—this generally makes for the best and most effective communication. It will require the training of a few selected individuals from each institution/organization. This may be particularly useful for street children, since their access to other media is limited and distrust of people in authority is likely to be strong, and
— Teachers—again some training will be necessary. This is obviously only for in-school/college groups. Some countries have adolescent/sex education as part of the curriculum, and messages on AIDS/HIV must be integrated into this.

Some of these, or a combination, can be used, depending upon the target audience, the situational analysis and a cost analysis. Among the settings or locales for conveying IEC messages, appropriate ones for this target group include:

— The classroom, for school and college students;
— Youth clubs;
— 'Video Parlours', which, in most places, draw a large number of young people; and
— Youth festivals, youth camps, sports events, etc.

6 2.6 IEC Materials Development

It is essential to develop appropriate communication tools to support the approaches that have been decided upon. IEC research inputs have already been indicated as being essential at the message design stage. Similar inputs are required in developing appropriate materials such as radio/TV programmes, posters and booklets. Pretesting, in particular, is a vital element of materials development.

When designing communication materials, experienced communicators should be involved. This is not something that should be left to medical experts or health workers. Further, the involvement of the target group (in designing the material) is essential and has been found to be very effective in terms of the final impact of the product. This particular target group (young persons) provides great scope for direct involvement in the development and even production—of materials. It is possible to tap student groups and to work through schools of art/communication/journalism, in particular, to evolve materials that are most appealing and suitable for the target group.

The materials produced must obviously be within the framework of the overall approach/philosophy and the messages identified for this specific target group. Special care needs to be taken to avoid any contradictions or ambiguities in the messages.

Full use must be made of textbooks for in-school/college groups. The materials developed for these books must be interesting, clear, and provide sequential graded learning. Since the 'printed word', especially in a textbook, carries great sanctity, this material must be thoroughly pretested to eliminate any possible misunderstandings or ambiguities.

6.3 Dissemination and Utilization

In examining the considerations outlined in the previous section, it is crucial to keep the target audience in mind In each country/situation, it is necessary to determine which message through which medium will most effectively **reach** (in this case) young persons.

Choice of the means of dissemination is therefore linked to the target audience and the message. Some channels for dissemination of messages include:

— Broadcast media. In many countries, the broadcasting organizations make some air-time available free of cost for social messages which may require strong advocacy efforts. Efforts need to be made to obtain such allocations everywhere. Care should be taken that spots or programmes aimed at youth are aired when young people are watching, which is usually during prime time. When free air-time is not possible, or more is needed, good planning is required to buy time in a cost-effective manner, trading off between costs and (target) audience size.

— Integration with on-going TV programmes/features. For example, some messages could be appropriately woven into a popular 'soap-opera'.

— Message dissemination through peer groups. NGOs can play a major role in this. Training of peer-leaders (mentioned above in the section on Training) thus assumes even greater importance. The possibility of organizing such groups is obviously higher for that segment of the target audience which is in school/college. However, attempts have been successful in organizing groups among street children and employed persons.

— Anonymous methods to gather queries from young people and disseminate accurate information. In some countries, schools have set up post boxes where students can place sensitive queries, to which answers can be given in a newsletter or in general discussions. Another method is to set up a telephone information hotline.

Curriculum. Where 'dissemination' takes place through the curriculum (in school or college), it is essential that the teacher does not shy away from confronting the issues. A discussion after each lesson is the ideal way of maximizing learning and aiding behavioural change by clarifying all doubts, etc. (see matrix presented in Table 40.1).

At the receiving end, utilization of media products is a vital, and unfortunately, much-neglected aspect. The impact of any communication is increased many-fold if it is discussed among receivers, if their questions are answered and if their doubts clarified. Steps must be taken to ensure this, either through inter-personal communication as follow-up, or through supporting printed material, where appropriate.

6.4 Monitoring and Evaluation

As discussed in the text of this document, it is essential to plan for monitoring and evaluation at the outset. Monitoring activities may include collecting reports from teachers or NGOs working with youth out of school, collecting data on the distribution of IEC materials and the airing of radio and TV spots aimed at youth, along with listener surveys. Evaluation can be accomplished if

Table 1. Matrix: Youth

Target group	Desired behaviour change	Approach	Media channel	Interpersonal channel (Networks)	Support services
Youth in school	Responsible sexual behaviour ↓ Drug use (injecting) # Condom use # Health care seeking behaviour	Mass media Peer education Curriculum development Co-curricular activities	TV, Radio Press Interpersonal	Schools School organizations Ministry of Education Ministry of Youth	Counselling Condoms STD services
Youth in college	# Responsible sexual behaviour ↓ Drug use (injecting) # Condom use # Health care seeking behaviour	Mass media Peer education Curriculum development Co-curricular activities	TV, Radio Press Interpersonal	Schools School organizations Ministry of Education Ministry of Youth	Counselling Condoms STD services
Youth out of school (urban)	# Responsible sexual behaviour ↓ Drug use (injecting) # Condom use # Health care seeking behaviour	Peer education outreach Mass media	TV, Radio Interpersonal Street theatre	NGOs Ministry of Youth	Counselling Condoms STD services
Youth out of school (rural)	# Responsible sexual behaviour ↓ Drug use (injecting) # Condom use # Health care seeking behaviour	Peer education outreach Mass media	Peer education Traditional media Street theatre	Rural outreach networks NGOs Ministry of Youth	Counselling Condoms STD services

{Cont.}..........

Street children	# Responsible sexual behaviour ↓ Drug use (injecting) # Condom use # Health care seeking behaviour	Peer education Outreach Mass media	Interpersonal Street theatre Traditional media	NGOs Department of Child Welfare Ministry of Social Welfare/Youth	Counselling Condoms STD services

TABLE 40.2. Matrix: Target Populations and Communication Approaches

Target group	Desired behaviour change	Approach	Media channel	Network	Support services
Brothel-based workers	Condom usage Seeking treatment for STD	Outreach Peer education	Target print and audio-video material Street theatre	NGOs Health workers Local GPs	Condoms STD services Counselling
Street sex workers	Condom usage Seeking treatment for STD	Outreach	Target print and audio-video material Street theater	NGOs Health workers Local GPs	Condom STD services Counselling
Madams of brothels	Condom promotion Condom usage	Outreach Peer education	Target print and audio-video material Street theatre	NGOs	Condoms STD services Counselling
Pimps	Condom promotion Appropriate treatment for STD	Outreach	Target print and audio-video material Street theater	NGOs	Condom STD services Counselling
Truck drivers/ transport workers	Condom use Appropriate treatment of STD	Outreach Peer education	Target print and audio-video material	NGOs Peers Trucking Association Ministries of Transport	STD services Condom Counselling
Men who have sex with men	Condom use Appropriate treatment of STD	Outreach Peer education	Target print material	NGOs	STD services Condoms Counselling
Migrant workers	Condom use Appropriate treatment of STD	Local media outreach Peers	Street theatre Traditional media Target print material and audio-video	NGOs Intercountry Cooperation Labour Unions Ministry of Labour	STD services Condoms Counselling

TABLE 40.3. Target Population and Communication Approaches

Target group	Desired behaviour change	Approach	Media channel	Networks	Support services
Injecting drug	Cleaning needles Condom use Appropriate treatment of STD	Outreach Peers	Targeted print and Audio-video material	NGO De-addiction programmes Prisons	Counselling STD services Condoms
STD patients	↑ in condom use ↑ in health care seeking behaviour ↑ treatment compliance	Interpersonal Mass media	TV Radio health workers	NGO s health Services	Counselling Condoms
General population	↑ inability to discuss ↑ sex and sexuality ↑ Seeking of information on STD/AIDS ↑ empathy for HIV and people with AIDS ↑ in condom use	Mass media	TV, Radio Press Billboard Exhibition Cinema slides	Associations Community organizations Workplace settings	Counselling Condoms STD services Information Services (Hotlines)
Policy-makers	↑ in support to AIDS prevention programme ↑ in understanding of communication needs	Mass media Interpersonal	TV, Radio Press Seminars Meetings		
Women	↑ in health care seeking behaviour ↑ in knowledge of STD & AIDS ↑ ability to negotiate sexual behaviour	Mass media Peer education outreach	TV, Radio Press Traditional media	NGOs Associations Existing government programmes Health workers Women's organizations	Counselling STD services

baseline data are collected on knowledge and practices. Key indicators of the desired behavioural change can be measured through repeat surveys. It is important to evaluate process and outcome if results are to be fedback into programme planning. Monitoring and evaluation must be planned before activities are conducted.

7. PLANNING A MASS AWARENESS CAMPAIGN

Mass awareness campaigns are recommended for reaching the general public with basic information on AIDS/STD, for articulating the general philosophy behind the overall programme, and for providing an umbrella message network for the entire programme. A mass awareness campaign is the utilization of all mass media channels (TV, radio, press, general print materials) to disseminate a sequence of basic messages on HIV/AIDS/STD in a co-ordinated fashion aimed at a loosely segmented target population. Often *ad hoc* media activities, such as individual TV spots, are mistaken for mass awareness campaigns. It is important that a campaign is recognized by the general population as a cohesive programme no matter which channel of the mass media is used.

Most national AIDS programmes do not have the infrastructure to develop such a campaign in-house and the development of the design and media plan is often contracted out to communications professionals/organizations. Understanding of the elements which go into planning a mass awareness campaign is, however, useful for a programme planner and a concise overview of the elements and steps necessary for an effective mass awareness campaign therefore follows.

Segment Target Population: A decision should be made on what segments of the general population should be targeted. For instance, if segmenting for youth, men and women between 15 and 49 is suggested, then messages directed at women, men, and youth in general should be developed.

Market Research: Before developing a campaign it is essential to conduct some rapid research among the identified segments of the general population to ascertain current levels of knowledge, general practices, sexual health care seeking behaviour and perceptions of AIDS and STDs. A combination of quantitative and qualitative data collection is recommended. Qualitative research should be conducted first, after which a broader quantitative study for a larger sample size can be implemented. The quantitative study can provide baseline data for future evaluation of impact. Marketing research firms and large social science institutions can be contracted to carry out this work. It is essential that the programme planner works closely with the contractor on questionnaire development and sampling.

Message Development: Specific messages for the segmented populations should be developed on the basis of the philosophy, the research and the availability of services.

Concept Development and Media Plan: The overall tone and theme of a campaign should be developed on the basis of the philosophy and the results of research. This will entail designing a logo and signature line or tune to unite the various media used. Some samples are 'Prevention is the only cure' with an identifiable graphic for use in all visuals. At this stage the mix of media will be identified ands for each audience segiment, a detailed plan for dissemination will be developed. This will include identifying appropriate air time and broadcast channels for TV and radio; identifying which press would be used for which segment listing out the support print materials which should be developed and where they would be disseminated; and sequencing messages. It is recommended that, for print materials, emphasis be given to visuals; even a literate audience will look at a visual before reading a text.

Professional advertising agencies, working closely with national AIDS programme staff, or other identified communications professionals should be recruited for the development of the overall campaign.

Prototype Development, Pretesting and Revision: Software for TV, radio, press advertisement and print materials must be developed in a cohesive fashion. It will be based on research, but will probably cover basic information on AIDS and materials to address the common misconceptions of each target group. For example, research among youth might show that they:

— have low levels of knowledge;
— perceive themselves to be not at risk;
— watch TV and listen to pop radio programmes; and
— do not read newspapers.

Based on this a decision could be made to develop TV and radio spots and a comic format brochure to disseminate in schools. A similar process would take place for each identified segment of population. All spots and materials. however, would share a common logo and signature line to identify each material as part of the campaign, reinforce messages and provide legitimacy for the information.

The overall concept and individual prototypes need to be thoroughly tested with the target audience. This can be done, for example, through focus group discussions, or through stopping people in the street or at a bus stop. If a large number of individuals do not understand the message, then it should be redesigned. After the pretesting process, revisions should be made and additional pretests conducted as appropriate.

Implementation: A campaign can run for a period of three months to one year depending on audience exhaustion and comprehension of the messages. All media materials should be ready and disseminated at the same time.

Monitoring: it is essential to carefully monitor the implementation and impact of the campaign to ensure that materials have been disseminated, and to assess audience participation through listener surveys, spot interviews, and analysis of letters and requests for information in an on-going fashion during the life of the campaign. If a particular material or software is clearly unacceptable, then it can be taken off the air immediately. An advertising agency will have the capability to professionally monitor the progress of the campaign.

Evaluation and Reprogramming: After the completion of the campaign cycle, a repeat baseline evaluation should be conducted along with a study to produce some qualitative data on the impact of the campaign. The data should be analysed and fed into reprogramming of the next cycle of the awareness campaign. Messages will change from straight information to more specific behavioural change messages based on the greater knowledge of the target audience. The next cycle of the campaign will probably tackle issues related to empathy for those afflicted and queries which have been raised in the first cycle. Awareness campaigns must be continuous.

Finally? a mass awareness campaign will begin the process of making people aware of the problem and the methods of prevention. It is only one component of an overall IEC programme and does not replace interpersonal approaches.

(This document was developed based on a consultation meeting held in WHO-SEARO, New Delhi during 20-22 March, 1994.)

41

Behaviour Change

(Summary Report of the Informal
Consultation on Behaviour Change:
a Central Issue in the Response to the HIV Epidemic
Dakar, Senegal, 12-15 December 1991)

The consultation was structured around six specific questions. This report summarizes the discussion around these questions and the responses.

Q 1. What behavioural and attitudinal changes limit the spread of the epidemic?

Q 2. What is the basis of our shared belief and hope that the epidemic can be overcome?

Q 3. How do the required changes come about?

Q 4. How can community-based organizations assist individuals and communities to change?

Q 5. How do programmes expand and develop to assist these changes to come about?

Q 6. How can these changes be documented and why do we want to do this?

Q 1. What Behavioural and Attitudinal Changes Limit the Spread of the Epidemic?

Behaviour change happens in the context of the individual, the group and the community. It is not just an event, but a process taking place over a long period of time, ranging from a stage of unawareness through awareness and trying out new behaviours, to reaching sustained change. Important facilitators of change include stories, role models and the support of the community and peer groups. Behaviour change is first of all a personal responsibility, but it is very difficult to achieve alone. Community support and help are essential for sustained changes in behaviour.

This process of behaviour change begins from birth and continues throughout one's lifetime. Individuals determine and shape their identities in relation to their immediate communities. Behaviour is a part of individual identity and is, therefore, strongly influenced by community values. People are constrained by their belief systems which reflect the community beliefs, and individuals need to learn how to explore alternative options. Individuals are able to change when and if the community recognizes that specific behaviours need to be changed and creates its own strategy to achieve this. But a supportive community atmosphere alone cannot always generate change: there is also the need for a positive approach to suggesting alternative behaviour (for example, young women may engage in sex to gain money or popularity, so alternative behaviour which also achieves these objectives needs to be identified). Resources may be needed to sustain behaviour change.

Q 2. What is the Basis of our Shared Belief and Hope that the Epidemic can be Overcome?

The influence of people living with HIV is a major factor in the belief that the epidemic will be overcome: respect for people with HIV is enhanced by their involvement with others working in the field and the way they have been able to teach others so much about the effect of the virus. The response of people with HIV has also reinforced the belief that human nature is essentially good.

There is evidence that people are able to change their behaviour and that communities are acting collectively to organize themselves to change, to care and to cope. We already know a great deal about the virus, and we have technical knowledge on how to prevent transmission. Lessons have been learnt from coping with previous epidemics. Stories of activities and achievements help to motivate and sustain others working in the field. There is increasing conviction of the need to support one another at the local, national and international levels. There is a great potential for change, compassion, consensus, involvement and collaboration.

Motivation also comes from a fundamental belief in people's capacity to change, and recognition that the response to the epidemic has reflected a range of human values such as trust, respect, dignity and solidarity. There is a strong desire for group survival, and recognition that there is no alternative to behaviour change. Concern for those affected and for the next generation was recognized as a major motivating factor.

Q 3. How do the Required Changes Come About?

Influences on an individual's capacity to change include: faith, religion, education, economics, and environmental influences. Some of these influences cannot be changed by the individual- such as family, time and place of birth, mobility, psychosocial dependence, peer pressure, and environmental changes. The media, membership in organizations involved in change, fashion and trends affect individuals. Traditional media (i.e. storytelling) are also an influence. Such factors can either be constraints or strengths in that they can either help or inhibit behaviour changes.

Working in the field of HIV is itself a factor in change. We are changing ourselves in the process of changing others. Organizations may need to change in order to accommodate our need to bring about change.

1. Personal Behaviour Change

Individuals in the group changed because they gained knowledge of the transmission and prevention of the disease, and because of various individual experiences of, for example, being infected, caring for someone who is infected, losing someone close or interacting with organizations involved with HIV.

They have received support and positive reinforcement from peer groups, family and friends. The desire to survive and the hope for a better future have both influenced individual behaviour, and this has included the re-evaluation of spiritual faith and values, which have in turn been able to sustain change. Finally, concern and respect for others have been important elements in determining behaviour.

2. Organizational Experiences

Change in an organization can be initiated by a variety of stimuli whose effects vary according to the type and situation of the organization, for instance:

The motivation for change may come from within the organization:

* Changes are driven by need and the recognition of need - projects run by an organization may move from simple to complex and from small to large as the people within the organization gain deeper understanding of the problems with which they work.
* Financial considerations may determine how programmes move. Increased resources may bring expansion or extension of services. Resource constraints may bring streamlining of activities or reorientation.
* Leadership determines how programmes progress. This may be through managers or through other influential individuals.

External influences can also result in change:

* Governments can be changed in response to community needs if they are identified and articulated.
* In certain communities in Africa, religious groups play a role which can be either a constraint on, or a catalyst for, change. In addition, some social and cultural agents can determine the way the programmes evolve.
* The severity of the epidemic and changes in the perception of its seriousness can lead to changes in programmes.

3. How is Change Initiated by People Living with HIV (PLWH)?

Individuals who are able to provide a role model by publicly avowing their status as HIV positive give others the courage to come out. But before change can come about, whether it is change in behaviour or the change in attitudes which allows people to be open about HIV infection, information is essential. This has to be available in the form of facilities for testing, supportive counselling and the development of the capacity in every individual to examine the options open to him or her. Changes in attitude are necessary before changes in behaviour at an individual or community level can take place.

Nomalizing HIV is necessary—exposing the myth of the hidden enemy and giving a human face to AIDS.

Active participation and leadership from PLWH is necessary in all our work. For this to happen, it is important to recognize that while PLWH are well, there is no distinction between them and anyone else. While they are sick, they need care and facilities, exactly the same as for any other illness.

However, while recognizing the vitas importance of role models and stories of people who are affected themselves, issues of confidentiality must be carefully thought through. PLWH need to be able to publicize their stories without losing their privacy. Loss of privacy often takes place at an enormous personal cost. Activist groups need to discipline themselves not to be casual about revealing identities.

In a discussion of openness about being HIV positive, the following points were made:

* There should be concern about the price of openness.
* It takes time to get a large enough number of people who will state openly that they are infected or affected.
* Openness should be planned and gradual; it needs a supportive environment.
* Secrecy also has a price, and a balance has to be found between the need for privacy and openness: an example

was given of a woman who died without having had appropriate treatment because her daughter did not know the nature of her illness.

* Secrecy can perpetuate the stigma attached to HIV, especially in relation to the media.
* If we recommend personal story-telling to people with HIV, we need a social contract to protect them from discrimination.
* Those who are not themselves infected with HIV can have stories to tell.

We are all potentially positive but public attitudes towards AIDS service organizations is often prejudicial and leads to a them and us syndrome.

4. Community Agents of Change and Role Models—how do they Initiate Change in Communities?

Community agents of change can be anyone who is motivated by:

* being infected or affected.
* caring for someone who is infected.
* knowing and understanding about HIV and its consequences.

Belief leads to conviction which leads to commitment which leads to change.

Change is affected by:

* modelling and using examples,
* sharing experiences and telling stories,
* challenging peers to take notice and act at every opportunity,
* organizing and supporting practical activities,
* facilitating community ownership, and
* changing the attitudinal environment within the community.

5. Interaction Between Communities: can this be a Catalyst for Change?

Belonging to a community is a prerequisite to change for individuals because of the esteem which the sense of belonging brings, and because of the support which the community provides. Change within communities involves the belief that change is possible.

Once communities have generated change, empowerment allowing obstacles to be overcome can follow. The dynamic which leads to change in a community creates the desire to carry the changre beyond the immediate community.

This can be carried out via a bridge to another community when there is an individual who belongs to overlapping communities; for example, the experience of the gay community in Malaysia was transferred to women's groups.

Some communities lack the sense of community identity to operate effectively. Established communities are able to help loose networks of people to become effective community members, and thus a base for change.

Comrnunities can act by example to other communities, proving that change is both possible and beneficial. The process of change is strengthening and desirable for that reason.

6. How do Communities Recognize that Change has taken Place and how do they use this to Sustain Change?

The tools currently used for looking at behaviour change are: seropositivity, clinical prognosis, levels of sexually transmitted infections and use of condoms. These are not necessarily valuable, because they measure factors which may not be related to behaviour change. By involving the community, it may be possible to make causal links. To do this, communities must be involved in the process of evaluating change. They need to be involved in determining indicators of change, identifying the information to collect, and at which stages of planning, implementation, measurement and evaluation. So far, monitoring behaviour change has not been done properly, and has not received enough attention.

Some of the indicators of change identified included:

* communities no longer condoning travel for sex;
* increased usage of condoms (but this can result in more sexual activity);
* villages becoming suspicious and unwelcoming towards strangers because they are thought to be to blame for the infection;
* marrying earlier—this is difficult because the bride price for young women is too high and because young men cannot afford any bride price; in one community the bride price was reduced;
* males have stopped running with the girls, i.e. having many sex partners;

* development of sex education in schools based on a concept of family life.

Q 4. How can Community-based Organizations Assist Individuals and Communities to Change?

Presentations from six of the participating organizations highlighted some of the ways in which behaviour change is initiated and sustained through community action. Brief descriptions of the organizations represented are attached to the end of this report.

1. **Counselling has a significant role to play:** The AIDS Support Organization, TASO (Uganda), reaches the community through counselling within the family, through the participation of the person with HIV. The communities identify themselves to TASO, and TASO is able to respond with training workers selected by the community to counsel and care. TASO is able to provide back up if the care cannot be managed within the community. This leads to community-based education programmes.
2. The same holds for Chikankata (Zambia), where the community itself is the initiator, and requests training and education. Two teams, one carrying out the home-based care programme and the other carrying out the community counselling training programme, build on the process of diagnosis and care in hospital, and an assessment of the appropriateness of home care. The community counselling team holds meetings with the community and initiates a file for each community, allowing for progress and strategies to be followed. Entry points to the community are from the experience of another community, from the acceptance of homebased care, or following recognition of the problem and the need to know more. WAMATA has observed an attitude change, in that people are becoming more willing to share information and experience; membership of the organization is growing.
3. The recognition that members of WAMATA (Tanzania) are HIV-infected brings about a change in attitude toward HIV and PLWH. Most of the counselling is done by volunteers and this is leading to wider participation in the community.
4. The Victorian AIDS Council (Australia) has found that education, carried out according to the principles of community development, has been successful in bringing about behaviour change and in involving a large num-

ber of people. Individuals are mutually supportive, and through campaigns with which they identify, come to participate in and control the services being offered. All the work has been done by gay men, but there has been no pressure for disclosure. Counselling facilities were available, but it was some time before these were used. The strength of the programme lay in the mutual support and respect for the people within it.

5. **Kitovu Hospital** (Uganda) has programmes covering hospital-based and home-based care. To assist behaviour change in the hospital itself, and recognizing that change is most effective in a group, a hospital community was established in order to encourage behaviour change in all aspects of life, including the spiritual aspects of change. The home-based care in the Masaka District, where there are high levels of sickness from AIDS, builds on community involvement to promote positive living and self-reliance. This includes income generation activities and focus group discussions.
6. **Women and AIDS Support Network, WASS** (Zimbabwe), has concentrated on the problems of women, particularly those who are in occupations where they are vulnerable to discrimination such as domestic workers. Change has been encouraged through close links and networking with other agencies and by drawing attention to some of the problems specific to women who are not protected by law(s) in their employment or in their relationships. Behaviour change which is positive for one individual may be detrimental for another, for example a second or third wife has no legal protection, and if her husband decides to return to monogamy, he can reject her.

The presentations highlighted the fact that communities need to define their own methodology and monitor their own progress. This depends on the capacity to agree within the community and through agreement to establish community norms which express what is acceptable to the whole community, developed through a process of discussion and consensus. Counselling, in various forms, is crucial to behaviour change - information is necessary before people can make choices. Research by outsiders may be irrelevant to the needs and experience of the community. Community organizations and communities need to set their own agendas.

Discussion brought up the following points:

1. Behaviour change is related to attitude change and it is difficult to evaluate attitude change; some indicators highlighted include:
   * Families are changing, getting involved with caring, and using the opportunity of having an infected family member to learn more about HIV.
   * Increasing numbers of people with HIV are coming forward to be educators.
   * Communities are becoming more open and involved.
   * People are joining organizations which are identified with infected people.
   * People are living longer with HIV and leading happier lives.
2. The discussion on research reflected the controversy of this issue.
   * Research should be action-oriented and participatory.
   * Research should always be accompanied by intervention.
   * Research has often been mistakenly seen as intervention.
   * Community-based care is a long-term process, but research results on this are demanded in the short term.
   * The importance of recognizing both the diversity of cultures in different regions and the commonality of regions was acknowledged. The need to present research in a particular way, in order for its value to be understood, causes frustration to community groups who know their work is valid but who have difficulty in getting it accepted as such. We all need to work towards legitimizing the research methods and the results coming from community groups. Terminology is important; for exarnple, anecdotes can also be case histories.
   * Research methods to evaluate behaviour change have not been acceptable to
     the scientific research mainstream.

Q5. HOW DO PROGRAMMES EXPAND AND DEVELOP TO ASSIST THESE CHANGES TO COME ABOUT?

Several differcnt stimuli to expansion were identified:

* Kilamanjaro Christian Medical Centre's, KCMC

(Tanzania), motivation came from individuals who were concerned about a need to know more and take action after they realized the high level of seropositivity in the community.

* Chikankata (Zambia) responded to requests from the community, following their realization that the traditional methods were not working and that more realistic approaches were needed.
* Programmes change if it is established that a strategy is not successful and that another must be developed.
* Increasing involvement of volunteers leads to a change in strategy because they represent community involvement.
* Community participation and involvement can change the direction or the plans of the programme.
* Evaluation may precede a decision to expand or alter direction.

Expansion may also be influenced by a need to complement services provided by governments, or by what other organizations are doing; it is important to avoid duplication. Equally, expansion may be affected by factors outside the control of community-based organizations: one example is that international NGOs can attract resources and staff from local NGOs, thus inhibiting their development.

Q 6. HOW CAN THESE CHANGES BE DOCUMENTED AND WHY DO WE WANT TO DO THIS?

Community organizations continually change, refine, revise and expand their programmes. They do this on the basis of observation, intuition, feedback. Their closeness to the community within which they were formed guarantees that this is a participatory process.

This is a process of continuing analysis, evaluation and redesign which occurs in response to (and in order to sustain) changes taking place in the community. This process can provide the basis of the documentation of change.

To overcome the epidemic, both attitudes and behaviour must change. This occurs through ongoing interactions between individuals and their communities.

Changes are taking place in attitude and behaviour. Both individuals and communities are changing. There is a need to record and share these processes. Systematic recording of processes needs thought and training. for the benefit of both community volunteers who play a crucial part within the community as well as professional workers.

Summary of Methods and Indicators of Change in the Community

Indicators of change are already being used informally by community organizations represented at the consultation. The indicators identified were illustrative rather than exhaustive. But they do identify ways in which change is being determined and identified, and this could form the basis of a more endogenous methodology.

Changes in Attitude

Change in attitude was seen as not only a vital first step in individual and community behaviour change, but also as a legitimate and very important end in itself in leading to an environment in which behaviour change is encouraged and supported.

Indicators of attitudinal change:

1. Establishment of HIV-related community organizations, which can be measured as:
   * Number of groups formed
   * Membership of such groups
   * Total membership
   * Involvement of people not themselves infected
   * Involvement of people not directly affected by HIV.
2. Involvement of people living with HIV (PLWH) in changing behaviour in the community, which can be measured by:
   * Number of PLWH trained as educators
3. Involvement of PLWH in decision-making at all levels, local to national, which can be measured by:
   * Consultation by decision makers with infected individuals and communities
   * Number of PLWH on management boards of community organizations, national HIV/AIDS committees, etc.
4. Acceptance of PLWH within communities, which can be measured by:
   * Number of families a) willing to care for their infected members and b) interested to find out more about HIV

* Number of PLWH prepared to:
  — tell their stories
  — become educators
  — participate on boards, in consultations, etc.

5. How community leaders talk about HIV/AIDS and PLWH, which can be measured by;
   * Language used
   * Concern and respect shown
   * Openness of discussions
6. Support for affected families, which can be measured by:
   * Number of people visiting an affected household
   * Care given to survivors—elderly parents or children
7. Talking about illness and death, which can be measured by:
   * Number of funerals where it is said that the person died of AIDS

Behaviour Change

The problems of research methodologies for measuring behaviour change are well known. However, communities can and do define their own strategies and targets, and can be helped to measure their own successes (or failures) against these. Doing this means identification of high risk behaviours (which is in itself an indicator of attitude change).

Indicators which have been observed or heard of by programmes at the consultation include:

1. Talking about change of behaviour, which can be measured by:
   * Reports to counsellors, educators, etc.
   * Information from men and women prepared to talk openly about how they have changed
2. Choosing to be counselled and tested, which can be measured by:
   * Attendance records for men and women at voluntary testing and counselling centres
3. Changing patterns of sexual behaviour, which can be measured by:
   * number of adultery disputes or divorce proceedings in traditional courts
   * Changes in sex-worker population
   * Changes in patterns of sex-worker clients.

Indicators of change in norms set by community:

Communities assist and sustain people in changing their behaviour and attitudes. Communities reach a consensus on strategies or behaviours which are acceptable or which are judged to achieve a certain aim. These changes in community norms often precede or accompany individual behaviour change. The monitoring may be done by the community as a whole or by individuals or organizations within it.

Indicators could include:

1. Acceptance of talking about sexuality and HIV infection, which can be measured by:
   * Education on sexuality and HIV in schools.
2. Changing of cultural practices which put people at risk, which can be measured by:
   * Number/proportion of spouses cleansed by non-sexual means.
   * Age of marriage and bride price.
3. Changing patterns of alcohol consumption, which can be measured by:
   * Opening hours of bars.
   * Number of people drinking in bars.
   * Sale records of alcohol in bars.
4. Communities seeking help for prevention and care, which can be measured by:
   * Number of communities requesting help
   * Number of families accepting home-based care for people with AIDS
   * Willingness to raise local funds for people affected
   * Identification by communities of high-risk behaviours
   * Identification by communities of behaviour-change indicators
   * Identification by communities of strategies for behaviour change.
5. Changes in community customs relating to sex and marriage, which can be measured by:
   * Greater stability of marriages
   * Resumption of teaching on taboos
   * Marriage patterns and pre-marital counselling

BEHAVIOUR CHANGE:

A Central Issue in Responding to the HIV Epidemic

Agenda for the Future

1. Carry back the message that behaviour change is a critical strategy for overcoming the epidemic.

   There is a need to influence governments and community groups to focus on behaviour change.

2. Incorporate the knowledge and insights of the informal consultation into the daily work programme of each organization.

   To do this, there is a need for increased understanding of the processes of attitudinal and behaviour change, as well as a need to learn from one another's experience in programme development.

3. Value the processes and knowledge by which individuals and community organizations identify needs in order to design, evaluate and redesign their programmes.

4. Feed back insights, intuitions, stories and research findings to communities, educators, outreach workers and programme managers.

5. Give value to what communities and their organizations are doing by documenting and sharing their experience.

6. Increase the sharing of experience among countries and regions.

   This can be done through the strengthening of existing linkages, the exchange of material, consultation, visits to other organizations and through meetings.

7. Bring about a partnership based on respect, trust and support between community organizations and governments.

   For communities and organizations to continue to function effectively, their initiatives must be complemented and supported by government policies and programmes. This requires a balance of support between government and community.

8. Establish a means or structure which would enable communities to share experiences, work collaboratively, provide credibility to community organizations, provide an agreed means of community representation at local and national levels and be a means of communication between communities and governments, particularly

in national HIV/AIDS programmes.

9. Create awareness that the resources needed to address the epidemic are already scarce, and that they must continue to come from within communities and nations. *Community initiatives always draw on community resources - volunteers, financial and political support. These form the basis of a self-sufficient response.*

   Community resources need to be complemented by government resources. This will require policies in support of community initiatives, the reallocation of national budgets and the selection of critical priority areas for supporting community initiatives. Communities can assist individuals in bringing about and sustaining behaviour change, but they may not themselves have the capacity to establish services requiring regular and sustained input of materials or technologies.

10. Report to one another widen six months on progress made in the implementation of this agenda.

Informal Consultation, Dakar, Senegal, 12-15 December, 1991

THE AIDS CARE AND PREVENTION DEPARTMENT THE SALVATION ARMY HOSPITAL CHIKANKATA, ZAMBIA

Chikankata Hospital has been implementing field-based AIDS care and prevention programmes since March 1987.

On-going home based care (HBC) is provided to an average of 250 patients, their families and their immediate communities each quarter. The team goes out three days a week and is committed to attending to the total needs of the patient. Two members focus on the physical, social and spiritual needs of the HIV-infected individual and his or her family while another concentrates on educating the family and the community on the facts about HIV and how to prevent its transmission. One of the team members travels with the Primary Health Care team to the schools in the catchment area twice a year to present the facts about HIV.

The objectives of the HBC teams are multiple. They visit people with HIV infection in their homes in order to assess their physical, psychological, social and spiritual needs, and to provide for these needs where possible. They carry out contact tracing. They carry out counselling and education within families and communities, providing personal support, and promoting sustained behaviour change through community counselling. They also assess the educational impact of AIDS management on people with HIV and their families. One of the team members is the school's educator. The team also tries to provide material support, giving milk. On occasion the hospital receives donations of blankets and clothes which are given out.

On the remaining two days of the week, a second team goes out to work with communities—clarifying facts about HIV, helping communities identify activities which put them at risk and coming up with strategies that will keep them from engaging in these high risk activities. This process is called community counselling. This is defined as an activity, focusing on groups and communities, which promotes responsibility transfer for behaviour change from others, including health care personnel, to the community.

Principles of counselling as applied in a one-on-one relationship have been transferred to counselling a large group or a community. After a community has been selected, the process of counselling communities, as in any counselling situation, follows the process of relationship-building, problem exploration, understanding and decision making, implementation and evaluation.

Different types of communities are concerned: kinship-based-village; occupation-based—industrial towns, commercial farms; religion-based—churches; and party systems-based.

Village health workers and other volunteers who are part of the PHC structure will be trained so that they will be part of the network working on AIDS care and prevention.

The aim of the home-based care and community counselling programmes is to transfer responsibility for care and prevention to the family and the community.

The hope for the future is to activate families and communities.

Families and communities need to have a sense that HIV is their problem and if it is going to be stopped, and if people are going to get the care they need to deal with being HIV+, it will because they, the family and community, have done something about it. Not because the hospital has done something.

The hospital's management plan consists of diagnosis/counselling; planned discharge; home-based care and hospital admission when required. Although the focus of this plan is to get the patient back into the home where he will be cared for by his extended family the hospital plays a vital part in diagnosis, stabilization and readmission for additional treatment.

From July 1989, the Chikankata AIDS care and prevention department has been conducting a five-day seminar each month.

The seminar is for health professionals and others who are currently involved in or need to start an AIDS care and prevention programme. The seminar provides an integrative approach covering such disciplines as counselling, clinical care, education, pastoral care and administration. The content is based on the practical, field-based AIDS care and prevention programmes at Chikankata.

WOMEN AND AIDS SUPPORT NETWORK (WASN)-ZIMBABWE

WASN was established in 1989 following the international Society for Women and AIDS in Africa (SWAA) conference held in Harare. It is a group of volunteers working on the fundamental principle that women will only be able to overcome consequences of HIV through improving their self esteem and confidence. It was recognized that people needed to change their attitudes and behaviour in order to stop further transmission of HIV infection. However, in many situations women were unable to make demands that their partners change their behaviour and felt helpless to prevent infection to themselves. They also wanted to publicly display solidarity with those of us who are PLWHIVs.

WASN works to share information about how HIV affects women, to encourage women as organized groups and clubs to support women living with HIV and AIDS, and to support each other in protecting themselves against becoming infected. They target organizations working with women so that the messages are carried through to more women than WASN can reach itself. Also it is desirable that the issues be included in more permanent fashion through programmes and curricula.

WASN analyzes the quarterly statistics released by the National AIDS Control Programme to emphasize the vulnerabilities of women in the AIDS epidemic. These figures encourage young school girls targetted by programmes to understand the consequences of early sex, and to be more assertive in refusing unwanted attentions. WASN published a booklet called 'Why Should Women be Concerned About AIDS?'. It emphasizes the importance of women talking to each other in all kinds of fora so that issues about sex, condoms, HIV and AIDS become less taboo. It also emphasizes women supporting each other rather than competing with each other.

Although legislation exists to protect the rights of workers in the formal sector, many workers in the informal sector are not covered. This includes women who work as domestic workers and child minders who are often dismissed if their HIV status becomes known. To organize employers, Women and AIDS Support Network organized phone-in radio programmes (the accessible media nationally) and print media articles on transmission of HIV—emphasizing how HIV is not spread by social contact.

WASN was concerned that women were often depicted as prostitutes in harsh judgmental images, shown as reservoirs of infection. This reinforced many male attitudes that HIV is a women's disease as it is caught from women, and women were blamed for spreading the disease. WASN makes input into several drama groups to encourage them to be more progressive and in particular to be more positive in the roles women play. They can be shown supporting each other, organizing to change attitudes and behaviour in the communities.

WAMATA (THOSE IN TANZANIA IN THE FRONT LINE AGAINST AIDS)

WAMATA began with FIVE families as a voluntary, non-sectarian and non-governmental grass-roots organization based on the spirit of solidarity, love and hope. Its mission is to provide medical and nursing home care, counselling and, to some extent, material assistance to people living with HIV. In its work WAMATA collaborates with the National AIDS Control Programme of the United Republic of Tanzania.

WAMATA provides a forum for grassroots-based organized action targeted at individual and community behaviour change; open and frank discussion of HIV as a socio-economic problem; sharing of experiences and knowledge about the epidemic among the members; planning, organizing and carrying out activities that not only comfort those living with HIV but also contribute something toward awareness of the need for individual and community behaviour change at least in the course of time of continued counselling work.

One of WAMATA's principle aims and objectives is 'To campaign against discrimination of HIV affected individuals and their families and involve the general public to institute and maintain behaviour change as a necessary step towards HIV prevention and control.' Its major activities are consciously based upon this objective.

WAMATA and other organs through campaigns, counselling, medical and home care activities have made it possible for positive and supportive attitudes to develop in the community towards those living with HIV. WAMATA members living and dying with HIV identify themselves as HIV positives. Some who were already terminally ill in 1989 have since sustained life, presumably partly because of the solidarity, support, care and hope they have been accorded by their organization (WAMATA). They are leading elements in the WAVIU (coined by the group living with HIV/AIDS to mean: People Striving to Control the Spread of the HIV Transmission).

WAMATA is involved in training of volunteer counsellors and provision of volunteer counselling, medical and home service. Indeed, most of the counselling and support is done by families and community members on a voluntary basis. Trained volunteer counsellors take on cases where the need for monitoring, supervision and follow up action has been identified.

WAMATA makes provision of material support to: HIV-affected families in need; children of HIV-affected families; and those affected families and individuals able, ready and willing to engage in income-generating activities.

WAMATA attempts to increase the participation of the wider community in the activities of the organization: in meetings, funding, publicity, etc.

THE AIDS SUPPORT ORGANISATION (TASO), UGANDA

TASO (The AIDS Support Organization) is an indigenous, non-governmental organization based in Kampala, Uganda.

In Kampala headquarters which houses training activities, support is given to the development and co-ordination of a community-based AIDS programme, and to the development of TASO and TASO-type activities in other areas. With its theme 'Positive Living with AIDS', TASO provides a package of counselling services to people with HIV and their families. The package includes counselling, medical support and day-centre activities. To strengthen its hospital/clinic-based service, TASO has initiated a community-based HIV programme.

TASO has established seven counselling centres in seven districts along the Trans-African Highway where high prevalence of HIV has been reported. An eighth centre is planned in Arua.

TASO has periodically undertaken a critical assessment of its work to deduce lessons learnt from its experience and determine the most suitable direction for the organization over the foreseeable future. The key task has been to balance the competing demands of helping as many people as possible and providing a high quality service of training and counselling.

To facilitate project planning and implementation, TASO has established a structure where, as an organization, it will concentrate on its role of training HIV/AIDS counsellors for TASO and other organizations, will directly administer two 'model' counselling centres (Mulago and Musaka), and offer technical and management advice and financial control to the other 6 affiliate centres.

TASO recognizes that HIV education and prevention is the best weapon available to fight against HIV infection and disease.

At the same time, TASO recognizes the need to care for those already infected. To meet these very demanding needs, TASO has approached the problem directly, through those infected persons. They are the entry point to the family and community. By involving people with HIV and those who are not infected (including those who think they are not infected) in the care of people with AIDS, TASO is offering not only AIDS care, but also HIV education and prevention. Face-to-face contact and practical experience are what counts.

In response to the enormous problems caused and aggravated by HIV, TASO has the following strategic board activities:

1. Training AIDS counsellors for TASO and other organizations to offer counselling services.
2. Offering counselling services to people with HIV and their families in all TASO-established counselling centres.
3. Complementing available medical service for PWA/HIV.
4. Promoting positive attitudes in families and communities toward people with HIV.
5. Building and strengthening community-based efforts in response to the HIV epidemic.

A total of 6,000 people with AIDS have received TASO services at these centres. TASO also supports primary education of 800 AIDS orphans, though over 6,000 have been identified.

Over 25,000 family members have received HIV information and education. And millions have been reached through the TASO video—Living Positively with AIDS - which has been distributed worldwide by WHO/GPA and other organizations.

KITOVU MOBILE AIDS HOME CARE AND EDUCATION PROGRAMME AND PASTORAL CARE AND COUNSELLING PROGRAMME, UGANDA

Kitovu Hospital is a Catholic, private hospital in Masaka District, Uganda. It has 185 beds, an out-patient department, a nutrition centre and a community-based health care programme. The hospital trains enrolled nurses and midwives.

In 1987, more than 60 per cent of patients in the general wards were HIV-positive, and the staff saw many children and adults with signs of HIV infection in the primary health care clinics. The AIDS programme at Kitovu Hospital was started in May 1987 as a part-time pastoral care programme. In October 1987 it became a fulltime programme, and it was decided to concentrate home care services on specific areas in Rakai and Masaka Districts.

The areas selected were chosen because they had the highest concentration of AIDS patients; people living in them could not visit the hospital because public transport was not available; the attitude of the local people to the team was one of openness and receptivity; the parish priest, health personnel, etc. had asked for help; and they were near enough to Kitovu for hospital vehicles to be used to bring patients to the hospital.

The AIDS programme consists of the following five interlinked components:

- hospital care;
- home visiting, including pastoral care;
- education in schools and villages;
- out-patient treatment;
- hospital pastoral care.

The main emphasis in the programme is on the Mobile AIDS Home Care Team and the Pastoral Care and Counselling Programme.

Clients are referred to the Home Care Team from the wards, the out-patient clinic and the Pastoral Care Programme. All persons with HIV infection and AIDS in the areas selected are eligible for home care.

Very ill patients and those requiring special aftercare are taken home from the hospital by the Pastoral Care and Counselling Team, which also visits patients who live near the hospital and who are too weak to come to the out-patient clinic.

Home care of persons with AIDS was chosen because it was known that people in the area prefer to die at home. In addition, it was assumed that the programme would make it easier to provide effective health education in the community.

VICTORIAN AIDS COUNCIL/GAY MEN'S HEALTH CENTRE, COLLINGWOOD, AUSTRALIA

The Victorian AIDS Council / Gay Men's Health Centre provides education, support, advocacy and other necessary services to people affected directly or indirectly by HIV. These services are provided regardless of gender, sexual preferences or health status, but the organization acknowledges that these services will be primarily designed to meet the needs of all gay and bisexual men in Victoria.

The organization is based upon the principles of community development. Policy and programming is designed by members of the community in conjunction with employees. Education strategies are designed acknowledging that sustained behaviour change is facilitated by peer support. Support services are designed to meet people's needs in an empowering fashion.

42

HIV/AIDS in South-East Asia

(Report of the Meeting of the National Programme Managers, New Delhi, 8-12, November 1993)

I. INTRODUCTION

HIV/AIDS continues to spread in South-East Asia. The infection is not only increasing among individuals with high risk behaviour but now starting to spread to the general population as well. The countries in the Region are gaining considerable experience in the planning and implementation of activities in the fight against HIV pandemic within the framework of their national or medium-term plans. These experiences must be shared. The National AIDS Programme Managers, during the eighth meeting in November 1992, discussed interventions targeted among individuals with high risk behaviour. From 8 to 12 November 1993, the WHO Regional Office for South-East Asia organized the 9th Regional Meeting of the National AIDS Country Programme Managers at New Delhi to share the country experiences on various areas of the AIDS programme. The objectives of the meeting were:

1. To review the implementation of AIDS prevention and care activities in the countries of the Region with a view to facilitating the exchange of experiences including the successes, constraints and lessons learned;
2. To identify policies, interventions and approaches from selected countries which have proven to be successful and discuss how these could be transferred and applied, with appropriate modifications, in other countries of the Region;
3. To select priority interventions and activities for the national AIDS control programmes to be included in the 1994-95 comprehensive work plan; and
4. To finalize the 1994-95 work-plan on activities to be supported by WHO;

Twenty-three participants from ten countries were present at the meeting. Representatives of international agencies such as UNDP, UNICEF, UNESCO, ILO, USAID and the Ford Foundation were also invited to participate in the meeting.

The meeting was opened by Dr. U Ko Ko, Regional Director, WHO, SEARO. After welcoming the Programme Managers and other participants, the Regional Director highlighted the dangers posed by the HIV pandemic in the South-East Asia Region. He invited the participants to use the workshop as a forum for exchange of country experiences and ideas for the prevention and control of HIV infection and to see whether such experiences could be replicated in their own countries. He urged the Programme Managers to think of programme priorities in the light of the limited financial resources available. The external financial resources are already shrinking, and hence efforts are to be made to raise financial resources locally and to make programmes sustainable. Mr. Bayani, Acting Resident Representative, UNDP, stressed on the need for all UN agencies to work together in assisting the countries of this region in combating the HIV/AIDS epidemic. He emphasized on the WHO/UNDP alliance to combat the disease and its relevance at this juncture to merge the technical and financial support for combating the pandemic which has already reached an alarming situation.

Mr. P. R. Dasgupta, Project Director, National AIDS Control Organization (NACO), was nominated as Chairman, Dr Wiput Phoolcharoen, Director, AIDS Division, Ministry of Public Health, Thailand, as Co-Chairman, and Dr U Myo Thet Htoon, Programme Manager, Myanmar as Rapporteur. The workshop sessions consisted of plenaries, general. discussion and group work,_. Background materials on relevant subjects were provided to the participants during the opening ceremony.

2. REGIONAL HIV/AIDS SITUATION AND EPIDEMIOLOGICAL SURVEILLANCE

2.1 Current Situation of HIV/AIDS in South-East Asia

In the South-East Asia Region, AIDS was first diagnosed in 1984 in Thailand. In most other countries, HIV was not diagnosed until 1986 or later. Since then, however, HIV infection has spread extremely rapidly and WHO estimates that currently there are more than 1.5 million HIV-infected people in the Region (Table 42.1).

Table 42.1. *AIDS and HIV infections in SEAR countries* (as of 30 June 1993)

Country	Reported AIDS cases	Estimated HIV Infections
Bangladesh	1	< 20, 000
Bhutan	0	< 300
DPR Korea	0	< 1, 000
India	336	1, 000, 000
Indonesia	31	< 20, 000
Maldives	0	< 100
Mongolia	0	< 200
Myanmar	47	1, 50, 000
Nepal	18	< 5, 000
Sri Lanka	24	< 1, 000
Thailand	1, 569	4, 50, 000
Total	2, 026	> 1, 500, 000

As of 30 June 1993, a total of 2, 026 cases of AIDS have been reported in South-East Asia. However, it is estimated that about 20, 000 AIDS cases have occurred till now. Thailand and India have reported the largest number of cases—1, 569 and 336 respectively - accounting for more than 95 per cent of the cases reported from the Region to date. Two countries, namely, Bhutan and DPR Korea, have not yet reported HIV infections (Table 42.2).

Trend data based on seroprevalence surveys confirm the alarming increase in HIV infection rates in selected high-risk populations. In Thailand, HIV rates of 0 to less than 1 per cent among Injecting Drug-Users (IDU) in Bangkok were found in various *ad hoc* surveys from 1985 to 1987. However, HIV rates increased sharply to 40 per cent by September 1988, and has now stabilized almost at that level. Rates similar to Bangkok were also seen in various other provinces of the country. This wave of HIV epidemic in IDU was followed by that among female prostitutes and, by successive waves of transmission, to male clients of the prostitutes, and from them to the wives and girl friends of these men in the general population. Nationally, the prevalence rates in June 1992 were 38.2 per cent in IDUs, 22.9 per cent in low-charge prostitutes, 5.7 per cent in male STD (sexually transmitted disease) patients and 1 per cent among pregnant women. Based on the currently available data, it is estimated that there are at present 450,000 HIV-infected persons in Thailand. The Thai working group projects that given that HIV transmission would continue, there would be 2-4 million cumulative HIV infections by the year 2000. In Myanmar, explosive increases in HIV seropositivity have been documented among IDUs—from 17 per cent in 1989 to 59 per cent and 71 per cent in 1990 and 1991 respectively. In addition, the rates

Table 42.2. *Number of HIV Positives Among the That male Population (low and high prevalence)*

Age Group	Population	Male Pop.	Prev. Low	Prev.+ Low	Prev. High	HIV+High
Less 5	5, 743, 000	2, 871, 500				
5-9	5, 802, 000	2, 901, 000				
10-14	6, 275, 000	3, 137, 500	0.1	3, 137.5	0.2	6, 275
15-19	6, 071, 000	3, 035, 500	0.6	18, 213	2	6, 0710
20-24	6, 071, 000	3, 035, 500	3.1	94, 100.5	3.5	1,06, 242.5
25-29	5, 125, 000	2, 562, 500	3.1	79, 437.5	3.5	89, 68,7.5
30-34	5, 125, 000	2, 562, 500	1.1	25, 625	1.5	38, 437.5
35-39	3, 600, 000	1, 800, 000	1.0	18, 000	1.5	27, 000
40-44	3, 600, 000	1, 800, 000	0.5	9, 000	0.5	9, 000
45-49	2, 261, 000	1, 130, 500	0.5	5, 652.5	0.5	5, 652.5
50-54	2, 261, 000	1, 130, 500	0.1	1, 130.5	0.2	2, 261
55-59	1, 434, 000	7,17, 000	0.1	717	0.2	1, 434
60-64	1, 434, 000	7,17, 000	0.1	717	0.2	1, 434
more 65	2, 240, 000	1, 120, 000	0.1	1, 120	0.2	2, 240
Total	57, 789, 000	28, 894, 500		2,56, 850.5		350, 374

among STD patients have registered an increase from 1.9 per cent in 1990 to 15.9 per cent in 1991 and from 8 per cent to 15.9 per cent among female prostitutes during the same period. About 1,50,000 persons are currently estimated to have been infected with HIV in Myanmar. Sequential infection was noted in Thailand starting with IDUs, and followed by female sex workers, STD patients and the community. This was also observed in Myanmar. In a study in the north-east Indian State of Manipur, none of the 2,322, IDUs seen from 1986 to 1989 were seropositive for HIV. However, the rate increased to 54 per cent during the period October 1989 to June 1990, and at present it is almost at the same level. Sequential infection, as observed in Thailand and Myanmar, is apprehended to occur in Manipur. In Bombay, the HIV seropositivity rate among prostitutes has increased from 2 per cent in 1988-1989 to nearly 40 per cent in 1991. Although there is evidence of increase in HIV prevalence among blood donors and women attending antenatal clinics, the rates are still less than 0.5 per cent. It is estimated that currently there are about one million HIV-infected persons in India.

Given the prevailing sexual behaviour and experiences in the three countries described above, there is a possibility of a similar scenario being repeated in other countries of the South-East Asia Region. Risk behaviour which promotes the spread of HIV, such as injection of drugs, male patronage of prostitutes, high rates of STD and low condom usage, are present in all countries. In view of the fact that heterosexual contact is the predominant mode of HIV transmission in the Region, that the rates of STD are high, and that there is considerable unprotected sexual activity, continued transmission of HIV in the general population appears inevitable. Predictions about AIDS tend to be unrealistic, but the current estimate of more than 1.5 million HIV infections in South-East Asia is nearly 12 per cent of the global total, while the proportion of reported AIDS cases is less than 1 per cent.

Furthermore, WHO estimates that while the annual number of HIV infections will peak in Africa by 1995, infections in Asia will continue to increase well into the early next century (Figure 42.1). The annual number of HIV infections by the year 2000 would far exceed that seen in sub-Saharan Africa. Given the mean progression time for initial HIV infection to develop into AIDS, now estimated to be ten years, it can be concluded that AIDS cases in the Region will continue to increase well into the next century, and close to two million cumulative cases of AIDS will occur by the year 2000.

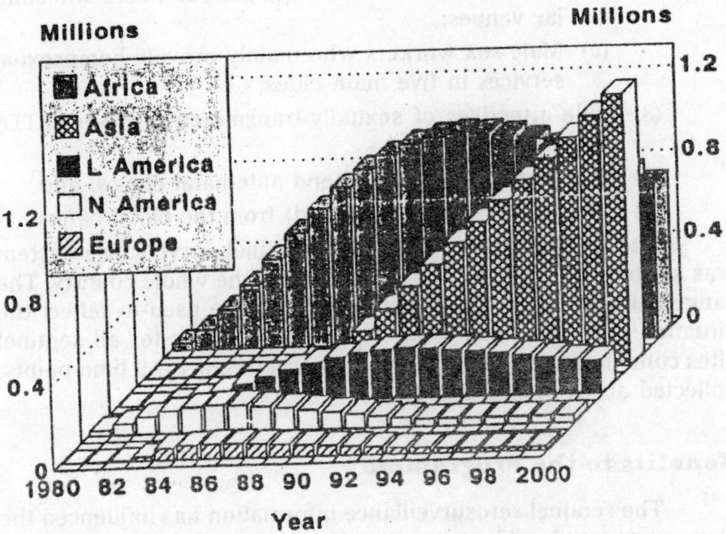

Figure 42.1. Estimated/projected annual adult HIV infections

2.2 HIV Sentinel Surveillance and Estimations in Thailand

The major objective of the HIV sentinel surveillance system in Thailand is to monitor high-risk groups in order to target intensified HIV intervention programmes and to provide early warning that the epidemic will soon reach the lower-risk general population. The latter assumes that high-risk groups are effective sentinels of future HIV infection in the general community. If this is true, local public health officials would have more time to organize control activities to safeguard the general public.

Surveillance Methods

The sentinel surveillance started in 14 of the country's 73 provinces in June 1989. Six months later the surveillance was expanded to 31 provinces, and again expanded six months later to include all 73 provinces. The semi-annual surveys are mainly focused on selected target populations in the city areas of the provinces, which include:

(1) Injecting Drug Users (IDUs) who attend drug abuse treatment clinics;

(2) Commercial Sex Workers (CSWs) which are subclassified as:

(a) Female CSWs in brothel settings;

(b) **Female** CSWs not based in brothels but in establishments such as massage parlours, bars and similar venues;

(c) Male sex workers who mainly provide homosexual services in five main cities;

(3) Male attendees of sexually-transmitted diseases (STD) clinics;

(4) Pregnant women who attend ante-natal clinics, and

(5) Blood donors (donated blood) from the blood banks.

The trends from the time the sentinel surveillance system was started in June 1989 are presented for the whole country. The ranges of prevalence and mean prevalence are used to reflect the situation at the national level. The median values for all sentinel sites combined are used to show temporal trends for 9 time-points, collected at six-month intervals.

Benefits to the Programme

The sentinel serosurveillance information has influenced the Government and public to realize the severity of the situation and to plan for action to combat the HIV epidemic. These are:

1. *Political will.* The evolving surveillance system provided information essential for taking rational action based on the prevalence of HIV infection in various segments of the society. The Thai Government established the National AIDS Committee chaired by the Prime Minister to respond to the HIV epidemic in 1991. The budget for the National AIDS Control Programme rose from 182 million bahts (approx. 7.2 million US$) in the fiscal year 1991 to 359 million bahts (14.4 million US$) and 1,125 million bahts (45 million US$) in the fiscal years 1992 and 1993 respectively. It will again rise substantially in the fiscal year 1994.
2. *Education for the general public.* Before 1989, the news on the AIDS epidemic in the country had never reached the first page of any newspaper. It was felt rumours about AIDS in the country would damage its image and hence the tourist industry. Since the last half of 1989, television and radio spots on AIDS have been aired on prime time. These spots warn the general public about the dangers of AIDS and explain exactly how to prevent it. The advertisements are explicit. In addition, the school curriculum on health education has been modified to include AIDS prevention messages.
3. ***Guidance in the development of the prevention programme development.*** **According to the results of the**

sentinel surveillance, over the last two years the IDUs and female CSWs have become the sources of HIV infection and are not the only high risk groups any more. The HIV epidemic has invaded the family; men, (pregnant) women, and their infants. Preventive actions, which focused on commercial sex activities such as the 100 per cent condom use programme, were changed to put the emphasis on the more difficult and complicated task of strengthening social norms to reject promiscuity and prostitution.

4. *Medical services safety.* In 1989, the Ministry of Public Health established the first decisive and effective intervention to prevent HIV transmission through blood transfusion. Since then, a total of 700,000—800,000 lots of donated blood are mandatorily screened for HIV antibody annually. Universal precaution techniques, practiced by public health providers, were strengthened through budgetary and technical support.
5. *Differentiating the action base on the epidemic pattern.* The epidemiological patterns of HIV infection in each part of the country are different. The northern epidemic wave has reached the family, while the north-eastern HIV epidemic is still confined to the IDUs and female CSWs. The southern and east-coast epidemics are spreading among the fishermen communities. The approach and response to these different epidemiological patterns should be strategically formulated by the local level, the so called provincial level.

Estimations of HIV Infection

The estimation of the number of HIV infected persons in Thailand is computed from the following data sources:

1. The demographic projection estimated by sex at five-year intervals from the National Statistics Bureau;
2. The donated blood surveillance;
3. The sero survey of military conscripts, and
4. Sentinel surveillance at antenatal care clinics.

The tables (42.2 and 42.3) seen here are an example of the estimation of HIV infected persons in early 1992. The projection of the population in each cell is derived from the census data of 1990. The estimation of male HIV prevalence is derived from the calculation of low and high prevalence. The low prevalence is derived from the distribution of the age specific prevalence rate from the

Table 42.3. Number of HIV positives among the Thai female population (low and high prevalence)

Age Group	Population	Female Pop.	Prev. Low	HIV+ Low	Prev. High	HIV+High
Less 5	5, 743, 000	2, 871, 500				
5-9	5, 802, 000	2, 901, 000				
10-14	6, 275, 000	3, 137, 500				
15-19	6, 071, 000	3, 035, 500	1.0	30, 355	1.96	59, 495.8
20-24	6, 071, 000	3, 035, 500	1.0	30, 355	1.82	55, 246.1
25-29	5, 125, 000	2, 562, 500	1.0	25, 625	1.82	46, 637.5
30-34	5, 125, 000	2, 562, 500	1.0	25, 625	1.12	28, 700
35-39	3, 600, 000	1, 800, 000	1.0	18, 000	1.12	20, 160
40-44	3, 600, 000	1, 800, 000	0.5	9, 000	0.64	11, 520
45-49	2, 261, 000	1, 130, 500	0.5	5, 652.5	0.64	7, 235.2
50-54	2, 261, 000	1, 130, 500	0.1	1, 130.5	0.1	1, 130.5
55-59	1, 434, 000	7,17, 000	0.1	717	0.1	717
60-64	1, 434, 000	7,17, 000	0.1	717	0.1	717
more 65	2, 240, 000	1, 120, 000				
Total	57 789 000	28 894 500				
Grand Total						404 028

donated blood samples. The high prevalence is derived from the sero survey of conscripts in 1992 and then proportionally adjusted by the age specific prevalence of the donated blood samples. The estimation of the female high prevalence group is derived from the age specific prevalence rate of the antenatal care clinic sentinel surveillance. The number of infected cases in each age group and sex are calculated and then combined to present the total number of HIV infected persons in Thailand.

3. EFFECTIVE INTERVENTIONS FOR HIV/AIDS PREVENTION

As experience with HIV/AIDS prevention increases in the Region, it is becoming possible to highlight what comprises the key elements of success for interventions to change the behaviour. These elements include the use of mass media, peer-to-peer approaches and condom programming, which National AIDS Programme should consider while planning their intervention programmes to change risky behaviour. At the district or local level, a need exists to develop interventions that address local needs and are tailored to local constraints. The district-level health of ficers who wish to develop locally-based interventions for HTV prevention or to assist non-governmental organizations in doing so should focus on organizational capacity and management, situation assessment, development and planning of the intervention and on monitoring and evaluation. The intervention activities should either motivate people in changing their behaviour or assist in changing the structure or environment that either puts people at risk or inhibits their ability to change.

Examples of innovative and effective interventions in South-East Asia are highlighted below:

3.1 Promoting Safer Sex Behaviour—Innovative Approaches Among Individuals with High Risk Behaviour

3.1.1 100 per cent Condom use Initiative in Thailand—an Update

Heterosexual intercourse is the most common mode of HIV transmission in Thailand. As of 30 September 1993, 75.5 per cent of 3 436 cumulative AIDS cases contracted the disease heterosexually. The most important factor relating to the rapid heterosexual HIV transmission is the sex entertainment industry. The total number of female sex workers in entertainment services in the whole country is estimated to be around 100, 000. They are the main sources of STD infection among male STD patients (i.e. over 96 per cent of male STD cases reported that they had contracted the disease from sex workers). Those infected acquired the HIV virus from their clients and then transmitted the virus to other clients who will further spread the disease to their wives and newborns. This trend is apparent from the increasing prevalence rate of HIV infection among sex workers, male patients attending STD clinics and pregnant women attending antenatal clinics.

Health education is the most important component in Thailand's AIDS programme. However, it is believed that the programme may be too slow to prevent effectively the spread of AIDS. Therefore, an effective programme to promote a higher degree of condom utilization is urgently required. In the past, efforts to promote condom use in Thailand relied mainly on information, education and communication activities. Reports from sentinel surveys showed that, as of December 1990, the average condom utilization rate among commercial sex workers was around 60 to 70 per cent and that among STD-clinic clients was under 50 per cent. As a result, the HIV infection rate among them still continued to increase.

It has been consistently observed that the majority of the sex workers want their clients to use condoms. However, they are unable to enforce such safety precaution regularly because a considerable number of clients refuse to use condoms. In some cases, even the owners of sex establishments pressure the sex workers to yield to the demand of their customers, that is to have sex without condom use. Therefore, increasing condom use within the sex industry was considered an arduous task.

In order to meet this challenge, the 100 per cent condom programme was initiated in August 1989 with the objective of promoting the use of condoms in sex establishments in Ratchaburi, a province in the central region, south of Bangkok. This will prevent heterosexual transmission of HIV among commercial sex workers and their clients, which will result in further prevention of HIV transmission to the general population.

Objective and strategies. The overall objective of the programme was to increase the rate of condom use in the sex establishments to 100 per cent. This is envisaged to be achieved through the co-operation of the government authorities and owners of the sex establishments in the province in order to instruct or require their sex workers to use condoms in all sexual encounters. If their customers refuse to use a condom, they are urged to withhold service and refund those customers' money. It is important that these measures be taken by all sex establishments in the area so that sex seekers will not be able to purchase sex services without using condoms in any sex establishment in the Province.

Methods of implementation. The programme began with a joint meeting between the government sector (comprises three main agencies: health, police and local administration) and owners of all sex establishments (both direct and indirect sex facilities). This was to declare the initiation of the programme in the Province.

In the meeting, the owners of sex establishments were educated about the severity of AIDS, the current AIDS situation in Thailand and in the Province, and problems associated with AIDS control. They were encouraged to prevent the disease by instructing or ordering their sex workers to use condoms in all sexual encounters and to withhold sex service to customers refusing to use condom. These measures were to be taken by all sex establishments in the area so that sex seekers will not be able to purchase sex services without condom use in any sex establishment in the Province.

Also, at this time, the owners were made aware of the methods of investigation into condom use among sex workers that would be employed as a part of the programme monitoring process. The penalties administered to those establishments found to be uncooperative included temporary and indefinite closure of their establishments by the police. Methods of follow-up and investigation of the extent of condom use among sex workers included:

(a) Questioning male clients attending STD clinics concerning the use of condom in recent sexual encounters with prostitutes and the location of these entertainment places.

(b) Collecting information from STD contact notification forms sent from STD clinics outside the area.

(c) Sending volunteers to randomly test the sex workers' level of adherence to the "100 per cent-condom-use-only" policy in the local sex establishments.

(d) Observing STD infection rates among sex workers receiving routine examinations at local STD clinics. According to the provincial STD control programme, sex workers are motivated to have regular weekly check up at minimum or no cost.

(e) Monitoring the number of condoms provided to each sex establishment in the area. The owners as well as the sex workers were also informed about the benefits resulting from their co-operation. These benefits included the maintenance of their previous level of income and the lack of detrimental consequences associated with HIV infection among their employee population.

Progress to date. The programme was satisfactorily run in the Province. The programme evaluation was performed by monitoring four factors which indicate progress and problems within the programme. These were (a) the prevalence of STD in the Province, (b) the prevalence of HIV infection in different target populations of each province from the sentinel serosurveillance, (c) attitude and practice relating to condom use among general population and groups at higher risk of STD infection, and (d) the provincial supply of condoms as well as the rate of condom use in sex establishments. The initial evaluation revealed satisfactory results especially in sex workers.

After successful implementation in Ratchaburi, the 100 per cent condom programme has been expanded to cover many nearby provinces since 1990. On 14 August 1991, the National AIDS Committee approved the nationwide expansion of the 100 per cent condom programme by issuing the following resolution: "The governor, the provincial chief of police and the provincial health officer of each province will work together to enforce a condom-use-only policy that requires all commercial sex workers to use condoms with every customer. All concerned ministries will issue directives that comply with this policy. In the case of Bangkok, the Bangkok Metropolis Administration and the Police Department are the operating agencies."

Since April 1992, all 73 provinces have reported the implementation of the programme to the Ministry of Public Health. It is still early to detect any decrease in HIV infection rate due to the 100 per cent condom programme. However, some promising results have been observed in most provinces. There has been *a marked increase in condom use in sex establishments* to a level as high as 90 per cent in June 1992. The *incidence of STD has decreased from* 6.5 per 1 000 population in 1989 to 4.48, 3.21 and 2.07 in 1990, 1991 and 1992 respectively. *The 1992 incidence is the record low in the last 20 years* (Figures 42.2 and 42.3).

Elements considered crucial for the success. The following are considered as key elements for the success of the 100 per cent condom programme:

— High level commitment.
— Reduction of political, legal and social barriers.
— Participation and co-ordination of all responsible parties.
— Facilitative social pattern of target population, i.e. organized form of sex establishments.
— Efficient STD control system.
— Efficient condom promotion programme as well as logistic management and quality control.

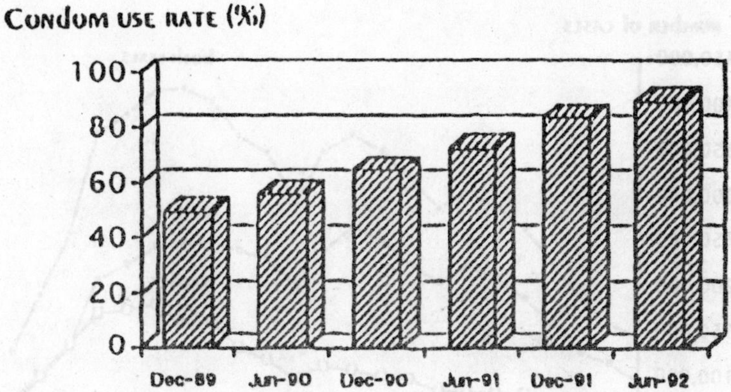

Figure 42.2. Trends of condom use rate among clients of sex-workers in brothel settings

— Benefit sharing nature of the programme.

— Lack of effective alternative strategies.

In conclusion, prevention of sexual transmission of HIV requires the active participation of both partners. However, such social and economic realities as poverty, inadequate education and subordinate social status may leave some individuals with little power or freedom to refuse intercourse or insist on the use of a condom. Sex workers in particular tend to be at higher risk of acquiring HIV infection through sex engaged in for economic survival. *The 100 per cent condom programme is an intervention to support and empower sex workers to be capable of controlling the action.* This will lead to the prevention of HIV infection among them and, thus, preventing the spread of HIV to the general population. With the implementation ofthe 100 per cent condom programme, the sexual transmission of AIDS will be greatly reduced nation-wide.

3.1.2 Peer Education and HIV Prevention Among Sex-Workers in Calcutta

In 1992, a community based sample survey of STD/HIV infections was carried out among the commercial sex-workers (CSW) of Sonagachi—a red light area in Calcutta. Sonagachi is one of the oldest and biggest red light areas in Calcutta having a population of 5,000 CSWs. The objectives of the study were to ascertain the prevalence of sexually transmitted diseases, to obtain

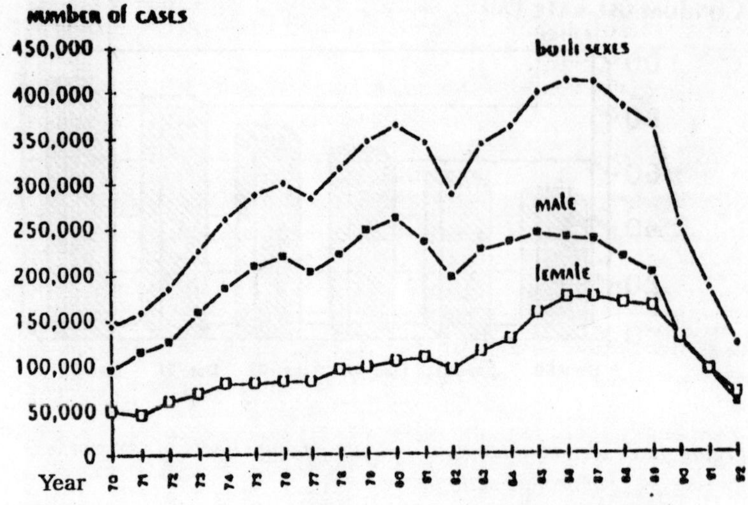

Figure 42.3. Case report of STDs by sex (Thailand, 1970-1992)

socio-economic information, to gather information about sexual behaviour and practices, to assess the extent of HIV infection, if any and to develop an intervention strategy of HIV/STD control. The survey was conducted jointly by All India Institute of Hygiene and Public Health and School of Tropical Medicine, Calcutta, 26 April to 6 June 1992. A sample of 450 CSWs were selected randomly and they were motivated to attend a clinic organized in the same area. CSWs were examined clinically to detect genital ulcers, genital warts, swelling of inguinal lymph nodes and signs of other STDs. Laboratory tests were conducted for four pathogens namely, *T.* pallidum by VDRL, TPHA & RPR, *N.* gonorrhoea - and *C.* albicans, by Gram stain and culture and *T.* vaginalis through wet mount in saline preparation.

An alarmingly high prevalence of STD was found among the CSWs. Seropositivity of syphilis was very high (62.97 per cent), followed by vaginal candidiasis (25.24 per cent), gonorrhoea (13.24 per cent), and trichomoniasis (11.11 per cent). It was also revealed from the study that about 81 per cent of CSWs are infected with one or more STD pathogens.

On the other hand, among 450 sex workers surveyed, 84.89 per cent were in the age group 15 - 29 years and about 84.44 per cent of the sex workers were found to be illiterate. It was also found that the majority of sex workers did not take any precaution against pregnancy. Clients of only 1.11 per cent of sex-workers were found to use condom regularly. Fortunately the HIV prevalence found among these sexworkers were very low (1.11per cent). Another positive aspect of this project was that during our survey work we were able to draw support from different sections of the community.

Methods of implementation. A batch of skilled field workers from a non-governmental organization assisted in the project and established good rapport with a large number of CSWs within a very short span of time. Though the study was completed by the early part of June 1992, the clinic continued to function as there was a great demand for the quality medical services provided by the project. The intervention programme of STD/HIV among the CSWs was started in September 1992 with assistance from NORAD, which is still continuing. Two non-governmental organizations, namely, Health and Eco-defence Society and Human Development and Research Institute, are active partners in this intervention programme. The programme components include early diagnosis and treatment of STDs, promotion of condoms and educational activities. To spearhead IEC and condom promotion activities, a batch of peer educators were identified and trained for a period of six weeks. The training curriculum included both technical and theoretical aspects of AIDS and STDs. They also received on an average 2-1/2 hours field training each day, six days a week for six weeks. At present there are 61 peer educators, who are the backbones of this intervention programme. House to house visit is the major communication strategy adopted in Sonagachi. Peer educators are divided in 12 groups. Seven of these groups are headed by one field supervisor - a social worker. Each group visits seven to eight brothels daily communicating with around 40-45 sex-workers and 5-6 "madams" (employees of the CSWs). They discuss different issues related to STD and AIDS, educate them regarding condom use with the help of flip charts and with other IEC materials and provide condoms according to the need and demand of the sex workers. They revisit the same brothel after a gap of six or seven days, assess the extent of condom use, collect information about non-compliance and complaints about quality of condoms.

Progress to date: At the start of this intervention programme, only 2,500 condoms were distributed throughout the month of September 1992. At present, roughly 62,000 condoms are being distributed to the CSWs every month, and it satisfies only 80 per cent of their demands. The use of condoms by the clients of the sex workers has been rapidly increasing as has been assessed by sentinel surveillance conducted in the month of May-June 1993 (Figure 42.4). The condom use has increased to 44 per cent compared to only 1 per cent about nine months ago.

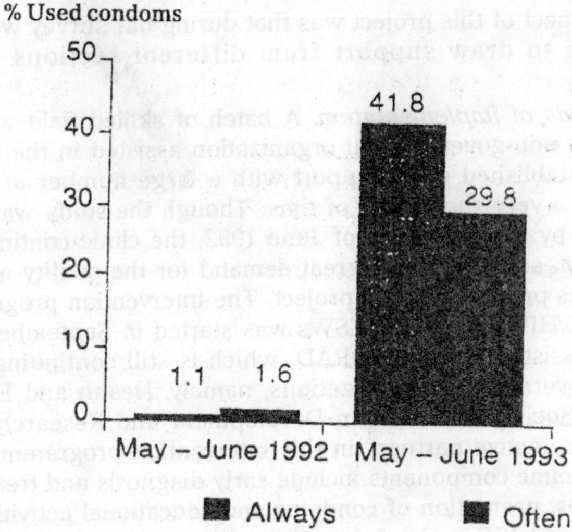

Figure 42.4. Peer education among commercial sex workers, Calcutta

It is true that the results placed above based on clinic attendance is not comparable qualitatively with the results of the community-based study conducted one year previously in the same population. However, it can provide some idea about the progress of activities in the area and it provides definite indication of changes in the sexual behaviour of clients. CSWs are being trained to develop skills to motivate clients on condom use through peer educators and field supervisors.

In the sex market, it is the buyer who dictates the norms and types of services that they would like to buy. So, various agencies involved in the trade need to be involved in the programme so as to motivate the clients to use condoms. At present, the intervention strategies include involvement of pimps, madams and landowners, and youth-club members. The twelve youth clubs of the area have been drawn into the fold of the intervention programme. Many youth-club members are actively involved in these activities. In fact both the clinics (one run in the morning and the other in the evening) are situated in the club premises. The morning clinic caters to 30-35 patients per day and the evening clinic (which is also attended by clients) caters to 15-20 patients per day. Through this clinic, we are providing medicine, counseling services, etc. Treatment is provided for all categories of illnesses. We provide the diagnosis of STD cases with laboratory support and also its management. These three-pronged activities have helped to increase the condom use of the clients and utilization of medical services by CSWs offered through those clinics. The impact of these activities is indicated by the decline in STD rates among the sex workers.

In conclusion, this project demonstrates the effectiveness of peer education in bringing about a behaviour change. *The commercial sex workers not only educate their peers and distribute condoms but provide the support necessary for behaviour modifications to occur.* The project also shows that implementation of such programmes among individuals with high risk behaviour can bring down STD rates and lead remarkably to maintaining HIV infection levels low. *Such programmes are essential and should be adapted for use in other parts of India and elsewhere.*

3.1.3 Targeted AIDS Campaign Among Transvestites in Indonesia

In Indonesia, studies show that upto 39 per cent of transvestites in many provinces are infected with syphilis, compared to less than 8 per cent of the prostitutes. During 1991/1992, HIV and STD serosurveys were carried out in 14 provinces with support from WHO. Results based on 18 194 individuals tested showed the STS (Serologic test for syphilis) positivity rates of 5.8 per cent among registered prostitutes; 7.5 per cent among unregistered prostitutes and 38.9 per cent among transvestites. A similar survey in 26 provinces conducted in 1992/1993, showed STS positivity rates of 7.7 per cent and 41.2 per cent among prostitutes and transvestites respectively.

Transvestites have a variety of occupations including hairdressing, beauty saloon management, entertainment, etc. As a matter of fact, they also engage in prostitution. Based on the above summary results, the Indonesian Public Health Association (IPHA) launched a health education campaign targeted at transvestites in Jakarta. A field study assessment of condom usage and availability among 59 commercial sex workers carried out in Jakarta in May 1992 by a consultant found that the transvestites in Jakarta were more likely to carry and use condoms when participating in penetrative sexual intercourse for payment than female and male CSWs in the city.

By the end of 1993, WHO-sponsored behavioural intervention projects—one in Jakarta to minimize HIV transmission among groups of Waria (transvestites) and the other in Surabaya by Perwakos (The Association of Surabaya Warias) to prevent HIV infection among transvestites had already been launched. These two transvestite projects are developed to be the prototypes of transvestite AIDS campaign, which can be replicated later in many other priority areas in Indonesia.

The objectives of these projects were to: (1) increase HIV/AIDS awareness and risk reduction practices among warias and their sexual partners (in Jakarta and Surabaya), (2) provide pre-test and post-test counselling for H1V seropositive and seronegative transvestites, their family members and partners, (3) provide a confidential HIV testing service, and (4) encourage the active participation of the waria community in preventing H1V transmission. Methods of implementation consist of training of peer group educators, designing and pretesting health education materials, condom promotion, establishing a clinic for Waria and outreach peer health education activities.

> **Results so far.** Under the project, 2,000 warias in Jakarta have already been given health education on HIV/AIDS. Blood samples from 500 warias in Jakarta and 400 warias in Surabaya were tested for H1V antibody, and in July a blood sample from one of the warias in Jakarta was found seropositive for H1V. The H1V seropositive waria was successfully persuaded to stop involving in prostitution and then become an owner of a beauty saloon. The important activities of the project are regular counselling, health services including laboratory examination (free of charge) and persuasion to change high risk behaviour/employment. Condom promotion is carried out through health education and social marketing. Each waria after having health education, including demonstration on how to use condom properly, is given 100 condoms. Whenever they need more condoms they can either buy them from condom sellers or request them from 1PHA. 1PHA has also launched a health education campaign targeted at transvestites.

An independent field assessment of condom usage and availability among 59 commercial sex workers (CSWs) carried out in Jakarta in May 1992 found that the transvestite CSWs in a location in Jakarta were more likely to carry and use condoms when participating in penetrative sexual intercourse for payment than female and male CSWs in the city. Moreover, the repeated observation that none of the transvestite CSWs would agree to unprotected receptive anal intercourse despite being offered twice the asking price (while all the male CSWs agreed to unprotected receptive anal intercourse at their initial asking price) highlights the marked difference in the attitude of these two CSW groups to condom use. There are anecdotal evidence to suggest that the transvestite CSWs were more knowledgeable and accept more readily safe sex practices. Another study showed that *condom use by Surabaya transvestites had increased from less than 5 per cent a year ago to 35 per cent in 1993, thereby demonstrating the effectiveness of the approach used among transvestites in Indonesia.*

3.2 PROMOTING SAFER SEX BEHAVIOUR: INNOVATIVE APPROACHES AMONG YOUTH

3.2.1 Universities Talk AIDS (UTA) in India: An Educational Experiment for Student-Youth

The National Service Scheme (NSS)—a student association for social welfare as part of its commitment to combat AIDS launched a project called "University Talk AIDS" (UTA) in 1991 in selected universities and colleges. The project has been designed and implemented by NSS with technical assistance from the World Health Organization (WHO) and the Ministry of Health and Family Welfare (MoHFW).

The objectives. The key objective of UTA was to raise awareness among university students of AIDS and STD. The project was directed towards creating desirable beliefs and attitudes towards AIDS and STD by providing accurate information on the subject and addressing the misconceptions that exist in the minds of the target audience. UTA's immediate objective is to raise the existing knowledge levels of university students and teachers on AIDS and STD. It was envisaged that the correct knowledge on AIDS and STD would slowly and gradually promote positive attitudes, which would, in turn, in the long run translate into a healthy and positive life-style. Thus, the long-term objective of UTA is to change the behaviour of today's youth.

Methods of implementation. In view of the communication objective of the Ministry of Health and Family Welfare, India, to reach appropriate information on AIDS to all young people in the age group of 15-30 years, the National Service Scheme identified the student community to be the primary target audience for the project. Positive attitudes among this target group could ensure a decelerated trend of students indulging in risk taking behaviour such as sharing of needles and syringes by drug users. The UTA programme is being implemented by the vast NSS network in the country. The key communication agents in the programme are the NSS volunteers. The project planners identified these volunteers to be both key informants and key influencers. They were identified as key informants or key communicators because this vast task force already existed in respective colleges and was engaged in implementing the other activities of NSS. Therefore, it was recognized that if this task force was trained on the subject, they could effectively reach out to the student and teaching community in their colleges.

The campaign was implemented step by step in the following manner:

Step 1: Establishing Project Objectives

The social marketing approach has been used to conceptualise and design the project. The UTA programme planners recognized that the first step was to equip the NSS student volunteers with correct information and knowledge on AIDS. To this end, four regional training workshops were organized in the third week of November 1991. These were organized at New Delhi, Calcutta, Baroda and Madras. All the four training workshops were initiated with focus group discussions. These focus group discussions were conducted by an independent research agency called Social and Rural Research Institute. This is a specialist unit of the Indian Market Research Bureau. The objective of conducting focus group discussions was two fold:

1. The organizers (NSS and WHO) wished to explore attitudes to AIDS, extent of understanding of the subject and attitudes to matters that have a bearing on AIDS such as sexual practices, use of drugs and safe sex; and
2. To provide an opportunity to the participants to recognize their own beliefs, attitudes, inhibitions and misconceptions.

The first objective was crucial because, if the communication was to have any favourable impact, it was important to ensure that the medium itself (in this case the NSS volunteers) was geared to disseminate correct knowledge and attitudes. Ideally, the entire training programme should have been devised on the basis of the feedback received from the group discussions. However, due to constraints of time, it was not possible to delay the training of the initial batch of volunteers. Nevertheless, the inputs of research were utilized for subsequent trainings.

Focus group discussions were extremely useful for the volunteers because they helped them to shed their inhibitions and exposed them to the type of difficulties they would encounter while communicating on the subject. It also triggered a process of evaluating their own perceptions and that of their "peer group". Such sensitization helps to create a favourable atmosphere for programme intervention, by overcoming the resistance of people to change. In the UTA programme, this process helped in sensitizing the participants to the reality of the AIDS threat that was facing India. Thus, in this manner the NSS volunteers could be effectively mobilized to initiate a dialogue with their "peer group" on AIDS and its prevention.

The participatory approach which was adopted during the training workshops also ensured an environment in which the volunteers could unhesitantly seek clarifications for dispelling their own doubts and mis-conceptions on the subject. In order to assess the similarities and differences among NSS volunteers and the non-NSS students who formed the bulk of the target audience, group discussions were also conducted among non-NSS students in all the four centres. This was necessary because it was important to know the frame of mind of the target audience before planning any communication intervention.

Step 2: Development of Campaign Strategy

The first phase of the UTA project focused on the development of the communication campaign strategy for the project. During the regional workshops, not only was information gathered about the knowledge, attitude and practice (KAP) of university students regarding sexuality and AIDS and awareness of HIV/AIDS generated among the communicators, but a series of targeted messages were also identified. On the basis of these messages communication materials were developed and designed for the project.

A unique approach was employed here. The communication materials were developed by the university students themselves. A nation-wide message and materials development contest was organized covering 65 universities across the country. After producing the initial draft of the materials they were pre-tested by the students themselves to ensure the efficacy of the materials. Based on the pre-test, necessary modifications were made to produce the prototypes which were again pre-tested and subsequently modified and refined. These materials were then collected, screened and judged at the state level in 20 states. A state-level ceremony was held at each of these venues to felicitate the winners, exhibit all the entries, involve the press and media to highlight the efforts of the students in the area of AIDS awareness and to generate interest among the general population. The prize-winning entries at the state-level were sent for the regional level competition where the two best entries were selected. A national ceremony was organized at New Delhi, where all the winning entries at the statelevel and the best eight entries (two from each region) were exhibited.

The material development contest was highly successful due to the following reasons:

1. Effective Communication materials were developed by the target group themselves. These materials were tested to ascertain that they actually conveyed what they were designed to convey.
2. The student community, i.e. the beneficiaries of the programme were mobilized and enthused .
3. A socio-anthropological content analysis of the communication materials was undertaken. This provided insights into the students perceptions about AIDS and

helped in identifying their biases and fears. This helped in identifying the existing perception and the desired perceptions.

Thus, the material development contest created a favourable tempo and environment for expanding the project activities. The participatory approach which was followed during the material development contest helped he creating a sense of involvement and "ownership" of the UTA programme. The empathy that was generated made the task of awareness generation and attitude change much simpler. Thus, the target audience was favourably disposed to further project intervention and this ensured a committed target audience.

Step 3: Implementation of Pilot Campaign

In order to sustain the tempo created during the first phase, NSS launched another countrywide mass awareness campaign entitled "AIDS AWARE college campaign". It was a week long campaign, which was launched last year on World AIDS Day. During this week a variety of activities were organized such as blood donation campaign, poster exhibitions, quiz on AIDS, public rallies and discussions, games and street plays. During this, demonstrations on correct use of condoms were also organised. The objectives of organising the World AIDS week were: (1) to assess the existent level of knowledge on AIDS/HIV, (2) to increase the level of awareness on AIDS/HIV, (3) it aimed at increasing the level of commitment of the target audience (University students) towards UTA, and (4) to create centres of consciousness on AIDS, thus providing launching pads for extending the coverage of UTA.

The objectives (3) and (4) were essentially directed at sensitizing and mobilizing students for playing a positive role both as receivers and providers of communication. This signifies the chain reaction where, over a time, the receiver of communication becomes the provider of communication. Thus, the requisite information reaches the entire target community. The UTA programme has various research components woven into it. This helps in both evaluating the performance of the programme and providing effective guidance and direction for the future. Thus, integrated targeted research has helped in ensuring pragmatism in the UTA programme.

Progress to date. During phase II of UTA, a evaluation study was also conducted. A brief questionnaire was given, both prior to and after the World AIDS Week, to the participants, to assess their level of knowledge and attitudes towards AIDS and related issues. This approach also helped in ascertaining the impact of the week-long campaign.

After the World AIDS Week, more than 200 colleges were declared "AIDS AWARE". In the UTA programme, specific criteria had been laid out for declaring a college "AIDS AWARE". In order to meet these criteria the colleges had to organize specific activities, and weightage was also given to the level of participation of its students he each activity.

The above approach ensured that messages were disseminated to the concerned target audience, through their active participation. It also created an atmosphere, where issues which were only joked about or were discussed in hushed tones could be discussed he the open. The momentum that had been set also helped the target audience to realize that AIDS was not distant. Therefore, it was in their own self-interest to know about AIDS and methods of its prevention. Moreover, the strategy of declaring colleges as being "AIDS AWARE" also helped generating a "sense of pride" and "ownership" of the programme among its students all of which went a long way in ensuring a more lasting impact of the communication intervention.

The first two phases of UTA covered around 250 colleges across 65 universities in the country. The target of covering 100 universities by 1994 and all the universities and higher secondary schools by 1995 has been set.

3.2.2 AIDS/STD Education in Schools in Mongolia

The reporting of the first HIV infected case in the country in 1992 provided an impetus for AIDS/STD education ha schools. In the absence of a cure for AIDS or a vaccine against HIV infection and in view of the increasing rates of STD among youth, education is recognized to be critical in prevention and reducing the transmission of both AIDS and STD in Mongolia. *Since considerable proportion of young people can easily be reached through schools, colleges and universities and may learn in the classroom the facts, values and skills they need to protect themselves from HIV infection, the Government, by issuing in 1992, decree No.18 entrusted the Ministry of Science and Education (MSE) and the Ministry of Health (MoH) with the task of integrating AIDS education within existing curricula in schools and postgraduate institutions at all levels.*

Objectives. The objectives of AIDS/STD education in schools are to impart appropriate knowledge, skills and attitudes to young people in order to form a basis for safe sexual behaviour that would permit them to protect themselves and others from infection before they have their first sexual experience, permit effective communication, responsible decision-making and the development of healthy human relationships.

Progress in promoting AIDS/STD education in schools. As part of the ongoing education reform programme, a new curriculum for the ten-year secondary education course has been developed by the Institute of Curriculum and Methodology under the National Pedagogical University and issued in 1991 by the then Ministry of Education. In 1992 the Ministry of Health submitted to the Ministry of Science and Education some proposals on a broad health education programme, including modules on HIV/AIDS/STD in the curricula of formal and non-formal (adults) education.

Keeping in mind the WHO guidelines, attention is paid in Mongolia to AIDS/STD education in schools by:

(1) developing a good curricula with substantial classroom time and environment for social and behavioural skills development,
(2) training teachers and preparation of guidelines and manuals,
(3) preparation and making available for children and students educational printed and audio-visual materials and textbooks,
(4) using all forms of education (mass or in target groups, formal or non-formal, use participatory or didactic methods, curricular or extra-curricular like role plays, etc.),
(5) creating an awareness on how AIDS is easily acquired, and the relevance of social, cultural, and behavioural contexts in the country,
(6) involving parents,
(7) monitoring and evaluating AIDS education, and
(8) ensuring that the subject can be taught.

Because of the new and sensitive nature of AIDS issues and their association with sexual behaviour, questions like what (content), how (styles), when (in what age) should be taught in schools with regard to AIDS/STD and who is to do it need a careful approach. The Ministry of Science and Education has decided to incorporate within the subjects "biology" and "physical education and health", the following modules in the existing (partly renewed) curriculum of secondary schools:

1. 4th grade (11-12 years of age): danger of HIV infection and AIDS to humankind
2. 8th grade (15-16 years of age): HIV/AIDS, STD, routes of transmission, role of immunity, ways of protection from HIV/AIDS/STD, anatomy and physiology of sexual organs
3. 8-10th grades (16-18 years of age): human relationships,

sexuality, healthy sexual behaviour, HIV/AIDS/STD and their prevention.

In October 1993, a one-day seminar was held for school teachers in charge of teaching "biology" and "physical education and health" in the capital city's secondary schools with the aim of providing information on global and country HIV/AIDS/STD situation and guidelines based on WHO recommendations in developing a curriculum for AIDS/STD education at the school level. In aimaks (provinces) and other cities, epidemiologists in charge of HIV/AIDS problems are assisting in developing and adapting modules on AIDS/STD education at local school level. Activities facilitating AIDS education in schools, such as preparation, printing and distribution of guidelines and manuals for school teachers, textbooks for children, conducting national workshops to train trainers of school teachers who will be responsible for AIDS education, have been included in the 1994 draft working plan for implementation of MTPII for AIDS Prevention and Care in Mongolia. These activities will be implemented by the Ministry of Science and Education in co-operation with the Ministry of Health keeping in mind WHO recommendations.

With regard to AIDS education at postgraduate institutions, lectures on the subject are being regularly given to students in order to sensitize and create awareness among them about HIV/AIDS/STD. Modules on etiology, pathogenesis, clhlical features, and consequences of HIV/AIDS have been aded newly to curricula of the National Medical University, National University and Pedagogic University. In some universities and colleges, some student organizations have started to deal with AIDS through condom promotion and promotion of safer sex behaviour.

3.3 CONDOM PROGRAMMING

3.3.1 Condom Social Marketing—a Major Priority

Social marketing is marketing through existing commercial outlets, a consumer good that fulfils a public health or a social need. It is subsidized by donors and/or governments to keep retail costs down and to increase access to the product by low income target audiences. Condom Social Marketing (CSM) is an approach that has been used in many developing countries to promote and distribute condoms for family planning, and for *STD/AIDS* prevention.

In South-East Asia, 396 million condoms were distributed in 1992 through CSM in 6 countries (Bangladesh, India, Indonesia, Nepal, Sri Lanka and Thailand), with India and Bangladesh contributing 67 per cent and 30 per cent respectively.

How Does Condom Social Marketing Work?

CSM is powerful because:

(1) people are more likely to use a condom purchased, even at low, subsidized prices rather than one that is given away free of charge by the government;

(2) it utilizes an existing distribution infrastructure of private retailers such as pharmacies, drug stores, food stores, hotels, and non-traditional outlets such as street vendors, bars, bazaars, barber shops, taxis, gasoline stations, vending machines and other;

(3) campaigns draw upon a wide range of communication techniques, including:

   (a) mass media advertising;

   (b) traditional media such as street theatre troupes and folk bands, especially in rural areas;

   (c) information, education and communication materials including comic books, leaflets, flyers, posters, videos and other;

   (d) face-to-face communication and peer outreach;

   (e) product promotion such as sponsored events, point-of-sale promotional items such as 2-for-the price of l or free samples of condoms; and,

(4) it uses public relations techniques to generate wide support among government and political leaders, the general public and the media.

CSM Increases Competition and Reduces Dependency on Public Sector Support

Marketing and product costs are subsidized so that condoms can be offered to consumers at a price that more people find affordable; while at the same time, some of government and donor costs of providing condoms are defrayed through revenue generated by the increased sale of the products.

There is a convincing evidence that condom social marketing promotional efforts stimulate the entire condom market. This means that other commercial condom marketers tend to increase promotion and advertising and sometimes even lower their prices in response to social marketing programmes. The increased competition enhances condom promotion and helps build a broader and more viable commercial condom market. CSM however tend more to be urban based, its implementation is initially costly, and serving rural areas is an expensive proposition.

In summary, *condom social marketing (CSM) programnle* channels providing broad access to attractive (commercially-developed), affordable (subsidized price) products for low income people at risk. While using private sector marketing techniques, CSMs are not-for-profit, socially-motivated programmes which generate income that can be used to offset the costs of operating the programme.

3.3.3 Condom Social Marketing in Bangladesh: Experiences from Family Planning

In Bangladesh, a country with 110 million people, the CSM programme has been in existence since 1974, funded by USAID and run by the parent organization Population Services International (PSI). CSM is a nonprofit-making concern engaged in providing low cost health and family planning products and services to lower income people. *The CSM has an extensive network reaching remotest parts of the country.* Four brands of condoms are being promoted and sold in the country. However, the public media such as television and radio have been prohibited from promoting condoms, and the words 'sex' and 'condoms' cannot be used in the television or radio broadcasting.

Despite such socio-cultural and religious constraints prohib iting condom promotion, particularly in the public broadcasting media, condom sales since 1983 have increased significantly, both in urban and rural areas; (but particularly more so in urban areas). The 25,000 family welfare centres and personnel of the non-governmental organizations account for nearly 70 per cent of condom distribution in the country.

3.4 STD PREVENTION AND CARE

3.4.1 STD prevention initiatives in Bhutan

Sexually transmitted diseases (STD) are a substantial problem in Bhutan. There has been reports of high prevalence STD he certain areas, and in antenatal clinic attenders the prevalence of STD and Chlamydia have been found to be quite high. Genital ulcers, urethral discharge and vaginal discharges are the most commonly seen STDs. The sluggish healtll-seeking behaviour of the people, especially among women, due to shyness and lack of symptoms, and lack of diagnostic facilities, are some constraints he assessing the actual situation, and contribute to the spread of the diseases. With the initiation of AIDS prevention activities ha 1988-89, STDs have come under the umbrella of AIDS/STD control programme. The programme is fully integrated in the existing health system, and there are no special STD/VD clinics

Strategies. The strategies that were adopted to strengthen the ongoing STD control activities included the establishment of the AIDS/STD control programme office, providing a management structure, and STD awareness activities targeted at the general population as well as special population groups such as students, armed forces and opinion leaders. Awareness campaigns focused on sensitizing about condom use and increasing awareness of how to prevent transmission.

Awareness activities were also intensified in high STD prevalent areas and border towns. In a high STD prevalent area, a mass education campaign was carried out to cover all the people. The campaign covered a gewog (block) with intensive information on STD/AIDS and their prevention. People in a locality were gathered by giving them prior information, and documentary and health education films were screened. This strategy drew a near 100 per cent crowd as films are a powerful media. After the gathering was fully settled and put at ease, slide presentations on STDs followed by condom promotion were carried out. The discussions that ensued clarified many issues and tried to clear the misconceptions people had about STDs. This mass education activity was also utilized to train the health personnel including health in-charge and village health workers in the district to carry out similar activities in their respective blocks. Therefore, the campaign not only aimed at educating the people about STD/AIDS but also trained the health personnel so that they could carry out similar activities in their areas, thus spreading awareness throughout the district.

Standardization of case management. A case management guideline based upon syndromic approach was prepared and distributed to all health facilities. The guidelines emphasize adequate and appropriate treatment, proper follow up and the importance of individual health education on disease transmission and risk reduction.

Training of health care personnel. To prepare the health workers for disease surveillance, management and prevention of STDS, almost all staff of the basic health units and a few hospital-based staff have been trained.

Research. A KABP (knowledge, attitude, behaviour and practice) survey and a Chlamydia prevalence study were conducted. A preliminary study to determine the prevalence of PPNG is under way. Pilot activities are being undertaken to improve the availability of condoms.

In conclusion, initiatives for the prevention of STDs in Bhutan have endeavoured to reduce the transmission of STDs and prevent the morbidity and mortality associated with it by establishing an integrated STD/AIDS control programme, extensive IEC campigns, standardization of management of STDs, development of laboratory capacity for early case detection and quality control, and training of health personnel to improve the quality of care.

Though no studies have been conducted as yet to assess the impact of the initiatives, *it is generally felt that the initiatives have succeeded in increasing the awareness about STDS, increasing the use of condoms, and reducing the incidence of STD in certain areas.* However, there are many constraints in further pursuing the achievements. It will be crucial to overcome these constraints for the success of the prevention initiatives in Bhutan, which include low literacy rate, lack of manpower resources, and lack of financial resources.

3.4.2 STD Control Activities in India

In India, a country with the second largest population after China, STD problem in the past has not been taken up as earnestly as it should have been. Precise information on the magnitude of STD as a public health problem is not available. It is however estimated that only 5 per cent-10 per cent of STD cases in the country take treatment from government STD clinics. No information is available with respect to the remainder of the STD patients who may be taking treatment outside government clinics.

In the first half of 1992, a number of STD baseline surveys were conducted in Jaipur, Madras, a rural area in Tamil Nadu, and in a red light area in Calcutta. In Jaipur 519 males were selected from transport and industrial workers, and 250 patients attending ante-natal clinics (ANC) for inclusion in the survey. On clinical examination 2.1 per cent of the males suffered from urethral discharge, while 0.8 per cent had a genital ulcer. Of the ANC attenders 58 per cent had a vaginal discharge, 27 per cent complained of lower abdominal pain, and 18.4 per cent complained of dysuria.

In Madras and Tamil Nadu study VDRL positivity ranged from 0.8 per cent among the industrial workers to 10 per cent in female remand prisoners, with relatively high rates in ANC attenders (1.74 per cent) and the rural population (3.3 per cent in females and 3.6 per cent ha males). The STD baseline study in a red light area in Calcutta was the first population based STD survey among sex workers, based on a cluster sampling technique. Not surprisngly, the study showed that only 25 per cent of the sex workers did not have any STD; 52 per cent suffered from a shlgle infection, while 23 per cent had two or more infections. A repeat survey was conducted in 1993-94, 12 monthes after a comprehensive intervention project had been initiated. The initial analysis of the results of the repeat survey showed that the prevalence had declined for gonorrhoea by 66 per cent, from 13.2 per cent to 4.4 per cent, for trichomoniasis by 31 per cent, from 11. 1 per cent to 2.5 per cent, while the VDRL positivity declined by 20 per cent. The HIV prevalence increased by only 53 per cent, from 1.3 per cent to 1.6 per cent. Antenatal-clinic attenders are in principle screened for syphilis. The prevalence of positive syphilis serology ranges from 1.2 per cent to 4.8 per cent in various groups of ANC attenders.

The policy adopted by the Technical Advisory Sub-Committee on STD for the control and prevention of STD, emphasizes the syndromic approach for the management of STD patients. A training module for "STD case management for first level doctors" is currently being developed. This module will form the basis for the training of first level doctors, in both the public and the private sector for STD case management. It is envisioned that the specialized STD clinics will play an important role in providing services for referral, training and supervision, and research. Monitoring of antibiotic susceptibility and the efficacy of the syndromic approach will also be done through these centres.

The existing guidelines for diagnosis, treatment and laboratory diagnosis of STD patients have been reviewed and "Simplified STD Treatment Guidelines" have been published. These provide treatment guidelines for syndromic management of STD patients. *In recognition of the fact that women have little access to non-stigmatizing services for STD care, an attempt is made to incorporate STD prevention and control in the existing family welfare services, as part of the reproductive health services.* A number of pilot projects are under development, to assess the feasibility, the cost and the outcome of such an integrated service.

One of the main strategies of the National Plan for the Prevention and Control of AIDS in India is the prevention and control of STD. Planning of STD control activities is a responsibility of the state AIDS officers, or where applicable the state STD officers. Plans have been received from a number of states, although not in all cases do these plans prioritize sufficiently for identified high-risk behaviour groups. A number of STD planning workshops have been organized, and further training will take place during the programme managers' training, which is planned for the second half of 1994. Technical assistance for the planning of state and municipal level STD control activities is provided from the centre, as is regular supervision. A management information system for the AIDS programme is currently under development. This includes a number of key indicators to monitor the implementation of the STD control component. An STD surveillance system is also being developed, with a first draft of an STD surveillance/protocol currently being reviewed.

3.5 BLOOD SAFETY

3.5.1 Blood Transfusion Services in Sri Lanka

In Sri Lanka, blood safety is one of the major activities in prevention and control of HIV/AIDS. All blood donations are screened for HIV, prior to transfusion. The blood safety is the responsibility of the National Blood Transfusion Services and the Central Laboratory for STD/AIDS control which come under the Ministry of Health.

Blood is declared as a drug in some parts of the Region, hence it must be carefully managed. Among important activities is provision of safe blood transmission. There must be a correct assessment of the demand and mobilization of the voluntary agencies for collecting blood through voluntary blood donation camps. Blood transfusion must be kept as a last resort and blood should be transfused only if it is a must to save life. Testing of pooled sera assists in cost-saving in Sri Lanka because HIV prevalence is still very low.

3.5.2 Rational Use of Blood in Nepal

Nepal Red Cross Society is responsible for providing the entire quantity of blood required for use by various hospitals and institutions in the country. The blood donation is a part and parcel of the activities included in the HIV/AIDS control programme and the blood donation is on a non remunerative basis. Prior to 1992, facilities for screening of blood were poor; after 1992, the programme embarked on a plan to go for universal screening of donated blood. Some of the policies and strategies which were formulated by the Kingdom of Nepal include:

1. Blood will be collected *only on* non-remunerative basis;
2. all collected blood meant for transfusion will be screened for HIV and VDRL;
3. Rational use of blood will be advocated and promoted throughout the Kingdom.

The government has started a targeted programme of regular training for medical personnel with regard to safe blood services through rational and judicious blood transfusions. These measures are expected to improve tremendously the blood safety situation in Nepal.

4. HIV/AIDS CARE

4.1 Development of Community and Home-Based Care for People with HIV/AIDS in Thailand

The concept of providing effective and humane care to people with HIV/AIDS must extend beyond the provision of acute, in-patient hospital care. Appropriate medical and social support services need to extend and include the community and families of people with AIDS. The characteristics of various difficulties and problems affecting AIDS patients might be divided into two types:

Underlying Structural Problems. The beginning of the AIDS epidemic is that of the silent HIV epidemic. The three modes of HIV infection may not be known equally well among all members of society, and certain groups may, by their very social status, be placed at greater risk of acquiring HIV infection. These individuals and clusters of groups may include isolated hill tribe villagers, low income urban slum-dwellers, illiterate and poorly educated hldividuals (particularly women), male and female sex workers, as well as injecting drug users. National efforts to reach out and inform all members of society about HIV/AIDS may first reach the higher to middle income groups, with greater access to information, communication and health services. Such underlying structural differences within the population place certain individuals at greater risk of infection. These same differences will also affect the delivering and availability of community care.

Problems associated directly with HIV infection: Persons with HIV will face additional problems, which may be classified into three stages:

1. *Asymptomatic stage:* During the asymptomatic stage, a person with HIV may face no new particular problem. However, should his or her HIV status become known to others, very real problems can soon develop. Healthy people with HIV may be tested without voluntary consent in many circumstances. In some countries, patients attending STD clinics as well as sex workers may be required to undergo mandatory testing. In other countries, medical staff may routinely test all patients. As a result of such testing, people with HIV may experience considerable fear and anxiety. These fears may include the fear of dying, social discrimination, loss of employment and rejection by friends and family.
2. *Symptomatic stage.* As HIV infection progresses to AIDS disease, individuals find it increasingly difficult to continue with daily-life activities. A person may no longer be able to work, and entire families may be placed into

economic crisis. Physical strength disappears and leaves individuals dependent on other care givers.

3. *Terminal stage.* At the final stage before death, PWAs require even more spiritual support and compassion. If they have children, they may also want someone to take care of their children.

The problems that PWAs face are complex and tend to become more severe as time passes. In order to provide care for AIDS patients and family, the services must be comprehensive and integrated at every level from household to community to institutional.

The care should include:

1. *Medical and nursing services:* in-patient and outpatient care, home nursing, hospice care, etc.
2. *Psychosocial support:* counselling, information and education, establishment of self-help groups, etc.
3. *Practical support:* social welfare services, housing, meals, transportation, recreation, child care, etc.
4. *Legal, ethical services:* protection of human rights, health and life insurance, access to medical care, etc.

The care should be continuously provided. At household and community levels, community based and home-based care should be provided.

Activities so far. To achieve the objective of establishing community-based and home-based care of AIDS patients he Thailand, efforts were made to compile ideas from experts in the area of community-based and home-based care among governmental and non-governmental agencies in early 1992. The idea was then translated into two projects. One was to develop a network of social services which will co-ordinate support for AIDS patients, and the second was to develop models of community-based and home-based care for AIDS patients in northern Thailand, where the epidemic is more advanced.

The first project which started in late 1992 for a six-month duration, emphasized the development and strengthning of networks among various social service agencies (public welfare offices, counselling clinics and the social welfare section in hospitals) in twelve selected provinces. Participating social workers realized the importance and need for providing care and social support to people with HIV and AIDS. It is shown that the project could provide services for 3,107 people with HIV/AIDS (3,670 service-episodes) during the study period. Among all episodes, 2,502 (68.2 per cent) were counselling, 1,050 (28.6 per cent) were financial support, and the rest were referral service and others. However, there is a need to train more social workers to increase understanding of the concept of confidentiality and counselling, as well as ways of assessing the problems of clients and home-visit techniques. One of the recommendations from this project was to allocate financial assistance for people with HIV and AIDS.

The second project focuses on the development of a manual on home-based care for AIDS patients. A workshop was conducted for representatives of 25 organizations (government and non-governmental) from the northern provinces. All participating agencies were requested to conduct a community-based and home-based care project in their local area. The project is going on. The feasibility will assessed and the lessons learned from each project will be studied at the end of this year. The home-based care manual will be evaluated. Training in and implementation of, community-based and home-based care will be expanded to cover more areas next year.

Other activities that will enable the possibilities of community-based and home-based care is to support non-governmental organizations working in the area of care. Since the beginning of the AIDS prevention and control programme, the Ministry of Public Heath (MOPH) has supported many non-governmental organizations working with AIDS patients, both technically and financially. Most non-governmental organizations provide comprehensive care in collaboration with other government and non-governmental organizations. The MoPH is also interested in setting up rehabilitation centres for AIDS patients who need basic physical and psychological support before returning back to the community. These rehabilitation centres will also serve as training sites for AIDS patients and their families. The first centre is expected to open early next year. Seven more centres throughout the country are planned to be opened during 1994-1995.

Obstacles. The major obstacle is the attitude of the public towards AIDS patients. There is still irrational fear of HIV/AIDS. Some groups of people do not understand and do not want to accept people with HIV/AIDS to live within the same community. The community-based and home-based care programme should also look into ways of changing the public attitude from fear, stigma and ignorance to acceptance, compassion and support for AIDS patients and their families. In this respect, educational messages now need to focus more on how to live with HIV/AIDS in society.

In conclusion, as the epidemic becomes more evident, *Thailand is beginning to develop strategies for communities to live with HI V and AIDS by integrating community-based and home-based care into the existing primary health care network.* It is important to acknowledge that community care requires an integrated joint effort by all concerned institutes, organizations and people. *In order to develop successful programmes to support people with HIV/*

AIDS, stigma and fear about HIV and AIDS must be overcome.

4.2 Development of Counselling Services in Myanmar

Myanmar's experiences of counselling services at the beginning have been very limited. Very few competent counsellors were available to provide the counselling service, and these were available only to the urban population, none of the non-governmental organizations worked in this area, and services were available largely in specialized service hospitals. However, since HIV/AIDS is now appearing in urban as well as rural areas, hospitals in both urban and rural areas have to provide the counselling services. The objectives of the counselling service in Myanmar are to:

1. provide psycho-social support for people who are infected with HIV:
2. provide information regarding the danger of high-risk behaviours in order to prevent them from becoming infected with HIV and to prevent transmission from them to the community.

The strategy for the development of counselling services in Myanmar included training of health workers especially in the areas where HIV/AIDS patients would most likely come for care; inclusion of counselling in the training courses of basic health workers so that they understand the importance of counselling. They can also, where possible, refer cases to a well-equipped hospital where specialists' services are available. The Government of Myanmar during 1992-1993 took the following steps in the development of counselling services:

(1) establishment of a counselling team and the AIDS prevention and control programme. The team conducts trahaing courses for people to become counsellors, and to monitor services provided to cases which were referred to the nearby referral centre;

(2) with financial assistance from WHO, several training courses for counsellors were conducted from September 1992 and during 1993; as well as an advance course for conllsellors who had undergone the counsellor's training previously;

(3) arrangements were made for counsellors to attend the monthly meetings to share their experiences and also get technical support from the experts;

(4) The Government issued directions to the department of health and superintendents of major hospitals to provide necessary support for counsellors to carry out their work.

In spite of these steps which the National AIDS programme

in Myanmar took for developing counselling activities, there still remain several constraints which need to be overcome. These include lack of money for conducting training courses, difficulty in selecting health workers who have the right attitude to undertake counselling, inadequate monitoring of the work being performed by the counsellors in the remote peripheral areas; and difficulties in distributing the health education material to counsellors in the rural areas.

5.PROGRAMME MANAGEMENT AND CO-ORDINATION

5.1 Multi-Sectoral Collaboration and Co-ordination:

Thailand's National AIDS Programme

As our understanding and knowledge has grown over the last decade in terms of the scope and impact of the HIV/AIDS pandemic, it is clear that the response to the epidemic transcends the responsibility of the health sector, thus requiring a multi-sectoral response. In recognition of this, Government of Thailand has taken decisive steps to encourage and enhance participation by various sectors and groups involved in AIDS work.

Collaboration among and co-ordination between various sectors and participating parties poses a great challenge for the country to facilitate involvement by all concerned parties in a way that will improve the overall national response to the AIDS epidemic as well as in making the most effective and efficient use of limited resources available to an ever-increasing number and wide-range of organizations becoming involved. The parties involved that are increasingly playing a more active role in AIDS efforts in Thailand include government ministries and offices, private sector, non-governmental organizations and multilateral and bilateral agencies (see Table 42.4).

Collaboration among various sectors and groups occurs through both formal and informal co-ordination mechanisms, which have been established and adapted to meet the rapidly changing nature of the AIDS situation in Thailand.

Formal-Co-ordination Mechanism and Structure. At central level, the National AIDS Committee (NAC) chaired by the Prime Minister with the Ministry of Public Health (MOPH) as the secretariat, serves as the national policy and broad co-ordination body of Thailand's National AIDS Programme. Included as members of the National AIDS Committee are representatives from all government ministries, special public agencies, non-governmental organizations, private sector and eminent experts. Sub-committees to consider various technical issues with regards to AIDS are appointed as appropriate and revised from time to time. AIDS policies are approved by the Cabinet and endorsed by the Parliament. These policies have been articulated within the Seventh Five-Year National Social and Economic Development Plan of the country and have been expounded in a Five-Year National AIDS Plan (1992-1996), providing the framework and guidelines within which HIV/AIDS activities are planned and implemented. The National AIDS Plan serves as an important co-ordination tool.

Each ministry has developed implementation plans for AIDS prevention and control activities consistent with the National AIDS Plan. In addition, each ministry has established an AIDS committee and assigned focal persons for co-ordination.

The provincial structure of the Ministry of Public Flealth and the Ministry of Interior plays a very important role he country-wide co-ordination. AIDS committees have been set-up at provincial and district levels, witil representation from local ministries, government and health offices and in some cases non-governmental organizations. They are responsible for developing AIDS implementation plans. STD/AIDS centres and clinics have been established at provincial and district levels and serve as co-ordination nodes for activities. At the primary health care level, village volunteers are active in disseminating AIDS information.

Thailand is currently in the early stages of a multi-sectoral planning exercise to revise the present Five-Year National AIDS Plan in order to develop further the implementation plan for 1995-1996, addressing the rapidly changing circumstances. In August 1993, all ministries, various government offices, non-governmental organizations, United Nations agencies and the private sector participated in a National Formulation Workshop of the implementation Plan for 1995-1996,organized by the National Economic and Social Development Board. This was a brainstorming exercise for various actors to contribute to an open participatory process by expressing views and experiences and to suggest revisions and additions to the current plan for consideration by a multi-sectoral working group. These inputs are being compiled and formulated into a policy framework which will include guidelines and measures to implement strategies. This plan will be endorsed by the National AIDS Committee and the Cabinet. A revised plan is expected by the end of the year in time to mobilize resources for the remaining two years of the Plan. Every ministry as well as non-governmental organizations will be requested to submit their plans/programmes for considerating the budget allocation from the Bureau of the Budget.

Table 42.4.
Role of Agencies in Prevention and Control of AIDS, Thailand

Agencies	Programmes			
	Public Information	Treatment and Care	Human Rights	Research and Evaluation
I Office of the Prime Minister	...	...	...	...
2. Ministry of Public Health	...	...	...	...
3 Ministry of Interior	...	...	...	...
4. Ministry of Education				
5. Ministry of Defense	...	...	...	...
6. Ministry of University Affairs	...		...	...
7. Ministry of Justice	...	...	...	...
8. Ministry of Finance	...	...	...	...
9. Ministry of Industry	...	...	...	...
10. Ministry of Transport and Communications	...	...	...	...
11. Ministy of Commerce	...	...	...	...
12. Ministy of Science and Tech. and Energy	...	...	...	...
13. Ministry of Foreign Affairs	...	...	...	...
14. Minisly of Agriculture and Co-operative	...	...	...	...
15. State Enterprises	...	...	...	...
16. Non-Government Non-Profit Agencies	...	...	...	...
17. Business Sector	...	...	...	...
Total	17	9	17	17

Notes: ... Most Involvement .. Moderate Involvement . Some Involvement

Informal Co-ordination Mechanism. In addition to the formal co-ordination mechanism and structure that exists, there are a number of informal processes going on which include a non-governmental consortium against AIDS in Bangkok, a northern Thailand non-governmental consortium, donors and United Nations agencies which all meet once a month, on a voluntary basis to be briefed and up-dated on the national AIDS policies, plans and situation in Thailand. These forums serve as an informal channel for groups to co-ordinate, share and exchange information on activities and resources. In addition, there is inter-communication and intra-communication, often through individual contacts with government, between ministries, non-governmental organizations, donors and United Nations agencies.

In the private sector, there is currently co-operation between businesses involved in the sex industry, the Ministry of Interior and the Ministry of Public Health in implementing the programme on 100 per cent - condom use policy. A more recent initiative is the Thailand Business Coalition on AIDS which was launched in September 1993 to educate and disseminate information about AIDS and to encourage businesses to adopt AIDS in the workplace policies for their staff.

Lessons Learnt. Strong political commitment by the Government is needed in order to mobilize all sectors to prevent and control HIV/AIDS. Substantial financial resources need to be set aside by the Government each year to sustain the momentum of efforts being carried out by public and private, non-governmental organizations as well as international agencies. Inter-collaboration and intra-collaboration/co-ordination among sectors and groups need to be strengthened and expanded.

The National AIDS Plan should be articulated within the framework of the National Economic and Social Development Plan. It provides the framework for long-term country-level co-ordination. The National AIDS Plan should be open for revisions and adjustments to address rapidly changing circumstances. As the epidemic expands, the plan leas naturally become broader and more inclusive of a diversity of groups which are playing increasingly active roles in AIDS prevention and control efforts in Thailand.

Financial contribution from multilateral and bilateral agencies to the National AIDS Programme tend to focus on their own priorities and interests. This may result in an unequal distribution of the assistance in certain geographical and programme areas. Financial commitments by multilateral and bilateral agencies are often of one-year duration creating short-term unsustainable activities for what is a long-term problem.

The Government of Thailand has made it a national policy to support the work of nongovernmental organizations by ensuring that a certain allocation of the national AIDS budget is made available to non-governmental organizations.

In conclusion, there are no blueprints for multi-sectoral coordination of the vast number of participating parties involved in AIDS efforts in Thailand. The country has recently embarked on a multi-sectoral planning process in order to formulate a revised National AIDS Plan for 1995-96, the fruits of which remain to be seen yet. however, experience has shown that in order to ensure maximum participation and co-operation by all groups, co-ordination must be done carefully and sensitively, and should be flexible and open to different views expressed by the various groups involved in the participatory planning processes.

5.2 National AIDS Programme Management: A Training Course

In order to enhance programme management at the national level, WHO has developed a training course which, like EPI, CDD and few other programmes. consists of modules. Each module addresses a major aspect of AIDS-programme development and contains exercises for the participant to practise what is leant. The titles of the 12 modules are:

1. Introduction
2. HIV/AIDS Problem, Control Activities and Target Populatioins for Preventicn
3. Interventions and Policies
4. Programme Prevention Priorities and Targets
5. Promoting Safer Sexual Behaviours
6. Condom Procurement and Distribution
7. Provision of STD Care
8. Prevention of HIV Transmission through Blood
9. Prevention of HIV Transmission through Injecting Drug Use
10. HIV/AIDS Care and Social Support
11. The National Plan
12. Monitoring and Evaluation.

On completion of this course, participants are expected to be able to plan, manage and evaluate a comprehensive national AIDS programme more effectively and efficiently. The Global Programme on AIDS has a supply of training modules for inter-country training. SEARO will be supporting such courses in 1994-1995. If countries are interested in conducting training they should approach the WHO Regional Office. WHO can supply sets of the modules and offer the assistance of trained facilitators/course directors at no cost to the country.

5.3 Evaluation of National Programmes and Prevention Indicators

Over the past decade, pressure for speedy and visible action against AIDS has often led national AIDS programmes to neglect evaluation. While evaluation may appear to be a luxury at first sight, it soon becomes clear that it provides a crucial resource for planning and implementing successful programme activities. Unless plans are made early enough for evaluation, programmes run the risk of facing unfulfilled expectations, frustration and disillusionment for lack of feedback on the effects of the hard work already carried out. Carefully conducted periodic surveys provide reliable information for long-term trends to determine the progress and future direction of the programme.

An evaluation package has been developed by WHO for use by national AIDS programmes. The package is designed in the form of a loose-leaf notebook in orer to allow for individual use and update of each section as needed. National AIDS programmes are assessed in a number of ways: first, through reviews of their implementation. Programme reviews provide a broad assessment of the national AIDS progrmme particularly of its management capacity. Second, to complement information provided by national programme reviews, a set of indicators describing the progress of activities has been developed in order to strengthen the capacity of AIDS programmes to conduct their own evaluation. The periodic assessment of these indicators is expected to yield information on the achievement of national targets. The information collected through the various instruments in the "methods package" will assist managers of national AIDS programmes in planning and reprogramming effective interventions.

Table 42.5. Methods for the Measurement of PIs

Methods	Population Survey/ Outlet visit	Health Facility Survey	Records	Sero-survey
PI 1. Knowledge of preventive practices	x			
PI 2. Condom availability (central level)			x	
PI3. Condom availability (peripheral level)	x			
PI 4. Reported non-regular sexual partners	x			
PI 5. Reported condom use with non-regular sex partner	x			
PI 6. & PI 7. STD case management		x		
PI 8. STD prevalence, women				x
PI 9. Reported STD incidence, men	x			
PI 10. HIV prevalence, women				x

A core set of indicators in the areas of prevention, care and support and reduction of socio-economic impact are needed to measure the progress of national AIDS programmes. As a first step, ten prevention indicators have been selected for their usefulness in monitoring the overall progress of the programme, their potential usefulness in the design of interventions and their relative ease of measurement. The areas covered by the prevention indicators are: knowledge of preventive practices, sexual behaviour, case management of STD, condom availability and use, and STD/HIV prevalence. The prevention indicators and their methods of data collection are shown in the list of prevention indicators in the table 42.5.

5.4 Budget and Financial Guidelines: Do's and Don'ts

Funds for AIDS programme activities are received from headquarters in instalments. Therefore, allotments actually received should be the guiding factor in implementation. WR's office while establishing obligations locally or sending request to the Regional Office (e.g. supplies and equipment etc.), should study the reports sent every month to ascertain whether adequate funds are available in the allotment concerned. If it is an approved activity *and* funds are available in the relevant allotment, it can be implemented locally or through the Regional Office (e.g. supplies and equipment). For the sake of convenience, funds are alloted by WHO Headquarters in BL 834—'All Local Costs'. However, the implementation should be done as per the workplan, and the funds can be reprogrammed by GPA/SEARO. Each activity or a group of related activities falling under one allotment should be assigned a separate sticker.

In the AFI system one sticker can be obligated under one allotment only. Obligation document quoting two allotments are received but with one sticker. Correct allotment reference should be mentioned on the transmittal letters. In many cases, the allotment reference given is GPA 001. In case of UNDP funded projects even the sublines should be mentioned. The amount obligated for programme support cost is not available for use. The Allotment Report (ACE 055) and the Obligation Report (ACE 026) being sent every month should be reviewed regularly. Timely review of unliquidated obligations would release funds for other activities. Feedback from countries is very important.

GPA Country Allotment Structure 1994-1995—vis-a-vis 1992-1993 (Comparison)

1. Allotment '200' (i.e., Staff Cost) and '290' (i.e. Liquida-

tion of previous year's obligations) will continue as in 1992-1993.

2. Instead of the present four allotments per country, i.e.

   210—Programme Management

   220—Health Education

   230—Surveillance and Control

   240—Laboratory Support

There will be only one allotment i.e., '250' with six categories in it.

1. All activities in the workplan are to be given an ARC (Activity Reference Code). Similarly, all obligations (except those under allotments '200' and '290' series) whether under DP, FX or RB funds will also have to be coded. Any clarification in identifying the appropriate Activity Reference Code can be obtained from TL/GPA's office/SEARO.
2. Existing flexibility provisions are being reviewed by WHO Headquarters and will be comunicated later.

GUIDELINES ON FINANCIAL MATTERS

1. Overall WHO/GPA Funds Controlled At HQ
2. IPF and Workplands for each country
3. Allotments
   - Receipt from WHO HQ
   - Availability of funds under different lines/components
   - Inter-line Transfers and Flexibility
   - SEARO
   - WHO HQ
4. Level of authority from implementation
   - Country Level
   - LCS/834
   - CSA
   - Short-term general service staff
   - Supplies and equipment (With delegation of authority)
   - Regional office
   - Supplies and Equipment
   - Short-term Consultant
   - Long-term staff
   - Group educational activities Etc.
5. Obligation
   - Government request
   - Conforming to workplan
   - Details of activity, budgetary breakdown and schedule of

payment

— Approval by the WR

— Approval by technical unit if not included in the approved workplan

6. Sticker

Obligations (One sticker per activity) Transmittal every week

(BFO's memo sea/bud/92/015 dated 30 January 1992 to WRs refers)

7. Payment for LCS

As per schedule or up to use 50,000. (Advance over this amount to be approved by regional office)

Sticker number and allotment to be quoted on the voucher cheque should not be in the name of an individual.

8. Submission of reports/accounts

No further advance under LCS should be approved for same activity if accounts for previous advance have not been submitted.

HOW TO IMPLEMENT LOCAL COST SUBSIDY?

LOCAL COST SUBSIDY

IF INCLUDED IN THE WORK PLAN (A)	IF NOT INCLUDED IN THE WORK PLAN (B)
	1. WR should request GPA/SEARO for technical approval 2. Should also indicate the activities which will be replaced to make funds avail able. 3. The procedure stated as in case (A) to be followed.

ACTIVITIES

WITHIN DELEGATION OF AUTHORITY NOT WITHIN DELEGATION OF AUTHORITY

If required funds are available in budget-line	Request GPA/SEARO for technical the approval/release of funds. Obligation to be established on Approval from technical unit
Obligations can be established locally, sticker assigned and funds released.	If Required funds are not available in the budget-line but are available in the Allotment. Suggest interline transfer while obligating documents if a part of the IPF remains to be received from HQ obligation can be established. Copies of allot. Notif. are sent to wR and monthly reports sent by bfo also indicate the sta tus of allotment received from HQ.

STICKER DOCUMENTS TO BE SENT TO BFO/SEARO ON WEEKLY BASIS THROUGH THE TRANSMISSION OF OBLIGATIONS

OTHER POINTS

I. Each obligation document/activity (Request for LCS) should be assigned a separate sticker. One sticker can be obligated under one allotment only.
2. The sticker and the allotment should be clearly stated on the obligation document/ Transmittal letter. In case of UNDP funded projects, even the sublines should be mentioned.
3. Obligations should be established and funds released closer to the dates of activity as per the time frame in the approved work plan.
4. Flexibility limits- 100 per cent within the allotment 20 per cent between allotments. 1994-95- Existing flexibility Y provisions are being reviewed by WHO HQ and will be communicated later.
5. Savings under "290" are not available for use.
6. Reports sent by BFO every month to the WRs should be reviewed carefully and observations thereon should be communicated to BFO promptly.
7. Any increase in allocation/budget for a country. Request should be sent to TL/GPA/ SERVO WHO will in turn take it up with GPA/HQ. Only on receipt of allotment notification funds can be obligated/release.
8. Amount obligated for programme support cost (PSC) is not available for use.
9. In 1994- 1995
   (a) The present four allotments per country i.e. 210,220, 230 and 240 will be replaced by one single allotment i.e., "250".
   (b) All activities in the workplan and all obligations (Except those under allotments "200" and "290" series) whether under DP. FX or RB Funds to be assigned an activity reference code (ARC).

6. CONSENSUS STATEMENT AND RECOMMENDATIONS

The assembled National AIDS Programme Managers, expressing grave concern regarding the continuing rapid progress of the HIV/AIDS epidemic in the Region, reaffirmed their commitment to the important goals of HIV/AIDS/STD prevention and control and reiterated the need to strengthen programme management, strengthen evaluation and monitoring mechanisms and using surveillance as an indicator for the progression of the epidemic. After reviewing the status of activities in each country and exchanging international, regional and national programme advances, the participants proposed the following recommendations for future national and regional action.

HIV/STD PREVENTION

Given the current status of the epidemic in this region, prevention programmes should remain the major focus of national programme activities:

1. Additional efforts need to be made in all countries to develop effective targetted interventions among high risk behaviour groups (injecting drug users, commercial sex workers and their clients, street children, etc.) including information, education, comunications, integrated STD service delivery and condom promotion and provision, utilizing community outreach approaches. Involvement of nongovernmental organizations and the private sector, particularly at the community level, are crucial in these efforts.
2. In the coming year ministries of health's ministries of education and other appropriate ministries should work co-operatively towards the integration of sex/lifeskill education into all levels of education (primary and secondary schools, universities, etc.), either as a part of the curriculum or co-curricular activity or both as appropriate, in collaboration with parent, teacher and student organizations.
3. Concentrated efforts need to be undertaken by the appropriate governmental and non-governmental organizations to develop effective education and intervention programmes targeted at youths out-of-school.
4. Comprehensive STD services, based upon the syndromic approach and including provision of effective, where possible, single-dose treatment, individual health education and counselling on risk reduction, treatment compliance, partner notification and condom use, and condom provision need to be integrated into existing health services, including primary health care services, MCH/FP clinics and non-governmental organizations/private health care services as a matter of priority.
5. National programmes should ensure that comprehensive condom programming strategies that address demand, supply and support functions are integrated into national prevention efforts, i.e., that plans and activities concerning research, IEC, appropriate distribution systems, logistics and training be co-ordinated to achieve national condom-related prevention goals. Condom social marketing programmes for disease control and family planning need to be developed and supported urgently.

6. Member countries should develop and adopt national policies for blood transfusion services, including voluntary donor recruitment and selection and the rational use of blood and blood products, in order to ensure a safe national blood supply.

CARE AND SOCIAL SUPPORT

(7) Member States should begin to plan for comprehensive programmes on HIV/AIDS care by establishing linkages within the government health and social welfare structures and between government and community based care programmes to ensure a continuum of culturally appropriate care from the hospital to tile holne for those suffering from HIV/AIDS. This should include developing collaboration with traditional health care systems.

8. Member countries should ensure a national policy against any form of mandatory testing (testing without informed consent), while undertaking to make anonymous voluntary testing witil counselling services available to the community.

9. Member countries should be encouraged to examine any legislation or regulations which discriminate stigmatize or infringe on the basic human rights of persons suffering with HIV/AIDS. Special policy guidelines to deal with the care and social support of marginalized populations suffering from HIV/AIDS such as sex workers, injecting drug users should be developed.

PROGRAMME MANAGEMENT AND CO-ORDINATION

10. All Member countries should develop, in an open participatory planning process involving all sectors, a national strategic HIV/AIDS plan as an integral part of the national health plan/development plan.

11. Member countries should ensure sustained political and financial commitment and support to the national AIDS programme through ongoing advocacy with opinion leaders, policy planners, politicians, the private sector and international and bilateral agencies.

12. Effective inter-sectoral and intra-sectoral collaboration should be ensured through the development of effective co-ordination mechanisms involving a broad-based multisectoral representation. This should include the private sector, nongovernmental organizations, religious

organizations and structures, local government structures, and international and bilateral agencies.

13. National AIDS programmes should strength their capacities to plan, implement, monitor and evaluate STD/AIDS programme activities through programme management training, including logistics management and training.

43

HIV/AIDS and STD Surveillance Data Management and Use

(Report of an Intercountry Meeting, Bangkok, 6-9 December 1995)

1. INTRODUCTION

The AIDS pandemic, which was first reported in 1981, has started making an impact in Asia. The region has recently witnessed the most alarming increase in the level of HIV transmission: there has been a three-fold increase in HIV prevalence since the end of 1993. As of mid-1995, 3.5 million people in Asia were estimated to be infected. In Thailand, 22,000 cases of AIDS have been reported so far, of whom more than 80 per cent have been reported since 1993, while India has witnessed an increase of 100 per cent in the number of AIDS cases reported between 1993 and 1994. Some countries still have a low prevalence; however, this situation could change rapidly.

Although the understanding of the virology, immunology and modes of transmission of the disease have increased significantly over the last 15 years, there is still substantial uncertainty about the actual extent and eventual impact of the HIV/AIDS pandemic in many countries of the South-East Asia Region. More complete descriptive data on HIV infection rates and sexual behaviours of people are of immense value in improving understanding of the dynamics and changing patterns of the pandemic. Continued efforts to collect surveillance data and use it to update estimates and projections are needed for mobilizing national response and sustained support against HIV/AIDS within individual countries. Such estimates are useful for advocacy and for planning impact alleviation programmes, including care of and social support for individuals and families affected by HIV/AIDS.

To discuss HIV/AIDS and STD surveillance, data management and use, an intercountry workshop was organized by WHO which was held in Bangkok from 6 to 9 December 1995. The objectives were:

(1) To review the progress in establishing and sustaining HIV/AIDS and STD surveillance systems in the countries of the South-East Asian Region, including the use of computer based information system such as EPI Info, EPI Model and EPI Map;

(2) To exchange experiences on the methods that could be used for making estimations and short-term projections on HIV/AIDS and STD using available data, and

(3) To make recommendation for further strengthening HIV/AIDS and STD surveillance in the countries of the South-East Asia Region.

The workshop, which consisted of plenaries, group work and practical exercises using computers was attended by focal points at country level of communicable disease surveillance programmes and of HIV/AIDS and STD surveillance as well as from WHO.

The participants were welcomed at the opening session by Dr. Jai P. Narain, Team Leader, Global Programme on AIDS, WHO/SEARO. The Regional Director, WHO/SEARO, in a message ready by Dr. M.J. Wysocki, Regional Adviser, Health Statistics, WHO/SEARO, emphasized on WHO technical support to countries, especially in the area of HIV/AIDS epidemiology and surveillance. In 1992, WHO/SEARO had conducted a workshop in Bali, Indonesia, on HIV surveillance which addressed the technical aspects of sentinel surveillance and recommended that all countries must have sentinel surveillance programmes to monitor the trends of the AIDS pandemic. It was now timely that the progress made in this direction was reviewed with a view to identifying areas requiring further strengthening. This workshop will, therefore, not only help in reviewing and improving the functioning of the existing HIV/AIDS programmes but will also provide a forum for participants to use computer based information and data management system, particularly for the purpose of making countryspecific estimations and projections, based on available epidemiological data.

2. AN OVERVIEW OF HIV/AIDS AND STD SURVEILLANCE

Public health surveillance is defined as the systematic collection, analysis and dissemination of data on the occurrence of a disease or condition in order to guide decisions towards its prevention and/or management. With regard to HIV/AIDS, it involves surveillance of HIV infection, of AIDS cases, and of other sexually transmitted diseases.

The main objectives of HIV/AIDS surveillance can be summarized as follows:

— to detect and describe the geographic, demographic and risk-factor distribution of HIV infection;
— to monitor the progression of the HIV/AIDS epidemic;
— to plan prevention activities and health and social services for persons with AIDS and HIV infection;
— to evaluate the impact of specific elements of national AIDS programmes.
— to estimate present and future impact of the pandemic;
— to provide comparative data on the global and regional scope of the epidemic; and
— to increase public and political awareness of the disease.

While AIDS case reporting reflects the transmission of the infection 5-10 years in the past and the current burden of serious HIV-related morbidity, HIV surveillance, i.e., the study of the prevalence of HIV antibody, permits monitoring of the current prevalence of the HIV infection. These two surveillance approaches are complementary and, therefore, indispensable components of the public health surveillance of the epidemic.

AIDS case reports, when complete, can provide information on the demographic and geographic characteristics of the populations affected by the epidemic and on the relative importance of the various exposure risks (important for prevention); they can measure the extent of serious morbidity associated with HIV infection (important for short-term planning of health care at national and local levels). Furthermore, AIDS case reports can be used to calculate earlier HIV infection patterns and tuture short-term projections of AIDS cases. Reporting AIDS cases also raises public awareness of the impact of the epidemic. Finally, international comparisons of AIDS case rate may be possible, provided case definitions and surveillance systems are reasonably compatible.

In the mid-1980s, after an antibody test for HIV became available, seroprevalence studies were undertaken in population groups with varying degrees of risk for HIV infection. At the same time, some countries attempted random surveys of the general population in order to evaluate the current HIV prevalence. It became clear soon after that general population surveys were costly and could give an inaccurate impression of HIV prevalence due to participation and selection bias, and the fact that groups at high risk for HIV infection are not randomly distributed in the general population. HIV serosurveillance in sentinel populations (sentinel HIV surveillance) is now routinely undertaken in most countries of the South-East Asia Region. This is the systematic cross-sectional surveying of the prevalence of HIV antibodies in selected populations which may be repeated at intervals over time. It is recommended by WHO as the principal method of data collection for detecting the presence of HIV infection and its geographic, demographic and temporal distribution and trends over time.

Populations particularly suitable for sentinel HIV serosurveillance are persons attending antenatal and sexually transmitted disease clinics, drug treatment centres, and other groups at high risk of HIV infection who have blood drawn for other purposes (e.g. syphilis serology). Clinic or health facility based sentinel HIV serosurveillance, which allows HIV testing by the unlinked anonymous technique is generally recommended. Unlinked anonymous testing refers to HIV antibody testing, after the removal of all potential identifiers, of sera previously obtained for other purposes. By this approach participation bias can be minimized.

Sentinel HIV serosurveillance does not involve randomized selection of sites, and therefore data from different sentinel sites should generally not be aggregated. While sentinel HIV serosurveillance can be used to monitor the HIV epidemic, it can, to certain extent, also be useful for estimating the present and future impact of HIV, or be used to evaluate the impact of a national AIDS programme.

The meeting concluded that assessment of the epidemic in any country depended on data from all available surveillance sources. Although AIDS case surveillance and HIV serosurveillance were essential elements of national AIDS programmes, additional sources of data, particularly on STDs when available, were extremely important when monitoring the epidemic and directing prevention and control programmes. Although not discussed further in this document, these data sources could include:

- the accumulated statistics on HIV infections resulting from diagnostic evaluation, counselling and testing services, and other public health activities;
- tuberculosis and mortality statistics;
- behavioural studies of risk factors for HIV infection;
- estimations of the sizes of populations at increased risk;
- special studies to determine the prevalence of AIDS or HIV-related illness he hospitals; and
- special studies to measure AIDS-related mortality.

3. ISSUES AND CONCERNS RELATED TO AIDS/HIV AND STD SURVEILLANCE IN SOUTH-EAST ASIA

3.1 Improving AIDS Case Reporting

The factors which influence the accuracy of AIDS surveillance system include the sensitivity and specificity of an AIDS surveillance case definition, completeness of reporting, and reporting delays. Therefore, every effort should be made to enhance AIDS case reporting through training of health care workers assigning responsibilities to individuals, putting in place standard operating procedures, and developing diagnostic and reporting guidelines, including use of uniform case definition for reporting purposes. Even in countries such as Thailand, completeness of AIDS case reporting is not more than 30 per cent.

The desired attributes of an AIDS surveillance case definition include ability to identify severe HIV-associated disease; high sensitivity and specificity; simplicity; and suitability for national and international comparisons. HIV diagnostic testing and other laboratory studies, including CD4+ cell counts, will strengthen some of these attributes (such as the ability to identify severe HIV-associated disease, the specificity and the sensitivity). However, they are not a requisite for AIDS case surveillance. AIDS case surveillance can be and is carried out successfully without HIV antibody or immunologic testing, and without complex laboratory procedure to diagnose opportunistic infection.

The WHO AIDS surveillance case definition formerly called provisional WHO Clinical Case Definition for AIDS, or "Bangui" definition, was developed in 1985 and is based on clinical criteria only. This was modified in 1992 by the WHO Consultation to Review the Priorities for Surveillance of HIV/AIDS and AIDS Surveillance Case Definitions. The new case definition does not require HIV antibody testing. Although some studies have shown that it may lack sensitivity, it is reasonably specific and widely used in countries with limited health infrastructure and limited clinical and HIV diagnostic capabilities. This case definition is feasible, inexpensive and has high predictive value in areas of high HIV prevalence. Limitations, however, include low sensitivity, lower specificity than other definitions which incorporate HIV testing, positive predictive value is very low where HIV infection prevalence is low and lack of accuracy related to tuberculosis. (Tuberculosis patients without HIV infection could be counted as AIDS cases because of similarity of symptoms and signs.)

It can, therefore, be recommended that in countries where HIV infection exists but HIV serology and other diagnostic facilities are not routinely available, should continue to use the WHO clinical case definition for AIDS surveillance. For reporting cases to WHO, the amount of data required should be kept as minimum as possible. These should include information on age, sex, transmission category and geographic location. Reporting should be made in the format provided by WHO South-East Asia Regional Office.

3.2 Adhering to HIV Sentinel Surveillance Methodology

Sentinel surveillance for HIV is developed primarily to monitor trends for HIV prevalence in selected populations, determine the geographical spread of HIV infection, and provide information for estimation and projection of all levels of HIV infection. While implementing HIV sentinel surveillance, the following methodological considerations should be adhered to by national AIDS programmes. (These are described in some detail in the WHO/SEARO publication "Carrying Out HIV Sentinel Surveillance —a Guide to Programme Managers").

— *Sentinel Site*: Selection of population groups or sites that are easily accessible. Implementation of sentinel surveillance does not require a random sampling of sites or groups but rather attempts to identify groups or sites from which good data may be consistently collected over a period of time.

— *Sentinel Populations:* Groups or sub-populations in which HIV prevalence will be monitored must be clearly identified. For example, pregnant women seeking antenatal care and military recruits are most likely to be representative of the generally sexually active population. If hemogram or syphilis screening is routinely performed, blood drawn for this purpose may also be tested for HIV antibodies. In low prevalence areas, HIV screening for surveillance purposes may be limited to sub-populations that engage in a behaviour that places them at high risk of HIV transmission. Common "higher-risk" populations include Injecting Drug Users (IDUs), Commercial Sex Workers (CSWs) and STD clinic attendees. In countries where blood donated for transfusion is routinely screened, these data are a convenient source of information. However, HIV prevalence information from blood donors may be biased in two ways. In settings where blood donors are paid, HIV prevalence levels are usually higher than in the general population. In situations where donations are voluntary and donor selection programmes have been implemented, HIV prevalence rates are frequently lower than in the general population. Because of the large sample size and the continuous nature of screening activities, with appropriate interpretation, HIV prevalence rates among blood donors provide convenient and valuable information on the progression of the HIV epidemic.

— *Sampling Duration:* To obtain the most valid measure of HIV prevalence, blood samples for HIV sentinel surveillance should be taken in less than a two-month period. In an epidemic period the calculation of HIV prevalence rates based on sampling periods of longer than two months may result in an artificially low rate.

— *Sample Size:* To obtain an acceptable level of precision of the calculated prevalence rate, WHO recommends a minimum sample size of 250 for "higher risk" and 400 for "lower risk" population groups.

— *Sampling Method:* To facilitate implementation, WHO recommends that consecutive sampling be used and that each individual be included until the desired sample size is reached. In some settings convenience sampling may be necessary.

— *Sampling Frequency*: Except in situations where transmission is thought to be explosive, WHO recommends that rounds of sentinel surveillance be carried out once every year (same months).

— *Testing Methodology:* To minimize participation bias, WHO recommends that, whenever possible, unlinked anonymous testing be used. In settings where unlinked anonymous testing is not possible (usually among certain "higher risk" population groups), testing should be voluntary, confidential and accompanied by both pre- and post-test counselling.

Implementation of sentinel surveillance is an intensive effort that requires training, support, supervision and co-ordination. Experiences from other countries in the Region show that implementation should begin with a few sites and easily accessible populations and, based on experience gained, the programme should be expanded to include other sites and sub-populations. Close supervision and monitoring is essential for implementation of a successful HIV sentinel surveillance programme. Data from HIV surveillance should always be presented in the form of rates rather than absolute number of persons detected with HIV.

3.3 Choosing an Optimal Surveillance Strategy

Each of the two surveillance methods previously discussed, "AIDS case reporting" and "HIV Sentinel serosurveillance", is important. For example, in areas where HIV infection is unrecognized or has been recently introduced, the main objective of surveillance may be to identify the areas or groups into which the infection is spreading so as to target prevention. In this situation, sentinel HIV surveillance of high-risk groups should take priority. Where HIV infection is already present and levels of prevalence are higher, the main objectives of surveillance should be to monitor the epidemic, to target prevention initiatives, and to plan health services. Sentinel HIV surveillance should be expanded to cover geographic areas and groups in which there is a risk of the infection spreading. In both situations (e.g. HIV infection recently introduced, or HIV infection at higher prevalence levels), AIDS case reporting should be undertaken and the choice of an AIDS surveillance case definition should be selected, based on resources and the level of clinical and laboratory diagnostic capability. Where resources are limited, the AIDS clinical case definition without HIV antibody testing may appropriately meet the surveillance goals. In countries where resources are less restricted, use of a more sophisticated AIDS surveillance case definition may be more appropriate.

It was stressed that other data sources on sexually transmitted diseases, sexual and injecting behaviour, socio-economic aspects, etc., should be used to supplement the information available from AIDS case reporting and sentinel HIV surveillance.

3.4 Initiating STD Surveillance

Surveillance of STD in the South-East Asia Region remains weak; there is a lack of reliable and accurate data on the prevalence and incidence of common sexually transmitted diseases in most countries. As a result, the magnitude of STDs and the trends cannot be quantified with any degree of confidence. The situation is further compounded by the lack of consensus on the approaches to be used to measure the disease burden and due to the inadequate laboratory diagnostic facilities available in most countries.

There is, however, a broad acceptance that collection and dissemination of surveillance data on STDs are essential to identify groups at high risk, establish realistic disease control objectives and evaluate the overall effectiveness of STD syndromic management and of HIV/AIDS primary prevention measures, as a good surrogate marker. Based on country reports, it is clear that the incidence and prevalence of STDs and complication rates are high in most countries of the Region. In Thailand, however, the incidence of STDs has been declining over the years.

The priority for the Region now is to establish a reliable but simple and practical STD surveillance programme using a standardized approach and format. In this regard, draft STD surveillance guidelines prepared by the American Regional Office of WHO were discussed with a view to adapting the same for South-East Asia. Consistent availability of reasonably accurate data on STDs will guide and assist STD/AIDS control programmes in evaluating the impact of control strategies, e.g., based on syndromic management of STDs and on IEC interventions targeted at individuals with high risk behaviour and in rationally planning for future strategies.

To assess baseline information, it would be useful to collate all available published and unpublished data and analyse them. Standard guidelines are needed to facilitate establishment of STD surveillance in countries, preferably based on and linked to the existing case reporting system. In men, surveillance should include reporting of grintal ulcers and uretheral discharge as syndromes from selected sites, while among women, STD surveillance should include report of VDRL/TPHA among antenatal clinic attendees and gonococcal cultures, where such facilities exist. *Monitoring of gonococcal antimicrobial susceptibility patterns should also form an integral part of STD surveillance.*

3.5 Using a Uniform Reporting Format

Uniform simple reporting forms should be used for reporting HIV, AIDS and STD data from periphery to control level within the country. For reporting of data to WHO, the amount of data required should be kept to the minimum possible. For example, AIDS case reporting should include information on age, sex, transmission category and geographic location. Format developed by the WHO Regional Office and provided to all national AIDS programmes should be used for reporting to WHO.

4. COMPUTERIZED DATA MANAGEMENT SYSTEMS

4.1 Analysis of AIDS Cases and Forecasting

The computerized data management system was introduced to the participants. It was emphasized that using computer systems for AIDS surveillance include the ability to enter, retrieve, delete and update data records using *Epi info* and an edit function to ensure data has been correctly entered and both summary and detailed analysis can be performed. The; summary analysis for reported AIDS cases should include cases by year and geographic area, and by age and sex. Information can be obtained in the form of line listing, histograms and pie charts. Detailed analysis of AIDS cases can include details on the clinical presentation and the modes of transmission. For HIV, the summary analysis should include the number tested for HIV, the number positive, the date of the sampling period, the geographic area or site, and the group tested.

Feedback should be presented to facilitate checking of data entered by data providers. Analysis and feedback should contain a comparison of information submitted by different providers. A report for communicating surveillance data to the WHO Regional Office should be generated and sent each quarter. (A prototype system illustrating the above was demonstrated and the participants practised entering data and producing reports.)

Epi Model, a microcomputer programme for making short-term forecasts of AIDS cases, was presented during the meeting. The three epidemiological assumptions necessary for a reliable forecast were discussed: the year widespread transmission began; the reference prevalence estimate, and the position on the epidemic curve. The year of widespread transmission is not necessarily the year the first AIDS case or HIV infection was detected, but rather the year when indigenous transmission reached the threshold necessary for continued local transmission. The reference prevalence level refers to the estimated number of adult HIV infections and not to the reported infections. The position on the epidemic curve is determined by taking into account the age of the epidemic, the likely peak prevalence level, and the annual distribution of observed AIDS cases and HIV prevalence levels.

4.2 HIV Estimation and Projection Methods

Because detection of HIV infection is limited by the sub-clinical nature of the infection and differential access to health care and HIV testing facilities, an estimation of the number of HIV infections is necessary to present a true picture of the extent of the epidemic. It is useful to set up a working group in each country which will be responsible for estimating HIV infections in the country. These estimates could be updated once a year based on available epidemiological data and using scientific methodology. Several methods of estimation were discussed in the meeting:

— *Enumeration:* Attempts have been made by some to use enumerated or detected HIV infections to estimate HIV prevalence. However, this leads to a gross underestimation of the level of HIV infections in a population. Individuals infected with HIV will develop symptoms and present for care only at the end-stage of the infection. Enumerated or detected HIV infections represent only the bare minimum. of the actual number of individuals infected with HIV; this also depends on the number of people and types of populations tested for HIV infection.

— *Population-based probability sampling:* A more reliable estimate of HIV prevalence could be obtained by probability sampling of the population. In many countries the prevalence is low and would require an extremely large sample. Because blood must be drawn, consent must be obtained and may lead to severe participation bias. If HIV is limited to "high risk" populations, access to these populations may be difficult. For ethical, logistical, financial and methodological reasons, WHO does not recommend that population-based sampling be undertaken.

— *Modelling:* If accurate information on transmission rates and behaviours that influence transmission are available, epidemiological models may be used to provide an insight into the dynamics of HIV epidemic. However, direct measures of HIV prevalence are frequently more reliable than estimates of the occurrence and distribution of behaviours influencing HIV transmission and are more easily implemented. The use of modelling to determine current estimates of HIV prevalence should be applied with care.

— *Expert judgement*—Delphi methods: in situations where data on HIV/AIDS levels, trends and distributions are limited, expert judgement can often provide a rough guess as to the likely range of prevalence. Knowledge of local situations and of infectious disease process (especially sexually transmitted diseases and epidemic theory) are an essential pre-requisite for involving experts.

— *Back calculation:* The number of incidents of HIV infection may be estimated using statistical back calculation. However, this method requires relatively complete AIDS case reporting over a period of time and is not able to estimate recent levels of HIV infection.

— *Extrapolation:* If a reliable estimate of HIV prevalence has been previously made, this estimate may be used to anchor future estimates for 1-3 years, assuming that there are no sudden changes in the populations effected. Long-term extrapolation should not be made and direct estimates from seroprevalence surveys should be frequently used to re-anchor the estimate.

— *Sero-surveys of sentinel populations* is often the most popular method of estimating the burden of HIV. It is well accepted that in many cases the most reliable estimate of HIV prevalence can be obtained based on seroprevalence studies of different sub-populations representing populations at different levels of risk. The HIV prevalence rate observed in different groups may then be applied to the population which the study group represents. For example, in epidemics where heterosexual transmission is predominant, HIV prevalence rates observed in pregnant women are generally applied to the sexually active population (usually aged between 15-49). in many countries, because HIV is not uniformly distributed throughout the population, separate studies for urban and rural areas may be necessary and the observed prevalence rates applied to urban and rural populations. If the epidemic appears to be confined to "high risk" populations, an estimate of the size of these groups is necessary. In general, such estimates may be made by applying the following formula:

$v = \sum (pi/ti)(Ri)$, where

v is the total estimate

p is the number positive in the group tested

t is the number tested in the group

R is the estimated size of the population for which the p/t may be applied. Care should be taken that the groups do not overlap. The meeting participants practised the use of above-mentioned methods with the help of computerized data management system, employing their own country specific surveillance data.

4.3 STD Estimates

STD estimates are important for programme development, management and evaluation. These are useful also to estimate the requirement of drugs and other resources as well as for general advocacy purposes. The first step in making specific prevalence estimates at country level is to determine the STD prevalence rates for syphilis, gonorrhoea, chlamydia and trichomoniasis, through a modified Delphi approach and after discussion with relevant experts in the country. Additional related information made possible through review of STD literature, library search and data from all available recent studies in the country supplemented by already available official STD prevalence figures can be shared with experts to obtain the best estimates of prevalence rates. Such data could include prevalence of positive serological test for syphilis among pregnant women or of gonorrhoea among women between 15-49 years.

By applying the estimated prevalence for each of the specific STDs to the mid-year population estimate of adults 15-49 year, it is possible to get prevalence or the number of STDs existing at any point of time that year.

The STD incidence can be estimated by discussing the estimated prevalence by average duration of infection. The latter, in terms of years, can be obtained roughly through discussions with experts and review of literature in each country. It needs information on the proportion of STDs that are symptomatic or asymptomatic, those who are treated and those who remain untreated, by sex. The exact methodology for estimating the duration seems complicated and is being refined.

5. RECOMMENDATIONS

The meeting made the following recommendations:

For Governments

1. Additional efforts need to be made in the countries of the South-East Asia Region to adopt and implement the standard protocol for HIV surveillance according to the guidelines given in the WHO/SEARO publication "Carrying out HIV Sentinel Surveillance".
2. The need for unlinked anonymous testing and the fact that initiating HIV surveillance in low-risk groups may be relatively unproductive unless a critical level of HIV prevalence among those with high-risk behaviour has been reached, should be kept in mind. In countries with mature epidemic, it would be useful to include military recruits also as a sentinel group to monitor HIV trends in the general population.
3. The HIV sentinel surveillance may be supplemented with elements of behavioural surveillance whenever possible and feasible.
4. The results of HIV surveillance in a country should be regularly reported to WHO/SEARO with the use of the format included in the publication "Carrying out HIV Sentinel Surveillance". WHO/SEARO, on the other hand, should provide countries with regular feedback.
5. Estimates of HIV prevalence, based on the results of HIV sentinel surveillance, should be made annually by a working group at national level. Wherever possible, computers should be used for data management and for estimation of HIV infections.
6. Countries should continue efforts to develop, in cooperation with WHO/SEARO, the standard AIDS case

definition and adopt the same while reporting AIDS in a standard reporting form. Every attempt should be made to promote reporting of AIDS cases and deaths to the National AIDS Programme, and to

7. When carrying out AIDS reporting for surveillance, all efforts should be made to ensure confidentiality at all costs.
8. Standard guidelines on surveillance of STDs should be developed in the Region, which could then be adopted for use by Member Countries. The work on the preparation of regional guidelines should be one of the areas of co-operation between national experts and WHO during 1996-1997.
9. In order to monitor STD trends, reporting should be based on syndromes; for example, among men, genital ulcer disease and urethral discharge should be reported, preferably from selected sites both in the public as well as private sectors. Among women, VDRL/STS routinely carried out at antenatal clinics should be monitored. In addition, at sites where facilities exist, data on gonococcal cultures should also be used for surveillance purposes.
10. These selected STDs should be reported on a monthly basis within countries, and to WHO on a quarterly basis. The WHO quarterly reporting form should be modified to include data on STD surveillance as well.

For WHO

1. WHO should continue to provide technical support to countries in capability building on HIV/AIDS and STD surveillance, particularly in the area of training.
2. WHO should draft guidelines on STD surveillance for use by Member Countries and finalize it in consultation with national experts.
3. WHO should provide feedback to countries on HIV/AIDS and STD surveillance on a regular basis.

44

Development and the HIV Epidemic

(A forward-looking evaluation of the approach of the UNDP HIV and Development Programme)

Bruce Parnell, Gro Lie, Juan Jacobo Hernandez, Cindy Robins

1. INTRODUCTION: THE UNDP HIV AND DEVELOPMENT PROGRAMME AND THE SPECIAL PROGRAMME RESOURCES

UNDP's HIV and Development Programme is engaged in responding to the HIV epidemic using approaches consistent with the adoption of the development paradigm of sustainable human development (Banuri *et al.* 1994, p. 21)*. It aims to build the capacity of people, communities and nations: building capacity to understand the ways in which the epidemic evolves through its interaction with human development, and the ways in which people can act in response to its causes and consequences.

During the fifth UNDP programming cycle (1992-96), Special Programme Resources (SPR) were made available to enhance the relevance, impact and effectiveness of UNDP's technical co-operation programmes. These resources were to be used to improve current procedures for, and approaches to, programme and

** The term 'sustainable human development' is used here because it summarises the purpose and approaches of the new development paradigm which is emerging as a result of dissatisfaction with traditional methods of technical co-operation. Sustainable human development has been defined in UNDP discussion papers as, "the enlargement of people's choices and capabilities through the formation of social capital so as to meet as equitably as possible the needs of current generations without compromising the needs of future ones"* (Banuri et al, 1994, p.2 1).

** SPR allocations 'INT/92/400 - Minimising the impact of HIV on development', and 'INT/93/401 Partnership programme to enhance national capacity to analyse and respond to the psychological, social and economic determinants and consequences of the HIV epidemic': these two allocations were evaluated simultaneously, and for the rest of this report are referred to as the singular, "SPR".*

project design, implementation and evaluation; and for exploring new catalytic and innovative approaches to development. The HIV and Development Programme (HDP) was allocated $5m for the cycle, subsequently reduced to $3.5m*.

The HIV and Development Programme was established in January 1992 to provide policy guidance to the organisation on HIV-related personnel and substantive issues, to co-ordinate all activities undertaken by UNDP in this area and to provide programme support to UNDP country offices and other units.

The establishment of the Programme was funded from UNDP's inter-regional programming resources, complemented by extra-budgetary support from the Netherlands, Australia and Norway. Since SPR funds could not be used for staff costs, the Programme has used extrabudgetary support, received in recent years from the United States of America and from Australia, for core costs: staff, communication, travel, translation and publications. The SPR was used to finance the activities undertaken and managed by this staff. This has been a constructive use of both sources of funding. The work of the Programme depends essentially on both sources of funds: without the capacity created by other sources of support, the Programme could not have used the SPR in the way it did. Therefore, although the stimulus for the evaluation came from the need to evaluate the use made of the SPR, the evaluation is of the approach of the Programme as a whole.

The HDP used the SPR to explore and enhance understanding of the ways in which the principles and approaches of sustainable human development can be applied towards developing understanding of, and effective responses to, the HIV epidemic. Its approach was based on a set of related understandings about the nature of human development, the nature of the HIV epidemic and the role of UNDP.

Based on these understandings, the HIV and Development Programme recognised that the HIV epidemic demands an urgent and effective response. However, the Programme recognised also that this response must take place in a context in which governments, development professionals and other agents of change find themselves facing new and highly complex phenomena. New knowledge and programming approaches are needed to develop effective responses to the multidimensional aspects of the epidemic. It was therefore decided to use the SPR resources to explore the possibilities of such knowledge and programming approaches.

This was done through a series of interrelated activities which addressed key areas of focus using improved methods of development practice, working in collaboration with the people whose lives are affected, and the organisations which support them, and with other individuals and agencies, including UN agencies, interested in developing sustainable responses to the HIV epidemic.

The approach used by the HDP recognised that the most effective responses would grow out of people's action within their own contexts: their own communities and their own countries. The approach was therefore based on capacity building, with an emphasis on the development of effective partnerships with those responding, in order to ground responses in people's shared experiences of the realities of the epidemic. The approach involved constant reflection based on the lives, dreams and hopes of those people struggling to respond.

Within the framework of this approach, based on the principles of sustainable human development and recognising the collaborative role of UNDP, a central question which was constantly explored through the HDP in relationship with its partners was, "How can we, together, move forward?

2. THE EVALUATION PROCESS

2.1 The Nature and Purpose of the Evaluation

The purpose of the evaluation was to review the use by the HIV and Development Programme of Special Programme Resources (SPR) at global, regional and national levels during the fifth UNDP programming cycle (1992-1996), and to consider what UNDP should be doing during the sixth programming cycle*. The evaluation was intended to be forward-looking, starting with consideration of what has been learnt through the HDP to date, but *aiming to generate further and deeper understanding of the practices* of sustainable human development as applied to the HIV epidemic, its causes and consequences.

Evaluation is a process inextricably linked to a sense of purpose, and there is no such thing as an all-purpose evaluation (Weiss, 1972). Evaluation processes should therefore relate to the needs and interests of the *users* of the evaluation. In this case, the people for whom the outcome may be of value and interest will not be limited to those defined in many evaluation texts as "key stakeholders". Along with UNDP, the *users of this evaluation* will include a range of people and organisations interested in learning more about how sustainable human development may work in their own and others' contexts: the partners, direct and indirect, of the HDP initiatives, staff of national HIV/AIDS programmes. UN agencies, NGOs, communities, consultants, academics and others

[3]The draft terms of reference for the evaluation are available on request from the HIV and Development Programme. The evaluation process was developmental in nature, designed collaboratively by evaluation team members and programme staff: the terms of reference were a starting point for this process.

affected by the epidemic. The evaluation process was therefore designed to elucidate lessons learnt through the approach of the HDP in ways which would also be of value to these users of the evaluation.

The evaluation was also designed to fit within a framework outlined in a UNDP discussion paper on guiding principles for evaluation (Benbouali, 1995). In relation to programmes of this nature, the paper notes that, "The development objectives are finally the results of strategic effects of many programmes/projects and efforts" (Benbouali, 1995, p. 2). A suggested means of enhancing understanding of such strategic effects is to concentrate on issues of *relevance* and *sustainability.* This makes such evaluation distinct from auditing and assessment, which focus on managerial and financial issues, and on measures of programme activities and performance as predetermined in initial decisions about programme objectives.

An emphasis on strategic effects is also central to the suggestion, outlined in a recent UNDP discussion paper on sustainable human development, that one of the indicators of sustainable human development is the extent to which social learning has taken place, as indicated by "... the emergence of new habits and routines (as) a critical indicator of social change" (Banuri, et a., 1994, p. 28). The evaluation explored the extent to which the HDP activities had enhanced such social learning, and hence capacity development, by exploring a broader range of critical indicators, more accurately described as the emergence of new *understanding* and *approaches,* as the concepts of *habits* and *routines* were considered too static to describe either the activities of the Programme or the Programme's intended strategic effects.

In line with the forward-looking purpose of the evaluation, and acknowledging the need for sustainable human development to grow out of people's lived experiences, the central issue of the evaluation process, reflecting the central question of the Programme itself, was "How can we, together, move forward?" In this case, the question was asked in relation to how we can use evaluation processes to generate a deeper understanding of the newer approaches to development practice.

2.2 The Evaluation Framework

It was important that the evaluation be conducted in a manner consistent with the dynamic, and even opportunistic, nature of the Programme. The world keeps changing, the determinants and consequences of the HIV epidemic keep changing, and the opportunities available to a low-budget programme operating globally also keep changing. So does understanding of what works best to promote sustainable human development. Therefore, it was important that the evaluation avoid a result of "locking" the Programme into a fixed *modus operandi.* For example, an evaluation with a linear logic which simply considered inputs, outputs, or immediate impact would have been inappropriate. Such an approach would require some sense of "fixing" the Programme as a static entity, clarifying what were the precise goals and objectives and measuring the outputs at just one point of time and in one context: the world as it was at one point in time.

Understanding the approach of the Programme as being based on a set of principles, from which arise methodologies and approaches, was therefore considered more accurate than attempts to define the Programme based on assumptions about clearly defined inputs and outputs. Early in the evaluation process, in July 1995, Programme staff developed a list of some of the concepts which the Programme was then using to describe its work and some of the concepts it was not then using.

The evaluation process was *interactive* and *iterative.* The *interactive* process involved working with the partners of the Programme, and others who use similar approaches in their own work, to develop together a deeper understanding of how the approaches work. The starting point was the Programme, but the evaluation enabled people to explore such issues with reference to their own lived experiences. This is consistent with the principle that, "The perspectives of and experiences of those persons who are served by applied programmes must be grasped, interpreted, and understood if solid, effective, applied programmes are to be put in place" (Denzin, 1989, p.105). The evaluation process was *iterative* in that it started with shared reflection about the nature of the Programme, went back into the field to explore how this understanding relates to people's lives, then returned to shared discussion about that, and so on.

The process was, in these ways, based on the qualitative research method of *interpretive interactionism* (Denzin, 1989). This method emphasises the need to *interpret* real-life phenomena in order to reduce complex reality to understandable and debatable notions. It suggests doing this in an *interactive* way, because deeper understanding about the meanings and significance of experiences and relationships arises when people reflect and engage in dialogue with each other.

Such an evaluation process meets two important requirements for the use of qualitative methodology:

1. The need to combine the collection of data with a rigorous interpretation of the significance ofthat data, as outlined by Patton (Patton, 1990, p. 423):

> ... we must be constantly moving back and forth between the phenomenon of the programme and our abstractions of that programme, between the descriptions of what has occurred and our interpretations of those descriptions, between the complexity of reality and our simplifications of those complexities, between the circularities and interdependencies of human activity and our need for linear, ordered statements of cause and effect.

2. The need to ensure that the people who conduct such interpretive analysis are those for whom the analysis is most important, as outlined by Denzin (Denzin, 1989, p. 25):

> Interpretive interactionism asserts that meaningful interpretations of human experience can only come from those persons who have thoroughly immersed themselves in the phenomenon they wish to interpret and understand.

2.3 The Evaluation Process: What was Done

Stage 1. Selection of evaluation team members

The evaluation team consisted of four people who are themselves affected by the epidemic. They are all engaged in responding to the epidemic in their own contexts, and have all been involved in promoting sustainable human development as participants in international networks, as consultants, or as long-term staff in development projects. In response to the second evaluation requirement above, the team members have all been partners of the Programme. They reflect a diversity of experiences of the epidemic and come from different global regions. Directly including more people from developing countries in the evaluation team was planned but was, ultimately, not possible. The nature of the evaluation process ensured, however, that many people from developing countries had direct input in both provision of information and interpretation of results. The evaluation team members were Bruce Parnell (team leader, from Australia), Juan Jacobo Hernandez (Mexico), Gro Lie (Norway) and Cindy Robins (Canada).

Stage 2. Selection of further participants in the evaluation process

Decisions were made about countries to which field visits would be made and criteria for selection of participants in interactive discussions and in workshops. These decisions were based on the qualitative research method known as purposeful sampling, as defined by Patton (Patton, 1990, p.169):

> The purpose of purposeful sampling is to select information-rich cases whose study will illuminate the questions under study. ... The logic and power of purposeful sampling lies in selecting information-rich cases for study in depth. Information-rich cases are those from which one can learn a great deal about issues of central importance to the purpose of the research, thus the term purposeful sampling.

The selection of evaluation participants was therefore based on determining which people were most likely to provide significant knowledge and insights which would contribute to a better understanding of how the approaches used work in practice.

The Programme had used a variety of new and innovative programmatic and organisational approaches to assist governments, communities and organisations, and the selection of evaluation participants had to reflect these approaches. Criteria for selecting participants were that they represented groups with whom the Programme worked in partnerships, people who were involved in networks responding to the epidemic, people who had participated in SPR activities, and people who were identified by Programme partners or other participants as being people who work in ways that are compatible with the approaches used.

The Programmers analysis had indicated that every facet of human, social and economic life can be affected by HIV and development, and that national responses must include collaboration between individuals, families, communities and governments. This mix was also reflected in the selection of evaluation participants, so that they included people from the governmental sector, non-government organisations, community groups, and grassroots movements as well as from the international community.

The three countries visited were Zambia, the Philippines and Mexico. These reflect a diversity of regions, countries with different experience of the HIV epidemic and its impacts, and countries in which the SPR has had varying levels of contact. A fourth country, Senegal, was visited by the evaluation team leader for the purpose of conducting a limited number of interactive discussions. This choice was made because, although the Programme has worked in Senegal, availability of partners at the required time meant that it was not possible to conduct the full range of evaluation processes in Senegal.

Stage 3. Interactive interpretation of the Programme's approach

The evaluation team leader worked with HDP staff in July 1995 to collate information about SPR activities and sustainable human development; to collectively reflect on the purpose, nature and approach of the Programme; to consider evaluation options; and to design a relevant evaluation process. A paper outlining the conceptual framework for the evaluation was prepared and distributed widely for comment amongst partners of the Programme and others interested in evaluation. It was developed as part of the evaluation process and was written with input from a number of people familiar with the work of HDP and evaluation methodologies to clarify the understanding of both Programme staff and evaluation team members.

Stage 4. Developing further understanding of the approach of the Programme

A planning workshop was held in Zambia in October 1995 for the evaluation team members, two members of the HIV and Development Programme staff and the UNDP HIV and Development national professional officer in Zambia, Margaret Mutambo. At this workshop, further consideration was given to the conceptual nature and approach of the HDP, with reference to selected publications on development practice, social change and evaluation which were tabled by workshop participants. The outline of the development practice framework for the HDP which is included in Section 4 of this report is based on the results of this period of the process.

The process of interpretive interactionism was applied to exploration of workshop participants' own experiences of development, the HIV epidemic, and the Programme. This ensured that all evaluation team members were familiar with the concepts and methodologies of the evaluation process. It also ensured that the evaluation team commenced development of a collective understanding of the nature and significance of the approach of the Programme and a shared understanding of issues to be considered during the country field visits.

Stage 5. Country field visits: interactive discussions

Interactive discussions were held with selected participants from each visited country. This dialogue differed from a usual interview format, in that those interviewed were able to talk freely about what mattered to them, but the interviewers from the evaluation team were also free to pursue issues they considered important; hence, use of the description, "interactive discussions", rather than "interviews".

The interactive discussions aimed to explore evaluation

participants' own experiences of HIV and development and any involvement they had with the Programme, and to engage with them in discussion about what approaches they find useful, regardless of whether or not their experience of those approaches was within SPR initiatives. The discussions explored issues through eliciting "thick description", as defined by Denzin (Denzin, 1989, p. 83):

> A thick description does more than record what a person is doing. It goes beyond mere fact and surface appearances. It presents detail, context, emotion, and the webs of social relationships that join persons to one another. Thick description evokes emotionality self-feelings. It inserts history into experience. It establishes the significance of an experience, or the sequence of events, for the person or persons in question. In thick description, the voices, feelings, actions, and meanings of interacting individuals are heard.

Stage 6. Country field visits. interpretive workshops

Interpretive workshops were held in each of the three primary countries visited in order to:

— provide a chance for people from each country to interact with each other in interpreting understanding of how various approaches work within their countries;
— provide a chance for larger numbers of people to participate in the evaluation process; and
— ensure that interpretations made by evaluation team members were able to be further considered by the people whose perceptions of relevance and sustainability were being considered.

Stage 7. Country field visits. review workshops

People responding to the HIV epidemic and development in each country usually do so working with National HIV/AIDS Committees, UN agencies and international donor agencies. To further ensure that the findings of the evaluation process were based in reality, and to ascertain the extent to which new approaches in sustainable human development are understood and supported (or not) by these agencies in each country, a short review workshop was also held in each country, and these agencies were invited.

At least some members of national HIV/AIDS committees in each country had been included in Stages 5 and 6 of the evaluation process. For this reason, very few also attended the first reporting back workshop review in Zambia, as this would have required yet further time commitment. Accepting this likely scenario, and in order to reduce the workload on those who had voluntarily offered to make the arrangements, it was decided that members of these committees should not be invited to attend the workshops in the Philippines or Mexico.

Many staff of UN agencies and international donor agencies attended the review workshops in each of the three primary countries. The workshops had a simple format, in which the nature of the Programme and the evaluation process was explained, the lists of concepts currently used and not used by UNDP were presented and initial interpretation of data by evaluation team members was presented for further discussion.

These workshops generated much interest, and dialogue ensued. Many participants indicated a good understanding of issues which were relevant within their countries of work, and demonstrated a keen interest in developing understanding of the interrelationships between the HIV epidemic and sustainable human development.

Stage 8. Commissioning of case studies

To complement information collected through field visits and consideration of published information, two case studies were commissioned to further explain the way the Programme worked in practice.

The first of these, entitled "Enhancing National Capacity Through HIV Action Research", was written by Catherine Hankins, a partner of the HIV and Development Programme, and two members of the Programme staff. It summarises what occurred and some of the key lessons learnt through this component of the SPR. The initiative aimed to enhance the national ability of people to find out what they need to know and to incorporate what they find into policy and programme design. This case study is included to provide insight into the practical ways in which a specific project was developed within the framework of the SPR, to indicate some of the lessons learnt through these types of processes and, consequently, to provide an example of the way the Programme evolved over time in response to lessons learnt. This case study is included in the text of this report, after Section 5.

The second case study, entitled "The Partnership Between the Salvation Army and the HIV and Development Programme" was written by Alison Rader and Captain Doctor Ian Campbell of the Salvation Army. It summarises the conceptual understanding about the nature of effective practices in sustainable human development which evolved over a long period of partnership between the Programme and the Salvation Army, and partnership between the Salvation Army's International Headquarters and its own partners in many countries. This paper's focus on development of conceptual understanding is deliberate, for two reasons. First, Salvation Army personnel and HDP staff reported that gradually enhanced understanding of development practice was one of the primary benefits to all parties engaged in this partnership. Second, evaluation team members felt it was useful to highlight specific lessons learnt through one particular partnership, as a typical example of the richness of what was achieved through an approach based on partnership. This case study is also included in the text of this report, after Section 6.

Stage 9. Interpretation of data

Collected data included information arising from shared discussions: discussions within the evaluation team and with Programme staff in the first four stages of the evaluation process, and discussions held with individuals and within workshops in Stages 5 to 7. In line with the processes of interpretive interactionism, this data was then collated, analysed and interpreted by the members of the evaluation team through a final workshop in New York over five days in November 1995.

This workshop followed an open-ended format, enabling development as it progressed and input from evaluation team members and Programme staff. Once again reflecting the interactive nature of the evaluation process, participation of others in this workshop was encouraged. At various stages, the workshop was attended by all HDP staff, by Gary Engelberg (a partner of the programme based in Senegal) and by Alison Rader of the Salvation Army.

During this workshop, the evaluation team identified the key concepts about which the evaluation process had led to deeper understanding, and shared information about what had been learnt about these concepts through the country field visits. The summary of understanding of how the Programme approach works in practice, which appears in Sections 5, 6 and 7 of this report, is based on this final workshop.

Stage 10. Report writing

The report was written following the final workshop. A brief report such as this cannot capture all that was learnt either through data collection or through the interpretive discussions. It is expected that further information about what has been learnt will be disseminated through the work and lives of the many people who participated in this process.

Selected notes made by evaluation team members during the data collection process are available on request from the HIV and Development Programme. These provide summaries of interactive discussions with evaluation participants, and thus enable richer insights into the ways in which the approaches of the Programme have worked in practice. Statements made in confidence are not available for distribution, but these constitute only a small proportion of the data collected.

3. THE SPR-FUNDED ACTIVITIES

3.1 Overview

The work of the HIV and Development Programme was guided by a set of related understandings about the nature of the HIV epidemic, the nature of development and the role of UNDP in the response to the epidemic. It took place in a context in which there was rapid and continuing spread of the HIV virus, no cure, and a potential for the HIV epidemic to impact on all aspects of human development.

The issues to be addressed were complex and various: moral, social, cultural, religious, psychological, legal, political, strategic and economic factors had to be considered. The programming responses had to be sustainable for perhaps many years to come, resulting in development of the capacity of individuals, communities and nations to adapt to the changing circumstances which may arise through interaction between the epidemic and the ongoing challenges of human development.

The HIV epidemic impacts on the broad range of human endeavour including social and economic development, welfare, education and training, employment, defence and law enforcement. The causes and consequences of the epidemic are closely associated with other challenges to development including poverty, unemployment, civil unrest, indebtedness and rural-urban movements. For example, HIV-related illness and death creates new poverty, deepens existing poverty and increases family and national indebtedness.

This interaction between the epidemic and development demands a multi-sectoral and interdisciplinary response, with collaboration between many partners: governments, international agencies, community based groups, NGOs, research institutes, private sector groups and, most importantly, the people directly affected.

The development of the Programme was based on a

recognition that UNDP's role is to assist developing countries to accelerate the process of capacity building within both governments and nations, through support for human resources development, institution building, strategic planning and management, good governance, and the promotion of sustainable human development. Thes development and dissemination of models and guidelines was considered of limited effectiveness. New knowledge and skills needed to be developed collaboratively, and new issues needed to be addressed as they were identified.

The Programme aimed:

to deepen understanding of the nature of effective responses to the epidemic, to determine what works and how, and what does not, and to take the best practices of development and apply them in this field; and

to increase UNDP's capacity to programme its resources more effectively and in this way to strengthen national capacity to develop an effective multi-dimensional response.

The elements of the approach adopted by the Programme were:

a continually deepening and changing *understanding* of the epidemic drawn from extensive and diverse experience in the response to the epidemic and in development practice;

an approach based on *capacity building:* the Programme tries to bring its expertise into processes of interaction which strengthen those values, processes, skills and behaviours which make it possible to establish an effective response.

an approach based on *partnerships:* the relation of partnership recognizes and respects the commitment and expertise that each partner brings to the work, accepts the importance of building consensus and solving problems across differences, is based on a set of ethical guiding principles and requires trust and respect; and

the continual *grounding* of understanding and of the approach, and the checking of these against the realities of the epidemic. In particular, this involves actively seeking and listening to the insights, reflections and experiences of the Programme's partners as well as following the developments in understanding and practice of individuals whom the Programme respects.

Such an approach requires extensive communication amongst all concerned and consultation with people in their own environment. The Programme found it was important that, wherever possible, the occasions and spaces made for discussion and learning should be where people themselves live and learn rather than in institutional settings.

The working principles of the Programme include the involvement of those directly affected by the epidemic in all activities and aspects of its work; gender sensitivity, representation and responsiveness; supportive partnerships with agents of change: individuals and community and non-governmental organisations; the strengthening of partnerships between the government sector and the community sector; sensitivity to ethical, legal and human rights issues; and the strengthening of partnerships across regional language groups.

The areas of focus of the Programme have arisen from these interactive processes. They include:

- # exploration of methodologies and instruments which can be used in national planning to minimise the social and economic consequences of the epidemic,
- # exploration of ways in which communities and nations can address complex and delicate ethical, legal and human rights issues,
- # consideration of the strengths and limits of initiatives directed specifically towards women,
- # developing understanding of how processes of social learning through research can be used in programme development,
- # ascertaining how networks can be supported and developed into sustainable institutional forms with the flexibility to accommodate to changing needs and circumstances,
- # exploring ways in which insights and lessons can be learnt and shared,
- # reflection on the role of language, images and metaphors in determining the nature of understanding and responses, and
- # consideration of ways in which fatalism and despair can give way to a sense of agency.

The HDP is thus clearly situated within the overall conceptual and operational framework of UNDP's work. It adopts approaches consistent with this framework and is based on concepts of sustainable human development, especially human survival; social capital formation; capacity building; social learning and partnership (see Banuri, et al. 1994); expertise (see Chambers, 1994); gender responsiveness; process consultation (see Joy and Bennett, 1994); strategic questioning (see Peavey, 1994); and governance.

Consistent with the principles of sustainable human development, the inclusion of the people whose lives are affected was considered essential and the Programme encouraged continual input from people directly affected by HIV and by development. This commenced with a workshop in New York in October 1992, in which a range of people directly affected by the epidemic worked with HDP staff, government officials, community workers, researchers and activists to develop general guidelines for the development of the Programme, including the identification of key issues to be addressed. The development of the Programme included ongoing interaction with these and other people, resulting in continual evolution of the Programme's approach, enhanced understanding of effective practices and the building of consensus on addressing a range of sensitive and complex issues.

The relationship between the approach of the Programme and recent advances in UNDP's understanding of the nature of sustainable human development was reviewed as part of the evaluation process, and is summarised in Section 4 of this report. The rest of this section (Section 3) provides a concise summary of the major types of activities which have been undertaken by the Programme. Although activities are described separately, the inter-connected nature of the factors which were addressed by the Programme means that these activities were not always discrete.

3.2 Minimising the Development Consequences of the Epidemic: Exploring Methods for Planning

With HIV prevalence amongst adults in some African countries now reaching 20 or 30 per cent of the adult population, there is intensified destruction of human and non-human capacity, and thus a new and critical need to find ways of addressing the consequences, not just measuring them. The HDP has supported many innovative processes in Africa and other regions to strengthen the capacities of governments, families and communities to mitigate these effects.

The first step in this process was a consultative meeting in Vienna in 1992 attended by other UN agencies, academics and people directly involved in their national responses to the epidemic. This meeting mapped out the main direction for SPR activities around minimising the development consequences of the epidemic, and defining processes which would enhance effective responses. It was agreed that a shift in balance was required, away from describing the consequences and towards developing types of understanding which would lead to strategies to address those consequences. Many activities followed, and there is space here for only a few examples.

— In collaboration with the International Institute for Applied Systems Analysis in Vienna, new computer software has been developed and made available at low cost to users. This makes it possible to access in a user friendly way the HIV data of the US Bureau of the Census, the largest data set available, and also to play interactive "games" which enable users to explore processes of HIV transmission and develop better undertanding of the dynamics of the epidemic. The software has been offered to UNAIDS to be used in furthering communication objectives.

— An unsuccessful attempt was made to strengthen the regional planning capacity in the Kagera Region of Tanzania through the inclusion of activities which addressed the effects of the epidemic. This is an area where there is an existing UNDP planning project and where HIV prevalence is very high. Important lessons were learnt from this experience about the processes required for gaining commitment to programme development, together with improved knowledge of the constraints which affect what is possible under conditions of widespread denial.

— Nicaragua is a country with low reported HIV prevalence in a region where other countries are already experiencing rapid spread of the epidemic, and where socioeconomic factors may enhance further rapid transmission of the virus. Attempting to induce more effective prevention by government and others, the HDP, in partnership with a national NGO, cosponsored a workshop and follow-up activities to enhance understanding of developmental aspects of the epidemic. This strengthened local capacity to undertake economic analysis, to measure the effects of the epidemic and to identify appropriate responses to the needs of those affected.

— A project was undertaken in several rural areas of Mexico, in collaboration with the National AIDS Programme and other partners including the NGO, Colectivo Sol. The project explored how to better use local structures and organisations, such as public libraries, to strengthen links between information providers and community-based service organisations such as health centres and women's groups. Important lessons were learnt about processes for building local trust as integral to and necessary for programmes relating to HIV prevention and care.

3.3 Capacity Development Through Research

An ongoing project explores how to strengthen national capacity to define, undertake and make use of research on the socio-economic causes and consequences of the epidemic. The project, in four African countries (Central African Republic, Kenya, Senegal and Zambia), has developed innovative processes to support national teams of researchers and others, working in partnership with National HIV/AIDS Programmes, affected individuals, researched communities and other potential users of data and analysis.

Research is now underway and important insights have been gained about how to best ensure that research is timely and relevant to programme needs. Activities which build on the lessons of the project are being developed in other countries and regions, including Myanmar and Nicaragua, with proposals also under consideration in Vietnam and Botswana.

This initiative is developing new approaches to technical co-operation, based on principles of process consultation which entail different relationships and use of new working methods between development partners. The SPR initiative has thrown light on how best to strengthen national research capacity through technical consortia; how to involve potential users throughout the research process; how to strengthen research skills and improve understanding of the ethical and development aspects of the epidemic; and how to ensure early discussion of, and improved methods for, the dissemination of research results and their effective use in programme development. *Case Study* 1 describes this project in further detail.

SPR funds are also being used to explore how the processes of research can be used to stimulate solutions as well as to increase understanding of problems. Research on families of children left without social and economic support after the death of their parents is being undertaken in a seriously affected area in the west of Kenya. The research methodology is designed to lead to processes of discussion and consultation within families and communities and with local government so that adequate support can be provided to these children. The findings are also contributing to national policy and programme development.

3.4 HIV and Development Workshops

Training materials and workshops have been developed focusing on the human, social and economic development dimensions of the epidemic. The workshops aim to increase awareness of the complex nature of the epidemic, to analyse approaches to strengthening community-coping responses and national responses, and to identify the policies and programmes required at all levels to respond to the epidemic. The belief that the epidemic can be overcome is central to the workshop.

The workshop is based on three principles:

— placing the psychological and socio-economic causes and consequences of the epidemic at the centre of the training: the analysis upon which the workshop is based focuses on identifying effective processes for reducing the impact of the epidemic on human, social and economic development and the impact of these factors on the spread of the virus;

— placing people at the centre of the analysis: people and their communities are central to discussions within the workshop, which focus on their expressed needs and concerns, their resources, their coping and survival strategies and their development aspirations; and

— placing hope at the centre of the response: people are changing their behaviour, families and communities are providing support and care for those affected, and communities, businesses and governments are developing strategies for preventing further infections and reinfection and for minimising the adverse impact of the epidemic.

The workshop is designed for senior government officials particularly from ministries of planning and finance, the productive sectors (agriculture, mining, industries, transport, etc.) and the social sectors, for senior United Nations officials and for the organisations of civil society. In addition to the workshop itself, shorter workshops on HIV and Development have taken place at national level for politicians, community organisations, NGOs, the private sector and others. National and inter-country workshops organised by UNDP include workshops in Australia, Austria, Benin, Botswana, Cameroon, Central African Republic, Chile, Cote d'Ivoire, Gabon, India, Jamaica, Kenya, Madagascar, Malaysia, Mexico, Morroco, Nicaragua, the Philippines, Poland, Senegal, Uganda, the Ukraine, the USA, Zaire, Zambia and Zimbabwe.

Many examples of flow-on effects from these workshops and the training materials used were reported during the evaluation process. Three training for trainers workshops have been held (Mombasa 1991, Agadir 1992, Kuala Lumpur 1994) and those trained have subsequently adapted and used the materials in many settings. The workshops have had an impact in enhancing people's understanding of what is needed and what is possible, on the development of effective strategies, in initiating the development of effective networks of people who may not otherwise have met, and in stimulating engagement amongst those who had previously not considered the epidemic relevant to themselves or their work.

In the Philippines, participants reported that they often use components of the workshop in their work in rural provinces, as they have found this an effective way to engage people's interest and understanding as a prelude to acting in response to the challenges of the epidemic. In two states in India, the training materials are being used by women sex workers working in red light districts to increase the understanding of their co-workers of the epidemic and of the need for a collective response. Already by 1993, over 500 groups of women sex workers had seen and discussed the module on The Unfolding of the HIV Epidemic. In rural Zimbabwe, the materials have been incorporated into village theatre productions aiming to increase awareness of, and a commitment to respond to, the epidemic. In Senegal, it was reported that the workshop had created an emotional as well as an intellectual engagement amongst many people who were already engaged in responding but who, as a result of the workshops, now did so more vigorously and with much greater personal conviction. Thus, the workshops have been able to address needs in new ways which people find directly relevant across international boundaries.

In many countries networks of NGOs have incorporated the development practice approaches and conceptual frameworks presented in the workshops into ongoing projects building local capacities to understand and respond to the epidemic.

3.5 Learning how to Learn from and with Others: Facilitated Study Tours

Exploration and testing out of new and innovative approaches to learning how to learn from and with others has been integral to the work of the Programme. One approach that has been developed, tested out and found to be effective is the facilitated study tour. This was first developed in response to a request from the National HIV/AIDS Programme in Djibouti for assistance in understanding and developing a community-based strategy to address the HIV epidemic. A multidisciplinary team from Djibouti, with participation from the Ministry of Health, counsellors, hospital administrators, the media, women's groups, community groups and lawyers, travelled first to Senegal. There the NGO, ENDA-Sante, ran a workshop to explore the lessons learnt to date about the centrality of the community response to the epidemic, including the importance of developing an appropriate legal and ethical framework to facilitate such a response. The workshop included visits to community groups and discussion with interested officials, researchers and activists in Senegal,

Following this workshop, the Djibouti team and the ENDA-Sante facilitators proceeded to Zambia and Uganda. They visited selected community groups and then spent an additional day in each country to reflect upon the relevance for their own country of what they had seen and learnt. The team prepared a paper summarising the lessons learnt and their applicability for effective programme design and development in Djibouti.

On their return to Djibouti, the team spent a week integrating their findings into the national HIV/AIDS plan and planning a pilot project to build national capacity to develop a community-oriented approach to the epidemic; to establish an appropriate legal, ethical and human rights framework for such an approach; to utilise existing resources for such an approach (including use of counsellors, local government structures and community leaders); to strengthen the trust between those individuals and families already affected by the epidemic and government and other community members; to delineate the roles and responsibilities of community organisations and government; and to develop participatory community-based monitoring and evaluation systems to capture the lessons and feed them into policy and programme development discussions.

The approaches used in the facilitated study tour resulted not only in stimulating the national authorities to rethink and redesign their HIV/AIDS strategies, but were supportive of building national capacity and fostering exchanges of experience and learning amongst many African countries.

Facilitated study tours were subsequently organised in response to requests from Swaziland, where the government wanted to explore and develop a national strategy for community- and family-based care and support, and from Vietnam, where the Vietnamese Armed Forces wished to strengthen their military HIV prevention programme and to develop stronger links between the military and civil society.

3.6 Ethical, Legal and Human Rights Networks

Networks of activists and professionals have been established and supported as a means of building capacity to address legal, ethical and human rights issues. These networks, in Africa, Asia and the Pacific and Latin and Central America and the Caribbean, draw their members from legal, governmental and academic institutions as well as from organisations of civil society. They are active in addressing the legal and ethical issues central to responses to the epidemic, and in the provision of services to those affected. Indirectly, they contribute to institutional capacity building and to human resource development.

These networks contribute to social capacity building through drawing together diverse groups of those interested or implicated to address issues of common interest. They broaden the base of discussion and contribute to consensus building within the community sector and amongst civil society, public and private sectors. They also advocate for law reform, changes in legal practices, the provision of appropriate services, policy and programme development, and they play a guardianship role in ascertaining the legal and ethical appropriateness of responses to the epidemic.

The value of the networking approach is evident in an example given by Attorney Manual (Manny) Goyena, a lawyer from the Filipino NGO, Alter Law. He talked in an interactive discussion with the evaluation team of how his organisation provided legal advice, but worked closely with other NGOs more able to be directly involved in social action. He had attended various regional meetings either in the law and human rights field, or as part of networking within the Asia-Pacific Council of AIDS Service Organisations (APCASO). He had been a participant at the first meeting organised by HDP for the Asia and Pacific region in Cebu, the Philippines, in 1993 and at the resource persons training workshop in Tarrytown, New York in April 1995.

Many people from the Philippines are now engaged as "overseas contract workers", working in other more wealthy countries usually for lower wages than local people. A recognised difficulty is their lack of rights within those other countries. Through the APCASO network, contact had been made between the Philippines AlterLaw group and lawyers in Malaysia. Together, the two groups are now planning proposals to address the rights of Filipinos working in Malaysia. Manny explained:

> We got [a lawyer] to meet with the Philippine NGOs working in Malaysia. So, we tried to define a model, file a test case. For example, the government now is just assisting people on the receiving end of complaints, but we're moving them to assist with initiating cases ... For example, with trafficking of women, ... because there are international syndicates, therefore responses have to be international.

Countries in which UNDP has supported networks and networking on ethics, law and HIV include, in Africa: Botswana, Burundi, Central African Republic, Cote d'Ivoire, Gambia, Ghana, Kenya, Rwanda, Senegal, South Africa, Uganda, Zaire and Zambia; in Asia and the Pacific: Bangladesh, Cambodia, China, Fiji, India, Indonesia, Malaysia, Myanmar, Nepal, Pakistan, Papua New Guinea, Philippines, Sri Lanka, Thailand and Vietnam; in Latin America and the Caribbean: Argentina, Barbados, Brazil, Mexico, Nicaragua, Paraguay and Venezuela; and in Europe and the Commonwealth of Independent States: Poland, Russia and the Ukraine.

In response to requests from NGO partners for capacity building and skills development in this area, a legal and ethical resource persons workshop was held in Tarrytown, New York, in April 1995. The focus of this workshop was on the use of process facilitation and strategic questioning skills in network building. Participants came from all regions previously involved in legal and ethical networking. A manual of the workshop materials is being produced on the use of process facilitation for network building to address legal, ethical and human rights issues.

3.7 Networking: Creating Spaces for Discussion, Support and Action

In a similar way, networks of people living with HIV and AIDS assist in both building capacity for representation and participation in policy and programme development, and in ensuring that expertise and commitment contribute to the strengthening of local and national responses. Such networks are important vehicles for protecting the rights of those affected and for providing protection and sanctuary. They enable those affected to enter into partnerships and provide the possibility of continuing organisational effectiveness even when illness and death affect individuals' ability to continue.

The Programme has provided a range of support to people living with HIV in their efforts to create national, regional and global networks, in advocacy of the principles of recognition and involvement, in the recognition of the particular expertise that living within the epidemic creates, and through involving them as partners in all its work.

It worked with the UNDP Regional Project on HIV and Development for Africa to assist with the creation of the Network of African People Living with HIV and AIDS (NAP+). It has been active in the formulation and implementation of the UN Personnel Policy on HIV and AIDS. Assistance has been provided to the Global Network of People Living With HIV/AIDS (GNP+) through provision of training in strategic planning and programme development. Support has also been provided to the International Community of Women Living With HIV and AIDS (ICW) to report on the lessons learnt during a pre-conference meeting held prior to the VIIth International Conference for People Living With HIV/AIDS, in Capetown, South Africa in March 1995.

In preparation for the Capetown Conference of People Living with HIV and AIDS, the Programme funded two GNP+ Board members to visit and work with groups of people living with HIV in Zimbabwe, Zambia, South Africa and Namibia.

The Programme has also worked closely with networks and organizations providing care and support to those affected. In particular, it has strong and continuing partnerships with ICASO, especially through its regional councils. It has also worked with the International HIV/AIDS Alliance and its national linking organizations.

3.8 Understanding Gender and HIV

The work of HDP addressing issues of particular relevance to women has focussed in two main areas: creating a greater awareness and understanding of the gender dimensions of the epidemic and developing more effective strategies to assist women.

From its start, the Programme has adopted the principles of gender sensitivity, representation and responsiveness to guide its work. It has sought an equitable participation of women in all its work and has played an important early role, especially through its publications and presentations, in drawing global and national attention to issues such as the epidemiology of infection amongst women, the susceptibility of young women to infection, the need for methods of protection that women can use in their socio-economic settings, the relationship between cultural and medical practices and infection rates amongst women, and the inequitable burden of care that communities and nations place on women.

Analysis of the way in which social and economic policies and institutions increase the effect of the epidemic on women led the Programme to an understanding of the causes of men's vulnerability to HIV infection and of their critical role in any strategies for women. A number of publications and presentations have addressed this issue.

There is now greater awareness of HIV infection rates amongst women and of the other ways in which the epidemic affects their daily lives but much more work is needed to develop effective approaches and practices to address these issues. The complexity of the analysis militates against narrowly focussed or single item responses.

The Programme has worked closely with women, and with organisations working with women, to increase understanding of how initiatives directed specifically towards women can help. It has also considered areas in which approaches directed towards men, or towards the contexts in which male-female relationships occur, are needed in order to better assist women and those they care about and for.

3.9 Civil-military Issues and HIV

It is estimated that HIV prevalence in military populations in a number of countries may be as high as 50 per cent. Reliable information on infection rates is scarce because of the enormous sensitivity surrounding the topic. This has strategic, political, social, economic and security implications at both national and global levels. In some countries security forces have begun to take action by working with national HIV/AIDS programmes. However, HIV within the military will continue to pose very difficult policy dilemmas both in branches of the military and in national contexts. Issues of concern include the effect on civilian populations, the ethics of mandatory testing, civil-military collaboration for prevention and care, and implications for peacekeeping operations.

Over the past few years, the HDP has been working in partnership with interested governments and institutions to explore civil-military issues around HIV. One outcome of these efforts has been the establishment of an international organisation, the Civil-Military Alliance to Combat HIV and AIDS, which now receives support from a number of UN organisations including UNAIDS and the World Bank, as well as from bi-lateral agencies including USAID.

Within this context, the HDP has been providing technical support and guidance to countries through facilitated study tours, missions and consultations. It has participated in meetings and training workshops of the Civil-Military Alliance and is represented on the Board of that Alliance. In December 1995, at the request of the Vietnamese Armed Forces, the Programme organised a facilitated study tour to enable them to discuss policy and programme issues with neighbouring Armed Forces and to explore ways for civil organisations and the military to work together. A group of senior military and civilian officials from Vietnam visited Thailand and the Philippines. The study tour was facilitated by a senior military doctor from the Papua New Guinea National HIV/AIDS Programme, a partner of HDP.

3.10 Learning, Advocating and Disseminating: Promoting more Complex Understanding and Action

The HIV epidemic is challenging accepted ways of understanding health and human development in our societies and demanding new forms of expertise and more integrated responses. It is raising conceptual, ethical and programmatic issues, many of which still need to be named, all of which need to be raised for discussion and exploration. The aim of the HDP publications and presentations has been to raise new or neglected issues, to encourage people to consider old issues in new ways, and to articulate the questions many of these issues raise about accepted ways of doing things.

The publications policy has been to keep papers brief, simply written and limited to issues not addressed, or not addressed from the same perspective, elsewhere. Authors are asked not to outline solutions but rather to stimulate the reflection and discussion essential for well-informed processes of change to arise within their own contexts. Publications have included issues and working papers, research studies, posters, statements of principles, training materials and a book.

Declarations drawn up at consultations and conferences organised by either the HDP or by UNDP's regional HIV and Development projects have been distributed in poster format, encouraging policy makers and practitioners to display them on walls of government offices, resource centres, clinics and other places used by people responding to the epidemic. These included the *Statement of belief on behaviour change as a central issue in responding to the HIV epidemic,* drawn up at an informal consultation hosted by the HDP in Senegal in December 1991, and the *Dakar Declaration of the African Network on Ethics, Law and HIV.* These short statements were widely distributed, both promoting and summarising new forms of discourse arising through sustainable human development responses to the HIV epidemic.

Many other issues were covered in papers which examined the multisectoral nature of the epidemic's socio-economic causes and consequences, and the development of effective, sustainable and compassionate responses. These papers cover themes relating to all the areas of the HDP, and titles include: *The HIV epidemic and development: the unfolding of the epidemic; The economic impact of the HIV epidemic; People living with HIV: the law, ethics and discrimination; Sharing the challenge of the epidemic: building partnerships; Young women: silence, susceptibility and the HIV epidemic; Children in families affected by the HIV epidemic: a strategic approach; The HIV epidemic in Uganda: a programme approach; The socio-economic impact of HIV and AIDS on rural families in Uganda.*

In order to diversify the voices of the HIV epidemic and to disseminate the lessons learnt thus far in developing countries, the HIV and Development Programme published a book entitled, *HIV and AIDS: The Global Inter-Connection* (Kumarian Press, 1995).

In order to ensure that the issues are accessible, the HDP has worked in a number of collaborative ways to ensure that its publications are available in a number of languages. It is working with Spanish-speaking and French-speaking HIV support organizations to strengthen their capacity to translate and distribute relevant HIV materials. The partner organization chooses material considered to be of relevance to the region and sets priorities for translation. It also identifies material for translation into English and other languages. The book, *HIV and AIDS: The Global Inter-Connection,* has been translated into Bahasa Indonesian, Bengali, Sinhala, Thai, Urdu and Vietnamese through a partnership programme with local publishing houses. It is presently under discussion for translation into French, Spanish, Japanese, and into Swahili by a consortium of people living with HIV or AIDS and government officials in Kenya and Tanzania. HDP materials have also been translated into Arabic, Russian, Chinese and Portuguese.

HDP materials are considered as public domain materials and it is made clear that they can be reproduced in whole or in part by any person wishing to understand and explore these issues further. HDP asks only for some acknowledgement and for suggestions for further papers and for comments on the series.

The HDP distribution policy is to distribute materials free of charge within UNDP programme countries, whenever interest is shown in receiving them. The materials have been widely distributed, in and outside of urban areas, to government and non-government organisations, to libraries and academic institutions. They have also been handed on from person to person.

The value of these publications in catalysing the responses to the epidemic of people in their own contexts was highlighted in comments made by Eduardo Nierras, an evaluation participant in the Philippines:

> My interest grew from my apprehension about the way HIV issues are gender and development issues. This leads to all sorts of understandings that people were, or are, trying to move towards, ... these papers showed me that other people were also thinking about these issues ...

4. UNDERSTANDING THE APPROACH IN THE CONTEXT OF EVOLVING NEW DEVELOPMENT PARADIGMS AND PRACTICES

The time is ripe for a thorough rethinking of development theory and practice. The costly mistakes based on the conventional modernisation paradigm and a top-down approach to development have to be rectified, and the right lessons must be learnt.

Perhaps the key lesson is that development starts with the people, and with their knowledge, culture and traditions as assets rather than liabilities. Unless this is taken as the point of departure, insensitive or impatient governments—and foreign donors— may easily destroy valuable social capital in the name of growth and "modernization."

Stefan de Vylder, development economist and practitioner (de Vylder, 1995, p.57)

These pleas for revision, made as concluding remarks to a recent UNDP discussion paper, provide a useful starting point for considering the association between the new approach to development and the HIV epidemic. The HIV and Development Programme explored the relevance of new development practices to the response to the HIV epidemic and, in turn, contributed to a better understanding of development practices generally, and specifically of UNDP's evolving approach to human development.

4.1 Key Lessons Learnt

This section is based on a review of selected literature on development practice and the nature of social change, and on interactive discussions which were held between evaluation team members and staff of the HIV and Development Programme. Consideration of what is now known about sustainable human development, capacity building and the role of UNDP led to deeper understanding about the way in which the approach of the HDP fits within the evolving framework of development practice and, in turn, has been able to contribute to development of this framework.

Discussions were informed by publications on the need for reappraisal of traditional approaches of technical co-operation in development, along with a recognition of the nature of the HIV epidemic. The HIV epidemic epitomises the need for new approaches to development practice because of the close association between the epidemic and human development, the continually changing nature of the causes and impacts of the epidemic in specific local settings, the fact that traditional approaches have mostly failed to reduce either the spread of the epidemic or to minimise its impact and, most importantly, because no one can claim to have expert understanding of what will work in all contexts to address the challenges of HIV and development.

The evaluation found that the work of the HDP is clearly situated within the conceptual and operational framework of UNDP's work, and that its approach is consistent with concepts used by UNDP. The Programme is contributing to the development of understanding of UNDP's evolving approach through learning more about what works in practice.

In particular, the Programme has put into practice the challenges of working in a way which catalyzes analysis and action by the people whose lives are affected. It has explored the implications of working to develop capacity through approaches based on partnership rather than dissemination of pre-conceived knowledge, it has learnt how to act as an agency which mobilizes people, and it has learnt how to be self-critical and self-evaluating.

The Programme's approach is situated within theoretical frameworks which help to guide these new approaches, and draws on understanding of social learning, strategic questioning and process consultation. Each of these frameworks emphasises the central role of transformation: transformation of individuals' perceptions and sense of personal empowerment, transformation of institutional approaches, and transformation of the roles of development practitioners. In these ways, the Programme has contributed to understanding of how sustainable human development works in practice, and of how such practice can contribute to more effective responses to the HIV epidemic.

4.2 Recognising the Need for New Approaches to Development and to the HIV Epidemic

Many development agencies, including UNDP, are re-considering what types of development practice may be effective in the context of current crises in meeting development needs (Banuri, *et al.* 1994). The imperative for change arises from a recognition that traditional forms of technical co-operation have been less than effective in meeting their objectives.

The report of a recent High-Level Seminar of the OECD's Development Assistance Committee, UNDP and the World Bank notes some current problems with technical co-operation (OECD/UNDP/World Bank, 1994). Though referring to development in general, some of these problems apply also to the field of HIV and development:

> Technical co-operation is donor driven ... Any single donor may be marginal, but in the aggregate, donors exert a powerful distorting influence on national processes of priority setting and resource mobilization and allocation.
>
> Technical co-operation has supported the monopolization of resources and power by governments ... (which) has not been compatible with social and economic progress.
>
> Within donor agencies there are short time horizons and pressure to deliver resources.

In facilitating responses to the HIV epidemic, top-down approaches based on what has been learnt in a few wealthy countries, and based on the need to be seen to produce quick results, are often the norm in developing countries.

Many programmes are funded by donors in a manner which assumes that people in various contexts simply need to be told "the truth" about the HIV epidemic; that the only sensible responses are use of condoms and treatment of those who are ill using expensive modern drugs which do not in fact save lives; that measuring the numbers of people infected is possible and is an essential component of an adequate response (at no matter what cost); and that tradition, especially religious beliefs and traditional medicine, is a hindrance in dealing with such a new phenomenon as the HIV epidemic.

The net result of such programmes, as widely acknowledged, is that responses to the HIV epidemic in many countries are ineffective in slowing down transmission rates, in reducing stigma and discrimination against those infected and those close to them, and in generating effective responses to the challenges the epidemic presents to human development.

The inadequacy of the application of classical approaches to technical co-operation to the HIV epidemic is further highlighted because so many of the problems which need to be solved are not yet fully understood by anyone, no matter how expertise is defined. For example:

- the epidemic in one country may be very different to that in another;
- the problems at one stage of the epidemic may be different to those at a later stage;
- the way the epidemic spreads is influenced by different development strategies, economic systems, and political situations;
- the possible range of responses to the epidemic depends just as much on personal and community-wide commitment to their resolution as on what may be externally viewed as necessary; and
- there are no obvious technical solutions, or even models of programme design, which are either entirely effective or readily transferable from one context to another.

How, then, can this be changed? What is required to generate effective responses to the challenges presented by the HIV epidemic in the context of development, or to the challenges of development in the context of the HIV epidemic?

4.3 Possibilities for Reform, and Implications for Addressing the HIV Epidemic

Partial answers to these questions may be found more readily in recent discussions about the nature of development than in discourse about the HIV epidemic. The OECD/UNDP/World Bank seminar suggested the following as part of an "Agenda for reform":

> On the donor side, there would need to be ... a commitment to provide support over longer periods with realistic time frames ... a different approach to the design of technical co-operation, with longer periods taken for a thorough analysis of problems and more extensive discussion of possible solutions, including the establishment of mechanisms for participation in decision making at each stage, and without donor pressure to regard technical co-operation as a necessary part of the solution to problems identified...On the recipient side, ... a strategic vision of the role of the public sector, governance, and the elements of an enabling environment for development.
>
> (OECD/UNDP/World Bank, 1994; see also OECD, 1991)

UNDP has responded to the challenges of this "Agenda for reform" through the development of more complex perspectives on human development:

> Sustainable human development is the enlargement of people's choices and capabilities through the formation of social capital so as to meet as equitably as possible the needs of current generations without compromising the needs of future ones.
>
> (Banuri, *et al.* 1994, p. 21)

The UNDP discussion paper in which this definition first appeared suggests that sustainable human development will result from new approaches within what it describes as "a new development paradigm". The HIV and Development Programme has explored approaches consistent with these suggestions.

Working within the framework of sustainable human development, the Programme has been based on a commitment to ensuring that solutions to the problems of HIV and development arise from:

— an enhanced capacity of individuals, communities and nations to understand the nature of the epidemic in their own contexts; and

— an enhanced capacity of individuals, communities and nations to find effective means to address those problems; which in turn depends on

— an enhanced capacity for people and organisations in all sectors (government, NGOs, the private sector, health and development agencies, religious organizations, and others) to work co-operatively and communicate with each other about problem definition as well as resolution.

No amount of technical co-operation can, on its own, enhance these capacities but it can facilitate necessary social change:

- — change in people's perception of their own roles and capacities in enhancing human development;
- — changes in the ways individuals and institutions relate to one another;
- — changes in the focus of analysis (from virus to people and their inter-relationships);
- — changes in the nature of what needs to be done, who needs to do it and where and how the impetus begins.

For these changes to be sustained, there needs to be a strong and widespread willingness to respond to the epidemic, and an external environment which enables such responses: an environment which encompasses cultural, policy-making, political and legal factors which influence people's abilities to understand and to act.

What, then, is the most useful role for an international development agency? How can effective development practice be applied within the HIV epidemic? Such questions cannot be explored independently of advances in understanding of development practice, nor of advances in understanding of the epidemic. The UNDP HIV and Development Programme complements the roles of many other UN, bilateral and NGO donor agencies working in development and in response to the HIV epidemic. The HDP therefore deliberately focuses on exploration of the association between HIV and development, and how more effective development practice can generate more effective responses.

The Programme is thus situated within the overall conceptual and operational framework of UNDP's work. Its approach is consistent with concepts used by UNDP, especially the concepts of sustainable human development, capacity building, social learning and partnership (Banuri, *et al.* 1994). Discussion about the new paradigm of sustainable human development has led to suggested guidelines, or starting points, for practice within this paradigm. The Programme contributes to this new discourse through having learnt more about what works in practice.

4.4 Learning to Move Forward, Along an Ever-Changing Path

A central question being constantly explored through the SPR is, "How can we, together, move forward?" Answering this questions leads to choices in the types of processes used, with the ultimate goal of assisting social change. Interim processes include identifying people and organisations who are social change agents, working with them and supporting them through partnership, and the facilitation of their networking with each other.

A useful framework to inform the nature of such social change processes can be found in a seminal work by Schon, *Beyond the Stable State* (Schon, 1971). Although written in response to crises in the welfare states of wealthy countries in the 1970s, the theoretical frameworks outlined by Schon have relevance for human development now.

Schon explores the nature of social change. He notes that the dominant model for diffusion of new ideas is based on the concept that, "A communicates to B what B does not know but A does". Like classical technical co-operation in development, which is based on the same model, this is inadequate to facilitate the range of innovations which are required to meet the complex realities of modern societies.

In what could now be seen as a forerunner to recent discussions on crises in development and in the international organisation of societies and nations, Schon notes that,

> Over time, we shift our perceptions on the problems that need solving. But institutions have an internal life of their own; consequently there are always mismatches between the institutional map and the problems thought worth solving.
>
> (Schon, 1971, p. 182)

The complex problems caused and/or highlighted by the HIV epidemic provide good examples of a proliferation of such problems. Just as the problems of human development are not solved just by the creation of good banking systems, so the problems of an epidemic driven by complex and dynamic social and behavioural systems are not solved by the improvement of medical or educational systems alone.

Schon's central thesis is that as such mismatches between problems and institutions becomes endemic, so do all sorts of responses, which vary in effectiveness and can in turn create their own problems. The net result is the loss of "the stable state". The challenge, then, is to find productive ways to deal with the consequences of the loss of the stable state.

The answers, Schon suggests, arise through processes of "social learning": a concept central to the newly defined human development paradigm. An imperative for effective change is the application of social learning to changing the nature of the state in general, rather than focussing on independent institutions. Failure to do so will result in endemic crises, as have now been identified in current discussions on development (Banuri, *et al.* 1994, pp.9-11; de Vylder, 1995, pp. 8-1 l).

Social learning requires an emphasis on process rather than

forseen outcomes, and on the generation of autonomous yet networked responses akin to the characteristics of social movements, rather than on the restructuring of individual institutions:

> The importance of this movement is not that it permits once-and-for-all redesign of institutions, but that it permits continual redesign of organisational elements within the framework of broad functional systems. Hence, the need for an internal organisation which can be continually redesigned without flying apart at the seams. Within the system, the foreground condition is not stability but change. Attention focuses on the process of transforming one structure into another rather than on the resulting structure.
>
> (Schon, 1971, p.184)

This is entirely consistent with the recent suggestion that, "UNDP must see itself as: (1) a catalyst and an advocate for social change; (2) an agency which mobilizes stakeholders in sustainable human development; (3) a supporter of potential partners; (4) a self-critical and self evaluating body; and (5) a promoter of institutions that enhance accountability and responsibility of all partners" (Banuri, *et al.* 1994, p. 7). It is also consistent with the approach of the HDP in that the Programme works in these transformational ways, is process-defined, and consciously works with, and promotes co-operation between, governments, NGOs, communities and individuals affected by HIV and by development.

Practical suggestions on how to bring about the required changes can be found in three critical components of the new approach to development which have all been drawn upon to directly inform the work of the programme: the need to start with people's own perceptions of their realities and to promote more actively the role of expertise which arises from lived experiences (Chambers, 1994); the use of "strategic questioning" (Peavey, 1994); and the culmination of a range of new approaches in a method of facilitation developed by Management Development and Governance Programme of UNDP and called, "Process Consultation" (Joy and Bennett, 1994).

4.5 Who Defines what is Real, and what is Needed?

The first of these was suggested in a paper prepared as an overview for a recent UNDP roundtable discussion (Chambers, 1994). Under the title, "Poverty and livelihoods: whose reality counts?", the author draws attention to the vast differences between the perceptions of poverty held by professionals and the perceptions experienced by the people who actually live in poverty. He suggests that the most valuable expertise in both understanding reality and knowing what changes are needed is the expertise which arises from lived experience. This understanding of expertise presents major challenges to those working in development and requires major changes in approach: "If poor people's realities are to come first, development professionals have to be sensitive, to decentralism and to empower, enabling poor people to conduct their own analysis and express their own multiple priorities" (Chambers, 1994, p.16).

The author notes that these challenges are not simple:

> The challenges are paradigmatic: to reverse the normal view, to upend perspectives, to see things the other way around, to soften and flatten hierarchy, to adopt downward accountability, to change behaviour, attitudes, and beliefs, and to identify and implement a new agenda; in sum, to define and embrace a new professionalism. (Chambers, 1994, p. 20)

Again referring to the need for a new agenda in development, this author suggests four pillars for a poverty agenda:

— analysis and action by local people, and putting first the priorities of the poor;
— the promotion of sustainable livelihoods (rather than simply economic growth);
— decentralization, democracy and diversity; and
— professional and personal change.

Such changes, he suggests, demand, "... altruism, insight, vision and guts" (Chambers, 1994, p. 28).

The scope of the changes required in development practice as a result of starting with people's own realities should not be underestimated. People's realities include not just perceptions of the world as it is, but also understandings of the ways it can be changed. These can lead to entirely new ways of defining and reaching programme goals.

4.6 Asking Useful Questions to the Right People

A second component of enhancing understanding of people's realities is the use of "strategic questioning" (Peavey, 1994). Strategic questioning is a process in which the person investigating and the person investigated become equal partners in a process of learning. One can find power in approaching a problem with the feeling of, "I don't know", or in allowing doubt into what is already known. Such attitudes open doors to new possibilities, through which both the listener and the person being questioned can realise change.

Strategic questioning is the skill of asking questions which will make a difference. It is characterized by six key features. In summary, strategic questions:

— are dynamic and create motion (for example, by asking, "How can we, together, move forward?");
— create options;
— can be a lever to reveal in-depth information;
— do not lead to "yes" or "no" answers;
— empower the person being questioned; and
— sometimes include "unaskable" questions which challenge assumptions and values.

4.7 The Central Role of Process in Building Capacity

Finally, a set of processes which have been adopted by the HIV and Development Programme is suggested in the guide, "UNDP Process Consultation: Systemic Improvement of Public Sector Management" (Joy and Bennett, 1994). This guide was developed to assist countries to face the challenges of building capacity for systemic public sector change and reform. It suggests that UNDP's role is to support that process by contributing resources and by, "... facilitating the sharing of experiences and insights in different areas of development" (Joy and Bennett, 1994, p. iii). In essence, the role of the external agency is to suggest issues to consider and processes which might be used to consider them, not to explain "realities" or to provide "answers".

Suggesting issues and processes is exactly what the Programme did, for example, with work in the legal, ethical and human rights fields. It would have been inappropriate and ineffective for the Programme to determine exactly what changes should be made to the legal and ethical environment in each country, because each country is different, as highlighted in the UNDP guide to process consultation:

> Client systems are not all in the same state of change-readiness or need: technical co-operation must start where the change programme is and support what the change programme needs next ... UNDP has a role in maintaining momentum not in providing direction. ... Action plans evolve with commitment; the client context is constantly changing and the UNDP programme needs to be responsive to and patient with this. ... Different forms of technical co-operation will be needed at different stages of a reform programme.
>
> (Joy and Bennett, 1994, pp. 3-5)

Consistent with the general approach of sustainable human development, the guide suggests a strong emphasis on working with processes rather than endpoints. It suggests that a further aspect of the approach required now, as used by the Programme, should be to explore the nature of the new development paradigm through simultaneous practice and reflection, rather than through desk-top programme planning followed by action: "New roles, and the new relationships they imply, are worked out and learnt by discussion and interaction" (Joy and Bennett, 1994, p. 37).

Importantly, the guide to process consultation also recognises the importance of the view of reality of an agency such as the HIV and Development Programme, recognising that there is room for outsiders to bring their own perspectives to problems, so long as those perspectives are offered in dialogue, not as "solutions" to which funding is tied. Such an approach was typical of the Programme's work in capacity building for undertaking research which would contribute to better policy and programming responses to the epidemic (see Case Study 1). The Programme's central role in this project was to ensure that an adequate range of people was involved in determining both research needs and methods, rather than a role of indicating what should be investigated through research.

4.8 Transformation as an Essential Component of Development

The UNDP process consultation guide affirms that "transformation" plays a central role in the new development paradigm. The central concern of the guide is with transformation of structures and processes, whereas the HDP staff are more critically aware of the need to enhance the understanding and practice of social change agents as a means of working towards this.

There is consistency between the guide and the Programme's approach in seeing transformation as something which will not happen overnight, in using processes which lead towards transformation rather than specifying the outcomes of that transformation, in recognising the central importance of developing relationships, and in continually grounding the programme in people's lived realities:

> There should be no attempt to specify all activities in detail, no pressure to complete every step within the timeframe stated or to hold inflexibly to what at first seemed the best sequence of activities. Expectations should be modified based on feedback from actual experience.
>
> (Joy and Bennett, 1994, p. 21)

4.9 The Evolving Nature of Sustainable Human Development

It is in this context that the Programme has worked, through developing, implementing and constantly evaluating new approaches through partnership with people in their own contexts. Indeed, the evaluation has been merely one more form of gaining the "feedback from actual experience" suggested in the above paragraph.

Most importantly, both the Programme and the evaluation are elements of a necessarily ongoing process of experimentation and learning. While much has been learnt to date, the path ahead is by no means certain, and there is a need for continual questioning in the context of ongoing partnerships with those whose lives are directly affected by the challenges of HIV and of development. The promotion of better understanding and more effective action in response to the HIV epidemic and development is at a stage which is typical of the field of sustainable human development in general:

> It is still too early to attempt a synthesis of the new theory of growth and development which appears to be emerging. The trend is clear, however: a more multi-disciplinary approach to development is gaining ground, signifying, among other things, more emphasis on people, ideas and institutions, and less on money and factories.
>
> (de Vylder S. 1995, p. 11)

The Programme has incorporated the need for continual learning with the need for urgent practice. In so doing, it has enhanced understanding of what is needed and has demonstrated that it is both possible and desirable to continue questioning the value of approaches as they are being implemented.

A final lesson, along the lines of what is now called "international best practice", may never be reached. This is because each country and each context within countries is different; the epidemic is evolving, and sustainable human development is itself a process, not an outcome. In the words of an evaluation participant from the Philippines, "International best practice is about starting a process." The most useful role for outsiders, then, may well be to help people to find their own effective processes. The development which results would then be relevant, sustainable and centred on people's most crucial needs.

5. DEEPENING UNDERSTANDING OF PRACTICAL IMPLICATIONS OF A SUSTAINABLE HUMAN DEVELOPMENT APPROACH

5.1 Key Lessons Learnt

This section is based on the results of interactive discussions held in the field between evaluation team members, partners of the Programme and others who have been involved in using similar approaches. It reports on issues of central concern to the evaluation.

It is one thing to say that new approaches are needed in development practice. It's another thing to build capacity in situations, like the HIV epidemic, in which no-one knows what will work, in which inappropriate development practices have sometimes already stifled the creation of effective local understanding and action, and in which the people whose lives are affected are often marginalised through poverty, cultural factors and lack of involvement in community and national decision-making processes.

In developing better understanding of what does work, it was therefore considered important that the evaluators go out into the field to engage in dialogue with the people whose lives are affected, and to not limit discussion specifially to the approach of just this one Programme. People were able to explain and discuss, with the evaluation team and with each other, what has worked to develop their own capacities, what has led to their own sense of creative engagement with the challenges of HIV and development, and what has resulted from these approaches.

Participants talked of their own experiences of capacity development. They often mentioned the need for the new approaches to proceed slowly at first, reporting that their own engagement and empowerment had arisen not from being told what to do, but through working in partnership with others who respected and encouraged gradual development of their own understanding, skills and actions.

Central to these processes was the concept of partnership. The evaluation process generated deeper understanding of what sorts of partnerships lead to capacity development. Key themes which arose through interactive dialogue are summarised here and explained in further detail in the text.

Many key findings centre on the nature of partnerships which build capacity:

— If development and maintenance of partnerships is genuine, then they will follow the usual patterns of human relationships

— Effective partnerships take time to establish and essentially involve two-way dialogue and development
— Effective partnerships are not always initiated or controlled by donor agencies or by central government authorities
— Effective partnerships allow all partners to make choices
— Effective partnerships acknowledge the contributions of all parties involved
— Effective partnerships are not always easy.

Others indicated some immediate effects of such partnerships:

— Inclusion of the people whose lives are affected in developing understanding and responses
— The development of 'safe spaces' which enable those included to discuss issues of central importance to them.
— The reflection and sharing of experiences, thus leading to understanding which would not normally be generated

Finally, a set of key findings indicated the longer-term results of the partnership approach to capacity building:

— Validation of people's own experiences and perceptions
— Development of empathy and deep understanding amongst the people whose lives are affected and thus amongst the people most likely to be able to work together to find effective solutions
— Experiences of solidarity which enable people to act together
— Empowerment and the releasing of energy, particularly amongst people who previously had felt disempowered and unable to either fully understand their own situations or act to bring about useful change
— Ultimately, effective and sustainable outcomes which result in long term and adaptable social change which addresses the challenges of HIV and development.

Following description of these key themes, a case study is presented which outlines the way approaches based on capacity development worked in practice in an ongoing project of the Programme to enhance national capacity through HIV action research. This case study demonstrates, from the perspective of the Programme, how the approach evolved, what was learnt about what works, what difficulties have been experienced through this practical experience, and thus what suggestions can be made for ongoing work by the Programme and others.

5.2 The Process of Capacity Building within the HIV Epidemic

The following sections highlight some of what has been learnt through the use of SPR about how the new development paradigm can be realised in practice. They are based directly on the data collected through personal interaction during the evaluation process: dialogues with individuals in the four countries visited, and interactive workshops.

Much information was collected in the form of narrative and "thick description". Of necessity, this section includes only the most significant findings, collated and summarised by the evaluation team after further dialogue and shared reflection ("interpretive interactionism". One important finding that is almost impossible to convey through a written report was the depth of feeling expressed by many evaluation participants about their involvement in responding to the epidemic. These included feelings associated with grief, loss and pain, but also included equally intense feelings of hope and confidence that they were, indeed, engaged in effective responses to the epidemic which are leading to worthwhile and positive changes. Many participants responded enthusiastically to the very idea of discussing processes which work, noting that such processes are often overlooked in attempts made to understand the global response to the epidemic.

Although grouped into sections in order to make the information more accessible, in reality there was much overlap between people's understanding of various concepts. The information is presented here as a further contribution to the discourse about the new development paradigm and its interaction with the HIV epidemic.

Central to discussion on sustainable human development, and to the work of the Programme, is the concept of capacity building. This was included in the list of "Concepts UNDP is currently using," which was used to generate discussion during Stage 5 of the evaluation process. The HDP aims to build capacity not just of individuals and organisations but of whole nations. Reflecting the need to commence with building capacity to understand, not just to act, the programme uses partnership and processes of shared problem solving, rather than skills transition, to develop capacity.

A crucial aspect of capacity building is that it builds on what is already there, even when existing capacity is not recognised by those who have it, as explained by John Musanje, from Zambia: "We need to mobilise the indigenous potential." The resulting enthusiasm expressed by evaluation participants who had been involved with the Programme is typified in the comment of David Chipanta, also from Zambia, that, "They (HDP) helped me see capacities that are dormant, such as the capability to listen, to change and to adapt."

What are the features of capacity building which generate understanding and more effective responses to the HIV epidemic? The next few sub-sections explain processes which people have found helpful in developing their own and their nations' capacities. Before these, the report addresses some more general aspects about the nature of capacity building within the context of the HIV epidemic.

5.3 Building Capacity to Respond in Different and Changing Contexts

A central feature identified by evaluation participants is that people and nations now require capacity to quickly understand and respond to changing contexts, not just to familiar or repeated situations. While some people noted that each stage of the epidemic presents different challenges, many noted also the evolving nature of their understanding of what is occurring and what is now required. Consider this quote from Roland Msiska, the former National HIV/AIDS Programme Manager in Zambia, reflecting on both his personal development of capacity and the way his programme now has to work:

> So, none of these deaths is the same. Each death raises different questions, different challenges. Each time you change, you become less dogmatic, more one who asks questions. ... Each death gives a different dimension to the epidemic. Yet we may have been dealing with the epidemic as if it's a single epidemic. There are different epidemics, moving around; they are constantly dynamic.

The changing nature of the epidemic and of emotional and cultural responses is not widely acknowledged, yet is an important feature of people's own perceptions of reality, and therefore affects their requirements in capacity building.

A corollary of the complex and dynamic nature of such capacity building is that capacity must be developed across institutional and state/community boundaries. This requires working with a range of institutions, as is reflected in the Programme's commitment to bringing together governments with NGOs, military with civil organisations, and researchers with users of research. In order that this work be effective, it simultaneously requires an emphasis on working with individuals, as noted by Carlos del Rio, the National AIDS Programme Manager in Mexico:

> Deep cultural changes have to occur, you need a societal response. Children must learn. Social realities must change ...

we need a deep effort ... But I have learnt that responses are personal not institutional.

The challenge of catalysing social change which grows from individual commitment can be met, in part, through working with individuals who act as social change agents. This can sometimes mean identifying people who already play that role, and sometimes mean drawing out the capacity of individuals to act as social change agents. This concept was well understood by many evaluation participants: individuals can catalyse sustainable human development within their own communities, through using processes similar to the concept of process consultations, as highlighted in a comment from Teresita Bagasao from the Philippines, who said that, "Being a social change agent is about asking questions."

The need for identifying and working with individuals who are potential social change agents was identified early in the Programme's development. The value of doing this was also a central theme in evaluation participants' comments about both their own and others' responses to the epidemic. The importance of individuals' commitment was highlighted in comments made by the National AIDS Programme Managers interviewed; from Zambia, the Philippines and Mexico. All three talked of the complexity of their jobs and the need to work across institutional and professional boundaries, of occasional or regular tiredness, but also of a strong commitment to their work; they had also noted varying levels of engagement and commitment from those with whom they work.

Another central requirement of capacity building is that of honesty, especially the honesty of being able to admit when simple solutions are not available or appropriate. Due to the complex and dynamic nature of the epidemic, it is not possible for any one individual or organisation to know how to deal with every problem that arises. During interactive discussions, for example, evaluation participants often responded very positively to being told that the Programme is questioning the nature of expertise. The general feeling was that so many of the problems which people now face are so new, so complex and so different to problems which can be addressed by one professional discipline or another, that there can no longer be "experts" in the traditional sense of the word. However, the nature of honesty and expertise is also relevant in a strategic sense: "Even saying, 'I don't have the answers', you have an answer", was a typical comment (again from Roland Msiska in Zambia). It expressed that working together with people to find answers can build capacity much more quickly than claiming that your own expertise is universally applicable.

Rather than focusing on skills transition, the Programme has found that capacity building arises from the development of shared learning through working in partnerships, as explained by Teresita Bagasao with reference to her own interaction with the Programme and the flow-on effects within her own work with NGOs in the Philippines:

> How do you consider agents of change? They can be experts and manipulate things. Or they can be experienced people but know that they're entering a different set of circumstances, so merge one's knowledge and experience with the country they're entering. That's the essence of partnership.

5.4 Characteristics of Partnerships which Develop Capacity

Consistent with the general approach of promoting sustainable human development, the role of the outsider in identifying social change agents is, to a large extent, indirect. The aim is not to go into other people's contexts (countries, communities) and identify individuals as social change agents but, rather, to establish partnerships which facilitate communities identifying and working with their own social change agents. A primary means of doing this is through bringing people together in groups and networks.

Thus, the first consultative meeting to discuss directions for the SPR, in October 1992, determined that a key element of the Programme should be, "To identify and to characterize the necessary and sufficient conditions for the development and maintenance of group and social cohesion". A primary reason for this was that, "The functional group—family, village, community, society—is the ultimate resource for behaviour change, for care and support, and for coping with the impact of the epidemic."

One method used to explore what is needed for development and maintenance of group cohesion was the development and maintenance of partnerships, commencing but not limited to partnerships between the Programme and those affected by the epidemic. Many comments were made by evaluation participants about the nature of those partnerships which develop capacity. Some of the recurring themes in these comments are summarised in the following points.

If development and maintenance of partnerships is genuine, then they will follow the usual patterns of human relationships. Sometimes partnerships will succeed without effort, sometimes enormous emphasis will have to be placed on maintaining the relationships, and sometimes they will fail. Ultimately, when partnerships work, they result in growth and changes amongst all partners concerned. These sorts of comments were made with reference to the Programme's relationships with its direct partners, to those partners' relationships with others in their own countries and in international networks, and to other partnerships which were identified by evaluation participants as examples of effective capacity building.

Effective partnerships take time to establish and essentially involve two-way dialogue and development. Capacity building does not work through patronising relationships, such as when donors have all the ideas and claimed expertise and involve local partners only in programme implementation. An example of this way of operating and the long term result was given by Peter Resurreccion, who works constantly across government/NGO boundaries in the Philippines, as he talked of earlier experience in the Department of Health:

> In the early years, foreign donor agencies came in and just did what they wanted. This led to me feeling like an admin person. I was just there to answer what they need ... and when they left, it all stopped.

In contrast to this, effective partnerships involve all partners being able to constantly question and challenge themselves and each other. Many participants reported that the HDP, and UNDP in general, often allowed this to occur. For example, Assistant Secretary Antonio Dujua, from the Department of Justice in the Philippines, noted that,

> UNDP doesn't foist things upon us ... they give hints, but don't say, "This is the way." And that gives us a sense of independence, with more room for creativity and productivity ... At the [UNDP] workshop on ethics, law and HIV there were people from many Asian countries. Each country has different legal systems and approaches, but the main objectives of the people at the workshop were the same. For example, trying to ensure that there would be no mandatory testing ... There were spaces where we could express ourselves, across cultures ... Some countries already had legislation. I came back here thinking that I could be able to push legislation.

The way effective dialogue can flow on from Programme partners to others was highlighted in comments made by staff of two Filipino NGO agencies which work to build the capacity of others in the Philippines through ongoing partnerships based on approaches identical to that of the Programme. These two people, from Kabalikat and Phansup (Philippine AIDS NGO Support Network) each noted that their own work reflects the way that Programme staff spend time "up front" in identifying potential Programme partners and in working to establish mutual understanding of roles and expectations before rushing into long-term partnerships. Such time consuming work does not always result in effective partnerships, but was reported to be an essential component of those which are effective. The results of such work are not always measurable using traditional measures of cost-effectiveness or project outputs, especially when time spent early on leads to decisions to discontinue potential, but in practice ineffective, partnerships.

Effective partnerships are not always initiated or controlled by donor agencies or by central government authorities. Participants in Senegal, Zambia, Mexico and the Philippines noted that many successful initiatives in response to the epidemic had commenced through voluntary activity, often starting with no clear idea of where their initiatives were heading, and receiving external funding only after difficult project development phases were complete. A few NGOs in the Philippines noted initial distrust of government involvement, claimed that successful initiatives almost always commenced with NGOs, and noted that when partnerships between government and NGOs work it is often because, in the words of one workshop participant, "NGOs have taken the pains to involve government." Hearteningly, some government workers in the Philippines also drew attention to this aspect of their partnership with NGOs.

Effective partnerships allow all partners to make choices. In provision of external assistance, there must be an ability for recipient partners to choose which aspects of that assistance they want, and what aspects of the external agent's experience they find useful. Partners of the Programme, especially those who had attended HDP workshops, reported that this was most often the case. Outsiders also need to be free to choose which partners they want to work with, but this may be complicated by the requirements of ongoing political challenges as, for example, when international agencies want to work with NGOs which are not close to their own countries' governments.

An important element of the importance of choice within partnerships was also noted by a participant from Senegal, when he talked about the importance of involving people with HIV but doing this in ways which enable them to choose when, where and to whom they come out:

> Yes, it's important to involve people with HIV in your projects, but also to look after them, not to leave them with a mess in their lives because you made them go public.

Effective partnerships acknowledge the contributions of all parties involved. Some participants reported that donors often assume that direction should be by them because they provide the funding, forgetting that the donation of time and expertise is a large expense for people living in poverty: "Donors and the community are both investing", said one participant, drawing attention to the need for both parties to determine the desired long-term outcomes of that investment. In contrast, effective partnerships engender mutual respect for the dignity and contribution of all involved.

Likewise, effective partnerships do not remain in the control of those who initiate them. This was highlighted, again, by Teresita Bagasao from the NGO, Kabalikat, in the Philippines:

> There is a role for encouraging networks. We have 100 groups doing their own thing. We still respond to individual organisations but we encourage links. Our vision is that we will just be one of those organizations, not the central one. Not necessarily running the show.

Effective partnerships are not always easy. Some partners of the Programme reported that on some occasions they felt they were being presented with rigid views of the epidemic and development, or that their own expertise was not always recognised. This reflects that processes to build consensus on shared senses of purpose, and mutually beneficial learning, must also be ongoing. Others reported difficulties in their ongoing relationships with each other, as when members of networks noted that it was not always easy or productive for NGOs and governments to work together, or even for NGOs from different countries to respect and work with each other. A few participants in the Latin American and Caribbean Council of AIDS Service Organisations (LACCASO) noted that this network had experienced difficulties but had overcome them over time.

5.5 Some Immediate Effects of Partnerships which Build Capacity

Partnerships are important not only for their own sakes, but because of what they achieve. Throughout all stages of the evaluation process, much was said about how working through partnership achieves relevant and sustainable responses to HIV and development. Comments of participants can be grouped in various themes, and these in turn can be grouped into themes about the immediate effects of successful partnerships and what people experience through these processes, leading to more powerful and sustained effects. Amongst the immediate effects are concepts of inclusion, the creation of space, reflection and sharing of experiences. The way people experience these processes is addressed in the next sub-sections.

Inclusion

Evaluation participants indicated the value of learning through interactive processes. However, such learning does not happen automatically whenever people meet together. An essential prerequisite to mutual learning is that all participants feel included.

Notions of expertise are important to this. In brief, if people feel that their own experience is valued by others, they will be more likely to talk about it and to share both what they have learnt and what they still have doubts about. This leads to others doing the same, and reflective dialogue helps in the development of solutions to newly identified problems.

The use of a wide range of available group processes, simulation games and other methods drawn from the fields of adult education and community development is important in these inclusive processes. While often used in local projects, the HDP has demonstrated their usefulness also in international networks and workshops.

It is important to include in sustainable development programmes the people whose lives are directly affected by the epidemic, to ensure that their experiences are valued, and to ensure that they feel able to contribute. A classic example is the inclusion of people with HIV in programme and policy planning. Promotion of this has been a feature of the UNDP HIV and Development Programme's work since the beginning. Recognition of its importance is now common on national HIV/AIDS committees and in many (but not all) international forums. However, this inclusion has often been tokenistic, resulting in people with HIV sitting in on committee meetings to which they have been invited at the last minute, not adequately informed of what is going on, and not included as equal partners in problem-solving within those meetings.

The HDP has explored ways to improve this situation, by promoting networks within countries, regions and worldwide so that people with HIV could share their experiences with each other before participating in wider networks, by inviting people with HIV to participate in all workshops and meetings held by the Programme, and by exploring within workshops various means of involving people with HIV in ways which enable them to participate and discuss their HIV status as and when they feel appropriate. The value of these types of initiatives was often mentioned by people with HIV who were involved in the evaluation process.

The issue of inclusion of people with HIV in workshops has led to much discussion amongst people with HIV, people involved in NGOs working in development, and other partners of the Programme. Gradually, it was reported, people are building up trust and understanding of how to make this work, by acknowledging that the answers are not simple but that they can be found through interactive processes.

Likewise, the Programme has promoted the involvement of others affected by the epidemic based on principles of including people affected and recognising expertise which arises from lived experience. Again, evaluation participants often acknowledged the importance of this.

The HDP evaluation process itself ensured inclusion of people whose lives are affected by the HIV epidemic, often to the surprise of those people themselves, because they are so often excluded. Reflecting a common experience of internalising lack of power, some participants in Mexico asked, "Why me? Why do you want to interview me?" One woman identified by HDP partners as being an active social change agent said her organisation was ".. just a grassroots organization", and asked, "Why don't you go to the big ones?" Constant experiences of exclusion result in a lowering of expectations about inclusion. The result is that the experiences of some of the people engaged in the most effective responses to the epidemic are often excluded from policy and programme development unless conscious efforts are made to invite their inclusion.

The lack of inclusion, or even active exclusion, of some people in many responses to the epidemic was also noted by many participants. Exclusion can be a damaging process which crushes hope and stifles the development of effective responses. Consider, for example, this statement by Eduardo San Miguel from Mexico:

> If NGOs do not revise or review their own approach to tolerance of opinions that are not their own, very little can be advanced. For example, the voice of those who are in the first circle around those with AIDS has to be listened to ... A female relative (of someone with HIV) at the national consultation had been talked down because someone said that the only people who are important are those with AIDS. That comment pleased the public, and left the woman discredited.

Another group not often included is the next generation. This is often reflected in countries in which it is believed HIV has a low prevalance: for example, when almost all HIV resources are spent on surveillance and education, with little interest in planning for future needs in care and support of people who are ill and the living dependants of those who have died. In contrast, a group of women in Zambia who are caring for the children of those who have died, a group called Kwasha Mukwenu, meaning "Help your friend who is in need", told evaluators that they are now teaching the older children how to care for the younger ones, in the conscious hope that their work will be continued in the years to come when they themselves are unable to continue providing care.

The Importance of Space in Enabling Inclusion

One immediate impact of effective partnerships is the creation of space in which people can think, feel, say and thus share things that are not always possible in the spaces of their everyday lives. The concept of space was recognised as an important component of inclusion. Again, simply being in one spot does not lead to people feeling included, or to them bringing to the sharing the things which may matter most to them. Two considerations are important here: first, having a space where people are free to talk undisturbed, and where time to reflect is deliberately allocated; second, creating a type of emotional space, in which people feel free to discuss some things they do not normally discuss. The requirements of such space, and the range of issues this enables people to address, are summarised in this quote from As Sy, the Executive Director of the African Council of AIDS Service Organizations (AFRICASO):

> Physical, geographical, places to meet ... but ... without being accused, discounted, excluded, assaulted; ideological space ... where you can feel safe to talk about sex, serostatus and human rights.

The use of space, like many other processes of inclusion, needs to be valued and cherished if it is to be effective. An example of this was learnt directly by the SPR evaluation team in Zambia. A workshop which had led to the telling of many important stories and the sharing of many emotions was joined after lunch by a few people who had not been there in the morning, and who held senior positions in government. The trust and the sense of sharing the same space which had been developed throughout the morning and continued during the lunch break suddenly disappeared, and discussion reverted to common bureaucratic and planning language, with little allowance for the importance of emotion or cultural insight. In retrospect, it would have been important to insist that participants attend for the whole day, or just for the morning, but that they could not arrive mid-way through the workshop.

Participants reported that one of the most effective uses of space is to allow people to bring their emotions into discussions: in the words of one participant from Senegal, allowing "... permission to feel." Despite the overwhelming significance of human emotions in enabling people to come to terms with and respond to the effects of the HIV epidemic, this is often not allowed, especially in international meetings. The assumption is, too often, that effective responses arise from scientific insight alone, and that emotions get in the way of good programming.

Likewise, discussion about religious beliefs is often excluded in policy making, on the basis that religion somehow interferes with rational responses to the epidemic. Thus, participants in Zambia and the Philippines reported that many outsiders had told them either to make special efforts to "get the church on our side" or, conversely, to make sure the church was not involved because it would interfere with the promotion of condoms. In both countries, efforts to include the church have proved of value.

Indeed, both communities and people's religious and spiritual beliefs were central to many of the evaluation participants' own experiences with the epidemic. What is often forgotten is that a faith community in many communities is the only institution which brings people together in groups. If group sharing is an essential component of developing capacity, then the involvement of faith communities is also essential. If action arises from understanding, then no action will arise if key components of understanding are denied: these include religious belief and spirituality, which are often intricately entwined with feelings of hope, empowerment and solidarity.

The importance of, and methods for, creation of space in which people can reflect on and share their innermost feelings and beliefs in relation to the epidemic was highlighted in an evaluation workshop in the Philippines. Discussion at one stage addressed the question of the extent to which Filipinos feel able to talk about sex. The experience of many participants was that Filipinos find this difficult, but this was challenged by a Catholic nun, who said that she had found that Filipinos like to talk about sex. Only when asked to explain how she enabled them to do this did she recount that such talk usually occurred, "... at the end of the second day of closed workshops." Thus, the evaluation workshop itself had created space for Filipinos to talk about the circumstances in which they could talk about sex. The result was that all participants learnt how to create space for this, by hearing from someone who regularly does so but perhaps did not realise how rare this is.

Reflection and Sharing of Experiences

Reflection, on one's own and others' experiences, was another immediate effect of working in partnerships which was reported by many participants. This was noted by Margaret Mutambo, from Zambia, as having obviously occurred amongst staff of the HDP:

> I don't think anybody can write what she (Elizabeth Reid, Director of the Programme) writes without reflection. The epidemic itself is something that makes you sit down and just think of things that are important.

The importance of reflection, and the types of insights to which it leads which are different from those which can simply be passed on as knowledge from one person to another, was also highlighted by Sr Marie-Luc, from Senegal:

> We don't have the answers, so we have to share. ... It's the entire being that's touched. People called upon to work in (the epidemic) ... have to feel all the implications of what it means. If all you do is campaigns and condoms, then you're missing the point. It becomes mechanical ... it is more multifaceted and profound ... it touches the individual in the most profound aspect of her being.

Like inclusion, reflection does not happen automatically, but can be invoked. Learning this through having participated in workshops which encouraged reflection was, in itself, an important lesson for Margaret Mutambo, from Zambia:

> Just bringing people together and giving them the chance to share, of course, with guidance. That is something that made me think, "I can apply that." People sharing, not something they have back in the office.

5.6 What People Experience as a Result of these Processes

It is the more powerful and sustainable effects of partnerships which lead directly to the types of understanding and action which are required for sustainable, adaptable and effective responses to the HIV epidemic in the context of human development. These include validation, the creation of social learning, solidarity, empowerment and the releasing of energy and, ultimately, sustainable and continuing social change.

Validation

One of the important effects of inclusion and sharing is the sense of validation that people attain and can give to each other. Validation is about making sure that people are not only included, but also that the value of their experience is acknowledged and affirmed.

Validation is important in any work which is attempting to redefine the nature of expertise. Expertise which arises from experience is not always valued, and people whose expertise arises from experience rather than formal education often internalise feelings of inadequacy and lack of expertise. The required validation need not come from external "experts" in a patronising way, but may more often come from people learning to value each others' experience. In Senegal, a number of workshops had been held based on the Programme's workshop in HIV and Development. Evaluation participants reported that within these workshops they had listened to one another and shared their understanding of what might work to bring about change. These processes had been very useful in validating not just their individual expertise, but also the power of sharing and developing that expertise together.

One seemingly ironic aspect of validation is the benefit some participants reported could arise from validating uncertainty. Sometimes, coming together with others to share understanding about the epidemic results in sharing doubts, uncertainties and even a sense of despair about what is occurring and what might be done. Rather than stifling responses, participants reported that finding that their own uncertainties were also being experienced by others was empowering, because it enabled people to see that the problems did not just rest in their own individual lack of power or insight. The sharing of uncertainty often leads to identifying ways to move beyond that uncertainty.

Developing Empathy and Deep Understanding

Many participants spoke about the importance to them of having developed the capacity for social, or community, learning through having first developed a deeper capacity for understanding the complex realities of the epidemic and its effects. Eduardo San Miguel, from Mexico, similarly talked about the nature of understanding which is effective in producing action:

> I've been trying to understand the epidemic in my own way. This has happened gradually. When you interact and you start listening to what people want to know, you have to think a lot, because when you ask questions around HIV and AIDS, you become vulnerable. To really understand, you have to ask concrete things, refer to specific experiences.

An important aspect of this was the acknowledgement that people must become engaged in understanding emotional aspects of the epidemic.

Solidarity

The sharing of experiences, amongst people within similar contexts, can result in important developments in people's ability to learn about and understand locally-situated realities in ways which may not always be understood, and certainly cannot be predetermined, by outsiders. The concept of solidarity which arises from sharing, and supporting each other through, difficult experiences was noted as important by many participants.

Solidarity was not always seen as solidarity in action; often, it referred to solidarity in hope. For example, Sr Marie-Luc, from Senegal, noted that she gained an important sense of encouragement in her work from people in France:

> Solidarity means you are not an isolated person, you can't stay in your corner, what touches our brothers touches us. A solidarity in sharing the misfortunes of others, individuals and nations. When I went to France last year and spoke about what we're doing here in Senegal, I told them you have to express solidarity with countries worse touched than France, and with less means than you have. Then, France sent me messages, documents, magazines, and the exchanges I have with those people ... we are carrying this together, it's not just one person. Solidarity means helping and giving of yourself ... to feel compassion for the problems that the other person is living.

Mary Kanene, from Zambia, noted that the evaluation process itself had provided her with a sense of solidarity, simply through allowing interactive discussion:

> It was a blessing ... through talking (with Cindy) I realised how much I really was doing ... I know that in my small things I can be of value. You don't have to stand alone on a hilltop to be able to access others who are in need.

Solidarity is not something which arises through transfer of skills, but it can be catalysed through programming approaches which promote the sharing of personal experiences. A powerful example of this was provided by Roberto Castro, a member of a research team in Mexico:

> We are studying coping strategies, but we also have to learn to cope with our own reactions to our findings. We are overwhelmed, sometimes it is too much ... Sometimes what we find touches some very, very personal experience. One person we interviewed told us about being abandoned by the family. ... When we discussed this, we moved from the interview experience to the experience of one of our team members. He had polio as a child. At the age of five he was attending a rehabilitation centre to train his movements. The children were picked up by a bus every morning and brought back at the end of the day. Once there was one child who was not met by his parents or anybody else. He had to be brought back to the rehabilitation centre. Later they found out that the family had simply moved, leaving the handicapped child behind. When our team member understood, he told his mother what had happened and the mother cried and cried. He realised he was so lucky to have a caring family. When my team member shared this story with me it changed my perspective. I used to think I was luckier than him since I had no polio, but his polio story had shown him that he was lucky to have a caring family.

The richness of understanding and empathetic feelings experienced by all members of that research team, as a result of the telling of this story, has helped them to develop a much better understanding of the way the epidemic has affected the people with whom they interact through their research, as Roberto explained:

> We are somehow understanding the complexity. A world in which people have very little control of their own fate. This way of looking at the world is very rooted in their everyday life ... Changing is possible, but difficult, and involves slow processes ... I would like to see that the insight we have gained through our research will have practical implications.

Empowerment, and the Releasing of Energy

Feeling that they are able to understand and respond to the challenges of the HIV epidemic and development was reported as centrally important to people's actual responses. Partnerships which lead to empowerment, which can sometimes be indicated by the presence of such feelings, are far more effective than those which build dependence. Anuar Luna, from Mexico, noted the close links between feelings of solidarity and feelings of empowerment: "The model is the tool, but the solidarity is the energy."

Programmes which work to build enabling environments, such as through changing attitudes and laws to make partnership between NGOs and governments easier, are therefore important. The means to develop enabling environments are many and complex, and require the interaction of numerous activities and the development of widespread understanding. Many participants reported that feelings of empowerment, feelings that they can act within their own environments, have come gradually and slowly developed through collective action.

Others reported that bursts of energy which enable them to respond to the epidemic are often associated with anger. Sara Longwe and Roy Clarke, from Zambia, were two such participants. They noted that a sense of anger at injustice and at patriarchal systems was an important motivating force, but that their anger at wider structural barriers was separate from the feelings they had working with people in their own lives. For example, Sara said that, "What gives me energy is to have one foot working in the NGOs and one foot in the grassroots." Roy acknowledged that he felt a sense of anger, "But at first when I felt anger it was a patriarchal anger: I am not having my wife treated like that! But later, I understood that the patriarchal reaction was a barrier to change."

A good example of how inclusive processes can be empowering was provided through a series of experiences related by Margaret Mutambo, the UNDP HIV and Development national professional of ficer in Zambia. She noted the value of processes of the Programme which enabled people within her own country to attend inter-country workshops in which they shared experiences with each other and with those from other African countries. The types of processes used within those meetings and workshops had resulted in her feeling able to act with strong commitment in response to the epidemic in Zambia. These processes, she said, were based on a recognition that everyone present had something to contribute, irrespective of levels of education or professional experience. Their very attendance indicated interest, and part of that interest was to learn. What the Programme had done, however, was to ensure that everyone also contributed to that learning, even in ways they had not expected themselves:

> Recognition of the person, not their skill. This leads to where you might not know you have something to offer until it comes out. Because there are some hidden skills that only another person can help you discover. They made clear that they thought I had something to offer. They did not know what that was, and I did not know what that was, but the workshop brought it out.

5.7 Sustainable Results: Responsive Social Change

The net result of partnerships, inclusion, solidarity and social learning is personal and social change which slows down the epidemic and minimises its negative impact. The importance of such change was often noted by HDP staff throughout the evaluation process, as was the interim step of change, or even transformation, of individuals and institutions.

The importance of transformation was also acknowledged by many evaluation participants. Transformation results in people feeling that they do understand enough to be able to act, that they want to take action, and that they are somehow "changed" as a result of that action. This was highlighted in comments by Anuar Luna, from Mexico:

> The [HDP] workshop gave me the capacity to see myself and others. This was my personal process: to discover the link between the personal and the global. The paper on strategic questioning also gave me a lot. In that workshop I felt the importance of meeting. I felt the global challenge and the importance for change, or deeply felt transition. The workshop was very, very important. ... We can influence many of the underlying problems of the epidemic. I think my life has changed in many ways. I have plans. I am enthusiastic. ... For me it was a long process to learn to think differently, to build a new way.

Evaluation participants reported various types of transformative processes which they found had been personally useful. Most often, these processes involved a combination of having lived through powerful experiences *and* having engaged in shared reflection about those experiences. As Roland Msiska, from

Zambia, said, "You go through these personal changes. Through a state of fear, to hope."

Thus, in workshops aiming to enhance understanding, processes which led to emotional responses had been very useful in generating commitment to responding to the epidemic. Likewise, people who said they had lived through traumatic experiences within the epidemic had found it useful to incorporate reflection on those experiences into general dialogue about policy and programme development. In turn, the involvement in policy and programme development had helped them to make more sense of their feelings of grief and loss.

Two particular components of the workshops on HIV and Development were mentioned by many participants, either as experiences which had led to changes for them, or as methods they use to help others understand various aspects of the epidemic. One is the simulation game, *Wilds fire,* originally developed for family planning situations by the Family Planning Association of New South Wales (Australia) and adapted for the Programme workshops. Another is an exercise called, *The Unfolding of the epidemic,* developed by HDP staff to enable people to understand the likely impact of the epidemic on individuals, families, communities and nations. Details of both exercises are available from the UNDP HIV and Development Programme. What is significant to this report is not those details, but a recognition that both of these exercises enable people to learn through shared reflection based on their own experiences, and both exercises enable learning at both an intellectual and an emotional level.

Some evaluation participants reported significant effects arising from a single interactive experience, such as a facilitated visit to a nearby country or participation in a single workshop. Transformation can result from single experiences which lead to feelings of, "Aha! Now I understand", or "Now I have changed." An example of this was the reaction of Santhi, from Senegal, to the exercise *Wilds fire:*

> You overcome your fear of AIDS. It's an adversary, but you've developed an idea of how it uses its tricks. So, it's no longer a fear of the unknown. It's transformation from not knowing, to being part of a network. I was the object of the transformation ... you suddenly realised anyone can get AIDS. ... You remember, "That bastard infected me!"

A participant reported in a final evaluation note of a workshop in Senegal that it had helped him to realise that:

> I thought I understood, but I didn't.
> I thought I was involved, but I wasn't.
> Things will be different from now on.

More often, participants reported that they had sensed changes in their own levels of understanding and commitment over time. This could come from continued involvement in a network, ongoing involvement in the development of training materials, or the repeated running of workshops for people in their own countries.

One person in Zambia reported the transformation he had experienced as a result of attending policy meetings on and off over a period of months during which a number of relatives and close friends died. The continual need to think about what should happen in national responses to the epidemic, interspersed with the intense personal experience of having people close to him dying, had resulted in an unshakable commitment to find better ways to help others respond to the epidemic. Similar experiences were reported by others working in UNDP, governments, NGOs or simply in their local communities.

Some government officials engaged in policy-making responses to the epidemic reported the importance of transformative experiences leading to changes in their perception of the significance of their work, and to a different type of engagement with their work in relation to HIV than what they had with other work. In helping to develop capacity, it is important to remember that government officials are also people who live in families and communities, and the importance of providing space for sharing of emotions and for validation of lived experience is as important for them as it is for others involved in responses to the epidemic.

The ultimate result of processes of capacity building is that people are able to further develop their own understanding and their own collective responses to the HIV epidemic and the challenges of human development. This was summed up well by Gary Engelberg, from Senegal:

> The virus is moving too quickly, so we need to involve people very quickly, ... I can't imagine knowing what's at stake and then not acting. ... That's the challenge, to get them to see what's at stake. Because it's dealing with procreation, love. Once people understand that, you just let them loose. You can create mutual support for those kinds of processes, follow up networks ... but what you have to create is a *mass movement* of people to stop the epidemic.

CASE STUDY 1: ENHANCING NATIONAL CAPACITY THROUGH HIV ACTION RESEARCH

Although the economic determinants of vulnerability to HIV at both the individual and societal levels are increasingly being recognised and studied, most attention so far in the social sciences has been focused on the impact of HIV, primarily in the industrialised world. The socio-economic impact of HIV on developing societies has been less well studied and understood. The HIV epidemic threatens social and economic development because, in contrast to other life-threatening infections which attack primarily the young, the aged and the infirm, HIV affects people responsible for the support and care of children, the elderly and extended family members, and it affects adults in their economically and socially most active years. HIV-related illness and death have the potential to deplete the labour force, undermine public sector capacity to govern, and lead to social and civil unrest.

At the macro-economic level, selective erosion of slices of the economy occurs as people with critical capacities such as bank managers, teachers, engineers or nurses become ill. Reduction in productivity and workforce depletions in key formal sector industries such as mining, tourism or agriculture can affect gross domestic product, export earnings and public revenue generation. Countries may then experience investment reductions in education and training which, combined with the loss of skilled labour, can lead to decreased output, skills, experiences, and aspirations with resultant further decreased investment. These macro-economic effects compound those of structural adjustment programmes in many countries (Lurie et al., 1995).

At the household level, reductions in earning capacity, increases in health related expenditures, the opportunity cost of time spent caring for the sick, and extra burdens placed on women threaten to substantially reduce household resources. Coping mechanisms may include changes in household composition and the modification of roles and activities within the family. Children may be withdrawn from school to assist with household duties or to enter the job market (Ainsworth and Koda, 1993, 50), cash crops may be abandoned in favour of subsistence crops that require less attention (Barnett and Blaikie, 1992, 89), traditional knowledge systems may be irrevocably lost and customary mechanisms for the care and support of orphans may be overwhelmed. Conventionally determined direct and indirect costs will clearly underestimate the real psychosocial, interpersonal, emotional, and economic consequences and costs of the HIV epidemic at the individual, household, community and national levels.

This case study describes and discusses the generalisability of a programme, currently underway in four African countries, which is aimed at enhancing the capacity of nation states to understand the threat that the HIV epidemic poses to their economic, social and political development and to respond effectively.

Extractive Research Approaches in Developing Countries

Research can provide information critical to formulating effective programming and policy initiatives that can increase the capacity of countries to meet the challenge of the HIV epidemic. To date, however, a good proportion of HIV-related research has not achieved these ends, which is not surprising given the long and notorious history of North-South research relationships. The approach used is the antithesis of local capacity building. Researchers from industrialized countries define a line of inquiry and then seek out local collaborators, both to ensure that the relevant approvals can be obtained and to provide on-the-ground assistance with the challenging logistics of data collection.

Following the operational phase, some data entry, verification and cleaning may be conducted locally but, more often than not, the information leaves the country with the industrialised country researchers never to be seen again. If and when the results are published, it is in the form of a scientific article, in a highly-rated journal priced beyond the resources of institutions such as the local university, let alone local collaborators. Local members of the research team are lucky to be included as co-authors, the standard gesture often being a simple acknowledgement of their help. Increasingly this approach is being rejected but it remains common.

Local Research Processes and the Link to Programming and Policy

The charges levelled at foreign investigators can also apply to the way local researchers behave. Indigenous scientists trained in industrialized countries, or in similarly-styled regional learning institutions, now form the elite cadre in developing countries. Following traditional approaches, topics and methodology may often reflect the individual curiosity of the researcher. In other, perhaps more common cases, research priorities and methodologies may be determined by donors with little interest in what is needed for more effective responses to the epidemic. Indeed, even in those unfortunately rare circumstances where local priorities are taken into account there is very little evidence that research is effectively used in the formulation of policy and programmes. For example, among 73 studies profiled in a directory of social and behavioural research on HIV and AIDS compiled in Zimbabwe in 1994, fully 71 per cent gave no indication that the results were being used in the formulation of programmes and policies (Misihairabwi et al., 1994, 23). Many studies conducted in developing countries are never published in local journals or even in the form of a final report and only exceptionally are results disseminated to the communities which were researched or to service providers and decision makers. It is unsurprising that in the conditions which prevail in many countries, where the norm has research being largely externally funded and determined, that local policy and programme needs are low on the agenda and that results are rarely translated into effective programmes or policy changes.

In addition to an evident opportunity cost to the *status quo,* ethical concerns are raised by issues of ownership of the data. At issue is whether research, particularly research addressing the cultural context and meaning of sexuality, will provide baseline data for programme development and evaluation or whether it will simply produce voyeuristic impressions and serve to increase the stigmatization of the community and its members.

Methodological concerns have been raised about the extractive research model and the tendency for quantitative questionnaire surveys to reflect the pervasive and tenacious assumptions of biomedicine about culture and behaviour (Schoepf, 1991). Ultimately, choice of methodologies, whether quantitative or qualitative, will depend on the nature of the research question being posed and should be based on whether the research findings generated by the chosen methodology will be informative and valid, and have the potential to significantly advance understanding and stimulate social change. Mobilising society will be essential for an effective response to the HIV epidemic and research which is capacity building is thus an important instrument in the process of strengthening social capital.

Capacity Building Through Research

Responses to the complexity of the HIV epidemic must be timely and must act to slow down the spread of the virus and provide support and care to those affected within communities. Research will play a critical role if results contribute to the development of effective HIV programming and policy and if the research process itself is empowering for research participants and their communities.

If research is to support the development of effective HIV programming, it should fit within a locally articulated plan of research needs and priorities, be timely and be affordable.

Moreover, given the urgency of the problems to be addressed through policies and programmes there has to be a reasonable likelihood that research will in fact yield results which can be embodied in effective responses to the epidemic. Small-scale, multifaceted, multidisciplinary projects may be more cost-effective than expensive large-scale ones and may furnish results more rapidly. The best way to ensure that such findings are used by those responsible for HIV programme development is to involve decision makers, programme developers, community activists and representatives from National AIDS Programmes (NAPs) from the outset of research design and continuously throughout the research process. The latter are critical partners since NAP staff know what research is being undertaken, planned or has been completed, and are the point of contact at the national level for bilateral and multilateral donors.

Individuals affected by HIV are central to a complex understanding of the nature of the epidemic and to the utilisation of eventual findings, and should be fully integrated into research processes from the start. Effective action-oriented research will involve people living with HIV and affected by HIV in the setting of research priorities, in the choice of research questions, in evaluations of the relevance of proposed investigations, in the research design phase, and in study conduct, analysis and dissemination of results.

Development is now understood as sustainable if it empowers people to take charge of their own well-being, if it builds on the strengths of local knowledge and values, and if an enabling environment is created at national and international levels which fosters and supports local initiatives (Banuri et al., 1994). In development practice the role of experts or donor agencies is increasingly understood as involving facilitation of processes for creating norms, values and practices that enable people and their organizations to gain greater control over their lives. In this paradigm, development is constituted by local sources of experimentation, of innovation, and of diversity fostered within a supportive macro-level institutional, policy and legislative environment.

At the heart of this new form of development practice is the recognition that sources of learning must be local in part so as to enable people to engage with "the global" on their own and better terms (Appadurai, 1990). For ideas and programmes to take root within communities, they must spring from within, they must be based on the realities of lived experiences, and they must be disseminated and defended from there. At the centre of this new development practice are concepts of consensus building, promotion of partnerships between the organizations of civil society and public institutions, human and social capacity building, ethical practice, and facilitation.

Participatory research initiatives can support and strengthen local processes of social learning and national capacities which transform social learning into policy and programmes. Community level responses empower participants, particularly infected individuals and communities, to identify their own needs and to ensure that chosen strategies can be implemented and maintained. It follows that researchers who are close to or part of affected communities are better placed than external teams to identify research themes and methodologies which are relevant and to ensure that their findings are of ultimate benefit to affected people, activists and organizations responding to the epidemic.

Programme Development: The UNDP Research Capacity Building Initiative

Based on a development approach of social learning and capacity building, the UNDP partnership programme was created to assist selected communities, academic institutions and countries to create capacity to undertake action-oriented research into the extent and nature of the psychological, social and economic causes and consequences of the epidemic; to analyse the data and findings in ways that would be directly relevant to programme and policy development; and to assist community organizations, programme managers, activists and leaders to assess and redesign their policies and interventions in light of the research findings. This work is being undertaken in Senegal, Central African Republic, Zambia and Kenya (Hankins, 1994, 1995a, 1996) as well as Myanmar (Porter, 1995) and Nicaragua. This case study focuses on progress to date in the African component, and includes discussion of the difficulties encountered and lessons learnt to date.

Programme Implementation Phase I of this pilot programme began in April 1993 with the formation of Country Groups in four African countries. Research topics were chosen, infrastructural support was provided, an inter-country training seminar was held in Senegal, research protocols were elaborated, technical support missions conducted, and presentations made to donors. Phase II, which focuses on the translation of data into programming and policy, was launched in August 1995 with skills building workshops for Country Group representatives, NAP managers, technical support partners, donors and African academics.

Phase I: From Research Needs to Raw Data

The four African countries evaluated for eventual participation in the Partnership Programme were chosen to represent both East and West Africa, francophone and anglophone cultures, and to provide a spectrum of HIV prevalence ranging from Senegal with the lowest rates at one per cent (Mbaye et al., 1993), Central African Republic at approximately ten per cent (Global Programme on AIDS, 1991), through to Zambia and Kenya in the ten to twenty per cent range for overall country HIV prevalence among adults (Hira et al., 1989; Kitabu et al., 1992; Mungai et al., 1992). Between April and June 1993, exploratory missions were conducted in each country, with NAP personnel, other pertinent government ministries, and key donors being consulted as to the relevance of such a programme. Their willingness to participate actively in the programme was assessed since neither the HIV and Development Programme in New York nor the HIV and Development Regional Project in Dakar would be directly funding any of the research projects developed within the initiative. Potential candidates for the multidisciplinary Country Groups were interviewed and asked to provide a written statement of why they wanted to participate. They were informed that the exchange being contemplated was one in which their time contribution would be balanced by new knowledge, skills and contacts. The Country Groups included a mix of senior and junior researchers, concerned community members, affected persons, institutional leaders and other users of research findings.

Country Group meetings were held to define priority areas for research and to draft initial proposals equivalent to letters of intention. A seminar attended by all Country Groups during September 1993 discussed principles, methodologies and ethical issues involved in psychosocial and economic research. It aimed to strengthen participants' awareness of the nature, determinants and consequences of the HIV epidemic and, in particular, to create a common conceptual framework for viewing HIV and development. The seminar paved the way for a collaborative effort among researchers from within and outside the region, and quantified the financial resources required to undertake designed studies and follow-up activities. Infrastructural support of $US5,000 was then provided to each team for research training, language courses and pre-pilot work.

In 1994, a technical assistance consortium of experienced researchers from within Africa, from other regions of the developing world and from elsewhere was established with the resultant diverse blend of researchers having both scientific expertise and experience working in partnerships of equals with others. Following this, technical support missions to Senegal, Central African Republic and Zambia focused on quantitative and qualitative research methodologies, economic theory and analysis, ethical issues, and presentation strategies. These assisted Country Groups to finalise their research objectives, determine appropriate research methodologies and study sample sizes, refine analysis plans, justify budgets, and prepare workplans. Fourteen proposals were prepared initially by the four teams. By early 1996 data collection had been completed in two projects and was underway in three others. Strong donor interest had been expressed in a further four projects and funding negotiations were proceeding. Research projects underway include evaluations of the management of HIV infection within the family, the socio-economic determinants of the HIV epidemic, the role of church groups in HIV/AIDS prevention and care, the socio-cultural factors associated with HIV prevalence, and the impact of AIDS in the business sector.

Phase I: Lessons Learnt

The lessons learnt during this pilot project are as relevant to Asia, and other parts of the world, where the socio-economic impact of the HIV epidemic is also being felt (Panyarachun, 1995), as they are to Africa. How well each step of the programme was implemented had predictable consequences for subsequent steps. Countries and their National AIDS Programmes had varying levels of commitment to the programme, some research teams were not well-balanced with respect to experience and motivation, stakeholders did not participate fully in the defining of research priorities, infrastructural funds were not disbursed in a timely manner, some members of the technical assistance consortium lacked process facilitation skills, and several local donors were reticent to fund projects. Some suggestions for avoiding these and other problems are presented in the discussion which follows.

Countries chosen should be those most likely to implement the programme successfully, to attract funding for research activities, and where the NAP and local UNDP offices have expressed interest. Although the partnership process is UNDP's responsibility, particular attention should be paid to ensuring that key individuals in the NAP comprehend what is being attempted and are prepared to integrate research projects into the NAP.

Country Groups have a tripartite composition of researchers (intergenerational and interdisciplinary), data users (government, civil society, professional associations), and members of concerned communities and affected individuals. The mix of disciplines and perspectives within Country Groups can be maximised by ensuring that those interviewing and selecting members have a clear understanding of the implications of the capacity building objectives for the choice of participants. Medical doctors, epidemiologists, survey sociologists, economists and other quantitative researchers should be fully complemented by anthropologists, ethnographers and others with qualitative research and strong conceptual backgrounds. In each Country Group, it is essential to have at least two representatives from infected and affected communities and their support organisations so as to reduce the possibility that illness will interrupt community representation or that token representation will lead to reduced participation due to intimidation based on hierarchy and position.

To minimise the tendency for Country Groups to define areas of inquiry on their own without outside consultation, a workshop should be held within each country to create a common understanding of the HIV epidemic and of the objectives of the programme. This should occur after the creation of the Country Groups and prior to any definition of relevant research tasks. Such a workshop could initiate a process of consultation with key stakeholders, such as representatives of both governmental and non-governmental organisations, community-based groups, donors, individuals and communities affected by HIV and others. Incorporating brainstorming sessions concerning the range of possible research topics, the workshop would help create top-level commitment to the process, and engender in the researchers a moral engagement for ongoing consultation and follow-through with key stakeholders and in particular with users of the research including the NAP and the Ministry of Planning. Although responsiveness to the needs of civil society is critical if social capital and social change are to be created it is important to be inclusive because the focus of each country's response to the epidemic is its strategy for HIV in which the National AIDS Programme plays a pivotal role.

Team building activities should incorporate a team-driven self-assessment of individual capacities and complementarities as well as of overall team composition, allowing for the possibility of adjustments. Team cohesiveness depends on several factors including leadership, team composition, personality factors, previous relationships, individual commitment and strategic replacement of members who leave the team because of lack of interest, conflicts of interest or new job responsibilities. Criteria for selection and procedures for choosing replacement members should be defined by participants at the first country workshop. Since both the personality and vision of the leader were found to be critical to team functioning and progress, selection criteria could be suggested at the time of Country Group formation. This may reduce the possibility that pre-existing local power relationships play the predominant role in the designation of team leaders. The underpinning philosophy is one of minimization of direction to the teams with emphasis on a process of technical co-operation which is based on principles of process consultation. This means providing guidance, challenging old ways of looking at things by raising new questions, offering expert information, analysis, and judgement while facilitating collective ownership in the design and implementation of new capacity building approaches to research, policy, and programme development (Joy & Bennett, 1994).

To avoid misunderstandings, it is important that the conditions of research participation be made clear from the outset. Team members are asked to make a personal commitment to exchange their time on a quid *pro quo* basis for capacity building without the possibility of either assured project funding or personal monetary recompense. Once a research project has been financed, direct payment of Country Group members or reimbursement to the employers of salaried individuals to cover time devoted to actual research work, such as the conducting of key informant interviews or participation as assistant moderators in focus groups, is justifiable.

The timing and objectives of a regional inter-country seminar should be carefully defined. The 1993 seminar succeeded in encouraging South-South collaboration and inter-country cooperation within the region and across language barriers but failed to meet some objectives, in part because often the definition of research needs had been carried out in isolation and, in part, because protocol development was well underway. Ideally, the initial inter-country seminar should follow country seminars and local processes of consultation for research question definition. Representatives of the Country Groups and of technical consortium members who have been involved in facilitating country workshops can usefully participate in the planning and programming of the inter-country one.

The establishment and maintenance of an appropriately skilled technical consortium were crucial to the success of the partnership initiative. In addition to specific technical back-up, more general support was provided for enhancing comprehension of the concepts of HIV and development and of the principles of research into the psychosocial and economic dimensions of HIV. Capacity to use research in programme design was strengthened by discussions identifying the linkages between research and policy and programme development. These in turn laid the groundwork for collaborative efforts among researchers, decision makers, affected communities, activists, and organisations responding to the epidemic. Down to earth advice on identifying and quantifying the financial resources required to undertake designed studies led naturally to the development of strategies for follow through at country level with donors and UNDP field offices.

Finding members for the technical assistance consortium with a broad understanding of both the HIV field and participatory development strategies, with appropriate scientific skills, and with personalities suited to a mutual learning process was challenging.

Constituting a technical support team composed of individuals who would complement each other in specifically addressing the needs of each country required consultation with numerous sources, evaluation of consultant capacity, performance appraisal of participants, and an element of luck concerning availability for specific missions. Facility in the language of the Country Group was obviously essential. The calibre of each technical support team had direct effects on the quality of the interactions between mission members and their country counterparts as well as on the overall benefits derived from technical visits, benefits which varied by country. Drawing on the specific expertise of members of the technical consortium, technical support missions provided assistance for three projects in Senegal, two in the Central African Republic, five in Zambia, and four in Kenya. Lack of time prevented assistance being given to most projects in the development of research instruments, codification manuals or interview guides as had been originally intended. Practically, Country Groups could choose two projects for external technical consultation which would provide the template for refinement by the research teams of any additional protocols.

The provision of supportive and facilitative technical assistance can tread a fine line between critique and criticism. Personality factors play a major role as does the experience of country counterparts and mission members in honest but affirming project review procedures. When most technical mission members come from industrialised countries and not all have training in process consultation principles and techniques, positive interactions may be hindered and traditional North-South one-way information transfer reinforced. Members of the technical assistance consortium must fully understand the implications of the programme's capacity building objectives for modes of interaction. The provision of specific training sessions designed to enhance the preparedness of consultants to participate effectively in the programme, combined with on-the-job training and performance appraisal, should be built into the programme. An emphasis on skill development with respect to process consultation (Joy and Bennett, 1994) and strategic questioning (Peavey, 1994) would help avoid inappropriate consultant behaviour during technical support missions.

To strengthen intra-regional ties, two of the three technical support missions included at least one member from a country within the region. As the programme matures two or more regional resource people should be used. As part of national capacity building, Country Groups should first assess whether technical assistance is available within the group and then if necessary seek assistance from other resources within the country. External technical support should be called upon only as a last resort although the provision of local assistance will also need to be facilitated to ensure that the programme's capacity building objectives are understood and respected. Technical support missions can reinforce the importance of qualitative research methodologies—such as focus groups, key informant interviews, and rapid appraisal techniques—in a synergistic blend with quantitative methodologies in the overall response to the epidemic. Technical support needs in the realm of qualitative research should be identified early so that technical mission composition reflects these needs.

As with all work undertaken by UNDP's HIV and Development Programme, the research capacity initiative is intended to be taken up and supported by UNDP country offices and other partners. Funding of specific protocols by UNDP was not an expected outcome of the programme since it would not have built local capacity to secure research funds. However, the local donor community often identified the research protocols as "UNDP projects" rather than acknowledging UNDP's role in a process of capacity building that led, *inter alia*, to the production of research protocols. Once such hurdles are overcome, donors who potentially may fund the actual research work should be involved early in the process to increase the likelihood that funds will be made available in a timely way. Expeditious financing of an initial project or of a pilot research activity, such as key informant interviews or questionnaire testing, significantly strengthens team cohesiveness and allows people to learn by doing.

The process of obtaining research funding commitments was facilitated by two factors. First, Country Group members who developed convincing formal presentations engendering donor confidence in the research teams' capacity found these to be effective in generating commitments from funders. Thus, an emphasis on refining funding presentation skills should form part of the technical support mission terms of reference. Second, Country Groups that created strong ties to the National AIDS Programme (NAP) and ensured that their work was perceived to be—and actually was—integral to the development of programmes and policies were more likely to obtain funding. The inter-relationships between NAPs and the Country Groups, and the priorities and interests of both parties should be the focus of formal and informal ongoing discussions throughout the programme.

Phase II: From Data to Policy and Programming

The first Phase II workshops, held in August 1995, focused on skills for the transformation of collected raw data into findings useful for policy and programme development. Participants included members of the Country Groups, NAP managers, technical support partners, invited African academics, and multilateral and bilateral donors. Workshop formats were derived from notions of partnership and shared responsibility for programming. Specific sessions considered a spectrum of issues, including processes to ensure continuing ownership of research by the communities involved, appropriate dissemination of research findings, research as empowerment, and strengthening capacity to use research in programming and policy. Skills building focused on facilitation, process consultation, strategic questioning, and development of performance appraisal criteria. Communication was enhanced and links forged between NAP managers and respective partnership programme Country Groups. Short and medium-term plans for in-country activities were developed through collective problem solving. The workshops highlighted the implications that capacity building approaches to research—aimed at stimulating social learning, building local research capacity and meeting the needs of programme managers, activists, and decision makers—have for technical co-operation, bilateral donor procedures, current practices of peer review and academic publication, and development practice.

Social Learning and Implications for the Provision of Technical Assistance

The UNDP partnership programme is based on the recognition that participatory research initiatives have the potential to support and create local processes of social learning which, when complemented by strengthened national capacities for thinking, reflection and analysis, lead to the transformation of social learning into policies and programmes (Banuri et al., 1994, 27). In addition to building local capacities for social learning, as this case study has shown, this UNDP initiative aims to create new approaches to the provision of supportive technical assistance. National teams and local communities take direct responsibility for establishment of research priorities and methodologies and for the development of ethical principles to govern the research. They set the conditions under which technical assistance is provided and determine the areas where their own research competence needs supplementation or strengthening. Technical assistance is then provided in a way that is both more complicated and yet more relevant and sustainable, with outside expertise fitted into local processes of social learning. The programme facilitates the drawing down of assistance from the best available external academic and development sources, national, regional and international. Currently this includes individuals from academic as well as national institutions in countries as diverse as Canada, France, the US, the

UK, South Africa, Zimbabwe, Senegal, Ivory Coast, Spain and Australia. The processes of learning and skills building occur within, facilitated from without.

The HIV epidemic provides the impetus for rethinking the role of outsiders, be they governments or others, in the creation of social change and in development practice. It poses a set of dilemmas for classical approaches to research and, since the issues it raises are the basic ones of development, research findings and processes will necessarily contribute to both development theory and practice. For research to play a critical role in the response to the HIV epidemic, communities, non-governmental organisations and community-based groups, as well as policy makers and programme planners, will have to come to view research as a useful tool for programming and forge mutually beneficial partnerships with researchers and donors. For the researcher, as for everyone, a new paradigm is required, one which Chambers (1994) describes as being people centred, participatory, empowering and sustainable. Much of the challenge is to give up power, to enjoy handing over the initiative to others so they can do more and in their own way, and to learn to value and enjoy these satisfactions.

References

Ainsworth, A. and Koda, G., 1993, 'The impact of fatal adult illness on school enrolments and attendance'. in Ainsworth, M., Koda, G., and Lwihula, G. (Eds.), Report of a Workshop on the Economic Impact of Fatal Adult Illness in Sub-Saharan Africa, The World Bank and the University of Dar es Salaam: Bukoba, Tanzania, 50-6.

Appadurai, A., 1990, 'Disjuncture and difference in the global economy', Public Culture, 2(2): 1-24.

Banuri, T., Hyden, G., Juma, C. and Rivera, M., 1994, Sustainable Human Development. From Concept to Operation: A Guide for the Practitioner, United Nations Development Programme, New York.

Barnett, T. and Blaikie, P., 1992, AIDS in Africa: Its Present and Future Impact, Bellhaven Press, London.

Chambers, R., 1994, 'Poverty and livelihoods: whose reality counts?', Overview Paper II, United Nations Development Programme, Stockholm, Roundtable, Change: Social Conflict or Harmony?

Global Programme on AIDS, 1991, Weekly Epidemiological Record, 66 (35), 257-9.

Hankins, C. (ed.), December 1994, Partnership for Capacity Building (Newsletter), HIV and Development Programme, United Nations Development Programme, Montreal, pp. 6-7.

Hankins, C. (ed.), August 1995a, Partnership for Capacity Building (Newsletter), HIV and Development Programme, United Nations Development Programme, Montreal, pp. 3-5.

Hankins, C. (ed.), February 1996, **Partnership for Capacity Building (Newsletter), HIV and Development Programme, United Nations** Development Programme, Montreal, pp. 6-7.

Hira, S.K., Kamanga, J., Bhat, G.J., Mwale, C., Tembo, G., Luo, N. and Perine, P.L., 1989, 'Perinatal transmission of HIV- 1 in Lusaka, Zambia', British Medical Journal, 299, no. 6718, 1250-2.

Joy, L. and Bennett, S., 1994, Process Consultation, Systemic Improvement of Public Sector Management, Management Development Programme. United Nations Development Programme: New York, 33-56.

Kitabu, M. Z. Maitha, G. M., Mungai, J. N., Plummer, F. A., Ndinya- Achola, J. O., & Temmerman, M. 1992, Trends and seroprevalence of HIV amongst four population groups in Nairobi in the period 1989 to 1991, VIII International Conference on AIDS, Amsterdam, PoC-4018.

Lurie, P., Hintzen, P. and Lowe, R.A., 1995, 'Socio-economic obstacles to HIV prevention and treatment in developing countries: the roles of the International Monetary Fund and the World Bank', AIDS, 9 (6), 539-46.

Mbaye, N., Diouf, A., Kebe, F., Diadhiou, F., Sarr, M., Fall, M., Sarr, M.A. N.G., Ba, D.S., Tall, N.D., Ouangre, A., Gueye, A., Siby, T., Boye, C.S., Mboup, S. and Kanki, P., 1993, 'Histoire naturelle de la transmission verticale VIH 1 et VIH 2 Dakar', unpublished paper presented to VIII International Conference on AIDS in Africa, Marrakech, Morrocco, Abstract M.O.P.046.

Misihairabwi, P., McChaven, N., Ray, S. and Weiss, E., 1994, Fostering Collaboration Between Researchers and NGOs on Women and AIDS in Zimbabwe, Women and AIDS Support Network and International Center for Research on Women, Washington, D.C.

Mungai, J.N., Maitha, G.M., Kitabu, M.Z., Plummer, F.A., Ndinya- Achola, J.O., Bwayo, J.J and Temmerman, M., (1992), 'Prevalence of HIV and other STDs in three populations in Nairobi for year 1991', unpublished paper presented to VII International Conference on AIDS, Amsterdam, PoC-4714.

Panyarachun, A. 1995, AIDS and Social and Economic Progress in the Asian and Pacific Countries, [Plenary Address] Third International Conference on AIDS in Asia and the Pacific, Chiang Mai, Thailand.

Peavey, F., 1994, 'Strategic questioning, an approach to creating personal and social change', in Peavey, F., By Life's Grace, Musings on the Essence of Social Change, New Society Publishers, Philadelphia.

Porter, D., 1995, Wheeling and Dealing: HIV and Development on the Shan State Borders of Myanmar, Study Paper 3, HIV and Development Programme, United Nations Development Programme, New York.

Schoepf, B.G., 1991, 'Ethical, methodological and political issues of AIDS, research in Central Africa', Social Sciences and Medicine, 33, 749-65.

This Case Study was prepared by Catherine Hankins, MD, MSc, FRCPC, a founding member, Group for Research to Action, McGill AIDS Centre, Montreal; Elizabeth Reid, Director, HIV and Development Programme, United Nations Development Programme, New York; and Des Cohen, Chief Economist, HIV and Development Programme, United Nations Development Programme, New York.

Acknowledgements

Catherine Hankins, Elizabeth Reid and Des Cohen wish to thank Sylvie Gauthier, Fiona Percy, and Mina Mauerstein-Bail. Co-ordinated by the Centre for AIDS Studies of the Public Health Unit of the Montreal General Hospital, now known as the Group for Research to Action of the McGill AIDS Centre of McGill University.

6. GROUNDING RESPONSES IN PEOPLE'S REALITIES: LISTENING TO HOW PEOPLE TALK ABOUT THE EPIDEMIC

The way people communicate about their own lives and the epidemic is an integral part of their own understanding, which in turn is the basis of action they take. Consideration of the language people use is therefore important to supporting the development of understanding and action. An example of the importance of this was noted by Dr Evelyn Gacad, the National AIDS Programme Manager in the Philippines. She referred to the fact that the recently developed National HIV/AIDS Strategy was written by Filipinos and included use of "Filipino English". This, she said, meant that people reading the strategy would recognise that it had been written by Filipinos, not outsiders, and that this would result in more widespread commitment to understanding and working within the principles outlined in that strategy.

6.1 Key Lessons Learnt

This section is based on the results of interactive discussions held in the field between evaluation team members, partners of the Programme and others who have been involved in using similar approaches. It focuses on developing deeper understanding of the way in which the language people use helps them to understand and act in their own contexts, and the way in which the language used in development practice can either enhance or hinder such understanding and action.

If development is to commence with people's perceptions of their own realities, and continue in ways which are consistent with their views about what is desirable and how change comes about, then it is important that they be able to bring their own understanding into the process. If development practice continues to be described and implemented using only the languages of technology, power, medicine, colonialism and social engineering, then there is little chance that different perspectives can even be described, let alone incorporated into the process. Yet this is what often happens in the global response to the HIV epidemic. Programmes are almost always described using words like "targeting", "intervention", "inputs" and "outputs": words which fit clearly into an overriding metaphor of social engineering, and which are not consistent at all with the underlying purpose of most of those same programmed which is to empower people to respond to the epidemic in ways which make sense within their own cultures and social realities.

Two issues were therefore apparent for the evaluation team. First, the need to create space for people to talk using their own chosen words and metaphors, to enable them to describe how capacity is developed in ways which make sense to them. Second, to engage with people in shared reflection about they types of words and metaphors which they are already using. As a result, some alternative metaphor systems could be identified in various contexts: metaphors which are different to the dominant metaphor of social engineering, and which may help explain how capacity development comes about when attempts are made to come to terms with what it means to work in genuinely collaborative relationships.

In this section, further background information is provided to explain why the use of language is so important, and how the HDP has attempted to address some language issues. Then, the results of interpretive discussion about the language people are using in the response to the epidemic are summarised, with some tentative conclusions made about the types of metaphors which arise when people talk from the heart about their own experiences.

Following description of these key themes, a case study is presented which outlines and explains the way the development of appropriate language and useful concepts became central features of one series of partnerships, commencing with but moving beyond the partnership between the Salvation Army and the HDP.

6.2 The UNDP HIV-Related Language Policy

A crucial component of the approach of the HDP has been the promotion of widespread discussion about the use of language in discussions about responses to the HIV epidemic. One example of this is the production of a document entitled, "UNDP HIV-related language policy". This document has been used in UNDP workshops and circulated amongst partners of the programme. The document suggests the use of language which is inclusive and which does not create and reinforce a "Them/Us" mentality or approach; which is drawn from the vocabulary of peace and human development rather than from the vocabulary of war; which uses descriptive terms which are those preferred or chosen by persons described; which is gender sensitive; and which suggests that terms used need to be adequate and accurate.

A simple one-page document, this language policy has had far reaching impact, perhaps because its basic purpose and the issues it outlined made immediate sense to the many people who have read it. It has been used all over the world, and evaluation team members have all either seen the document or heard of its use in sparse and unrelated networks, including the HIV and Development Network of Australia, the Global Network of People Living with HIV, the Philippine National AIDS Council's committee on policy development, and networks of NGOs in rural areas of Senegal.

6.3 Noting the Emergence of New Forms of Discourse

The UNDP HIV and Development Programme has expressed concerns about the dominance of particular types of language in public discourse about HIV, drawing attention to the way in which some uses of language can limit understanding, but also noting the emergence of new forms of discourse which are more optimistic and empowering to those affected by the epidemic. These include use of, "... a language of processes rather than interventions, of people as responsible actors rather than as manipulable objects of interventions" (Reid, 1994). The approach of the HDP, using the inclusive and empowering processes outlined in Section 5, has enabled people to bring their own experience and understanding into programming responses. The language they use provides a good example of how such processes lead to deeper understanding. In planning the evaluation process, evaluation team members and Programme staff members identified language issues which the evaluation team decided to consider, centring around the use of metaphor in discussions about HIV and development.

6.4 Understanding the Role of Metaphor as a Means of Understanding Reality

The every day language of people, within many languages, is pervaded by the use of metaphors, to such an extent that these metaphors influence the way people understand the world. This has been documented and explained by Lakoff (Lakoff, 1992). An example provided by Lakoff is that metaphors such as, "Love is a journey" enable us to understand all sorts of complexities about love, which may otherwise remain an abstract concept which is very difficult to understand. Such metaphors may be primarily used in literature. However, there are more complex, more pervasive metaphors which are infused into our every day understanding.

Put together, these result in "systems" of metaphorical use which influence not just our understanding of single concepts, but also the relationships between many different concepts.

Use of metaphorical systems, rather than just single metaphors, is a feature of many discussions about HIV. The most dominant and obvious metaphorical system is the system of the metaphor of "social engineering".

6.5 The "Social Engineering" Metaphor

Within the metaphor system of social engineering, an example of a single metaphor is the use of the term, "expert". The idea is that an "expert", just like an engineer working with a mechanical system, can learn all there is to know about a particular situation, through observation, and then change that situation, through some sort of "intervention", to make the whole thing "work better". No one says that social systems are mechanical, but an unconscious implication of use of this metaphor is that the methods used to fix machines can, by and large, be transferred to the field of human development.

Such simple use of metaphors may appear harmless enough. However, when they are put together within an overall metaphorical framework, they come to dominate the ways people think about particular situations. Again, referring to programming responses to the HIV epidemic, consider the following terms, which appear again and again, and think about how they may influence the way people think about the epidemic:

input
output
analysing the situation
fine tuning of programmes
programming
measuring effectiveness
targeting
intervention
expert
control
testing

There would be no problem with use of these terms within a metaphorical system of "social engineering" if they enabled better understanding of different situations and if they led to more effective responses. The problem is that use of this particular metaphorical system has been so pervasive that it has led to exclusion of other ways of talking about the HIV epidemic. As one participant from Zambia noted, "They used these methods to deal with smallpox. Now they're trying to do the same with HIV. HIV is far more complex than smallpox, but the language they use does not acknowledge that". The result is that the use of this metaphorical system has limited the development of effective responses to the epidemic.

The way in which use of this metaphor has worked against the inclusion of many people's concerns within an epidemic intricately linked with culture and values was highlighted by Eduardo San Miguel, from Mexico:

> Social engineering does not refer to social relations. It seemed to be very technological, market oriented, reflective of state intervention versus participation in activity, with a high role for hierarchy. Authority without taking anybody into account.

Language consistent with this metaphor was most often used by participants responding to the list of "Concepts UNDP is not currently using". Common reactions to this list involved recognition that these types of terms were often used by funding agencies, and often led to forms of project proposal writing and reporting which conflicted with participants' own experiences in working with people in their own contexts. Some participants noted, for example, that they have to work with people in one way and report back to international agencies in another way.

6.6 How do People Talk about the Epidemic?

The evaluation team paid close attention to the way people are talking about the epidemic, in order to see if it was possible to identify aspects of emerging new types of discourse which are being used in people's everyday experience of responding to the epidemic. This process involved listening to the language people are using and considering whether there are some alternative metaphorical systems already in use. Through these sorts of listening processes, of which the evaluation was merely a simple example, a more comprehensive understanding of use of language may evolve, helping to connect the processes used in development assistance with the realities of people's lives.

Using interactive processes, the evaluation identified some recurring metaphors which seemed to form metaphorical systems, centering around concepts of "farming", "war", "building", and "family". Importantly, use of different types of metaphors seemed to vary between countries. This may reflect different cultures, but also may arise from different experiences of the epidemic.

6.7 The "Farming" Metaphor System

Many participants in Zambia used words and expressions that are often associated with farming. For example:

> We are planting the seed of love in these children so that they will grow up and be caring persons. We know that not all seeds will grow, but we have to put our faith in the future of these children. They will also be the ones to take care of our children when we die.
>
> *(Rose Mwitelela from Kwasha Mukwenu, a community based programme for care of children whose parents have died as a result of AIDS).*
>
> It is like growing something: it doesn't take a day. You must be prepared to wait. you need to nurture and care for the tree to yield fruits which you may never yourself get to see. *(Sister [Dr.] Auxillia Bupe Ponga, D.O.R., Director of Women and Development, National Commission for Development Planning).*

Farming in African societies is often done by women, and is connected to sustaining life through providing food for family members. It involves responsibility, care, patience, knowledge, attentiveness, and being sensitive to the surrounding environment (changing weather conditions, droughts, floods, access to water, etc.).

Farming in the African context means interaction with natural surroundings, and an understanding of interdependence. It also means that even if you have to put in a lot of work, the product of your work will not come immediately, but the product of your work may be essential for surviving. Farming is not linear: it is not a question of putting in the seed and waiting for the result. Conditions change and responses must change accordingly. Farming follows certain cycles and is process-oriented. Note the similarities with approaches in sustainable human development, and with the approaches of the Programme.

The responses to the HIV epidemic of the women quoted above centre around responsibility, care, flexibility, and the changing of responses after taking into account many different circumstances. The responses were future-oriented and illustrated hope in what many other people would see as the most grim of circumstances.

The Programme works with concepts that form an integral part of a farming metaphor, such as "nourishing", but it has not consciously used this metaphor. Many of its initiatives involve similar understandings of the importance of preparing the ground, planting seeds of hope, and following up with nurturing processes rather than use of control and reporting mechanisms.

6.8 The "War" Metaphor System

Some words used by evaluation participants can be used within several metaphors. This illustrates the importance of interactive exploration to identify patterns of meaning behind use of words. Words that are used within the metaphors of both social engineering and war include, "targets", "operations", "interventions" and "they". Some other words used in a metaphor system based on war are:

> fight, barriers, conflict, battle, resistance, shield, targets, power, power-imbalance, hostility, invasion, enemy, oppression, submission, victim, win.

Within the war metaphor the perception of the *enemy* varies. The enemy may be the virus. Often, however, the enemy is perceived to be the HIV-infected person, either as the one who destroys others or as one who is already infected, degraded, made unworthy, demoralized through being victimized and thus no longer one of 'us':

> ... the first time I opened up to those pastors' wives, I saw a judgemental spirit. ... There are words still being used that should be removed. "Victim!" ... so people put a label on you. *(from a Zambian HIV-positive woman who is active within the church and who works voluntarily in hospitals helping people with AIDS).*

Other people may also be seen as enemies:

> Don't come near me because I am going to get it from you (the homosexuality). The attitude of many of my colleagues is that homosexuality is "vampirism". ... Social images of sexuality as the unnameable and filthy are reinforced by prejudice and intolerance ...
> *(Eduardo San Miguel, the National Commission on Human Rights, Mexico).*

Amongst people engaged in effective and voluntary responses to the epidemic, the perception of the enemy is often very different to that in the above quotes:

> ... The conflict is really a struggle for dominance and a struggle for resisting dominance ... of course we meet resistance, but we soldier on ... AIDS is a crosscutting issue. This is really about fighting the patriarchal structure. And if this is not recognized in the response to the AIDS-epidemic we will have no movement forward!
> *(Sara Longwe and Roy Clarke, private development consultants, Zambia).*
>
> There is a danger with the use of metaphors. Sometimes we use them firmly without reflecting on them. I realize I am

always fighting. I am constantly talking about breaking the walls of the ghetto, about tearing down barriers. I am thinking and functioning within the war metaphor and this is the first time I have stopped to reflect on it. The NGO's in Mexico are also fighting between themselves. This discussion has been really valuable for me. I discover that I don't always need to fight, that actually a lot of the NGOs and others involved in responding to the epidemic can communicate and co-operate and have a lot in common in spite of the diversity.

(Irma Rosado, ASPANE, participating in the workshop in Mexico).

6.9 The "Building" Metaphor System

The metaphor of building was used in several ways amongst evaluation participants, and was particularly noticeable amongst evaluation participants in Mexico. It is used to illustrate construction and creation processes, as processes involving collective action and solidarity. The building is often seen as a home—providing sanctuary and protection. The metaphor of building was also used in the context of constructing barriers:

If you are a caring person you get a lot of satisfaction seeing that people get out of distress. When facing a challenge you can see that you are one of the builders—that also gives you energy.

(John Musange, Family Health Trust, Children in Distress Project Manager, Zambia).

In Mexico, exploration of the building metaphor revealed that building was associated with traditions of neighbours and friends helping each other in building homes. It evokes such associations as "solidarity", "reciprocity", "mutuality", and "belonging in a community".

When discussing people's decisions about when to discuss being infected, concepts like "coming out" and "out of the closet" were used in association with the concept of building. Interactive reflection in the workshop in Mexico revealed that coming out can make you vulnerable because it could put you in the open with no protection, with no shelter, with the risk of losing belonging. Use of the metaphor helps make clear some connections between the issue of "coming out" and the issue of "enabling environments".

6.10 The "Family" Metaphor System

Language centring around the concept associated with "the

family" was often used by participants in the Philippines. This was not observed during the workshops held in the Philippines, but was identified during later interactive processes when evaluation team members who had visited the Philippines reported back to others. Hence, use of the metaphor has not been discussed with participants in the Philippines, and its inclusion here is very tentative, aiming to provoke discussion rather than to draw conclusions.

Use of this metaphor was typified in discussion about the fact that many successful projects started with very humble beginnings, with no clear understanding of long term goals or even general directions. People simply, "... came together" to explore what they might do. People work together, support one another, and grow together, just as children grow within a family. There was a strong sense of nurturing new developments in a caring way in the Philippines. For example, many NGOs which have worked successfully on issues around the epidemic in Manila are now engaged in encouraging the development of NGO initiatives in other regions of the country. This work was often reported as using similar approaches to those used by the Programme. For example, the use of validation was important. One NGO worker drew attention, for example, to the importance of what she called,

> The principle of acknowledging small successes. For example, with kids learning to walk the one or two steps when they don't fall. So they glean some satisfaction when they start to move. Think maybe three or six months later what they'll be doing.

6.11 The Use of Inclusive Processes in Enabling People to Share their Understanding

This discussion on metaphors is included as an example of the way the inclusive processes explained in Section 5 create the opportunity for people to bring in their own understanding of reality, and to develop effective responses based on that understanding.

The language people use is but one indicator of their understanding. Inclusive processes enable the sharing of ideas using language which the people involved relate to and understand, and also the development of responses to which people feel committed because they are based on their own choices. Limiting the way people speak about the epidemic, even when this occurs unconsciously, will almost certainly hinder the development of effective and sustainable responses.

Active listening, the promotion of dialogue as a means of developing shared understanding, decision-making, and consensus are therefore important components of new programming practices in sustainable human development. Such processes are based on mobilizing the expertise of all involved rather than on the notion of "experts" coming in from outside and determining what responses should be developed within specific contexts.

CASE STUDY 2:
THE PARTNERSHIP BETWEEN THE SALVATION ARMY AND THE HIV AND DEVELOPMENT PROGRAMME

"Sharing Experiences Means Extra Space for Mutual Growth"

Introduction

Not all organisational interactions are healthy—those of the UN system and non-government organizations can bring to mind situations of awkwardness, tension, competition and exclusion.

Occasionally that is not so—the reflections of conversations, key events, key lessons learnt through organisational sharing of the UNDP HIV and Development Programme (New York) and the Salvation Army International Headquarters (IHQ) (through the IHQ technical assistance team) recall a healthy experience of mutual learning expressed through:

* Informal discussion.
* Regional and national co-operation with a focus on local programming.
* Participation of the Salvation Army in UNDP formal processes, e.g. SPR.
* Participation of UNDP in Salvation Army processes, e.g. International conference on HIV, Leysin, July 1991; participatory evaluation of the work of the international technical assistance team, Ottawa, Canada, September 1992.

The values that underscore co-operation need to be identified not only because they are crucial to organizational collaboration, but because mutual learning is essential for an effective response to the HIV epidemic. No longer do communities and organisations have the luxury of time to "play games", to be "territorial": the problem is too big for all of us combined, let alone any organisation trying to do it alone.

The values for effective co-operation include a willingness to share, to listen, to learn from the other, to be enabled in personal and organisational development because of the influence of the other, to be secure in sharing, to recognise the common foundation of sensitivity to the personal and community voice of suffering and of the search for hope, the need for a commitment to an ethic of care, and to a belief that changc is possible. These values are expressed and developed in a context of belonging rather than separateness. They are the cement which holds together the foundations of programme development at local, regional and international levels. Complementing these values are the use of key concepts which include the link of care to prevention, and community involvement in social change.

How have values been shared, concepts formed, and programmes developed in more effective ways because of the co-operation between the two international organizations?

1. Zambia 1988

Picture the Chikankata AIDS team, frantically integrating daily work with evening planning and late night writing, entertaining, hosting, being hospitable to constant visitors, all of whom seemed to want to come at the weekends because that was when they had spare time!

Occasionally the visitor was not ordinary, but somehow communicated an insight.

Such a visitor was Elizabeth Reid (of UNDP). She came as an analyst, as a human being, as a person enmeshed in the emotions associated with the impact of the virus on a person and a family. She seemed to see something different, and what was so implicit to the implementing team was named by her.

She saw that the person with HIV had been placed fairly and squarely in the middle of circles of concern—that the person mattered and yet the person was in relationship with others.

She saw an attempt to articulate, at that stage, the link between the care of a person and the positive motivation towards protection and prevention by and in affected others.

The key values observed appeared to be:

1. Care is necessary for human dignity, encouragement and development.
2. Care links with motivation of affected others towards prevention and positive development through change.
3. Programme implementors don't have to be interventionists but can be participants.
4. Outside experts need to live the rhetoric—they need to sit with others, listen, absorb, sense, reflect, and learn.

These values were the basis of the Chikankata programme, characterised by the word "integration".

This concept of integration implied the interlinkage of many disciplines; the community voice was linked with the national voice in policy development; and, in a most basic sense, the integration of a care process with a prevention response came from within the motivation and initiative of people rather than relying primarily on external interventions (which were popular at the time).

2. London 1990

Ian Campbell, appointed by the Salvation Army to be Medical Adviser to the Salvation Army, finds his way to London and, within the first few days of arriving in February 1990, is in contact with "the network".

One early link was with UNDP New York, out of respect for relationship, as well as the felt need in Ian to find out what was going on internationally and to strengthen the process of international linkage of the Salvation Army.

The values and concepts expressed by the Salvation Army at that time with respect to AIDS had been more clearly articulated as "transferable concepts"—care linked to prevention; community related to belonging; change relating to attitudes, behaviours and environment; decentralised approaches embracing the notion of teamwork and linked to sustainability; the search for and discovery of hope; normalization meaning the realistic recognition of living with HIV/AIDS; and others.

A facilitator group had formed to develop programme and concept transfer internationally through the Salvation Army system.

Elizabeth Reid and Mina Mauerstein-Bail (of UNDP) together encouraged the identity that was being expressed by the Salvation Army. In a visit to the Salvation Army International Headquarters, including an interaction with the Commissioner, Bramwell Tillsley (second in command of the Salvation Army internationally), the statement was made by Elizabeth Reid that, "It is not our job to shape you in the UNDP image but to affirm you in your own identity, as the best way to help the international response to AIDS."

The values expressed by UNDP included the following:

* Unity in diversity—but a common belief that social change is possible.
* Respectful affirmation that religious belief is the key to effective living in many people's lives and in the identity of many faith organizations.

One *key concept was inter-organisational sharing as a means of strengthening identity and performance.* This has been the foundation for informal and formal interaction since 1990.

3. Leysin, Switzerland, July 1991

By agreement of the General, the first Salvation Army international conference on AIDS was held. This proved to be a catalytic event to a sequence of programme design, support and evaluation, and organisational sharing. This sharing is currently inclusive of 30 countries, with 50 community-based programmes still emerging, some of which can still be directly related to the Leysin conference.

A key feature of conference programme design, by the international technical assistance team, was the inclusion of other organisations to underscore the value of mutual learning.

The values expressed by the Salvation Army and by UNDP (represented by Mr. Wally N'Dow, then the UNDP Resident Representative from Central African Republic, subsequently in Tanzania, and now the Assistant Secretary-General of HABITAT, and Secretary-General for the HABITAT II Conference, June 1996) were that inclusiveness is valuable, and that inclusiveness is of direct benefit to work because of its influence on programme planning and development.

Wally N'Dow, a Muslim, was stimulated by the conference, and clearly felt that he belonged. An indicator was seen at the conclusion when he gathered everybody together, holding hands, and led the group in a song. He felt free to share his own faith background with another faithbased organization. The common ground was of response, in a spirit of service and facilitation, to the intrusion of HIV/AIDS. The common vision was the opportunity for community development, change, and hope.

4. Senegal, November 1991

Informal Consultation on Behavioural Change. Through a process of interlinkage between the UK NGO/AIDS Consortium, the Salvation Army, Save the Children (UK) and UNDP (New York), a reflection happened on the process of behaviour change. An influential and succinct statement on behaviour change emerged as the product of the work of 16 local programme teams, and of a facilitation process formed by inter-organisational sharing. This was in itself an indicator of successful sharing of values and concepts, and was ahead of its time because so many unusual boundaries were crossed.

The meeting in Senegal seemed to have that quality of reaching out into the future. A significant shift was felt in development of consensus about the concept of "*community*".

The Salvation Army view for some time had been that people are interconnected in relationships in community—people are "autonomous" and yet that does not mean that they work alone. Their decisions are influenced by others and the intricacy of the community process for seemingly simple actions should never be underestimated. Apart from a statement on the influences on behaviour change, this was another major outcome of the Senegal meeting, but it was subtle in that the connection between the person and community relationship had already been discerned mutually by UNDP and the Salvation Army. Perhaps it was more distinctively observed by Elizabeth (of UNDP) at the meeting, particularly through informal conversation in lunch hour times and after hours with people such as Roy Mwilu and Noerine Kaleeba. The meeting formed the environment for productive healthy mutual strengthening of learning, particularly the interconnection between community belonging and change.

5. Other Connections

In betwen these "major events", informal visits to New York, warm connections at regional and international meetings continued ...

6. Washington, June 1992

The US Congressional Forum on HIV/AIDS. An opportunity for influencing US policy on funding? A time for talking between people belonging to organizations? Politics?

Ian (of the Salvation Army) presented on "Care and traditional values in relation to responses to AIDS and HIV", with reference to the Chikankata Hospital experience of connecting care to prevention. Elizabeth spoke on "contracts" between people—using a different language but reinforcing the shared values and concepts contained in the former conversations and experiences. She spoke movingly of contracts between persons, men and women, communities and nations, linking this to development, positive change and hope.

The key value affirmed was that people develop through relationships, not by power and conflict. The key concept strengthened, which is crucial to effective programme development, was that people in the intimacy of their relationships need to respond as relational beings and as people in groups, as well as being persons functioning as individuals.

7. Berlin, July 1993

"HIV/AIDS and Military Populations", a UNDP supported

initiative, examined creatively the role of military populations in responding to and perpetuating the epidemic.

Another type of "military"—the "Salvation Army"—was creatively incorporated by Elizabeth Reid and Mina Mauerstein-Bail (of UNDP), probably as an effort on their part to increase the representation of values and concepts that go beyond the prevailing images associated with military populations.

Instead of seeing military populations as isolated units, the reality is that they connect to civilian populations in times of war and peace, through sexual activity, and through family and community life. The meeting did not ignore the accentuation of the risk environment provided by military populations in times of instability and civil war.

The key value shared indirectly and directly was that people in "groups" are actually not isolated in those groups— in this sense "targeted interventions" need to be very strategic and linked to the recognition that people in groups are also in other relationships.

The key concept underscored by this exploration of linkage to the wider community was that people who define themselves as being within a very select community or group are actually a subgroup of a wider community.

This is crucial to effective programme development because it is clear that through targeted interventions alone, marginalisation often increases for people who are commercial sex workers, truck drivers, youth, military people, religious people, etc. It is still commonly the case that targeted interventions are named as the only practical way forward. Even if other strategies are named, there is often a tendency to rely on targeted interventions as the priority, and in isolation from other relationships, because this appears to be easier.

8. Community Response

After Ian's visit to Zambia, Zimbabwe, Uganda and Kenya in May 1994, the emerging distress felt within families and communities impacted Ian (of the Salvation Army) with a sense of urgency that there needed to be a definitive reflection on processes of behaviour change. He wrote about this to Elizabeth (see letter).

Elizabeth responded to Ian's letter with her own letter—there was evidence of an instinctive perception of the real issue, beyond the words, of personal family and community impact that was way ahead of anyone's ability to name (see letter).

A key value being expressed was, "We do not know what we think we know." The epidemic teaches us that it is impossible to say that we have arrived, and that the best we can do is to share together, looking at relationship variables, real people, real experiences, real behaviours. This will give some opportunity to stretch out to touch the meanings associated with the epidemic, most of which are felt non-verbally and often missed by most people.

26 May 1994
London, UK

Dear Elizabeth,

I will be in New York for the afternoon of Wednesday, 8th June.

I hope it will be possible to see you even briefly. It will be important to share experiences gained through the mission just completed to the Congo, Zaire, Zambia, Kenya and Uganda.

The linkage of care in the home to change through and by the community is more clearly affirmed. At field level, systematic home visits by a team can be linked through 'confidential sharing' to community mobilisation for support and change.

Every household in the Chikankata catchment area is now listed, by the initiative of the community. Although it is not yet established, the view is emerging that every house can be visited on a systematic basis when there is someone who is sick and every house can be included now in a present and future plan for neighbour support and visitation. These two extra elements of neighbour to neighbour support and inclusion of a future need, expressed now, are two simple but very important elements of a workable approach to management at field level in high prevalence places.

Organisations like the Salvation Army are ready made for this sort of involvement but catalytic funding is needed in low, medium and high prevalence countries to normalise the process of home visits, community involvement and change. It seems to me that this can take anything from six months to several years, and that it can happen in low prevalence areas (e.g. Mizoram, India) as well as high prevalence areas (e.g. Chikankata, Tshelanyemba Hospital).

The team at Chikankata tried to describe both 'community pain' and 'hope'. The pain is reflected by serious disposition in people, lessening or disappearance of wailing when deaths happen, and adjustments to counselling processes that include, for example, recognition that though one person of a couple to be married might be sero-positive, they may still go ahead if they know what the future might hold because otherwise how can love be found and expressed? Also the recognition has dawned that the loss is accumulative and that it is only just beginning. The hope, as we said a year or so ago, is both concrete and mysterious—people can care for each other, but at the same time, the mystery of belonging energises people and motivates them to care, to love, and to be realistic.

Definition of hope is an important theme to spread around the world, because as people find capacity to cope, they can become disabled by the increasing accumulative loss and pain.

I know you know these things but I felt you should be the first to have a reflection letter on my return (today is the first day in the of five)..

We (Alison and I) look forward to seeing you and/or Mina, if possible.

Yours sincerely,
Ian D. Campbell
Captain
MEDICAL ADVISER
The Salvation Army

---

30 May 1994
Rosedale, Australia

Dear Ian,

It was such a pleasure to hear from you. Particularly since, as usual, we seem to be seeing and thinking the same things. I have recently had two brief trips to Zambia. How desolate that country will be one day. Unless... Both times I got out into the villages but the second trip I went down to Livingstone to see the work of three UN Volunteers working to strengthen community based responses to the epidemic.

One of the images that I will long carry with me was sitting in the courtyard of an urban health centre in one of the poorest compounds talking to the home-based care team that one of the volunteers was training and working with. When we arrived, it was the day of their normal weekly meeting, none of the women were yet there. We were told that they would be late since they had gone to a nearby compound to collect food for the work that they had been doing in a public works programme. This food, we were told, was all that many of them had to keep going. They were all volunteers from the surrounding compounds. They all had families of their own and each day was a struggle for survival. Yet they volunteered. And to do what must be one of the most depressing works of neighbourliness that exists: offering solace with little if anything in the way of physical support to the (mainly) AIDS dying.

The system was, usually, that when the neighbours heard that someone was sick, they told or sent a message to the Counsellor attached to the Health Centre. After she (almost invariably; in the home-based care team, one man had been trained but had not ever shown up after — this needs some reflection) had visited the house, she would add the family to the list for the care team. With a system such as this, the carers are not helping the HIV infected, but only the dying, the terminally ill. And usually those who are caught unawares by the dying, without preparation. The team told me that often they find the whole family starving, with no thought having been given to how those surviving the dying person will survive. The team has little to offer. Mostly they do not even have soap to wash the sick and themselves afterwards, no disinfectant, no food tor the starving or protein supplements for the weak, etc. (This lack of support needs to be addressed within the programme.

But what they do have is extraordinary. They have courage and compassion. By just turning up and crossing the threshhold, they challenge, and encourage, the rest ofthe community to do likewise. They ensure that the family is not humiliated and neglected but rather remains part of the community. They help start the essential process of changing attitudes towards the HIV infected and dying. Once inside, they bring concern and care. They are someone to talk things through with. For everyone, the sick and the well, the spouse with her or his fears and the children with their fears. They take over, for at least two short periods each week, the care of the sick, the cleaning up of the diarrhoca, the washing up, the making of the beds, etc.

Who are these women? What motivates them to do this? I do not know the answer to the latter question for that would have required more time to listen to and understand the answers than I had there. But I asked them who they were. Mothers all of them, as I recall. At least one recently widowed. All of them having trouble coping themselves, few of them with much education, all of them searching for ways to earn a little extra money. I wondered ifithe answer to the second question included an element of what you call a future need, an investment in the care of others now in the hope that there will be someone there to care for you when your turn (inevitably, one feels is the extent of the despair) comes. I talked about these women at the recent SWAA regional conference in Zambia.

Thus, even in this micro example, one sees the linkages from care to change through and by the community, to a network of concern and compassion that links present giving to the possibility of future needs, to a process of community mobilisation, that you talk about in your letter, an approach,that I too believe can be put in place in both low and high prevalence areas.

In many ways the UNV programme and the Salvation Army are similarly placed: at community level, where these processes of care and change must be set in place. At present, the Salvation Army has the critically important advantage of your team there to give them guidance on how to do it well. The UNVs need similar support if they are to do it effectively and sustainably. There are others also that we must identify.

The uniqueness of the Chikankata and similar programmes is that the person at the centre of this process is not always terminally ill, the condition with which they went to hospital may have been treatable, and so the teams work with both the HIV infected well and with the dying. In the former case, the person may be well enough to start planning for his or her illness and death, to start planning for their children's future, to start to pass on their knowledge to others. There is an urgent need, in Africa in particular, to help people to start talking about all these things, to ensure that they have access to voluntary counselling and testing services, so that the testimony of the infected and well can be heard, their needs addressed and the quality and length of their life lengthened so that they can continue to nurture and raise their children and to contribute productively to the economy. Apart from anything else, Africa cannot afford to lose prematurely their knowledge and skills and their children need them to be there with them for as long as possible.

The other issues that you raise are ones that concern me deeply. The terrible pain, loss and grieving associated with this epidemic and the fact that it is cumulative and that the future will be much worse than the already often unbearable present. And the deep need to be able to continue to love and to express that love, even if the loved one is infected. Remember Berlin. Although we must do everything in our power to try to ensure that loving someone is not an inevitable death sentence for the spouse and a curse for the children of this love. We must make sure that such people can talk through this choice, have access to good quality and affordable condoms and that the psychological and emotional problems associated with using them in every act of lovemaking during the relationship can be talked through. (I revised and expanded some of my Berlin thoughts on this recently, in Mombasa, at the first conference of the Network of African People with HIV and AIDS. The reaction of those attending, men and women each in their own way, has given me much food for thought).

Your words and insights on hope are, again, critically important. This, and the associated emotions of empathy, compassion, laughter, respect, love, empowerment, etc., that is, the will to live, are all that will carry people through the terrifying trauma and pain that this epidemic carries within itself.

How much ofthe afternoon (and evening?) of June 8 can you and Alison give to me/us? There is so much to discuss. If the Regional Bureau is in agreement, I would also like you and Alison to meet with the team doing the evaluation of the Africa Regional Project which will be in town that week for their briefing. For these are the ends of the Project. How can one evaluation progress towards them?

I am very much looking forward to seeing you. Thanks for writing down your thoughts and reflections and sending them to me. I was touched. Some of your observations brought tears to my eyes.

Being in Australia, by the way, is wonderful. Love,

Elizabeth

9. Regional Inclusion

The Salvation Army international team co-ordinated a series of regional workshops focused on "concept analysis ", beginning in November 1993 in Zambia (for Africa), September 1994 in the Philippines (for East Asia and the Pacific), Bangladesh in February 1995 (for South Asia) and Bolivia in August 1995 (for Latin America).

With each of these workshops, it was possible for UNDP (New York) to allocate a small funding grant to support the work of the international team which, in most cases, was the catalyst to other organizations giving funding sufficient to meet the needs (e.g. a $5,000 grant for the meeting in the Philippines stimulated other donors to provide the rest of the funding amounting to $75,000). Perhaps of more significance was the inclusion of people from other organisations and locations.

For example, the inclusion of people from Bulgaria, Poland and Russia (2 from each location, representing national and non-government responses) proved to be a major creative element stressing the process of inclusion at a meeting attended by people responding to AIDS and HIV from villages in Papua New Guinea, from the Marshall Islands, and from Salvation Army administration levels in other countries of the region.

But the *conceptual foundations of care, community, change, hope and sustainability* were shared effectively, across culture and language, and so it was possible to find convergence as well as to acknowledge divergence. The programme development culture of eastern Europe superficially appeared to jar with the ethos of the meeting; and yet the necessary struggle to find common ground was probably key to accelerated learning by all the participants.

Of significance was the recognition of the *value of spirituality and faith* in motivating people to respond, within organisations, to the challenges of the epidemic. There is a strong faith tradition in Eastern Europe and in South-East Asia. This congruency, itself a reflection of the congruency of respectful recognition of identity between the Salvation Army International Headquarters and UNDP New York, was a strengthening feature of the meeting.

Madu Balu Nath, of the UNDP HIV & Development project in Delhi, acknowledged similar values in her participation in the Bangladesh meeting. She spoke of the need to work from the inside out, of participation with community spirit, and of listening to community voices as a means of guidance in the response to the epidemic.

For example, Juan Jacobo Hernandez of Colectivo Sol was able to say, at a moment of crisis and creative development involving a former Salvation Army officer who is HIV positive and who was also a participant, "The Church has AIDS. The Salvation Army has AIDS. Thank you God." He prefaced his comment by saying he had never prayed before.

Around this time Elizabeth began to speak of the need for a gathering of religious leaders and the Salvation Army team is supportive of that approach, willing to participate and facilitate— a future challenge.

It is a sobering thought to recognise that the intimacy of life is expressed through relationship, which in turn is expressed sexually, emotionally, and through the exploration of the meaning of 'soul' which finds its expression in various forms of prayer.

There is a language of hope forming—based, for example, on the acknowledgment of the need for intimacy and health of relationship; and of terrible loss that is not just happening now but awareness as to the awful knowledge that the past and the future are being lost in the present. This is loss of community memory. Yet hope is yearned for, sensed, claimed, and expressed in the poorest of circumstances. People feel it in caring with each other; in working together for change now; in simply being able to talk in new ways; and in still believing in a future, unseen and unfelt, yet it is there.

10. National and Local Interaction

The horror and hope of Rwanda is unmatched. In April 1995, it was possible for the International Salvation Army team to support the Salvation Army work in development through agriculture, health and pastoral care by advising on how that work could be interlinked with response to HIV and AIDS.

It was recognised that HIV/AIDS is an entry point to the fragility and capacity of life and this is no more true anywhere than in Rwanda which is searching for its "soul" through the visible process of reconciliation.

As in other countries, a visit to the UNDP office, encouraged through correspondence from Mina Mauerstein-Bail to the UNDP Resident Representative in Kigali (as had happened previously with Bangladesh, Uganda, etc.), paved the way for mature interactive mutual learning between the two organizations, ... at country level.

The values represented included recognition of the role of an international structure to help facilitate within the organisation so as to make it receptive to the "stranger" at the doorway. Cultivation of a spirit of inclusion and mutual learning was the service of UNDP, New York, and the result was affirmation in the mind of the Salvation Army team in Rwanda that HIV/AIDS is a development and reconciliation issue.

Summary

Inter-organisational sharing is not just about sharing information and holding on to personal identity no matter what—effectiveness is determined by *shared values*, that embrace respect; affirmation of the other identity given that it is founded in genuine compassion, and a capacity for strategic action embracing both care and change; a culture of mutual learning, of facilitation, of service, of listening in to community voices, of sitting within the suffering without ever believing it is possible to provide for it entirely; and participation in the search for hope. These values are crucial to the "common ground" of conceptual reflection for effective programme development.

The key concepts for the Salvation Army include the interlinkage of care to prevention, belief that change is possible, community as circles of belonging and participation; sustainability depending on the interlinkage of the person in community to care and prevention. Hope is related to all these factors.

There is an obvious congruencey with UNDP's ongoing exploration and reflection on conceptual foundations. Different language may be used, but there are nevertheless similar foundations.

These are based, perhaps for both organizations, in a mixture of organisational identity, experience, instinct, and the personal values of those involved. These are related to personality, character and experience, yet they alone do not provide a common ground for learning—it is their linkage to conceptual definition and, in turn, to patterns of action that helps draw the organisations together informally and formally in a continuing exploration of the unknown, the unfelt and the unseen.

Perhaps the most powerful, positive, interlinking factor is the mutual recognition that the epidemic has outstripped us in its negative impact. There is a curiously powerful common background for people of the Salvation Army International Headquarters technical assistance team and the people involved in HIV and Development, New York—experiences of suffering, of participation, of positive change; and a capacity for conceptual reflection indivisibly linked to these experiences. These are the elements that are most important to forming the common ground that is essential for effective organizational sharing.

This Case Study was prepared by Captain Dr. Ian Campbell and Alison Rader of the Salvation Army, HIV and Health Programme Development Team.

7. SOME ISSUES RELATING TO THE NATURE OF CHANGE WITHIN DEVELOPMENT PRACTICE

Recent practices of technical co-operation used by UNDP and others have an inclusive, process oriented approach. This approach is characterised by use of the concepts of partnership, shared reflection on lived experiences, the gradual evolution of people's understanding and ability to act, and a collective development of effective responses which cannot be pre-determined but which are, almost by definition, relevant to the lives of the people who develop them and are thus more likely to be sustainable.

The dominant model of development which guides development and HIV-related practice generally uses an approach characterised by use of analysis of situations through externally designed research, and programming based on interventions or disseminations. These programmes aim to change people's behaviour and determine the possible range of effective responses according to pre-conceived and measurable predictions of outcomes.

The evaluation found that the proponents of the effectiveness of the new human development paradigm, and those who are most able to explain how it works, are most often those whose lives are directly affected by the epidemic and who have themselves been through transformative experiences. They often expressed a quiet yet confident hope that the processes with which they are working will continue to result in effective responses to the challenges of HIV and development.

Those working within a less process-oriented approach expressed the most pessimism and the least belief in forward movement. In the absence of finding effective "models" which work and which are replicable, they were unable to capture the sense of forward movement which was evident amongst people who were acting within a paradigm of inclusion and participation.

7.1 Key Lessons Learnt

This section is based on the results of interactive discussions held in the field between evaluation team members, partners of the Programme and others who have been involved in using similar approaches. It explains some implications arising from the way in which changes are occurring in development practice. These changes affect what is happening in the field, as described here from the perspectives of those whose lives are affected.

While discussions take place amongst high level international organisations about the need for new approaches to development practice, and changes take place in the field within specific development projects, many individuals and organisations now feel çaught between two paradigms: the traditional approaches of technical co-operation, which still dominate the understanding of many middle level bureaucrats in funding and programming agencies, and the newer approaches of sustainable human development, which are being applied in ways which make sense in their daily practice.

Thus, there are important difficulties which arise from the experience of being caught between two very different, and often seemingly irreconcilable, approaches. Such difficulties are intensified because even some agencies which are involved in the development of new approaches, including UNDP, are not yet reorienting their programme planning, management and evaluation processes in ways which clearly support such changes.

7.2 Problems with Interaction Between Different Types of Development Practice

The fact that process-oriented approaches to HIV and development are taking place within an international climate in which most programming responses to HIV and development are still based on practices derived from a more directive paradigm presents problems. These problems include the following:

(i) Since the approaches of the sustainable human development and capacity building are still being developed and explored through processes of social learning, it follows that they are not widely understood, not clearly articulated even by those adopting them, not accepted by all UN or donor agencies, and not consistently applied.

(ii) For this reason, many people are using one approach amongst the people who are affected by the epidemic and whose understanding and action they are supporting, but having to account to funding agencies, or donor countries, using the language and appearing to use the practices of the other paradigm.

(iii) The sustainable human development approach requires changes to many current practices of technical co-operation. It requires important shifts in the roles and practice of many individuals and organizations, both in donor and recipient countries. Many individuals and organizations are resistant to such change.

8. CONCLUSIONS AND RECOMMENDATIONS

The UNDP HIV and Development Programme (HDP) used the Special Programme Resources (SPR) to explore and enhance understanding of the ways in which the approaches of sustainable human development can be applied towards building capacity to understand, and to effectively respond to, the HIV epidemic. The evaluation process was exploratory and forward-looking, aiming to generate further and deeper understanding of the nature and approach of this type of programming.

Key findings of the evaluation were:

— that there are many people now engaged enthusiastically in what they themselves consider to be effective and sustainable responses to the HIV epidemic within their own contexts;

— that these people themselves affirm that the approaches used within the Programme, and similar approaches used by others, have enhanced their understanding and responses to the epidemic within the context of human development; and

— that the way these approaches have been described, developed and articulated by the HDP have validated and enhanced their own capacity, and thus helped answer the central question of, "How can we, together, move forward?"

In essence, it could be said that the work of the Programme

was based on an inter-related series of active and reflective processes which were used to catalyse further active and reflective processes in responding to the HIV epidemic. Using approaches which evolve from its understanding of development practice, the Programme worked with people committed to responding compassionately and effectively to the epidemic to help catalyse such reflective processes. Those processes began to challenge commonly held assumptions about what drives the epidemic and what may work to slow it down, and to shift the focus of attention onto the processes of social change which will lead to effective community and national responses.

The types of process-oriented approaches explored through the HDP are:

— based on human interaction, and the facilitation of processes;

— necessarily slow at first because they must grow from shared understanding and consensus building which, in turn, must evolve as real human relationships evolve within the context of lived experience; but

— lead to more effective, adaptable and sustainable responses in the long term because they build on capacity which already exists and thus create strategic effects which continue beyond the participation of the Programme, without resulting in dependency relationships with donors or technical advisers.

In effect, the processes of inclusion and partnership draw out people's understanding of both what is occurring within their own contexts and of their capacity to respond. An important strategic effect of these approaches, as described by evaluation participants, is that the people who are involved as direct partners of UN or donor agencies which use these types of development practice themselves use similar approaches in their interaction with others in their own countries and in regional networks addressing specific concerns. Thus, their own practice extends the effects of the individual programme under consideration. The evaluation was, in effect, another component of this ongoing evaluative and action-focussed approach.

Understanding of sustainable human development is still evolving as the nature of effective development practice is being explored on many fronts. The HIV epidemic, varying in its evolution and its effects in different countries, and at different stages of the epidemic within countries, presents particular challenges to any fixed understanding of what may work to catalyse effective responses to it. The problems addressed with certain responses today will be different tomorrow, or in different contexts. Therefore, new processes must continually be created to enhance understanding and to develop effective responses to new problems based on processes of social learning *which arise from within* communities and nations.

Such processes do not end with the drawing together of lessons learnt through one programme such as the SPR. This is important because, even though many of the practices of the Programme are now being adopted by other agencies, approaches based on the need to enhance understanding of the nature of effective processes and partnerships are not. While it is important that the lessons learnt through the Programme are shared and disseminated, it is equally important that the processes which led to these lessons themselves continue, both in UNDP and elsewhere. This is very different from the nature of lessons learnt through many other types of research or programming: in this case, understanding and practice must continue to evolve simultaneously through use of inclusive processes and continual questioning.

The evaluation has highlighted that approaches consistent with the principles of sustainable human development are taking place within a world in which development practice is often characterized by the mores of traditional technical co-operation. Approaches for the achievement of sustainable human development which include shared reflection, inclusion, and the conscious use of processes to allow scope for a range of possible outcomes, are beginning to be adopted. Traditional technical co-operation is driven by donor preferences, and characterised by use of external experts and use of quantitative measures to ascertain effectiveness in meeting predetermined objectives or outcomes. It is less concerned with capacity building or with the discourse of partnership or participation.

The differences between these two approaches lead to different types of practice. However, the differences are not often acknowledged, as highlighted by some reported experiences of evaluation participants. The result is that many people seek to promote social learning through using the project design processes, reporting, measuring procedures and language systems of traditional forms of technical co-operation. Conversely, it is possible for people to change their use of language but not practice. However, both the Programme and the evaluation process found that it is possible for people and agencies to shift their understanding and practices from traditional approaches to those described in Section 5. This occurs more easily when the reasons for, and the approaches of, sustainable human development are articulated, explained and communicated interactively, allowing people space to consider the relevance of these approaches within their own contexts.

That this is necessary was highlighted through one of the

findings of the evaluation process: those people approaching the HIV epidemic using approaches consistent with the framework of sustainable human development demonstrated more hope, confidence and forward movement than those working within alternative approaches.

It is important now to ensure that the lessons learnt through the HDP are shared amongst the people whose lives are affected, and disseminated within UNDP, other UN agencies and the international development assistance community. What is required is a more widespread *understanding and adoption of the approaches of sustainable human development* within the context of the HIV epidemic.

Thus, there is a need to share the lessons learnt within the HDP using approaches consistent with the Programme itself. That is, in ways which enable a wider variety of people affected by HIV and development to be involved, and which facilitate reflection about the relevance of these approaches in various contexts and the sharing of ideas about possibilities for changes in development practice.

For the people directly affected, this requires use of approaches to sharing what has been learnt in ways which are inclusive, and which create space for such sharing and further network development. The very nature of what has been learnt leads not to a set of ideas to be disseminated so much as a series of processes to be invoked.

For UN and donor agencies, this requires that approaches to sharing what has been learnt incorporate processes which enable critical reflection on the possibilities for changes within current development practice. Changes are required, for example, in the processes used for research, training, policy and strategy development, programme design, reporting procedures, and evaluation methods. These changes, in turn, require changes in skills required, and therefore in methods used for staff development and for future selection and training of staff and consultants. Ultimately, changes will be required in the management practices of UN and donor agencies, particularly changes which will enable the inclusion of the people whose lives are affected in determining priorities and aproaches to be used in programming.

UNDP has a particular role within the new joint cooperative programme, UNAIDS, and the current evaluation process indicates two key challenges:

1. There is a need to ensure ongoing association between the evolving understanding of effective approaches in sustainable human development and the evolving understanding of effective responses to the HIV epidemic. This

will be most likely if there is an ongoing direct association of UNDP with development of responses to the HIV epidemic.

2. In order that UN Resident Co-ordinators can effectively undertake their function of co-ordinating the support of UN agencies to national responses to the HIV epidemic, there is a need to ensure that UNDP in-country staff, the Resident Representatives and staff of other agencies understand the ways in which the approaches of sustainable human development can enhance understanding and lead to more effective action in response to the HIV epidemic.

Recommendations are based on the lessons learnt through the HDP and the deeper understanding of the approach which has arisen through the evaluation. They are based on the need to ensure that the processes of social learning generated through the SPR continue amongst individuals, communities and nations affected, and also within the UN system. The adoption of these recommendations will enable ongoing sharing of what has been learnt amongst other people and agencies who are, or who are interested in, developing similar approaches. Such sharing will ensure more widespread adoption of approaches which promote responses to the HIV epidemic which are grounded in people's lived experiences and evolve in ways which build upon existing capacities.

Recommendation 1: That UNDP share what has been learnt through the HDP with the people whose lives are directly affected by the challenges of HIV and development. This sharing must take place using processes which enable and encourage the involvement of people who are not normally part of development networks, and using processes such as workshops and network development which enable inclusion, reflection, sharing and the development of ongoing partnerships within nations and within regions.

Recommendation 2: That UNDP share what has been learnt through the HDP with UNAIDS, other UN agencies and with bilateral and NGO donor agencies. This sharing must take place using processes, such as workshops, which enable interactive discussion and reflection on current development practice within the HIV epidemic, and which lead to the development of new approaches in project design, management and evaluation practices. This sharing must not be limited to those staff or agencies already engaged in responding to the HIV epidemic.

Recommendation 3: That UNDP take active steps to ensure an ongoing association between evolving understanding of approaches in sustainable human development and evolving understanding of effective responses to the HIV epidemic. This could commence with a series of related planning workshops at country, regional and global levels, in which UNDP staff and others develop means to ensure such an ongoing association. These methods may include new approaches to staff development and new methods for interaction between UNDP staff and others engaged in responding to the challenges of HIV and development.

Recommendation 4: That UNDP, in association with UNAIDS, support UN Resident Co-ordinators in co-ordinating UN agency support for national responses to the HIV epidemic, by ensuring that Resident Representatives are educated about both the association between HIV and development and the nature of approaches to sustainable human development which facilitate enhanced understanding of, and effective responses to, the HIV epidemic.

REFERENCES

Banuri T. Hyden G. Juma C. Rivera M. Sustainable human development: from concept to operation, a guide for the practitioner. New York, UNDP, 1994

Benbouali A. Evaluating success and assessing performance: a draft discussion paper. UNDP Office of Evaluation and Strategic Planning. Internal paper, New York, UNDP, July 1995.

Denzin N K. *Interpretive interactionism.* Sage, *1989,* Newbury Park, California.

Chambers R. Poverty and livelihoods: whose reality counts? An overview paper prepared for the UNDP Stockholm Roundtable on Global Change, 22-24 July 1994.

Joy L. and Bennett S. Process consultation: systemic improvement of public sector management. New York, UNDP, 1994.

Lakoff G. The contemporary theory of metaphor. In: Ortony A (ed.). Metaphor and thought. Second edition. New York, Cambridge University Press, 1993.

OECD/UNDP/World Bank. Report of the High-Level Development Assitance Committee/UNDP/World Bank Seminar 1994: "Improving the effectiveness of technical co-operation in the 1990s". OECD/UNDP/World Bank, 1994.

OECD. Development Assistance Committee: principles for new orientations in technical co-operation. Organisation for Economic Co-operation and Development, 1991.

Patton M. Q. Qualitative evaluation research and methods. Sage, 1990, Newbury Park, California.

Patton M Q. Developmental evaluation. Evaluation Practice, 15(3), 1994, 311-319.

Peavey F. Strategic questioning, an approach to creating personal and social change. In: By life's grace: musings on the essence of social change (pp.86-111). New Society Publishers, 1994, Philadelphia, Pennsylvania

Reid E. Approaching the epidemic: the community's response. AIDS Care, 6(5), 1994, 551 -557

Schon D. A. Beyond the stable state: public and private learning in a changing society. Temple Smith, 1971, London.

Speth J. G. Foreword by the administrator. In: Banuri, *et al.* Sustainable human development: from concept to operation: a guide for the practitioner, New York, UNDP, 1994.

de Vylder S. Sustainable human development and macro economics: strategic links and implications. UNDP, 1995.

Weiss C. H. Evaluation research: methods of assessing programme effectiveness. Prentice Hall, 1972, Englewood Cliffs, New Jersey.

45

HIV Co-ordination at the United Nations

Ms. Elizabeth Reid
Director, HIV and Development Programe, UNDP
to the Co-ordination Segment of ECOSOC relating to HIV and AIDS

---

13 July, 1992

Mr. President, Distinguished Delegates, Colleagues,

On behalf of the Administrator of UNDP, Mr. William Draper, I welcome this opportunity to address you.

The UNDP statement on this agenda item is available and was circulated in advance as requested by delegations last week. This statement directly addresses the issues relating to the co-ordination of HIV-related policies and prograrnmes from UNDP's perspective. Since it is available and because Dr. Merson's forceful statement has also covered many similar issues, I will not directly summarize the statement. Rather I would like to take this opportunity to respond to the request of the delegations of the United Kingdom, Argentina, Canada and others to identify some of the relevant issues and problems and to outline possible strategies to address them.

Mr. President,

There are, I believe. two important characteristics of the HIV epidemic which need to be acknowledged and understood for they affect and determine the nature of the response to the epidemic.

Firstly, the epidemic is at one and the same time both a crisis and an endemic condition. It is a crisis because the speed of spread of this virus can be so awesome. Infection rates in adult populations can, and have, increased from two per cent to 25 per cent in only a small number of years, before people are even aware that they are surrounded by infected family and friends, before they are aware that their communities have been invaded. This fact alone should be sufficient for it to be viewed as a disaster, albeit too often invisible in its early stages, as much in need of an immediate response as the invasion of one country by another. For war nowadays rarely has the toll in human lives that this virus is causing.

That it is an endemic condition may best be simply illustrated by the fact that, even if in seriously affected countries there were to be no further cases of infection as from today, the pain and trauma of the deaths of those already infected will continue for the next twenty years and the social and economic repercussions of their deaths will continue on for decades and generations after that. We know thav nowhere in the world is the spread abating or even slowing down. Each day of continuing spread adds to the duration ot its devastating impact.

Both dimensions, the epidemic as crisis and the epidemic as endemic, need to be recognised. Each has its own appropriate responses.

Secondly, the epidemic manifests itself both as a specific problem out also as a pervasive one. Its specificity is revealed in increasing numbers of people, mostly healthy, productive young men and women, getting sick and dying. The response of the first decade of the epidemic addressed this quality of the epidemic.

However, as is argued in the UNDP statement, the repercussions of these deaths will permeate and affect every facet of human life and national development, more so in seriously affected countries where men and women are infected in more or less the same numbers. The causes and the consequences of the spread of the virus embrace poverty and wealth, disempowerment and influence, deprivation and development, trust and bad taste; the very way we are as human beings.

Both of these dimensions of the epidemic, its particularity and its ubiquity, must also be recognised. Each of these too has its own appropriate responses.

Thus this epidemic is conceptually slippery: at once a crisis and an endemic condition; at once a specific issue and a permeating one.

Mr. President,

These two characteristics of the HIV epidemic impose a set of imperatives upon us:

* the imperative of an effective response;
* the imperative of a sustainable response; and
* the imperative of a co-ordinated response.

The prerequisite of an effective response is a common understanding of the nature of the epidemic, which takes into account its above two characteristics, and a shared vision of the way forward. This we do not yet have. This should not surprise us for the epidemic is a new and complex phenomenon for which there is no likeness in living memory, not one drawn from war, not from disease, not from natural disasters nor from man-made ones, including poverty.

This is not to say that we are blindly groping. As the Secretary-General's report (E/1992/67) states, we are doing what we know needs to be done while we search for new and more effective ways to respond. The more we share a vision of an effective way forward, the more co-ordination will naturally follow.

Both WHO and UNDP have placed high priority on this quest: through expert group meetings, informal consultations, the exchange of experiences, the documentation of successes and through informal exchanges between communities and governments, among donors and within the United Nations system. UNDP has developed and piloted a workshop designed to reach a common understanding at country level of the nature of the epidemic and of effective approaches to its many facets. Such an understanding is an antecedent condition for co-ordination.

At global level, the recent proposal for a Global HIV/AIDS Co-ordination Forum was born from the same analysis.

The second imperative, that of a sustainable response, means that while the required human and financial resources must be available for identified effective responses, these responses must also be ranked in order of effectiveness since resources, whether of individuals, communities, nations or of external support agencies, are limited.

The commitment and contributions of affected individuals and communities have yet to be recognized or valued but they are extensive. They lie at the heart of a sustainable response to this epidemic but in most cases they need to be supplemented by further human and financial resources. The closeness of these individuals and communities to the problems and needs created by the epidemic ensures that the responses are appropriate. Similarly, governments are increasingly allocating resources to the epidemic.

Thus priority must be given to strengthening national capacity to ensure that these resources, and that of the external support agencies, are used in the most effective manner. There is not time and there are not sufficient resources for ill-conceived, inappropriate and ineffective responses. The selection must be ruthless for the demand on resources will continue and increase inexorably for decades. Communities and governments must have the ability to monitor assess and evaluate their interventions and to modify, redesign and expand them.

Where the response to the epidemic is effective and sustainable, hope is brought into being that the desolation and distress of this epidemic can be restrained, a hope that can turn back the tides of fatalism and despair.

Mr. President,

Only one other requirement then remains for a co-ordinated response: there is a need for mechanisms to ensure that the search for affective and sustainable policies and interventions is an ongoing process. Such mechanisms are needed among the community groups responding to the epidemic, between such groups and government, among government ministries, between the public and the private sectors, among external support agencies, especially within the UN system, and between donors and countries.

These mechanisms must be flexible for different countries have different capacities and different needs. A variety of approaches to co-ordination have been established. They need to be rationalised and strengthened. The United Nations Resident Co-ordinator has a critical role to play in ensuring that this occurs at country level.

Mr. President,

UNDP, with its understanding of the complex dynamics of human development, can assist in bringing about a common understanding of the nature of the epidemic and a common vision of the way forward.

Further, UNDP, with its relation to the United Nations Resident Co-ordinator, will be a critical player in the process of creating mechanisms for dialogue, collaboration and co-ordination.

Finally, UNDP, with its extensive presence at country level, its neutrality and its experience in a broad range of sectors and programmes, is a resource to be mobilized for national capacity building to ensure that this imminent threat to human survival, human rights and human development can be overcome.

Mr. President, Distinguished Delegates, Colleagues,

On behalf of the Administrator of UNDP, Mr. William Draper, I welcome this opportunity to address you under this agenda item designed to provide an overview of trends and prospects for the world economy and their implications for development.

The UNDP statements on agenda item 3 (b) touched briefly on the characteristics which distinguish this epidemic from other diseases but also from war and from natural and man-made disasters. T. refer the distinguished delegates to this statement and will not take up this aspect of the epidemic now.

This epidemic is occurring at a time in history when not only economic and political trends are causing concern but also i a period of quite unsettling social change itself affected by current economic trends.

Firstly, the structures of family life are changing. In all regions of the world, fewer women marry today than in 1970 and fewer women are having children. More than 30 per cent of households in the world are headed by women but at least a quarter of the women heading households in developing regions are elderly.

Secondly, since the 1970s, women's share in the labour force has been rising and it is anticipated that it will continue to rise. Almost everywhere women are working more outside of the household while at the same time the household remains a major place of work for women. The proportion of men who are economically active is down everywhere. Whilst women's share in the labour force is rising, the proportion of women and of women headed households below the poverty line is increasing.

While women's lives in families are changing, there is little evidence that men are undergoing comparable change.

This weakening of family structures is occurring at the same time that in most countries of the world investment in social support systems to families and employees has dropped significantly.

Women's survival is increasingly an issue of serious concern. Women outlive men almost everywhere but they are still in the minority in many developing regions because of higher rates of female mortality. There are not as many women as men in the world. Indeed in many countries, there are fewer than 95 women for every 100 men. Women's survival is already threatened by gender selective abortion, female infanticide, the criminal neglect and abuse of young girl children, the unacceptable extent of the death of women during pregnancy and in childbirth and other threats to women's lives. These deaths are avoidable; the social and economic distress caused by them should not be being borne.

These socio-economic trends pre-date the HIV epidemic. The epidemic will exacerbate them and in turn will itself be fed by them. The structures of family life will be further and radically changed as parents die dcattering households. Extended family support systems may have burdens placed on them that they are unable to bear. Yet families provide nurturing, care, companionship and security to their members. They act as buffers against crises and form an important part of the basis of community coping strategies. It is imperative that social policy frameworks be established so that these family structures are strengthened and supported if we are to live through this epidemic.

The survival of women is being further threatened by their increasing rates of HIV infection. Already, one in every 21 women in Africa die from childbirth related causes. Add to this the current estimate of one in every 40 women in Africa being HIV infected. Both these causes of death are preventable wherever they occur in the world. The economic and social dislocation caused by this wanton slaughter or women will not be able to be home either by households or by nations.

None of these trends can be addressed in isolation. They are interwoven and interrelated. Perhaps this epidemic will be the catalyst which will force us to action. However, for our response to be effective and sustainable, we will need to forge a number of social contracts or partnerships.

The first social contract must be between men and women.

This epidemic and its impact will never be overcome unless men and women can forge a true partnership of mutual respect and trust and of equitable sharing of the burdens caused by this epidemic, the burdens of sadness, pain, care and support. Women alone cannot stop the spread of the virus and women alone cannot bear the burden of its personal, social and economic consequences. Men must be involved. A social contract must emerge, and soon, to face these challenges together, as husband and wife, brother and sister and as partners, friends and colleagues.

Secondly, there must be a social contract between the affected and the not yet directly affected.

The infected and those close to them are amongst the most powerful agents of change in the world today. They can give us glimpses of how we can peacefully co-exist with the virus, of how we can become empowered through the trauma and the tragedy of the epidemic. Within the desolation of this epidemic, they give us snatches of laughter and happiness. They can help us explore and better understand the nature of intimacy, desire and sexuality in the age of the virus.

But these insights of the affected will not be shared, this gift will remain ungiven, if, in the sharing, the affected are stripped of their self esteem and dignity, subjected to humiliation and discrimination, left alone in a hostile limelight without support and companionship.

This is a critical social contract: the opposite of the Them/Us mentality which has sadly too often characterized perceptions of and responses to the epidemic. There is not other in the shadow of the epidemic. We are all there.

The social contract, therefore, must enable the creation of a supportive milieu that encourages the affected to speak out, tell their stories, reflect on their lives and hopes and help us all to live peacefully with this epidemic.

The third social contract must be between communities and government.

The responses of affected communities provide us with the hope that the epidemic can be overcome and the inspiration as to how this can come about. These responses are universal. Wherever the virus has spread, communities have responded, to provide care and support to stop further infection, to assure the rights of the affected, to minister to spiritual, emotional and physical needs.

But individuals, families and communities cannot carry this epidemic alone. There must be a social contract, a partnership between governments and affected communities. Governments must provide an enabling environment that will noursh and sustain these responses. This enabling environment must include national policies that acknowledge the centrality of community responses, a body of legal and human rights laws that respect the principles of non-discrimination and respect for the rights and dignity of affected individuals, mechanisms for interaction between government and communities, and assistance, as required, for programme design, delivery and financing by communities.

The need for additional resources for this epidemic is frequently mentioned. Whilst it is clear that external resources are needed, it is important to stress that the first financial resources that are mobilized to respond to this epidemic are those of individuals, families and communities. This remains unrecognized and unquantified. We must name this and quantify it for sadly this is the way that most people recognize value.

These resources-peoples' volunteered time, the food, meals and insights they share, the transport provide, the labour contributed, the funds raised- lie at the heart of a sustainable response.

Yes, the resources must be supplemented. They are not without end; they themselves are depleted by the epidemic; they are not, always or usually, sufficient. The communities know what additional resources, human or financial, they need for sustenance and growth. They need to be empowered to be able to define their external support requirements, select them, manage them and account for them in appropriate ways whether these resources come from national or international sources.

Mutual trust and respect is a sine qua non for a social contract between communities and their government. This may not be easy for either but it must come about.

The fourth social contract must be a global economic contract.

As the epidemic deepens, its devastating impact on all aspects of human life and national development is becoming better understood. Certain nations may be brought towards the threshold of destitution. Will there be a global economic contract? Will the world community provide the foreign direct investment in the education and health of people and in the technological development of these nations? Will there be global social safety nets to allow nations rendered poor by this epidemic, and the poor within them,. to survive.

The free working of the global market tends to increase the disparities between rich and poor nations and rich and poor individuals. At the national level, governments try to offset such tendencies by redistributing income through systems of progressive income tax and by supplementing this with social safety nets to prevent people from falling into poverty and absolute destitution. No such systems exist at present at the global level.

The closest the world comes to a global safety net is the current system of development assistance. However, this system is fatally flawed, firstly in the inadequacy of its extent. Secondly because its allocation at present is unrelated to levels of poverty. South Asia, for example, receives $ 5 per person. India has 34 per cent of the world's absolute poor, yet receives only 3.5 per cent of total aid flows. Countries that invest more heavily in military expenditure receive more aid than those with modest investments.

If overseas aid is to be able to serve as a social safety net for the world's poor, it will have to be based on principles requiring that aid should be directed to priority concerns for human survival and human development.

These four social contracts or partnerships are essential to an effective sustainable response to this epidemic.

We now know well the main areas for programme focus in response to the epidemic. These are behaviour change, the care, support and treatment of those affected and, as the epidemic deepens, the maintenance of the basic infrastructure of communities and nations: water supply, electricity, road maintenance, financial institutions, education and health systems and so on.

Our strategy for the immediate future must be to bring about the social contracts or partnerships which will enable us to achieve these programme ends.

UNDP is committed to helping forge these social contracts and to working actively with communities, nations and the international community to identify and strengthen effective, sustainable policies and interventions.

46

World AIDS Day, 1 December

Today, the international community rededicates itself to fighting the world-wide scourge of HIV/AIDs, to combating fear, ignorance and prejudice, and to providing new hope for the millions of people around the world living with HIV.

HIV/AIDS is a global problem. No country or region is immune Today, some 22 million people are living with HIV/AIDS, while the total number of world-wide AIDS related deaths has reached 6 million. These are appalling statistics, but there is nothing inevitable about the global spread of HIV.

In the developed world, the success of prevention and sex education programmes, and awareness campaigns among intravenous drug users have demonstrated that rates of HIV infection can begin to be arrested and addressed with positive results.

In the developing world, the challenge remains greater. Over ninety per cent of all new HIV infections occur here, and programmes to prevent the spread of the infection have so far met with limited success. In addition, new anti-virus therapies and treatments remain extremely costly and beyond the means of the vast majority of AIDS sufferers in the developing world.

The United Nations has taken a lead in promoting vital education and prevention programmes, and is working closely with Member States and local populations on the ground. The Joint United Nations Programme on AIDS, launched on 1 Janurary 1996, marks an important step forward in the global fight against HIV/AIDS. The Programme, in partnership with Member States, is working hard to promote greater co-operation and co-ordination in the field, and to develop new policy initiatives and mobilise new resources at the global, regional and country levels.

Above all, this initiative emphasises the growing partnership between the United Nations system and individual people living with HIV. The Programme seeks to be inclusive in its dealings with affected communites and individuals throughout the world.

The challenge of World AIDS Day is to translate understanding and awareness of HIV/AIDS into positive action and more effective and co-ordinated public policy response around the world. Today, more than ever, the global challenge of HIV/AIDS demands an informed, considered and generous response from us all.

47

Challenges for UNDP in A Changing World 1990-2000: Social Trends

Ms. Elizabeth Reid
UNDP, New York

The last two decades have seen the emergence of a number of social trends which will converge in the coming decade, fomenting a period ot rapid social change. This decade may well become known as the white water decade with the development community at times feeling that it is being swept out of control down its rapids.

If people are to be placed at the centre of development during these changing times, the social context of development will be as important as its political, economic and administrative contexts.

I wish to look briefly at some social trends relating to family structures, gender and the HIV epidemic, which I believe, will affect the fabric of our societies.

THE STRUCTURES OF FAMILY LIFE ARE CHANGING?[1]

Families provide nurturing, care, companionship and security to their members. They act as buffers against crises and form an important part of the basis of communities' coping mechanisms.

In all regions, fewer women marry today than in 1970 and those who do spend less of their lives married and fewer having children.

In Africa, the proportion of women in the 20 to 24 age group who have never married increased between the 1970s and the early

'80s from 25 to 33 per cent. A similar but less pronounced trend occurred in all other regions except Asia.

In all regions, similar but less pronounced trends occurred among:

* teenage women
* men 20-24 years
* women and men 25-44 years.

This trend for both women and men may be significantly reinforced during the 1990s by the HIV epidemic.

Up to 30 per cent of households are headed by women. At least a quarter of the women heading households in developing regions are elderly.[2]

The Latin American and Caribbean region has the highest number of countries where more than 20 per cent of households are headed by women:

Barbados (44), Chile (22), Cuba (28), Dominica (38), El Salvador (22), French Guiana (31), Grenada (45), Guadeloupe (34), Guyana (24), Honduras (22), Jamaica (34), Martinique (35), Netherlands Aptilles (30), Panama (22), Peru (23), Puerto Rico (25), St. Kitts & Nevis (46), St. Lucia (39), St. Vincent/Grenadines (42), Trinidad and Tobago (25), Uruguay (21) and Venezuela (22). Africa has 8 such countries; Asia and the Pacific, one.

The proportion of both women headed households and households headed by elderly women and men could significantly increase in the 1990s in countries seriously affected by the epidemic.

Extended family support systems may have burdens placed on them that they are unable to bear in high incidence areas.

Infection is clustered in families. It is highly likely that both husband and wife may die, leaving the elderly, children and other household members without means of support. Where the adult population is seriously affected, the reliability of traditional support systems may be threatened.

The proportion of women and women-headed households below the poverty line is increasing. Poverty accelerated the spread of the HIV epidemic, particularly for women for whom sex work is often the only available coping strategy. In turn, the epidemic deepens poverty, destitution and homelessness.

Increasingly divorce is instigated by women.

In Europe three-quarters of all divorces are instigated by women.

Since the 1970s, women's share in the labour force has been rising and it is anticipated it will continue to rise.

Almost everywhere women are working more outside of the

household while at the same time the household remains a major place of work for women.

Women everywhere retain primary responsibility for household work, even when they have economic responsibilities inside and outside the household. Men in developing regions generally do even fewer household chores than men elsewhere. The proportion of men who are economically active is down everywhere.

While women's lives in families are changing, there is little evidence that men are undergoing comparable change.

This weakening of family structures is occurring at the same time that in most countries of the world investment in social support systems to families and employees has dropped significantly. If these trends continuez alternative sources of nurturing, care, companionship and security will have to be found for we cannot live or develop as human beings without them.

WOMEN'S SURVIVAL WILL INCREASINGLY BE AN ISSUE OF SERIOUS CONCERN THROUGH THE 1990s

Women now outlive men almost everywhere but they are still in the minority in many developing regions because of higher female mortality.

There are not as many women as men in the world (2.65b out of a total 5.3b—1990). Indeed in many countries, there are fewer than 95 women for every 100 men. All of these countries except two are in the Asia and Pacific and West Asia regions.[2]

Women's survival is threatened by:

- Gender selective abortion, female infanticide and the criminal neglect and abuse of young girl children. The Indian economist, Amartya Sen, argues that there are 100 million missing women in Asia in our generation.
- Maternal deaths and disability. One million women die each year of reproduction related causes, mainly illicit and unsafe abortions and obstetric complications. Over 100 million women become disabled or suffer a disabling illness each year as a result of complications in pregnancy.[3]
- Ninety eight per cent of all maternal deaths and disabilities occur in the developing world.
- In Africa one in 91 women will die in pregnancy or childbirth.

  In Asia: 1:54

  In Latin America: 1:73

  In Northern Europe: 1:10,000

Other threats to women's lives include: bride burning, dowry deaths (estimated at 1 every 12 minutes in India) domestic violence and the HIV epidemic.

These deaths and disabilities arc wanton and avoidable. The extent of the loss of productively active women is unaffordable. The social cost and distress caused by these mother's deaths and women's disabilities are unbearable. The demand for changes will increase throughout the 1990s.

FOR THE REMAINDER OF THE 1990s, THE SURVIVAL OF PEOPLE, BOTH MEN AND WOMEN, AND THEIR SOCIAL, POLITICAL AND ECONOMIC INSTITUTIONS WILL BE OF INCREASING CONCERN.

The HIV epidemic has been visible now for over 10 years. However, our understanding of the epidemic and its implications for human survival and human development is still in its infancy.

Yet this epidemic has totally permeated our societies.

WHO/GPA estimates:

— globally, one in every 250 adults is infected;

— in sub-Saharan Africa, 1 in every 40 adults, women and men, is infected.

The epidemic spreads with alarming rapidity wherever the conditions for spread are present.

In one African country, the incidence of HIV infection in the urban adult population has doubled each year in the last four years:

1987: 0-3 per cent adults infected
1988: 6-8 per cent
1989: 10-12 per cent
1990: 22-24 per cent

A similar rate of spread has been identified in Thailand where infection rates among compulsorily drafted military recruits have risen from 2 per cent in 1989 to 6 per cent in 1990.

The incidence of modes of transmission varies with the social context.

WHO/GPA estimates:

* Globally, 60 per cent occurs between women and men
  15 per cent between men
  15 per cent through injecting drug use
  10 per cent all others
* In Africa, 80 per cent between men and women
  10 per cent perinatally
  10 per cent all others

These figures indicate where programming priorities must lie if the epidemic is to be stemmed.

The characteristics which distinguish it from other diseases include:

— the long period between infection and onset of illness, on average 10 years in developed countries, possibly less in developing countries;

— the majority of those infected are adult men and women; people with significant numbers of dependents and in their economically most productive years;

— the associated epidemics, tuberculosis, for example, which is now a serious problem in most affected communities:

— the fact that once a person is infected, and the overwhelming majority of people are unaware that they are infected, he or she is infectious for life and unless precautions are taken can transmit the virus to others.

The epidemic is not randomly distributed. It is clustered in households, geographically and occupationally.

In Thailand, the highest number of known cases of infection occurs among construction site workers (36 per cent). In the Central African Republic, 22 per cent of those infected are students.

Whenever people move, the virus moves, particularly where the movement is of single people.

Thus, spread of the virus is facilitated by:

— transport systems

— labour markets

— formal and informal teaching patterns

— seasonal labour

— warfare, destabilization, mandatory and other forms of civil unrest.

The conditions of spread are exacerbated by urbanisation poverty, and migration.

This epidemic will, as it spreads and deepens, force us to rethink approaches to national planning and development assistance. At the same time, the epidemic will undermine national capacity to plan, manage and deliver in countries with high infection rates in urban areas.

Virtually everything we do as planners and agents of development will be affected. The epidemic and its impact will have to be factored into everything we do.

Both economic growth and the mechanisms for redistribution will be undermined. The epidemic will reduce private and public savings. At the same time, demands for public interventions and expenditures will rise, for example, in health, housing, social security and food subsidies. Productivity will be reduced through illness and deaths, particularly of skilled and experienced personnel.

Redistributive mechanisms such as credit and social investment schemes, employment creation schemes, education and training will need to be rethought as mechanisms to address critical needs and to improve the human condition.

There will be immense costs to communities and nations. The early illness and death of the active labour force will generate a need for replacement social investment at a time of shrinking public and national resources. The anguish of the illness and deaths of so many young adults will be difficult to bear. However, an understanding of the extent of the personal, social and economic costs will strengthen the demand for effective prevention programmes, the most effective way of minimising the adverse impact of the epidemic.

We cannot assume that there will be sustained large scale resources transferred to seriously affected countries. The resources and responses will need to come from within communities and nations.

If the 1990s is a period of rapid social change with many trends amplifying the adverse consequences of other trends, then our programming and procedures will need the flexibility to respond and there will be an even stronger imperative for effective programmes. We will be held to account and judged on the extent to which we contribute to human survival find human development.

We need to learn to apply research findings directly to programming. Let me give a few brief illustrative examples, conscious that the brevity will distort the complexity of social situations.

Studies show the following:

— There is no correlation between improving women's socioeconomic status and reducing maternal death and disability.

An improvement in women's social and economic lives is essential for human development. Howevers maternal death and disability can be reduced only by an analysis of direct causes and the establishment of a programme to address them. The methodology for this and the range of direct causes are known.[4]

— The return on investment in women's education is consistently higher than the return on educating men.

Studies in Malaysia show that the net return to education at all levels of wages and productivity is consistently 20 per cent higher for girls and young women than for boys and young men.[2]

The World Bank is now reflecting this in its programming in certain countries by offering financial assistance to parents who allow their female children to go to school.

— Increasing women's income leads to a spread of benefits to all other household members, which does not occur with increases to men's income.

These data have been available for some time but have not, to my knowledge, been taken into account in programme development. Investing more in opportunities for women in education and in formal and informal opportunities for work is far more than an investment in women. It is an investment in their families and communities. It is an effective way to assist people out of poverty. It is a *sine qua* non for human development.

— Women are assiduous and prompt with credit repayments.

Experience with credit schemes in all regions show that defaults in repayments by women are consistently held to less than 2 per cent. One study of women's loan repayment behaviour in Ahmedabad, India, showed that most defaults were because of maternal deaths and disability.[4]

— Information alone rarely changes sexual behaviour.

Information, education and communication (IEC) are necessary but not sufficient to change behaviour. An evaluation of a well designed IEC programme for the prevention of further transmission of the HIV virus showed that 98 per cent of the sexually active population knew accurately how the virus is transmitted and how transmission can be prevented but only 5 per cent had in fact changed their behaviour to prevent themselves from becoming infected.

— Securing the blood supply will have only a slight impact on reducing the rapid spread of the HIV epidemic.

A secure blood supply is critical to retaining people's faith in modern medical services. However, a number of approaches to modelling the epidemic have shown that the resultant impact on the spread of the epidemic under most known circumstances is minimal.

It should be noted that today's data are not necessarily tomorrow's. The social context must be monitored since the situation is not static. For example, Jamaican data indicate decreasing participation of boys in secondary education. Such trends should trigger the establishment of a monitoring system and a response to prevent the range of possible serious consequences of such a trend.

The convergence of these social trends has implications for

the restructuring of the United Nations system. We cannot afford any longer to assume that knowledge and technology can be transferred or technical advice given without regard for the cosial context. Just as they cannot be divorced from the economic and political context. Social analysis must form an integral part of the situational analysis upon which all forms of assistance are based. Diarrhoeal diseases cannot be addressed outside of the context which gives rise to the problem and within which the solutions will be found. Grain storage technology must be accepted by the communities within which it is being introduced and must be suitable to their needs and circumstances. There are many such examples and they are all familiar to us.

Yet the system as presently structured does not facilitate achieving these basic necessities. The context of change is best known by nationals and national capacity must be strengthened to demand a multi-disciplinary and integrated approach. The UN system must be able to respond. This will require a change in the way of the Specialised Agencies or a new role for DIESA. UNDP's advantage is that because of its network of field offices, it is close to and better placed to understand the social context within which human development takes place.

NOTES

1. Coote, A. et. al. *Changing Family Structures.* Report of the Institute of Policy Studies, London 1991.
2. United Nations Statistical Office. *The World's Women 1970-1990: Trends and Statistics.* United Nations, New York, 1991.

   2. Op. cit.
3. Jacobsen, Jodi L. Women's Reproductive Health... *The Silen Emergency,* World Watch Paper 102, June 1991. World Watch Institute, Washington, 1991.
4. Forward Looking Assessment of the Prevention of Maternal Mortality and Morbidity in the Context of the Safe Motherhood Initiative, UNDP, 1991.

   2. Op. cit.

   4. Op. cit.

###